Nutrition Basics

FOR

Better Health

AND

Performance

Second Edition
Revised Printing

Liz Applegate, Ph.D.

University of California–Davis
Nutrition Department

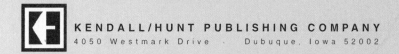
KENDALL/HUNT PUBLISHING COMPANY
4050 Westmark Drive · Dubuque, Iowa 52002

All figures are reprinted by permission of Liz Applegate, Ph.D.

Copyright © 2004, 2006 by Liz Applegate, Ph.D.
Revised Printing, 2008

ISBN 978-0-7575-4986-1

Printed in the United States of America
10   9   8   7   6   5   4

Contents

Dedication

In memory of my mother — her patience and strength were enduring.

Acknowledgments

This second edition of *Nutrition Basics for Better Health and Performance* reflects a growth in both content and clarification from the first edition. Creation of this book took numerous dedicated and supportive individuals who had the vision for its completion and were willing to see every last detail through. An individual instrumental in the completion of this new edition is Sandra Samarron, the head Teaching Assistant for the past few years. Sandra expertly reviewed the text and contributed significantly in clarifying concepts throughout the book. As a suburb instructor, Sandra also recognizes the importance of integrating material consistently. I thank her for all she has done for this book, as well as the course.

Deep thanks also goes to Marlia Braun, my former Teaching Assistant for several years, who has helped tremendously on the first edition and assisted in the preparation of this new edition. She has excellent insight into students' perception and interests in nutrition. Marlia has also made putting together the figures, tables and charts doable—no small task! I would also like to warmly thank my trusted assistant, Tahlya Cox, who has patiently worked with me and Kendall-Hunt in the preparation of this second edition. Without Tahlya, completing this monumental project would not be possible!

As you look through the text, note the wonderful diagrams and artwork, which were created by artist Steve Oerding, Mediaworks Information and Educational Technology, UC Davis. His expert work has given me the opportunity to put concepts and ideas in nutrition to life. What once were mind-boggling topics have now become enjoyable as well as understandable for the students. Thank you so much Steve. I also thank the Regents of the University of California for giving permission to utilize these illustrations.

The folks at Kendall-Hunt also deserve tremendous thanks. Frank Forcier, my editor, and Becky Ruden, my former editor at Kendall-Hunt, both had vision and worked hard to bring this book to publication. Also, Amanda Smith and Colleen Zelinsky took tremendous care to ensure accuracy and kept the project moving gracefully. The back cover recipe ideas, which are delicious and good for you, were inspired by a creative, patient, and enduring friend—thanks Jeff. Finally, my thanks as well as appreciation go to the thousands of energetic, inquisitive students I have had the honor to instruct at the University of California, Davis. Over the years, these students help shape the delivery and content of the course material and continue to inspire me to reach for my best as a teacher. Thank you all.

About the Author

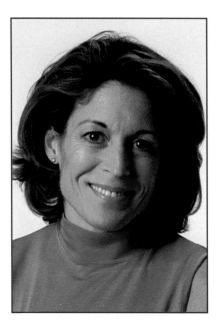

Dr. Liz Applegate, a nationally renowned expert on nutrition and fitness, is a faculty member of the Nutrition Department at the University of California, Davis. Her enthusiasm and informal style make her undergraduate nutrition classes the nation's largest with enrollments exceeding 2,000 annually. She received the *Excellence in Teaching Award* from the University of California, as well as the ASUCD *Excellence in Education Award.*

Dr. Applegate is the author of several books including *Bounce Your Body Beautiful* (Three Rivers Press 2003), *Encyclopedia of Sports and Fitness Nutrition* (Three Rivers Press 2002), *Eat Smart Play Hard* (Rodale Press, June 2001) and *Eat Your Way to a Healthy Heart: Chocolate and 99 Other Foods to Help Your Heart* (Prentice Hall Press, 1999). She has written over 300 articles for national magazines and is Nutrition Editor and Columnist for *Runner's World* magazine. Dr. Applegate is on the editorial board of the *International Journal of Sport Nutrition and Exercise Metabolism.* She is a Fellow of the American College of Sports Medicine, and a member of the Sports and Cardiovascular Nutritionists, a practice group of the American Dietetics Association. Frequently she serves as a keynote speaker at industry, athletic, and scientific meetings.

Dr. Applegate appears as an expert on international, national and local radio and television shows including *The Early Show* and *Good Morning America*, as well as health segments on the *Discovery Channel, CNN* and *ESPN.* She is frequently quoted in *Shape, Vogue, Men's Health, Better Homes and Gardens, USA Today, LA Times, Washington Post,* and other national print media.

She is a consultant for U.S. Olympic athletes and is the team nutritionist for the Oakland Raiders.

Web: *http://nutrition.ucdavis.edu/Faculty/applegate.html*
    www.lizapplegate.com

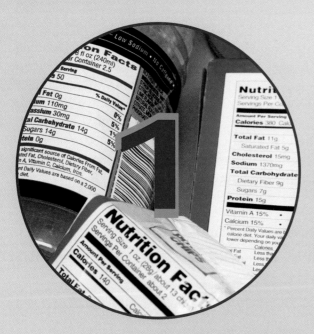

Speaking of Nutrition . . . Some Basics

Welcome to the world of nutrition. Taking this class means you have an interest in your health and fitness. And I applaud you for wanting to take charge of your body—learning about what your body needs for optimal health for today and a lifetime. Your food choices impact your performance today as well as set the stage for health and disease prevention later in life.

In this course you will learn that while many people tend to categorize foods as "good" or "bad," such as carrots and oranges versus burgers and fries, that all foods fit in your diet. Some do provide you with an array of substances better for your health than others, but eating and living well is about making balanced choices. During this course you will have the opportunity to assess your food choices by completing the Diet Project. As you learn about the roles of protein, fiber, fat, vitamins, and more in your body, you can compare how your diet rates with recommendations for optimal health, and then learn how to best meet your needs through foods and understand where supplements may be an option.

Before we can explore specifics about what's best for you to eat, a few basics must be introduced. So let's get started!

WHAT ARE NUTRIENTS, THEIR BASIC FUNCTIONS, AND HOW MUCH DO YOU NEED (THE RDA)?

How much food do you eat in a year's time? Or, what about the amount of food you may eat over the next four decades? Like many college students, you most likely average about 1 million calories a year or in 40 years almost 100,000 pounds of food.

1

So where is all this food going? What could your body possibly be doing with such a tremendous amount of food energy and material? This food and energy goes into making you and maintaining your "appearance." Every day your body renews itself—making new cells, tissue, hair, and more. In fact, take a look in the mirror. Even though you look the same as you did a year ago (perhaps you may have a new hair color or style, or ear piercing), you are not the same person. You actually have an entirely new skin surface, newly remodeled bones, and fresh lining to your intestinal track. In fact:

- About 1% of your blood cells are new every day.
- The cells in your intestine renew themselves every three to five days.
- Your skin is sloughed daily (which is some of the dust in your dorm room or apartment!).
- You're busy growing new body hair daily.

Nutrition Bite

Fun fact about your hair—you grow over 350 miles of hair in a lifetime!

The food that you eat supplies you with the parts and fuel—**nutrients**—needed to keep up this type of rebuilding and renewing schedule. Food supplies nutrients that:

- provide energy
- serve as building materials
- help to maintain or repair body parts

There are six classes of nutrients (all totaled there are 50 nutrients):

1. Proteins
2. Carbohydrates
3. Fats
4. Minerals
5. Vitamins
6. Water (a single nutrient in a class by itself)

All six classes of nutrients are present in the body but in differing amounts or percent of your body weight as follows:

1. **50–60% water**—males generally have about 60%, and females have 50% due to differences in body fat and muscle content.

2. **15–25% fat**
   - Desirable levels: 15% for males and 22–25% for females
   - Body fat levels influence body water content because fat tissue is very low in water content (about 23%) compared to muscle or brain tissue (70%).
   - As body fat increases, body water decreases; as body fat decreases, body water increases. This explains why most males have a higher percentage of body water than females.

3. **18–20% protein**—males have more than females due to higher lean or muscle mass.

4. **4–5% mineral**—the body's mineral content is primarily in bones and teeth. This varies by gender (males have higher levels than females) and race (blacks have more than whites, which have more than Asians).

5. **Less than 1% carbohydrates**—storage of carbohydrates in the muscles and liver is vital for fuel during exercise and rest (especially for the brain).

6. **Less than 1% vitamins**—very trace amounts exist in each cell.

Nutrition Bite

Is there a best body fat level for athletes?

Here are some numbers for body fat in collegiate athletes (see Figure 1.1). And as you'll see in Chapter 7, there is not a perfect or ideal body fat that depicts optimal health but rather ranges.

Foods, as well as the body, contain all six classes of nutrients in varying amounts. Must you eat all 50 some nutrients, or only some?

PERCENT BODY FAT VALUES IN ATHLETES

	MALES	FEMALES
Basketball	7–12	18–27
Distance Running	3–8	8–18
Gymnastics	7–12	16–22
Soccer	4–10	14–25
Swimming	5–12	10–20
Tennis	12–16	15–22
Nonathlete, avg.	15–16.9	20–26.9

FIGURE 1.1

Essential nutrients are those nutrients:

● the body either cannot make or

● cannot make at a rate sufficient to meet your needs.

● They are therefore required in the diet.

For example, calcium is a mineral that originates in soil (rocks), gets into plants that cows eat, and then gets into milk, and eventually gets into our bodies. We are incapable of making calcium, so we must get it from the food we eat.

On the other hand, water is made every day in our bodies as we metabolize food for energy. However, we only make about a cup each day, which falls short of the several cups we need. Therefore, water is essential in the diet.

How Do Nutrients Function in the Body?

1. **Energy**—Only proteins, carbohydrates, and fats (the macronutrients) contain potential energy. Elements, primarily carbon, are connected to each other via chemical bonds that are much like tiny stretched rubber bands, when let go, the energy is released. The energy released from chemical bonds is measured as calories. (We'll learn more about this in Chapter 3.)

2. **Structure**—Nutrients such as protein and calcium are the building material and structure for bone and teeth.

3. **Regulation**—As regulators, nutrients help manage and oversee many processes in the body such as building new hormones, regulating fluid balance, or catalyzing a reaction such as enzymes, which are made of protein. Regulatory nutrients are much like traffic lights that help regulate the flow of vehicles on busy streets.

How Do We Express Our Nutrient Needs or Requirements?

An arm of the government—the Food and Nutrition Board—takes on the task of determining and setting nutrient requirements. These standards are called **Dietary Reference Intakes (DRI),** used by health professionals and others in establishing nutrient intakes for planning and assessing diets for healthy individuals. Under this umbrella term of DRI, there are five separate nutrient standard values, of which the **Recommended Dietary Allowance (RDA)** is one. You are probably familiar with or at least heard of this term before. In this course we will make reference to the RDA, what it means, how the RDA for a given nutrient is determined, and how best to meet your need. While the other nutrient values are important in the world of nutrition, in this course we will not utilize these except for making reference to the Tolerable Upper Intake Level or UL. This is the highest level of daily nutrient intake that is likely to be safe and not pose any adverse health effects to most people in the population. But dietary or supplement intake exceeding the UL for a certain nutrient, such as iron, may present some health problems. As we will cover in the topic of supplements in Chapter 9, not only can we get too little of a nutrient, but excessive intake through foods that are fortified with nutrients such as vitamins as well as supplements pose health risks.

A Closer Look at the RDA

The RDA is the daily amount of nutrient considered adequate to meet the needs of nearly all healthy people in the population (about 98% of us). The RDA is NOT a minimum amount nor is it an average need but instead a generous value. And the RDA is set based on scientific information.

- The RDA has been determined for protein and other nutrients (vitamins, minerals, etc.).

- The RDA is established for several age groups, gender, and physiological states (pregnancy and lactation).

- The RDA is designed to be an average over several days. (In other words, you don't have to meet the RDA each day, but instead averaged it over several.)

- Adjustments are made when setting the RDA based upon several factors that we will highlight as each nutrient is covered, such as the quality of the diet (as in protein covered in Chapter 2), bioavailability (as with minerals covered in Chapter 8), and losses due to food preparation (as with vitamins covered in Chapter 9).

You will not need to memorize each RDA (except for protein) but instead know what goes into setting the RDA and what it means to you.

Ever wonder why you still function even though you haven't eaten all day, or why your body's internal temperature hovers around 37 degrees Celsius or 98.6 degrees Fahrenheit despite freezing or scorching temperatures outside?

The reason is actually more of a concept or process called **homeostasis.** This is the maintenance of relatively constant internal conditions (such as body temperature and blood sugar levels) through the efforts and control of many systems in the body.

The concept of homeostasis will be emphasized throughout this course to help us predict as well as understand why our bodies respond and perform the way they do. For example, once you grasp the concept of homeostasis, you will soon understand why taking large amounts of a particular supplement such as vitamins or amino acids (components of protein) will not drastically change or alter the way your body or cells work so as not to upset other systems in your body.

Let's use the example of body water content to help understand homeostasis as well as learn more about the nutrient water. Recall that about 50% to 60% of your body weight is water. Figure 1.2 depicts the fluid inside and outside the body cells; the distribution of body water is determined and controlled by several factors such as hormones, the action of the kidneys, and the mineral and protein levels in body fluids.

You needn't ever worry about your body water level as fluid homeostasis is regulated well. On average a typical person takes in about $2\frac{1}{2}$ liters of fluid daily and loses the same (see Figure 1.3).

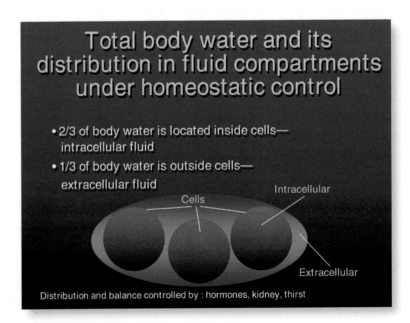

FIGURE 1.2

FLUID BALANCE			
INTAKE:		**OUTPUT:**	
Fluid	1.2 liters	Urine	1.5 liters
Food	1.0 liters	Stool	0.1 liters
Metabolic	0.3 liters	Sweat and breath vapor	0.9 liters
	2.5 liters		2.5 liters

FIGURE 1.3

On your final, you will be asked to define homeostasis and give an example of a nutrient under homeostatic control. By the end of the course, you'll surely have many ideas for your answer.

INSIDE WORK—THE PROCESS OF DIGESTION AND ABSORPTION

How do we process food and prepare it to enter our bodies? Our bodies accomplish this task through the process of digestion and absorption. **Digestion** is the process by which food is broken down into a form that can be absorbed by the intestine. **Absorption** is the process of moving nutrients into the body or bloodstream. Digestion occurs in the digestive tract, which begins at the mouth and is 26 feet long. Visualize the digestive tract as "outside" your body; that is, the digestive tract is a tube that runs through your body but the contents (if you swallow a golf ball, for example) are not really inside of you. Absorption only occurs when the food (its components) is transported from the small intestine into the circulation.

Figure 1.4 illustrates the digestive tract (with each part identified) along with some of the accessory organs, collectively called the digestive system.

There are two parts or types of digestion.

1. **Physical digestion:** the moving and grinding of food. This starts in the mouth with chewing, though you do not have to chew your food (despite that mom told you to chew your food well before swallowing) to completely digest your food. Once you have chewed (or just swallowed) your food, the bolus (swallowed food) moves down your esophagus into the stomach where it is "blenderized." The stomach, which has a 4-cup capacity, is much like a blender (strong muscles) that makes a smoothie out of your swallowed food.

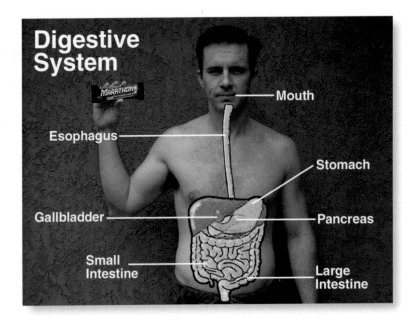

FIGURE 1.4

2. **Chemical digestion:** the chemical breakdown of food through the use of digestive enzymes (actual breaking of chemical bonds in foods). This process starts in the stomach with a majority occurring in the small intestine. The digestive enzymes needed to break these bonds are secreted by the pancreas into the small intestine. Once the process of chemical digestion is complete, the food has been digested and the process of absorption occurs.

Absorption is the process of taking these small food fragments from the small intestine and transporting them into the blood. The surface of the small intestine is where absorption occurs. The surface of the small intestine, as shown in Figure 1.5, is designed for maximum surface area. The folds, the folds on these folds called villi, and then hair-like structures on villi called microvilli all contribute to a tremendously large surface area that allows the nutrients an opportunity to be taken up into the

Nutrition Bite

The surface area of your intestinal track would cover about a third of a football field!

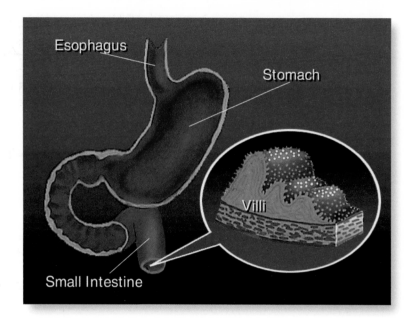

FIGURE 1.5

body and eventually into the circulation. Figure 1.6 illustrates villi and microvilli structures and the placement of capillaries that allow for transport of absorbed small food units into the body.

However, some food is not digested and absorbed. These items, such as fiber (or if you happened to swallow a food wrapper), move into the large intestine where the body extracts water and minerals, and prepares

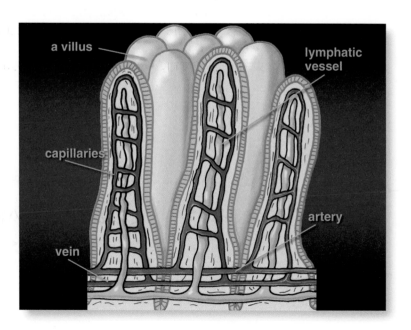

FIGURE 1.6

the remnants as stool. The stool then represents material that never got into the body in the first place, but only passed through the digestive tract. Along the same thought, you might have wondered what urine represents. This is metabolic waste, which is substances such as excess sodium that the body (kidneys) have filtered from the cells, blood, and elsewhere and sent out in the urine.

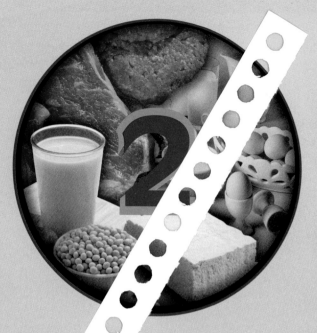

Protein—
The Versatile
Nutrient

No doubt you have good feelings about protein—usually thoughts of muscle strength and good health come to mind with protein. For millions of dieters, high-protein diets have become a way of life in an effort to shed unwanted pounds. In this chapter on protein, you will see how vital this nutrient is for an array of duties in the body including immune health, muscle strength, and recovery along with the truth about high-protein diets as a means to lose weight.

In this chapter we will cover four major areas regarding protein:

▶ How protein structure makes each protein different from the other and affects their function.

▶ How the body processes protein and its building blocks—the amino acids.

▶ The consequence of protein deficiency—how much protein you need and the impact of exercise and other factors on protein requirements (along with whether protein supplements are needed).

▶ How to meet protein needs and make healthful food choices (meat vs. vegetarian diets).

UNDERSTANDING PROTEIN STRUCTURE AND FUNCTION

The word *protein* means "primary." Early scientists of the 1700s and 1800s knew that a source of protein was vital for life. In those early days of nutrition, scientists believed that there was one single substance "protein" and that this substance contained the element nitrogen. These early researchers also knew that the element nitrogen was in the air that both humans and animals breathe but that a dietary source of nitrogen (thus protein) was vital for life. During this time scientists also knew that nitrogen was unique to protein.

By the 1900s scientists discovered that rather than one single substance, there were many, even thousands of different proteins, all of which contained the element nitrogen. Different proteins were discovered in the human body such as proteins in the blood and protein in hair, while other unique proteins were discovered in foods such as in eggs and beef. How did all of these proteins differ from each other? A look at protein structure will explain these differences along with getting us on our way to understanding why we need protein, how much we need, and how best to meet that need.

Chemical Structure of Protein

We will use two examples in discussing the chemical structure of protein: a protein in food that you might eat such as beef, and a protein found in your body such as a blood protein. Figure 2.1 shows these two proteins.

- Notice that each protein exists as a three-dimensional shape, much like a rope folded up in a specific way. This 3-D shape is different for each protein, whether in food or in the body, and as we will learn, the shape of each different protein is designed to suit that protein's function (such as carrying a vitamin in the blood, which is why this protein has an opening or dish-like shape).

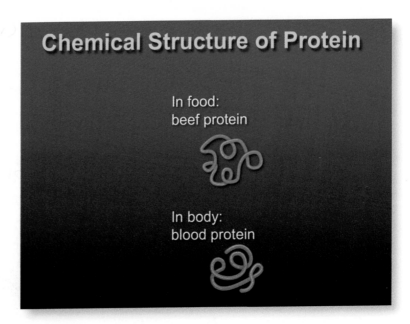

FIGURE 2.1

- If we snipped a piece from each of these 3-D structures, upon close inspection, we would find that rather than a rope, the protein is made up of a chain of linked subunits—hundreds of them.

- These subunits are called amino acids, as shown in Figure 2.2. There are 20 different amino acids reflected in Figure 2.2 as different colors and numbers. Amino acids are linked together by peptide bonds.

Nutrition Bite

You may come across the term peptides *when looking at protein supplements over the Internet or in a store. This term is used to describe a few amino acids joined together. Peptides are essentially small fragments of a protein, and offer nothing special over eating proteins whole from foods.*

Amino Acid Structure

Now let's take a look at what makes up an amino acid, and very importantly, how amino acids differ from one another.

Elements that make up amino acids (and other nutrients) follow certain rules when it comes to making chemical bonds. The four elements that make up amino acids are: carbon (C) with four bonds, oxygen (O)

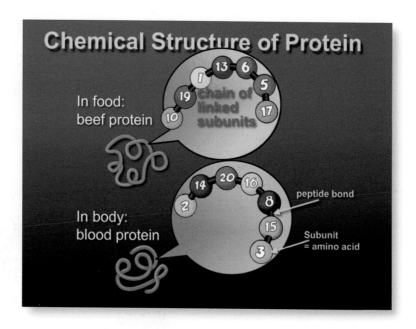

Chemical Structure of Protein

In food: beef protein

chain of linked subunits

In body: blood protein

peptide bond

Subunit = amino acid

FIGURE 2.2

with two bonds, hydrogen (H) with one bond, and nitrogen (N) with three bonds. In Figure 2.3 illustrating a generic amino acid, the amino group (N) and the acid group (i.e., COOH group) are identified. Every amino acid has both of these chemical groups.

The R group pictured over the middle carbon represents a chemical group (rather than an element with the abbreviation "R"). There are 20 different R groups—20 different chemical groups. This means there are 20 different amino acids, each with their own name. A few examples are shown in Figure 2.4.

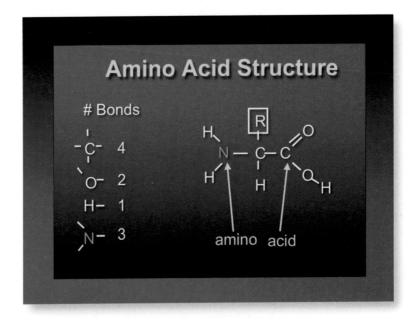

FIGURE 2.3

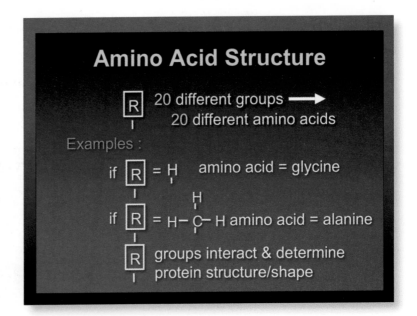

FIGURE 2.4

- Many of the amino acid names sound the same and often end in "ine." In this course we won't worry about their names, but instead will differentiate between amino acids by referring to them with the numbers 1 through 20 as shown in Figures 2.2 and 2.5.

- Each R group has specific chemical properties. Some R groups may like to interact with a watery environment, while others might be attracted to other R groups. This is very important when it comes to a protein's 3-D structure and function.

- Upon inspection of one protein (beef) compared to another (blood), we notice that the sequence or order of amino acids differ, as shown in Figure 2.5. This in turn determines how a protein is shaped. R groups interact with other R groups down the chain and fold up depending upon the sequence of amino acids in the protein chain.

- In the beef protein example, note the sequence of amino acids. Amino acid #10 interacts with amino acid #17. This interaction causes the chain to fold, creating the loop on the right. This R group interaction dictates how the protein folds. Because each protein has a unique sequence of amino acids, this makes the shape or structure of the protein unique.

- How was the amino acid sequence determined for a specific protein? We will discuss this more in another section, but each cell in animals and in plants comes equipped with a set of instructions (genetic material) that determines what proteins each cell (cell type) makes. So in a cow's muscle cells the genetic material instructs what protein to make (unique amino acid sequence). In the case of a cow, muscle contractile protein is made. We in turn

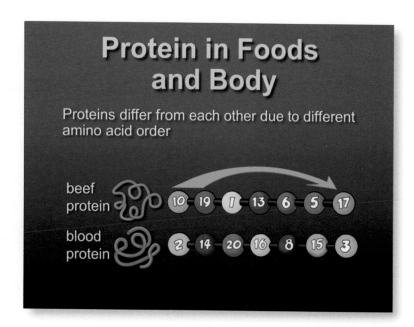

FIGURE 2.5

eat this protein when we eat beef (among many other types of proteins found in beef).

Amino Acid–Protein Analogy

I like to use an analogy—letters of our alphabet spelling words—that helps to clarify how amino acids' sequence determines shape and shape determines function of a protein.

- Amino acid order is like spelling a word (the order of letters).
- Folding of the amino acid chain into a 3-D shape (structure) is like the pronunciation of that word (since the letters in that order follow phonetic rules).
- The protein structure is like the meaning of the word.

Use this example of seven letters shown in Figure 2.6 and you can see how letter sequence is vital to the word meaning just like amino acid order is vital to protein shape and structure.

- Just as words can have more than one of the same letter, such as the words "pepper" or "school," proteins also can have duplicate (or more) of a given amino acid. Also, proteins vary from one another on the profile or amounts of each of the 20 amino acids.

Amino Acids—Are They All Essential or Just Certain Ones?

- Of the 20 different amino acids, nine are essential—they can't be made in the body and are needed in the diet (supplied by foods that

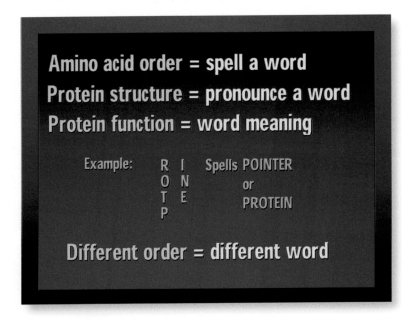

FIGURE 2.6

contain those nine essential amino acids in the food's protein). These amino acids are referred to as the essential amino acids or EAA for short. The reason is primarily because the R group on these nine essential amino acids can't be made by our metabolic machinery.

- The other 11 amino acids are called nonessential amino acids or NEAA for short. These do not need to be in your diet since you have the ability to make the NEAA from other components in your diet (carbon from fat or carbohydrate, for example). But you do need a source of nitrogen in your diet to build a NEAA. Remember those early scientists proved that protein was the vital supplier of this element.

This brings us to two important reasons why protein is needed in our diet:

- A source of EAA
- A source of nitrogen (needed to make NEAA)

Function of Protein

Recall the three basic functions of nutrients: structure, energy, and regulation. Protein is a versatile nutrient and performs all three.

1. **Structure**

   - Bone: minerals, calcium, and phosphorous are deposited on a protein honeycomb-like structure to make bone.

   - Connective tissue: a structural protein called collagen acts much like glue that holds us together—literally keeping teeth in the gums, blood vessels intact, and joints held together. Collagen makes up about 25% of the protein in the body making this structural protein of great significance. (Collagen will be discussed in Chapter 11 when vitamin C is covered, because this vitamin is needed to make healthy collagen.)

2. **Energy**

   - Protein (specifically food protein) possesses potential energy in its chemical bonds. This energy is released in the form of heat or calories (more in Chapter 3) and this energy can be used by the body.

   - There is no storage of protein or amino acids. This means that all protein in the body is actively working. So using functional tissue for a source of energy means that protein loses its ability to do its job as that protein. This contrasts with fat and carbohydrate, which are stored as fuel reserves.

3. **Regulation**   Thousands of proteins perform regulatory roles in your body from building a new strand of hair to helping your cells regulate water level. Here are a few examples of protein in a regulatory role:

- **Hormones:** Some hormones are made of protein, but not all. Insulin, a hormone made by the pancreas, is involved in carbohydrate homeostasis.

- **Enzymes:** All enzymes are made of protein and these are chemical catalysts that facilitate or allow a reaction in the body to occur. For example, to build a new muscle protein, an enzyme is needed to bring together the amino acid building blocks and form the muscle protein.

- **Immune system:** Specialized cells which fight off infection, are built with protein.

- **Fluid balance:** Special proteins in the blood and inside cells keep the fluid balance at the delicate one third outside of cells and two thirds inside of cells.

Think about these important regulatory roles for our discussion of protein deficiency. Would fluid balance be maintained or would an infection be a risk for a person not getting enough protein?

PROCESSING PROTEIN IN THE BODY

Now let's take a look at how your body processes protein from its digestion to its use inside cells for protein synthesis. Follow what happens to a sample meal, consisting of a glass of soy milk and a turkey sandwich, as these food proteins are digested.

Protein Digestion

The proteins pictured at the top of Figure 2.7 (representing the mouth and throat) are from the soy milk and from the turkey sandwich (though there are other proteins in these foods). These proteins have different 3-D shapes (different proteins) and thus different amounts of the 20 amino acids.

- The physical digestion of protein begins in the mouth with chewing the food and mixing it with saliva. But, there's actually no need to chew your food at all or for a certain number of times (maybe your mom told you to chew your food seven times before swallowing). The rest of your digestive tract can handle unchewed food although swallowing slightly chewed food is more comfortable.

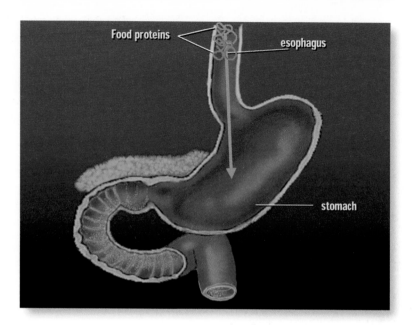

FIGURE 2.7

- Once swallowed, the soy milk and turkey sandwich travel down your esophagus and land in your stomach for the remainder of physical digestion. Here in the stomach, the food is "blenderized" much like a smoothie. Also, special cells in the stomach secrete acid and this mixes with your soymilk-turkey smoothie (see Figure 2.8).

- The acid disrupts the R groups of the amino acids in the strand of protein. This causes the protein structure to denature, or unfold, as shown in Figure 2.9. This is the beginning of chemical digestion for protein.

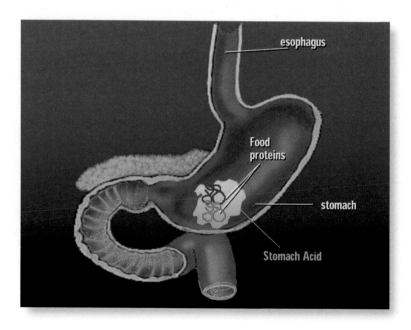

FIGURE 2.8

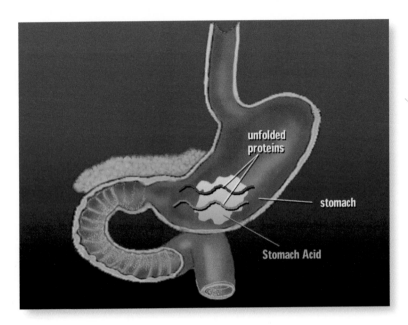

FIGURE 2.9

- These unfolded strands of protein then move into the small intestine where a digestive enzyme from the pancreas is secreted to complete chemical digestion (Figure 2.10). This enzyme, protease (*hint:* "prot" = protein; "-ase" = enzyme), chemically breaks the peptide bonds releasing individual amino acids into the small intestinal space, as shown in Figure 2.11.

- Both EAA and NEAA are present, thousands and thousands of each. The intestinal track cannot tell which amino acid came from which food.

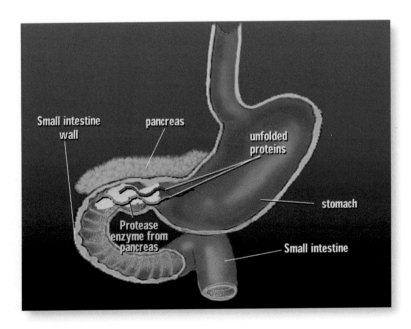

FIGURE 2.10

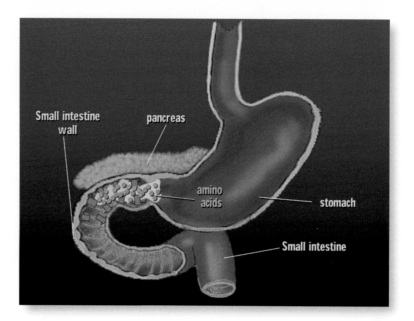

FIGURE 2.11

● Additionally, intestinal track cells are sloughing off and being digested along with the food. The proteins from these cells are also digested in the same way (see Figure 2.11).

● **The end product of protein digestion is individual amino acids from food and from digested intestinal track cell protein.** These individual amino acids are absorbed through the wall of the small intestine (see Figure 2.12).

Now let's take a look at how your body uses these absorbed amino acids.

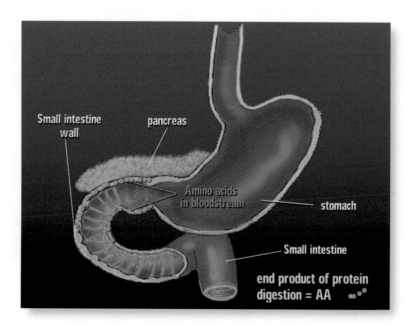

FIGURE 2.12

How the Body Uses Protein

After the meal of soy milk and a turkey sandwich is digested in amino acids, and assimilated (absorbed), these new amino acids are now surging through your blood vessels heading off to muscle cells, liver cells, and even eye ball cells for use.

Figure 2.13 indicates how the body (each cell) uses amino acids. We will build on this diagram as we continue to discuss the options for amino acid use by the cell.

- Inside a body cell (such as liver or muscle cell) consider the mix of EAA and NEAA as a "bucket" of amino acids. Based upon the set of instructions that a specific cell has (for example, a muscle cell has instructions to make contractile protein; and a liver cell may have instructions to build a fluid balance protein), the cell pulls the amino acids needed to build the proteins it is instructed to make out of the "bucket." The cell will make only what it is instructed to make (i.e., type of protein) and only in the amount needed. This means that, even if the bucket is "overflowing" (loads of amino acids because of extra protein in the diet), only the amount of protein needed will be made. (Remember homeostasis?)

- Also, the right profile or proportion of amino acids must be present in the "bucket" to make the protein. If a particular NEAA is missing from the bucket, the cell has the ability to make that amino acid if given a source of nitrogen, which would come from other amino acids. If a particular EAA is missing, the protein will not be made. A substitution with another amino acid in the chain would mean that the strand of amino acids would fold up differently due

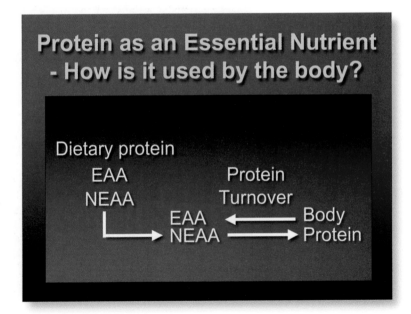

FIGURE 2.13

to the R groups and thus the structure and function would be different. Back to the alphabet–amino acid analogy, putting the wrong amino acid in would be like creating a typo instead of a word.

- Take another look at Figure 2.13. The amino acids are made into a protein, and then they break down again. Amino acids ⇆ protein implies that proteins are being made, and then broken down again to their building block components, and then made into other proteins again, and so on. Why would the cell do this? It seems like a waste of energy.

The process of **protein turnover** (see Figure 2.14) is a very good thing because it allows us (our bodies) to make more of a protein that we might need immediately and less of another protein that is not quite crucial at the time. Here are some examples.

- If you were to swallow a rock or sharp object with your food and damaged your intestinal track, it's nice to know the damage would be repaired in about three to five days since this area does turnover quickly. If you didn't repair yourself in a timely fashion, then your intestinal track damage may impair your ability to digest and absorb food and subsequently get the nutrients you need to stay healthy.

- If you get sick with a serious illness such as chicken pox, you would want your body's immune system to rise to the occasion and kick the virus, rather than just produce a set number of immune fighters which may not be designed to fight this specific infection. In the meantime, your body can make less of other proteins such as the enzymes that break down alcohol. You probably won't be drinking much when you are sick!

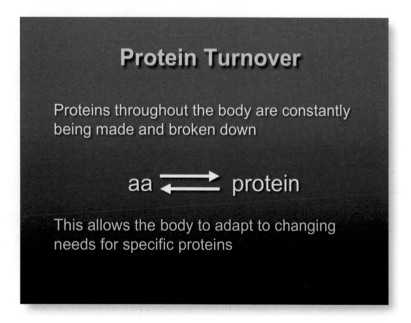

FIGURE 2.14

The rates at which some proteins turnover are shown in Figure 2.15. Make note of the high turnover proteins which are affected more dramatically than slow turnover proteins during protein deficiency. Which condition—intestinal trouble versus brain damage—would a person more likely recover from once adequate protein was consumed?

● Not all proteins turn over; some are lost to the body. These are known as the "dead-end" proteins because the body doesn't get them back after they are made. These include the proteins in hair, skin, nails, and stool (from unabsorbed dietary protein and sloughed off intestinal cells). Think of these dead-end protein losses as a hole in the bottom of a water tank, where water leaks out steadily. The water must be replaced to keep the fill line constant. In your body, dietary protein must be consumed to replace these dead-end protein losses.

● Let's now complete the diagram by adding Figure 2.16 and look at what happens with amino acids when we have an excess—in other words, our "bucket" is overflowing. We've already established that with excess amino acids, more proteins are NOT made. So what happens to the excess?

As shown in Figure 2.16, the nitrogen is stripped off the amino acid, leaving what is called a "carbon skeleton." So now we have two items to track: **nitrogen** and **carbon skeleton.**

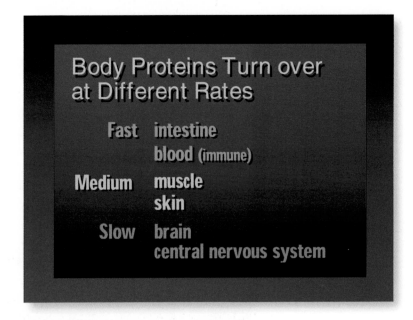

FIGURE 2.15

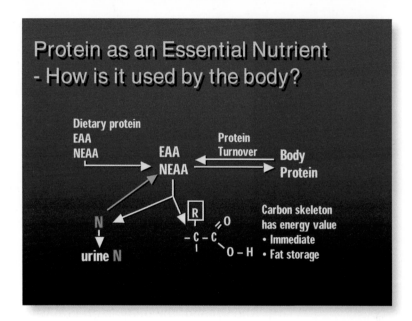

FIGURE 2.16

Nitrogen: The option is there, as the arrow indicates, that the nitrogen could be used to make a nonessential amino acid. But since amino acids are in abundance, the need to do this is unlikely. Instead, the nitrogen must be removed because it is a toxic substance that the body wants to get rid of soon. In the kidneys the nitrogen is transformed into a substance called urea, which is then excreted in the urine. It costs calories to do this process but the body is willing to put in the extra cost since nitrogen is a toxic substance. So, if you have consumed more protein than what you need, you will excrete the excess nitrogen in your urine.

It's important to point out that you always have some nitrogen (urea) in your urine at all times, not just if you are consuming extra protein. This is because at any given moment in time, a cell is pulling the nitrogen off to use the carbon skeleton to make another amino acid or some other substance.

Carbon skeleton: This "skeleton" of an amino acid contains potential energy in the chemical bonds. This energy can be utilized immediately, that is, broken down with the chemical bonds being broken and heat released—your body can extract about 4 calories for every gram of amino acids/protein (more on this in Chapter 3). But what if you weren't in need of immediate energy? This potential energy in the carbon skeleton does not go to waste. Instead, with a bit of chemical magic, the carbons are rearranged into fat. This means that **amino acids or protein eaten in excess of need can be converted to and stored as fat.** Since most Americans exceed their protein needs (our "bucket" is overflowing) and many don't exercise or expend enough calories, the carbon skeletons go to fat (remember, the nitrogen goes to the urine).

Does Taking an Amino Acid Supplement Make a Difference?

With what you've just learned about amino acid, their use by the body and how your cells treat excess amino acids, let's take a look at adding more to the mix. Many people take an amino acid supplement in hopes of improved muscle weight gain, or perhaps another benefit touted on the supplement label. Now that you know how amino acid metabolism works, you can decide whether an extra of one or more amino acids will make a difference in protein synthesis.

Refer to Figure 2.17. If a person takes an amino acid supplement, eaa_3 for example, this ends up in the "bucket." The amount in supplements is quite small, and the extra will go virtually unnoticed. But more importantly, will extra of an amino acid increase the amount of protein being made? No extra protein will be made for two reasons. First, extra of one amino acid does not mean more of an entire protein will be made (similar to saying you could spell more words if you have more of the letter "e"). And second, the body is programmed to make a certain amount of each protein (remember homeostasis?) so no extra will be made. Now what do you think—is taking this supplement of amino acids helpful?

Key Concepts about Protein

It's time to pull a few items together to make sure we have a good understanding about key protein concepts.

- Each protein has a unique order or sequence of amino acids.
- There are 20 amino acids. Nine amino acids are essential, and all 20 are found in your body proteins and food proteins. Each protein has different proportions of each of the amino acids.

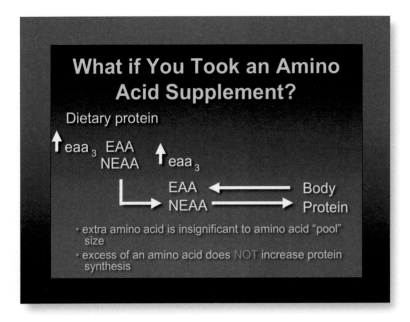

FIGURE 2.17

- Proteins in the body turn over.
- There is no storage of protein or amino acids in the body.

PROTEIN DEFICIENCY AND REQUIREMENT

In this section, we'll take a look at what happens when too little protein (or insufficient EAA) is consumed as well as how much protein is required and what factors, such as exercise or severe illness, impact protein needs.

Protein Deficiency

Before we can discuss protein deficiency, we need to review a few things about growth stages. Intuitively, you might agree that protein deficiency in a young child would have a different impact, more severe, compared to an older child or an adult. This has to do with the impact of growth on protein needs.

Stages of Growth

The first stage of growth occurs during fetal development up to the first 18 to 24 months of life. Growth during this stage is accomplished by an increase in the number of cells in an organ and tissue. For example, the brain increases in size due to an increase in cell number, as shown in Figure 2.18, therefore, nutritional status is very important at this stage in life. Inadequate intake of protein or other nutrients such as vitamins can lead to permanent damage or stunted growth (permanently reduced height and stature).

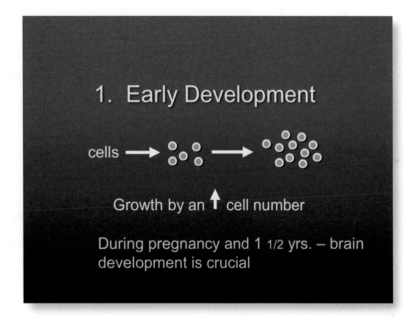

FIGURE 2.18

During this later stage of development pictured in Figure 2.19, growth occurs mostly by an increase in cell size. This stage occurs in children and teens, while there is still some increase in cell number during these years. The results of a nutritional deficiency at this stage is not as devastating if proper nutrition is provided soon.

Consequence of Protein Deficiency

High turnover proteins (recall those with a high turnover rate) will be affected most dramatically with protein deficiency. These high turnover proteins rely on a constant supply of amino acids.

Protein deficiency during early development results in:

- mental retardation
- reduced growth or stunting (permanent)

In young children, teens, and adults protein deficiency results in:

- **Edema**—retention of fluid, giving a puffy swollen appearance. Proteins involved in fluid balance are not being made, so that fluid leaves the inside of cells and moves to the extracellular space giving a swollen appearance.

- **Intestinal problems**—diarrhea and poor absorption of nutrients. Without sufficient protein, the individual cannot keep up with the rapid turnover of intestinal cells (every three to five days). The intestinal track surface becomes smooth, and with the reduced surface area, nutrients are not absorbed so diarrhea results as water is drawn into the intestinal track.

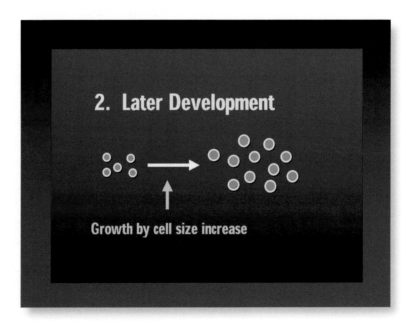

FIGURE 2.19

- **Distended abdomen**—fatty liver and fluid retention cause the belly to protrude. Fluid buildup in the abdominal cavity causes a distended abdomen. Also, the liver is unable to make proteins necessary to package up fats and send them out into the bloodstream. The liver then builds up with fat and enlarges. This is seen in alcoholics because of a poor diet and alcohol interferes with liver function (more on this in Chapter 10).

- **Infections**—eye, lung, and skin infections develop due to reduced immune response. Without adequate protein, the immune system becomes weak and invading bacteria and viruses take hold. Often, people with protein deficiency succumb to these infections.

Conditions seen with protein deficiency:

- **Kwashiorkor**—this means "the evil spirit that infects the first child after the second child is born." This condition occurs in young children (usually in underdeveloped countries) that are weaned from breast milk at about 9 months of age when the mom becomes pregnant with a second child. The weaning food given to this first child is generally low in protein and the child becomes very sick by the time the second child is born. Often this first child has edema which then progresses to an emaciated look.

- **Protein-calorie malnutrition**—severe wasting of muscle and fat as the person is starved for total food or energy. The body breaks itself down and muscle wasting appears.

Protein Requirement

The time has come to figure out your protein requirement. This method is going to involve just a bit of math in a three-step process. In the end, you will know your RDA for protein.

Why do you need protein?

- source of essential amino acids

- source of nitrogen (to make NEAA)

Three-step process to compute the RDA for protein:

1. Compute the minimum amount of protein needed for an average person.

2. Adjust this figure to account for population variability.

3. Adjust this figure for quality of protein in the diet.

Start with an average adult, male or a female (who is not pregnant or lactating because these factors would alter protein needs), weighing 70 kg (about 155 pounds). How much protein does this person need every day?

Recall that the body is like a tank with a leak of water—how much water do we need to put in to cover water losses? Now think of our body and the protein we lose every day—hair, skin, nails, urine, and stool. These losses could be collected (very tedious) and used to calculate how much minimum protein is needed to cover daily losses. The amount of nitrogen in these items is measured since nitrogen is unique to protein—nitrogen is our marker for protein.

Nitrogen Losses Reflect Protein Needs

This average male or female loses nitrogen daily that we can measure—let's say that it is 5 grams daily. This value must be converted to grams of protein per day (and this would represent the "leak" in the tank). To do this we are going to make a conversion of grams of nitrogen to grams of protein. We will use a factor of 6.25 grams of protein for every gram of nitrogen. (This factor comes from the fact that 16% of the weight for all proteins is nitrogen. So 100 grams of protein has 16 grams of nitrogen or divide 100 by 16 and you get 6.25 grams protein/gram nitrogen. *Note:* This is only a conversion factor and has nothing to do with your RDA for protein!)

For Our Average Male and Female

$$5 \text{ grams nitrogen} \times \frac{6.25 \text{ grams protein}}{\text{gram nitrogen}} = 31 \text{ grams protein}$$

This means that 31 grams represents the minimum amount of protein these two people weighing 70 kg would need each day ("leak" in their tank). There's a catch though. The protein needed must be perfect protein, protein that supplies all nine EAA in the amounts needed to make body proteins. Only two proteins meet this description: human breast milk protein and egg white protein. Thus, this 70 kg man and woman must eat 31 grams of egg white protein daily to cover their protein losses/needs.

STEP 2

In this step we take into account variation in the population. Let's take into consideration that not everyone is average, that is, not everyone loses 5 grams of nitrogen daily.

As shown in Figure 2.20, the need for protein falls on a distribution curve. So to meet the needs of *nearly all* people in the population, let's

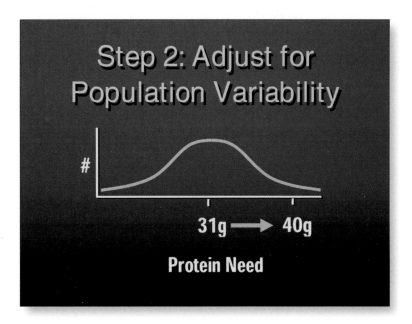

FIGURE 2.20

add to 31 grams and push it up to 40 grams of perfect protein daily. This amount of perfect protein should meet virtually everyone in the population who weighs 70 kg. (By the way, we got the number 40 by adding two standard deviations to the average value.)

STEP 3

This final step takes into account that we eat a mix of proteins each day rather than just eating egg white protein. Food proteins contain all of the 20 amino acids and the nine essential amino acids. But various food proteins have these nine EAA in different amounts.

We'll be discussing protein quality in the next section. For now, let's say that if we gave egg white a quality score of 100, the protein in most people's diets would score about 70 (peanut butter, milk, fish, soy, beans, etc.). This ratio of 100 to 70 is used to adjust the 40 grams to 56 grams per day for a 70-kg adult male or female. This means that a 70-kg male or female could meet their protein needs on 56 grams of proteins from a variety of sources.

But since not everyone weighs 70 kg, we need to express this as a requirement based on 1 kg of body weight, in a way that all of us can use:

The RDA for protein for adult men and women is 0.8 grams protein/kg body weight per day

This value represents the amount of protein from a mix of food sources that should meet the needs of nearly all healthy people in the population. Also, this amount is averaged over several days and does not represent a minimum value.

Let's use the RDA for protein in a calculation. How much protein does a 50-kg woman require?

$$50 \text{ kg} \times 0.8 \text{ g/kg per day} = 40 \text{ g protein/day}$$

This value represents the amount of protein that should be more than adequate for her from a variety of sources.

A QUESTION FOR YOU

Her 50-kg male friend requires more protein. True? False?

False! Protein requirement is not a function of gender, so he would require the same amount.

Factors That Change Protein Needs

The RDA for protein above is for an adult man or woman. As you might expect, the protein needs for a child, teenager, and pregnant or lactating woman are different. How does injury, illness, and exercise impact protein needs?

1. Growth

The RDA for infants is about 2 grams of protein/kg body weight per day. This is much greater than the RDA for adults due to the infant's rate of growth compared to that of an adult. Consider that each day a growing baby is ending the day with more cells than it started with (so, of course, the need for more protein). Look at the numbers in Figure 2.21 to see how the protein requirement changes with age as growth rate slows down. *Note:* The only time there is a gender difference is during the late teen years, due to differences in growth rate. Girls are finished growing by approximately age 15 or so, while boys continue to grow and therefore need more protein.

The table in Figure 2.21 expresses protein needs based on body weight or what's referred to as relative protein needs. Don't confuse this with the overall protein need of a given individual expressed in grams per day. With this in mind, who requires more protein: an infant who weighs 10 pounds or an adult weighing 150 pounds? The adult would need more simply because he or she is so much larger than the baby. But if you were asked who needs more on a relative basis, the infant would (2g/kg versus 0.8 g/kg).

RDA FOR PROTEIN BASED ON AGE	
AGE (YR) RDA	PROTEIN G/KG BODY WT
0–0.5	2.2
0.5–1	1.6
1–3	1.2
4–6	1.1
7–14	1.0
15–18	0.9 male
15–18	0.8 female
19 +	0.8 male/female

FIGURE 2.21

2. Pregnancy and Lactation

Over the course of a pregnancy, a woman typically puts on about 22 to 27 pounds of body weight. Much of this weight gain is due to an increase in blood volume, and an increase in her fat stores, uterine size, and breasts along with the weight of the baby. If this is all taken into consideration, a woman needs 25 grams of extra protein daily above her RDA.

Lactation or breast-feeding requires additional dietary protein as the mother produces milk (protein source) for the newborn. An extra 25 grams per day is needed for a lactating woman.

3. Injury and illness

Remember that the RDA meets the needs of nearly all *healthy* people in the population. What about people who are sick with a severe illness such as pneumonia—do they need more protein? Or if a person is injured such as with burns or extensive surgery, how are protein needs impacted? These are individual situations that alter protein needs and must be considered. A health professional such as a physician or dietitian could assess the protein needs for an individual who is seriously ill or injured. When you get sick with a cold or flu, your protein needs are not dramatically altered so there's no need to worry about eating more protein during those times of illness.

4. Exercise

The RDA for protein is computed for a person who is NOT engaged in regular, vigorous exercise such as weight lifting or running.

Studies show that people who engage in regular exercise for about an hour daily need more than the RDA for protein. The amount over the RDA depends upon many factors such as the type of exercise—its duration, frequency, and intensity.

For weight-training athletes or those involved in contact sports such as football, muscle mass increases. There is also some muscle damage that occurs during impact exercise. Research studies show that an extra 0.4 g/kg body weight or 50% above the RDA is needed.

For endurance athletes (runners, triathletes, and cyclists) another situation occurs. Protein contributes a small amount to total energy use—about 10% overall. For the average person not participating in these types of sports, protein needs would not be altered. But consider that some of these athletes train for hours every day. This translates to an increase in protein needs of about 0.4 g/kg body weight or 50% above the RDA.

Since many athletes take in more calories than a nonathlete, they typically get enough protein and there is no need to supplement to get this amount. However, for some athletes who have difficulty making good food choices, a protein powder mixed with juice or made into a smoothie is a good way to meet protein needs.

Protein on Food Labels—The Daily Value for Protein

Now that you know your personal protein requirement based on your weight, how can you use that information to make food choices based on the Nutrition Facts food label? As you might guess, food manufacturers couldn't list everyone's protein requirement on the label—it just wouldn't fit! Instead, what is used for a point of comparison is the Daily Value for protein. We'll be learning more about the Daily Value, or DV for short, in future chapters. The DV is set for a variety of nutrients such as protein, fat, saturated fat, fiber, and more and is based on an average consumer taking in about 2,000 calories daily. The DV is a suggested intake for good health and the prevention of chronic disease. (More on this in Chapter 6 when we cover fat and heart disease.)

The Daily Value for protein is 50 grams. This means that the average consumer eating approximately 2,000 calories daily needs about 50 grams of protein. Food labels list the amount of protein in a serving of the food, as shown in Figure 2.22. Food labels are NOT required to list the percentage this product provides of the DV for protein unless a specific claim is made on the label in regards to protein such as "excellent source of protein."

However, you can calculate what percent of the DV a serving of food provides with some simple math. Here's how it's done for a serving of cheese casserole (see Figure 2.23).

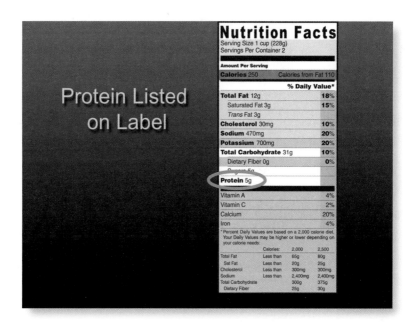

FIGURE 2.22

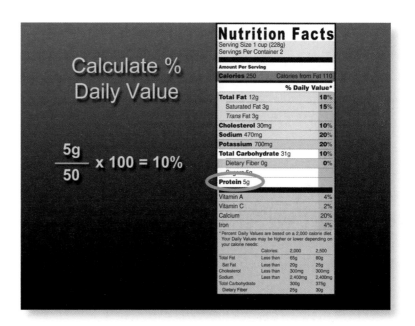

FIGURE 2.23

Using food labels or the chart on page 38, which lists the protein content of several types of food, practice calculating the percent of DV. Many foods such as canned tuna, chili, and others provide a substantial amount of the DV for protein.

FOOD, SERVING SIZE (SUGGESTED ITEMS)	GRAMS OF PROTEIN
milk, low-fat, 8 ounces	8
soy milk, 8 ounces	7
refried beans, 1 cup	12
yogurt, low-fat, cup	13
lentils, dry, 1/4 cup	13
Thai Fish Curry	17
soyburger, a 2-ounce patty	18
skinless chicken breast, grilled, 4 ounces	20
canned tuna, 3 ounces	22
beef chili, 1 cup	24
PowerBar Plus Protein	24
smoothie (Jamba, w/protein)	25
fast-food items • Pizza Hut Veggie Lover's, pan, medium 12″, 1 slice • Taco Bell Burrito Supreme • McDonald's Chicken McGrill • Burger King Whopper	 10 17 26 29

MAKING PROTEIN FOOD CHOICES

Now that you know how much protein you need, and that food proteins (like body proteins) differ in their amino acid content, let's consider making protein choices. Since food proteins differ in their amino acid profile, do you think that the protein in peanut butter would meet your need for protein as well as egg protein? Intuitively you might say no, and you're right. This is what protein quality is all about, and understanding this can aid us in making choices from including meat in the diet to adopting a vegetarian plan.

Protein Quality

Food sources differ in the quality of protein present. All proteins contain the EAAs and provide a source of nitrogen. But, as mentioned before, proteins differ in the amount (or proportion) of each of the essential amino acids they provide. It's the EAA content of a food protein in relationship to our need that determines the quality of a food protein.

The quality of a food protein can be assessed directly (measuring the EAA content of the food protein) or indirectly (assessing the growth of a laboratory animal eating a diet that contains the test protein). We will cover two protein quality tests—one indirect and the other direct. First, we need to provide some definitions used in discussing protein sources.

Complete Protein

- Complete protein contains all nine essential amino acids.
- The essential amino acids are present in proportion to need.
- The food protein is digestible.

Examples of complete proteins:

- beef
- fish
- egg
- poultry
- dairy
- soybean (soy products)

Egg protein and human breast milk protein are complete proteins and are perfect; that is, they're the best complete proteins you can get. In general, animal sources of protein are complete and when you think about it, many animal proteins are similar to our own proteins (muscle or flesh, for example), which would mean that essential amino acid profiles would match our needs fairly well. Soy protein is the only plant protein source that is complete. So tofu, soy burgers, and other soy foods are good-quality protein sources.

Incomplete Protein

Incomplete protein does not contain all nine essential amino acids in amounts proportional to need. Examples of incomplete proteins are shown in Figure 2.24.

What if you only eat incomplete protein sources? Many vegetarians do this. It is certainly possible to meet your needs for EAA but you must use some care. More on this later.

GRAINS	BEANS (LEGUMES)	NUTS	SEEDS
oats	kidney	peanuts	sesame
wheat	garbanzo	cashews	sunflower
barley	navy	almonds	pumpkin
rice	pinto	walnuts	

FIGURE 2.24

Protein Quality Tests

Protein quality tests measure either indirectly or directly EAA content. Let's take a look at two protein quality tests: Protein Efficiency Ratio and Chemical Score.

1. Protein Efficiency Ratio or PER

This is an indirect measurement of EAA content. In this test, growing laboratory animals such as rats are fed a diet containing the protein in question, corn protein for example. Each day, weight gain is measured and the amount of food (protein) eaten is determined. The PER is a ratio of weight gained to protein eaten.

$$PER = \frac{\text{weight gained}}{\text{protein eaten}}$$

A high PER would mean that the protein was utilized (meaning, good EAA content) and the animal grew well. A low PER would mean the EAA content was poor because the animal's growth was not good. Some PER values are shown in Figure 2.25.

As you may notice, complete proteins have a high PER and incomplete proteins have a low PER. Does this fit with our definition of complete and incomplete proteins? There are a few limitations using the PER quality test.

- The PER does not reveal which EAA might be in low amount in the protein.

- Also, how well a laboratory rat grows on a specific protein may not reflect how well a person might utilize the test protein.

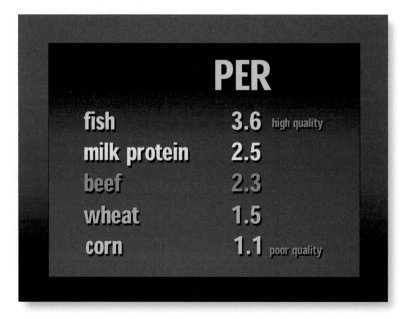

PER

fish	3.6	high quality
milk protein	2.5	
beef	2.3	
wheat	1.5	
corn	1.1	poor quality

FIGURE 2.25

With these two things in mind, measuring protein quality may be better assessed using a direct measure of EAA content.

2. Chemical Score

This protein quality test is a direct measure of essential amino acid content. The protein to be tested is put into a machine that can tell you how much of each amino acid is present and what the relative percentages are, that is, percent by weight. These percentages are then compared to the percentages found in our "gold" standard egg white protein. This is chosen because egg white's essential amino acid content best reflects our need for the nine essential amino acids.

For simplicity, only five of the nine essential amino acids are listed in Figure 2.26 for egg white and our test protein from white flour. This is done to save space, but in a true chemical score test, values of all nine essential amino acids would be listed.

In Figure 2.26, the amount of each of the EAA as percent by weight is listed for egg white and the test protein. Also, thrown in to test your understanding of protein quality is the value for glycine, a nonessential amino acid. Don't be fooled by this because if you follow on with the calculation for chemical score and don't omit the glycine, you will obtain the wrong number. Ask yourself, do we care how much of a NEAA is in a food protein? Does this impact the quality? No to both of these questions! So be sure to cross out this value for the NEAA, glycine.

FIGURE 2.26

CHEMICAL SCORE		
AMINO ACID	EGG WHITE	WHITE FLOUR PROTEIN
lysine (EAA)	7.0	2.1
methionine (EAA)	5.6	4.0
leucine (EAA)	8.6	7.0
tryptophan (EAA)	1.7	1.1
valine (EAA)	6.6	4.1
glycine (NEAA)	2.2	0.5
Chemical Score = 30		

The next step is to compute what percentage of each EAA of our test protein white flour compared to egg white protein (see Figure 2.27).

The **chemical score** of a protein is the lowest percentage computed—in the case of white flour protein lysine has a value of 30 (30 percent of the lysine content of egg white). If glycine had not been canceled out, then the score would have been computed as 23, which is incorrect since this NEAA does not impact the quality of the protein.

The score also tells us which EAA is in the lowest amount relative to our need. This is called the **limiting amino acid—the essential amino acid in a food protein in the lowest amount relative to need**. All incomplete proteins have one or more limiting amino acids.

Most grains (flour, barley, rice) are limiting in lysine and most beans (legumes such as kidney and black beans) are limiting in methionine. This actually is great when combining these sources of protein in vegetarian meals and diets because grains and beans compliment each other and form a complete protein. (More on this in the next section.)

Is Protein Quality an Issue for Children and Adults?

How big of an issue is protein quality when you make your daily food choices? To answer this, we need to look at how much of your daily protein needs must be as the essential amino acids. (Recall that you need protein as a source of EAA and a source of nitrogen.) As you might imagine,

CHEMICAL SCORE

AMINO ACID	EGG WHITE	WHITE FLOUR PROTEIN	%
lysine (EAA)	7.0	2.1	$2.1/7.0 \times 100 =$ **30**
methionine (EAA)	5.6	4.0	$4.0/5.6 \times 100 = 71$
leucine (EAA)	8.6	7.0	$7.0/8.6 \times 100 = 81$
tryptophan (EAA)	1.7	1.1	$1.1/1.7 \times 100 = 64$
valine (EAA)	6.6	4.1	$4.1/6.6 \times 100 = 62$
~~glycine (NEAA)~~	~~2.2~~	~~0.5~~	
		Chemical Score = **30**	

FIGURE 2.27

the EAA needs for an adult would be different than that for an infant or child because of growth.

- **An adult needs only 0.09 g of EAA/kg of body weight or 11% of the RDA for protein as EAAs.** This means that the other 89% can be any amino acid since they all supply nitrogen. If you wanted to meet your need for EAA by eating an incomplete protein source exclusively, this could be done. You would need to eat, for example, one loaf of bread (grain protein) to meet your need for EAA—a doable but boring diet. Nonetheless, you could eat a loaf of bread in one day, but this is not the case for a young child.

- **Infants require 0.7 g of EAA/kg of body weight or 40% of their RDA for protein as EAAs.** Why the big difference? Infants are making new proteins every day above those that are just turning over as an adult would. (We are in maintenance.) Could an infant meet their need for EAA by eating one incomplete protein source exclusively? If it takes four loaves of bread to meet the EAA need of a 1-year-old child, it would be impossible to get such a small child to eat so much! So feeding an incomplete protein source as the exclusive protein source would not meet the child's needs. Instead, a complete protein source would be better. Any suggestions? How about breast milk, or if the child is old enough, fish, soy, beef, or dairy products would all be good choices.

Vegetarian Diets

Now with a good understanding of protein quality, let's take a look at vegetarian diets. Perhaps you are a vegetarian, or considering adopting a vegetarian meal plan. This section will help you put together plant sources of protein that will meet your need for protein, particularly EAA.

Humans have long been meat eaters. In fact, we have teeth designed for tearing flesh (canine teeth) and others (molars) for grinding nuts, berries, and seeds. Vegetarian diets arose in biblical times for religious reasons. Today people choose vegetarian diets for a variety of reasons—religious, ethical (in objection to slaughtering of animals for meat), economical (animal sources of protein are typically more expensive than plant sources), or for better health and environmental (animal protein requires use of greater resources such as fuel and land compared to an equal amount of vegetable protein).

The health benefits of vegetarian diets have been known for some time and research studies show that vegetarians tend to have lower risk for a variety of diseases related to diet such as heart disease, certain cancers, and obesity. But vegetarians also tend to lead more healthful lives overall—exercising more regularly, not smoking or using drugs or engaging in other safe lifestyle habits such as wearing seatbelts more often. So some of the health attributes of a vegetarian diet may be due to other healthy practices other than diet.

As you go through this course, you may opt for more vegetarian meals or even choose to be a vegetarian as a way to eat more fiber and key nutrients that promote good health and to cut back on saturated fats. Strict vegetarian or "vegan" diets include no animal products in their diets. Other forms of vegetarianism include "ovo-vegetarian" (eggs are eaten) and lacto-vegetarian (dairy is consumed). People may also consider themselves vegetarian if they include chicken or fish but no red meat, but these are not forms of vegetarianism.

The issue for vegetarians is paying attention to combining protein sources in order to complement incomplete proteins. For example, if you combine grains and legumes, you will get enough of the limiting amino acids (lysine and methionine, respectively) as shown in Figure 2.28. Eating soy on a regular basis also ensures that you will get ample EAA since this is a complete protein. If you're planning on including more vegetarian meals in your daily fare, check out the vegetarian menu provided on page 45 to give you some ideas.

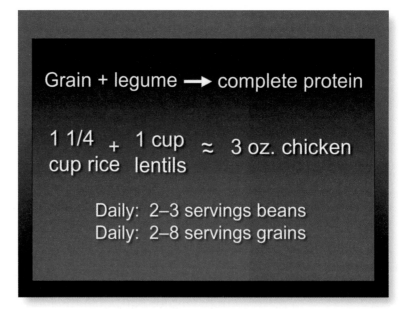

Grain + legume ⟶ complete protein

1 1/4 cup rice + 1 cup lentils ≈ 3 oz. chicken

Daily: 2–3 servings beans
Daily: 2–8 servings grains

FIGURE 2.28

Vegetarians

To get all of the nutrients you need from non-meat sources, just follow this food plan.

Breakfast

- ½ cups nine-grain cooked cereal topped with 1 ounce chopped almonds
- ¾ cup blueberries
- 2 tablespoons honey
- 8 ounces soy milk

Morning Snack

- 2 ounces trail mix (raisins, dried papaya, pumpkin seeds)

Lunch

- One bean burrito (1 cup black beans, ½ cup rice, 1 ounce soy cheese)
- ¼ cup salsa
- 1 cup fruit salad

Afternoon Snack

- One banana spread with 2 tablespoons peanut butter
- 8 ounces cranberry juice

Dinner

- Spinach pasta with "meat" sauce (1 cup spinach pasta, ¾ cup red sauce, two (soy) veggie burgers crumbled into sauce)
- 1 cup steamed broccoli
- 1½ cup dark greens tossed with 1 tablespoon olive oil vinaigrette
- 1 ounce dark chocolate

Calories: 2,500; Protein: 92 grams; Carbohydrate: 413 grams; Fat: 26% calories

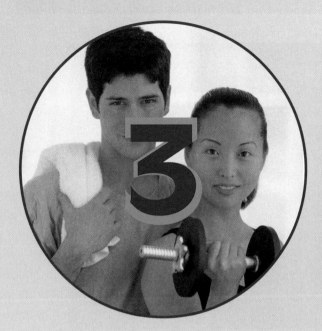

Calories— The Energy Basis of Nutrition

With our first nutrient under out belt, we must divert a bit and discuss the topic of energy. You undoubtedly have tossed around the term *energy* before, often in conjunction with feeling low "energy" or describing a person's demeanor as high "energy."

In this course **energy** means the ability to do work: either metabolic work (building a protein in a liver cell for example) or physical work (moving furniture or running). During our discussion of energy, we will cover two areas:

▶ The energy value of foods—how it's measured and how to calculate what amount of energy is in the food you eat.

▶ Your energy requirement—how much energy you need to support your metabolism and other activities.

ENERGY VALUE OF FOODS

Several scientists took up exploring the energy value of food centuries ago. One in particular, Lavoisier, made the comparison between how much energy is released when a carbon-containing food (such as bread, vegetables, butter, or meat—these all contain the macronutrients carbohydrate, protein, and fat) is burned and how much energy is released when an animal eats this same food. (See Figure 3.1.)

The carbon in the food, in the presence of oxygen, is burned and gives off carbon dioxide (CO_2) and heat. Our body's metabolism, or that of an

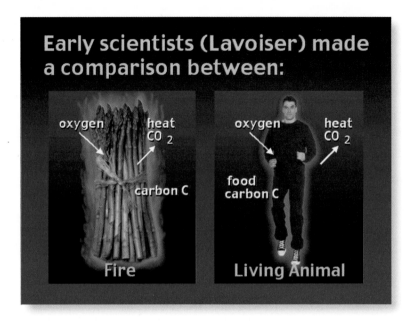

FIGURE 3.1

animal, can be thought of as similar to the burning of food. The carbon in the food is combined with oxygen and the chemical bonds are oxidized (or burned), releasing their potential energy as heat.

When we eat food, we (1) break chemical bonds in the macronutrients protein, carbohydrate, and fat; (2) release the energy in the form of heat, and (3) release the carbon as CO_2. (See Figure 3.2.)

Rather than just referring to energy released as "heat," let's give it a unit of measure: the **Calorie.**

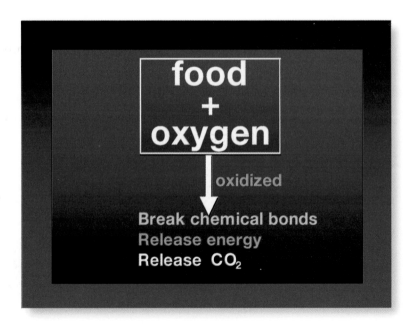

FIGURE 3.2

A **Calorie** is the heat needed to raise 1 liter of water 1 degree Celsius. You may have taken a chemistry course and learned about a calorie being the amount of energy needed to raise *one gram* of water 1 degree Celsius. Chemists use this much smaller unit of heat energy. But in nutrition, a Calorie is 1,000 times the size of a chemistry calorie. You needn't worry about making any conversion because at all times when the term calorie is used in this course, on food labels, and on calorie expenditure charts, we are referring to the nutrition calorie. Sometimes I use the abbreviation kcal or kilocalorie to signify calorie. (This simply means 1,000 chemistry calories and is scientific lingo but you should still read kcal as "calorie.")

Now let's figure out how much potential energy or calories are in carbohydrate, fat, and protein. A specially designed machine, as pictured in Figure 3.3, called a bomb calorimeter, is used to determine the potential energy or calorie value of foods. This clever machine consists of a small container where the food in question rests ready to be burned with an ignition wire. A larger chamber of water maintained at a set temperature surrounds the smaller container. Once the food is ignited and burns, heat is given off and the water heats up. From the change in temperature in the water chamber, the number of calories in the food can be calculated. This value represents the total potential energy released from the food and is displayed in calories (or kcal) /gram.

Here is the potential energy in the macronutrients. (You needn't memorize these numbers.)

Carbohydrate	4.2 kcal/gram
Fat	9.4 kcal/gram
Protein	5.7 kcal/gram

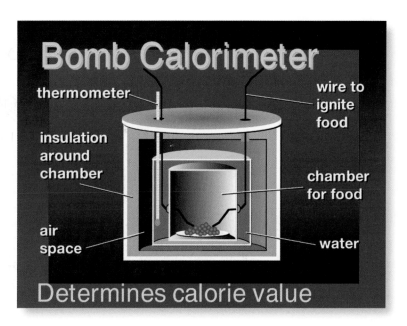

FIGURE 3.3

Do you think our bodies are efficient as a bomb calorimeter machine? Our bodies actually are unable to extract all the potential energy; we lose some due to indigestible losses (after all, the machine doesn't have to chew and digest the food) and metabolic energy losses (with protein energy metabolism only).

The amount of energy that is physiologically available to us from the macronutrients is slightly lower than the total potential energy.

Refer to Figure 3.4. Some portion of the carbohydrate we eat, about 5%, is not digested and absorbed and will be lost in the stool. (Thus, your stool has some potential energy due in part to undigested carbohydrate.) You are left with 4 kcal/gram of carbohydrate, which is the **Physiological Fuel Value** for carbohydrates. This is the amount of energy your body realizes or gets when you eat 1 gram of carbs.

Refer to Figure 3.5. As with carbohydrates, a small portion (5%) of fats are not digested and absorbed and go into the stool, which represents a loss of potential energy. Thus, fat has a Physiological Fuel Value of 9 kcal/gram.

Matters get a bit more complicated with protein because the element nitrogen is part of the amino acid structure. This nitrogen must be disposed of through a means that costs the body calories. Refer to Figure 3.6. We start with 5.7 kcal/gram and we lose in the first step about 10% of the energy due to indigestible losses (some vegetable sources of protein—remember the incomplete proteins, which are not well digested).

If an amino acid is used for energy or converted to fat for storage, the nitrogen must be taken off. Can we just let the nitrogen hang around and use it later? No, nitrogen is toxic and we need to get rid of it right away.

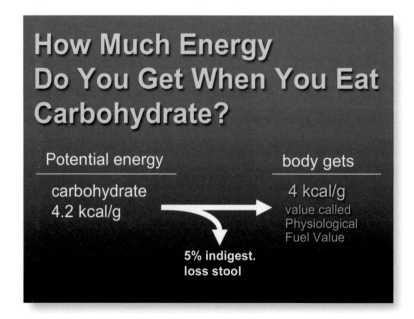

FIGURE 3.4

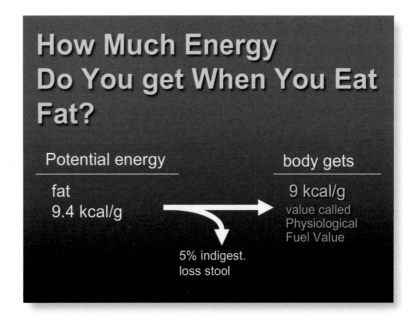

FIGURE 3.5

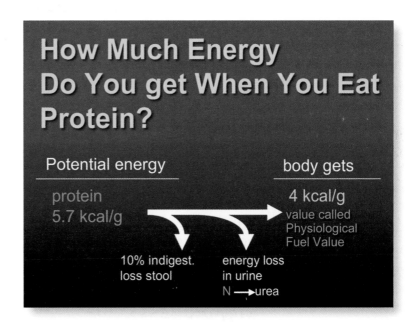

FIGURE 3.6

Our bodies must make urea (which cost calories) as a vehicle for nitrogen to leave the body via the urine. This means that your urine has metabolic waste from the breakdown of protein, a loss of approximately 20%. In addition, 10% of the protein consumed is not digested or absorbed which also represents a loss of energy in the stool. We started out with a potential energy of 5.7 kcal/gram and end up with 4 kcal/gram as the Physiological Fuel Value for protein.

Figure 3.7 shows the Physiological Fuel Values for the three macronutrients. (These are also the values that appear on food labels.) These

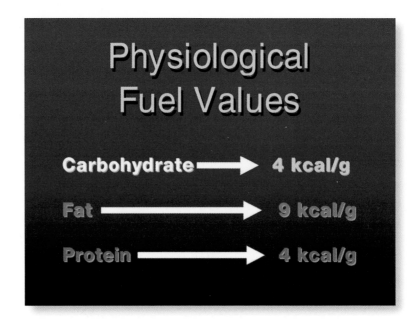

FIGURE 3.7

values are very important for you to learn. You will use them in calculating the calorie value of foods as well as what percent of the calories in a food or meal come from either carbohydrate, fat, or protein.

Let's put these numbers to work and calculate the number of calories in a food like a hot dog with a simple three-step process.

1. Note the number of grams of carbohydrate, fat, and protein there are in each turkey hot dog.

2. Multiply each by its respective Physiological Fuel Value. (Make sure you also write down the units of kcal/gram.)

3. Add up the resulting products to get the total available energy (kcal/g).

One turkey hot dog (wiener only!) contains:

Carbohydrate	1 gram	×	4 kcal/g	=	4 kcal
Fat	16 grams	×	9 kcal/g	=	144 kcal
Protein	7 grams	×	4 kcal/g	=	28 kcal
TOTAL				=	176 kcal

What if you wanted to know the percentage of calories from fat in a turkey "dog"? Simply divide the number of fat calories by total calories and multiply by 100 to get a percentage.

$$\frac{144 \text{ fat calories}}{176 \text{ total calories}} \times 100 = 82\% \text{ fat calories}$$

Wow!! Looks more like a "fat" dog. There are other types of hot dogs available, reduced-fat, soy, and other versions that are lower in fat. As you'll learn in later chapters, keeping total fat intake to less than 30% of the total calories helps reduce risk for chronic disease such as cancer and heart disease.

You can also calculate the percent of calories from carbohydrate and protein. On your diet project, you'll be doing exactly that as well as doing these types of calculations on the exam.

Here are a few final notes on calorie value of foods:

1. Calories in a meal are additive.

- This means the calories in your hot dog get added with calories in the bun, condiments you may use, along with a soda and chips you may also eat with your hot dog.

- This also means that there is no such thing as a "negative calorie" food (regardless of what your friends may tell you). For example, chewing celery does not provide you with negative calories.

2. Water, cholesterol (a fat-like substance present in foods in a very small amount), vitamins, and minerals all have NO calories. Remember, only the macronutrients, protein, carbohydrate and fat, can be burned for energy.

3. Fiber, which is an indigestible carbohydrate, cannot be broken down in the intestinal track and therefore is excreted in the stool. Thus, fiber has no available energy to us; however, fiber is very important as we will learn in the next chapter.

On food labels, total calories are listed per serving. Calories contributed by fat are also listed. Both total calories and fat calories are expressed as physiologically available energy, not total potential energy.

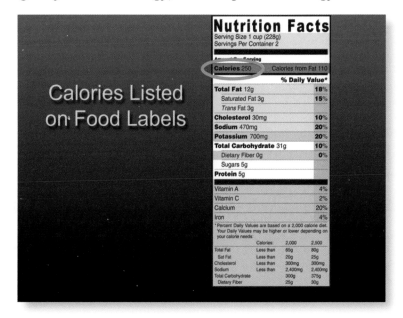

FIGURE 3.8

DETERMINING ENERGY NEEDS

Now that we know the definition of energy and how much energy is in food, let's figure out how many calories (or how much energy) you need to support normal body functioning.

Your daily energy needs reflect the sum of three components:

1. Basal Metabolic Rate (BMR)

- This is the amount of heat/energy/calories needed to keep basic body functions going such as your heart beating, lungs breathing in and out, as well as your liver doing its maintenance duties. The **BMR** is measured in a person at rest, no food or fasted for about 12 hours, without exercise or strenuous physical activity for 24 hours (hard workouts cause your metabolism to rise), and in an environment (room) where the temperature is neutral.

- The BMR is typically the largest component of daily energy needs and values usually fall between 1000 to 2000 calories daily.

2. Thermic Effect of Food (TEF)

- This is the amount of energy needed to digest and assimilate food.

- The TEF represents the smallest component of your energy need and values usually fall between 50 to 200 calories.

3. Activity

- This is energy needed to perform any activity above the basal metabolic rate—sitting, standing, jogging, taking notes in class.

- The activity component is usually equal to or less than your BMR, depending upon your movement during the day.

Summary:

- Component 1 + 2 + 3 = the total energy requirement for adult men and women who are NOT pregnant or lactating.

- For children, you must also compute a fourth component, the amount of energy needed for growth.

4. Growth

This energy need component supports the cost of building new tissue as well as the actual cost of the material that makes up tissue such as muscle or bone. We will not be computing this in class but you need to know that growth must be taken into consideration when determining a child's energy requirement.

Fat Gain or Loss

Before we move on to computing energy requirements, let's consider what happens if a person is over or under eating. That is, what happens if you consume in excess of your energy needs or less than your energy needs? This would mean that you are not in energy balance (calories in = calories out) and that the excess calories (calories in > calories out) would be stored as fat, and weight would be gained (more on this in Chapter 7). And if you were in a calorie deficit (calories in < calories out), the deficit would be met by taking calories out of storage (fat), thus weight loss.

The number to compute weight gained or weight loss is 3,500 calories per 1 pound of body fat gained or lost (in excess or deficit). We will use this number later in a calculation so you can see how works. (See Figure 3.9.)

Now let's compute the three components of your energy requirement.

Computing the Calorie Cost of BMR

The amount of energy you need to maintain basic bodily functions depends upon several factors: body weight, age, gender, and body surface area. A University of California Davis professor some years ago determined the relationship of body surface area to BMR. Computing BMR based upon body surface area would take some doing and a bit too complicated for us. So in this class, we will use a very simple method based upon body weight and gender:

Males: 1 kcal/kg body weight per hour
Females: 0.9 kcal/kg body weight per hour

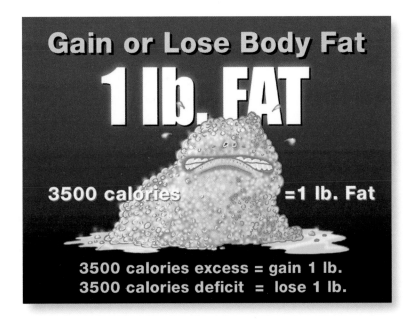

FIGURE 3.9

Men have a greater BMR per unit of body weight because of body composition differences (more lean or muscle tissue, which costs more to maintain, than women who have proportionately more body fat, which is a much less "expensive" tissue to maintain). Here's a sample calculation:
What is the BMR for a 55 kg woman?

$$0.9 \text{ kcal/kg} \bullet \text{hour} \times 55 \text{ kg} \times 24 \text{ hours/day} = 1188 \text{ kcal/day}$$

Her BMR falls right into the range 1,000 to 2,000 given earlier. (It's important for you to double-check your number to make sure you did the calculation properly and always include the units.)

Factors That Alter the BMR

There are several factors that can change how many calories you burn just to maintain your basic bodily functions.

1. **Age.** You guessed it, getting older puts a damper on your BMR. After about age 20, your BMR drops about 2% to 3% for every decade. So a 60-year-old would have a BMR that was about 12% lower than in her twenties. This drop in BMR with age is mostly due to a decline in activity that in turn leads to a loss of muscle mass with age, since muscle requires more energy to maintain than fat tissue. But you can hedge off this slump in BMR by maintaining muscle through resistance exercises such as calisthenics or weight lifting. And it's never too late to boost your muscle mass—even a 90-year-old can get buff!

2. **Fasting.** When you skip eating altogether, your BMR drops about 10% to 20% within 24 hours. This is a smart response by your body as it tries to conserve energy. Think back to prehistoric days when cave people went without food for days because it was scarce. Those people who could survive by slowing their BMR passed on their genetic material. (Low and behold, we are their descendants!)

3. **Exercise.** Participating in physical activity boosts your BMR. The effect is variable and may last only 30 minutes to as much as 24 hours; it depends upon the type of exercise—its intensity and duration. The more vigorous, the greater the BMR boost. After exercise your body recovers, rebuilding proteins, storing up more carbohydrate fuel and other general recovery duties. This all costs calories, which shows up as a greater BMR. The amount may be a mere 25 calories or over 250 calories daily. No matter what the boost in BMR, exercise is great to do and good for you!

Nutrition Bite

Many supplements sold on the Internet and in stores claim to "rev up your metabolism" (or BMR). One supplement sold as a skin patch delivers the mineral iodine, which is a component of the thyroid hormone responsible for setting the BMR. But remember homeostasis? Extra iodine doesn't mean the body will start wasting calories. Truth be told, these supplements fall short on their claims.

Computing Calorie Costs of Activity

Estimating calorie costs of activity can be done several ways.

1. **Time and activity method:** Activity costs are based on total time spent in each activity multiplied by the caloric cost of that activity. (Check Figure 3.10 for some values.)

$$\text{time (min)} \times (\text{kcal/min} \times \text{kg}) \times \frac{\text{kg body weight}}{} = \frac{\text{kcal spent on activity}}{}$$

This method is tedious. You have to keep very good records or carry a tape recorder to document every single activity you perform during the day. While this method is used in research, we won't be doing this in class because it's so tedious!

ENERGY EXPENDITURE DURING VARIOUS ACTIVITIES		
	MALE 70 (KG) **KCAL/MIN**	**FEMALE 55 (KG)** **KCAL/MIN**
Basketball	8.6	6.8
Cycling (10 mph)	7.5	5.9
Running (7.5)	14.0	11.0
Sitting	1.7	1.3
Sleeping	1.2	0.9
Walking (3.5 mph)	5.0	3.9
Weight lifting	8.2	6.4

FIGURE 3.10

2. Activity profile expressed as a percentage of BMR: This method categorizes a person into one of four activity profiles. Each profile represents a percentage of the BMR that would then be added along with BMR and TEF to estimate the daily energy requirement. The four activity levels:

CATEGORY	% BMR
Sedentary	+ 30%
Light	+ 50%
Moderate	+ 70%
Strenuous	+ 100%

Which category best fits you?

Sedentary: typical student, lots of sitting (studying), watching TV, computer time, maybe exercise two to three times per week, ride bus to campus. Any job held is not very physical—a desk job, for example.

Light: more daily movement, not much sitting, bike or walk to school, exercise three to four times weekly. Any job held has some walking, stair climbing, and other movement involved.

Moderate: very active days, workout four to five times weekly. Active job that involves being on feet hours a day—child care, for example.

Strenuous: major stud! Exercise vigorously most days of the week, little sitting. Physically demanding job such as landscape.

Let's compute how many calories a 55 kg woman would burn on activity with a moderate activity level.

1. Calculate BMR

$$55 \text{ kg} \times \left(\frac{0.9 \text{ kcal/kg}}{\text{body weight}} \times \text{hour} \right) \times 24 \text{ hours/day} = 1188 \text{ kcal/day}$$

2. Activity = 70% of BMR

$$0.7 \times 1188 \text{ kcal/day} = 831.6 \text{ kcal/day needed to support activity}$$

Once you compute your calorie cost of activity, the number should either be equal to or less than your BMR. (If the number you get is greater than the BMR, go back and check your work.)

Computing Calorie Cost of Thermic Effect of Food (TEF)

The energy needed to digest and assimilate food is generally between 5% and 10% of the daily calorie intake. Fat and carbs take around 5% for processing while protein costs 10%. In our calculation, we'll use 5% of calorie intake needed for TEF. The best estimate of total calorie intake is the sum of BMR and activity.

Let's compute how many calories are needed for TEF for a person with a BMR of 1,000 kcal and activity level of light or 500 kcal daily.

$$\text{BMR} = 1{,}000 \text{ kcal/day} \qquad \text{Activity} = 500 \text{ kcal/day}$$

$$
\begin{aligned}
\text{TEF} &= 0.05\,(1000 + 500) \text{ kcal/day} \\
&= 0.05\,(1500 \text{ kcal/day}) \\
&= 75 \text{ kcal/day to digest and assimilate food}
\end{aligned}
$$

Double-check your math. TEF should fall between 50 and 200 kcal/day.

Computing Total Energy Requirement

Now let's put everything together and calculate the energy requirement for the following person. Let's go through the example in Figure 3.11 step by step: BMR, then Activity, then TEF, and finally add these three components together to determine the energy requirement.

1. BMR

$$0.9 \text{ kcal/kg} \times \text{hour} \times 52 \text{ kg} \times 24 \text{ hours/day} = 1123 \text{ kcal/day}$$

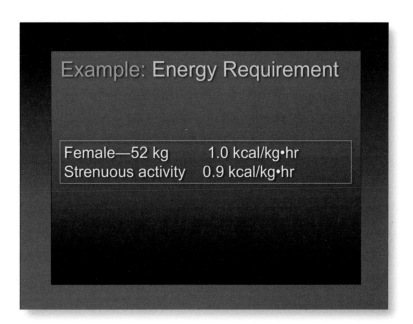

FIGURE 3.11

2. Activity

Strenuous activity level = 100% BMR = 1123 kcal/day

3. TEF

0.05 (BMR + Activity) = 0.05 (1123 kcal + 1123 kcal) = 112 kcal/day

4. Total Energy Requirement

BMR + Activity + TEF or (1123 kcal + 1123 kcal + 112 kcal)
= 2358 kcal/day

At each step, double-check your numbers. Is the BMR within (or near) the range of 1,000 to 2,000 kcal/day? Is the Activity value in keeping with the BMR? Is the TEF between 50 and 200 kcal/day?

Now ask yourself, do all women who weigh 52 kg have the same energy requirement? The answer is NO. Not all 52 kg women have this activity level. Energy needs must be computed based on activity level as well as body weight and gender.

Computing Total Energy Intake

Now let's add a twist: gaining or losing weight and how this impacts computing energy intake for a person.

Let's compute the energy intake for the example in Figure 3.12. In this example, we now must account for the fact that this man is overeating or gaining weight at the rate of 500 kcal/day. This will impact the TEF (more food, therefore, a greater cost of digesting and assimilating the food). Follow the same sequence as the first example, but now account for the gain.

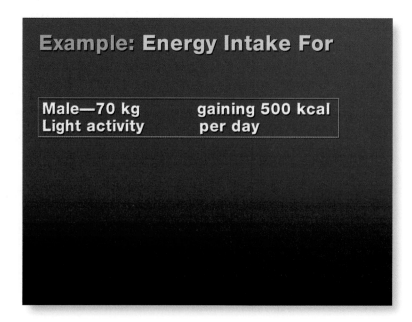

FIGURE 3.12

1. BMR

$$1.0 \text{ kcal/kg} \times \text{hour} \times 70 \text{ kg} \times 24 \text{ hours/day} = 1680 \text{ kcal/day}$$

2. Activity

$$\text{Activity} = 50\% \text{ BMR}$$
$$= 0.5 \, (1680 \text{ kcal/day}) = 840 \text{ kcal/day}$$

3. Gain

(We now add in the gain—which is equivalent to the amount he is overeating—the number of calories in a double-decker fast-food burger each day!)

$$= 500 \text{ kcal/day}$$

(*Note:* Even though he is overeating and technically gaining weight, do not adjust his body weight in computing the BMR.)

(*Note also:* If he were losing at the rate of 500 kcal/day, you would simply subtract the 500 kcal = −500 kcal/day.)

4. TEF

$$5\% \, (\text{BMR} + \text{Activity} + \text{Gain})$$
$$0.05 \, (1680 \text{ kcal} + 840 \text{ kcal} + 500 \text{ kcal}) = 151 \text{ kcal/day}$$

(*Note:* If he were losing weight, the loss would be subtracted, thereby lowering the TEF.)

Remember to double-check all your numbers to see if they are reasonable.

5. Total Energy Intake

$$\text{BMR} + \text{Activity} + \text{Gain} + \text{TEF}$$
$$(1680 \text{ kcal} + 840 \text{ kcal} + 500 \text{ kcal} + 151 \text{ kcal}) = 3171 \text{ kcal/day}$$

This is his energy intake, NOT his energy requirement. Why not? Because he is overeating exceeding his energy requirements.

How much fat would this man gain in one week?

$$500 \text{ kcal/day} \times 7 \text{ days/week} = 3500 \text{ kcal/week}$$

This translates to 1 pound of fat gained in one week. (Recall that 3500 kcal = 1 pound fat.)

You now have mastered two important concepts surrounding energy:

1. Energy value of foods

2. Computing our energy requirements

Go practice your new skills on the diet project or these sample problems.

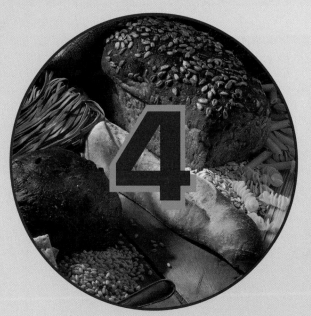

4 Carbohydrates —The Energy Nutrient

Following our discussion of the energy value of foods and energy requirements, the second major nutrient—carbohydrate—follows logically. Known primarily as the "energy nutrient," carbohydrate-rich food provides the majority of calories in your diet.

In this chapter, we'll cover four major areas for carbohydrate:

▶ Carbohydrate structure and food sources

▶ Carbohydrate digestion

▶ Understanding the power of fiber

▶ Carbohydrate energy metabolism and the impact of exercise

CARBOHYDRATE STRUCTURE AND FOOD SOURCES

The word *carbohydrate* means just what it says: "hydrated carbon," or simply carbon with water attached. Most carbohydrates come from plants— apples, potatoes, wheat, and sugar (from sugar cane plant or sugar beets). (The exception to the plant carbohydrate rule is the sugar found in dairy products.) Plants are able to make carbohydrates by trapping the sun's energy by means of photosynthesis.

As shown in Figure 4.1, plants take up water from their roots, CO_2 from the air along with the sun's energy (solar energy) and combine this to form

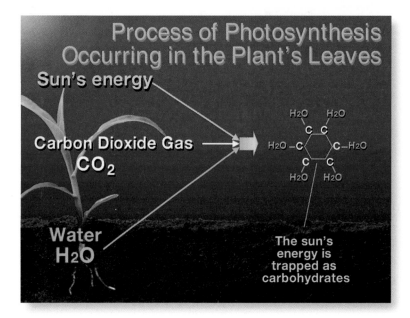

FIGURE 4.1

carbohydrate, which the plant then stores (potato, apple, etc.). Ask yourself where the CO_2 came from? (Recall from Chapter 3 that CO_2 is exhaled in your breath when foods are oxidized during energy metabolism.)

The sun's energy is now trapped as potential energy in a carbohydrate unit. We will cover how this energy is released in more detail later in this chapter. For now know that this energy represents carbohydrate's major function in the body—energy source. About half of your calories come from carbohydrates. Carbohydrate energy is specifically necessary for brain function and during high-intensity exercise.

Now let's take a closer look at carbohydrate, specifically its structure.

Carbohydrate Structure

The three levels of carbohydrate structure, which are all present in foods and in your body, are: monosaccharides, disaccharides, and polysaccharides.

1. Monosaccharides

The most basic structure of carbohydrate is a six-carbon ring with water attached to each carbon. "Mono" means "one" and "saccharide" means "sugar."

There are three different monosaccharides, all with six carbons but with slight variations on the arrangements of the attached water and chemical bonds. Monosaccharide food sources are referred to as **simple sugars** or **simple carbohydrates.**

Rather than looking at the detailed chemical structure, each monosaccharide is represented with a symbol. (See Figure 4.2.)

Be familiar with food sources of monosaccharides.

As noted above, the monosaccharides are part of the next levels of structure—disaccharides and polysaccharides.

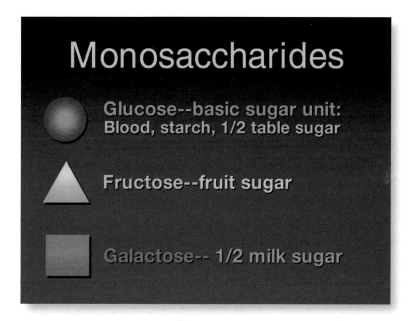

FIGURE 4.2

2. Disaccharides

With disaccharides, the sugar rings are joined together—"di," which means two. Like monosaccharides, food sources of disaccharides are referred to as **simple sugars** or **simple carbohydrates.** There are three disaccharides of significance in your diet: sucrose, maltose, and lactose.

- Sucrose is one glucose and one fructose molecule joined together. (See Figure 4.3.) Food sources include cookies, candy, soda, or anything made with table sugar, corn sweetener, and other forms of sucrose such as brown sugar (white sugar with a small amount of molasses), powdered sugar, and crystallized sugar or "sugar in the raw."

- Maltose is two glucose molecules linked together. (See Figure 4.4.) There are very few food sources of maltose. It is a breakdown product of starch (a polysaccharide found in potatoes, pasta, etc.) during digestion. In fact, if you chew a piece of bread for several minutes, the maltose will begin to be released in your mouth (more on carbohydrate digestion later) and this tastes

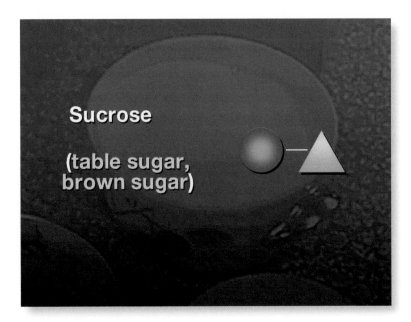

FIGURE 4.3

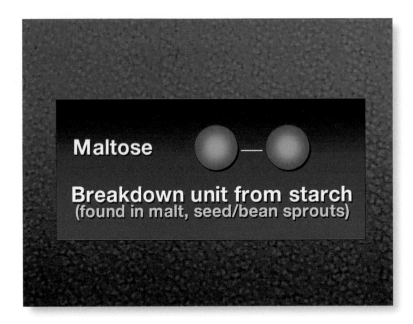

FIGURE 4.4

slightly sweet, almost nut-like. Bean and other seed sprouts contain maltose. Maltose is also added in the making of beer (malt) and is used as a flavoring agent in some foods.

● Lactose is one glucose and one galactose molecule linked together. (See Figure 4.5.) Known as milk sugar, lactose is found in dairy products such as milk (including human breast milk), yogurt, ice cream, and cheeses. Lactose is one of the few sugars made by animals and hence, found in some animal products.

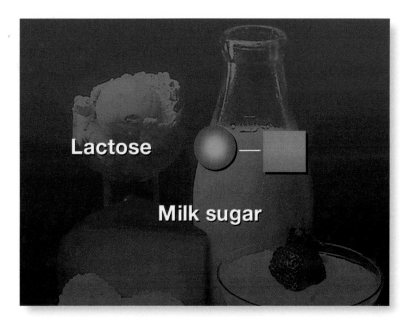

FIGURE 4.5

What's Honey?

- Honey is a supersaturated solution of sugars and water made by bees from their collection of nectar from flowers. As shown in Figure 4.6, honey is a mixture of fructose, glucose and some sucrose.

- Honey versus table sugar: Gram for gram, honey is sweeter tasting because of the fructose content. Per teaspoon, honey has more calories than table sugar (20 vs. 16 calories per teaspoon). However,

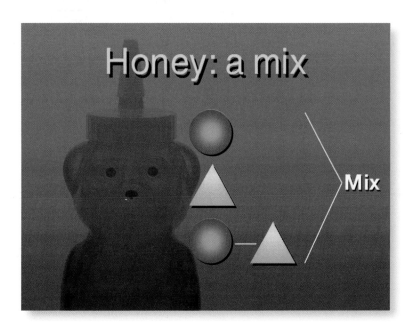

FIGURE 4.6

honey is a solution of sugars and more carbohydrate is present per teaspoon than table sugar.

- Since honey is collected from plants, it contains very small amounts of substances called antioxidants that may have health benefits. (We'll cover more on this in Chapter 9.) Research is ongoing to determine if any extra nutritional benefits result from honey. Most likely, the amounts of antioxidants are so small that a teaspoon of honey here and there in your diet provides no nutritional advantage over table sugar. For centuries, however, honey has been known to have healing properties that fight bacterial infection in skin wounds such as burns and ulcers. Special compounds are present in honey from the small amounts of bee saliva that act in combating infection.

Nutrition Bite

How much honey does a bee make in its lifetime? About an eighth of a teaspoon, that's all! So next time you enjoy some honey on a slice of bread, think about the effort that goes into that delicious bite.

3. Polysaccharides

As you might guess, polysaccharides are many simple sugars (six-carbon rings) linked together. Polysaccharides containing foods are also called **complex carbohydrates.** We will cover three polysaccharides: starch, fiber, and glycogen.

Starch

- As shown in Figure 4.7, starch is made up of hundreds of glucose units linked together in a straight chain, or a branched chain as shown.

- Starch is the most common polysaccharide in food. It comes from plant foods such as grains (wheat, rice, barley, oats), foods made with these grains (pasta, bread, muffins), and vegetables (corn, potatoes). Starch is also in unripe fruit (which you probably don't eat); during the ripening process, this starch converts to fructose, explaining the sweet flavor of fruit.

Fiber

- Shown alongside starch from a potato for comparison in Figure 4.8, fiber is also made up of hundreds of glucose units. But the linkage between glucose units is different (at a different angle than the

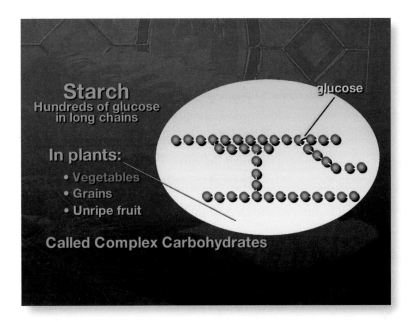

FIGURE 4.7

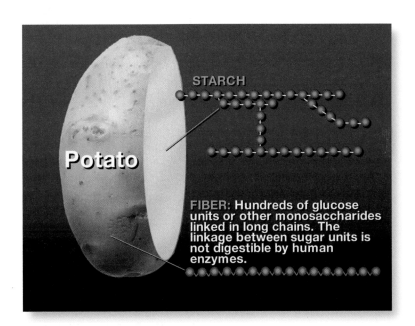

FIGURE 4.8

chemical linkage in starch); this simple difference makes fiber indigestible for humans because we lack the enzyme to break this chemical bond. Since this fiber is not digested, and it is too big to be absorbed, the fiber passes through our intestines into the stool. Thus, we end up losing a source of potential energy. Despite this loss, fiber has a number of health benefits that will be discussed in another section of this chapter.

● A group of animals called ruminants can break this bond in fiber. Cows, sheep, and other ruminants can digest fiber (with the help of bacteria in their stomach, which actually makes the enzyme to do the job). These animals can get much of their nourishment from grasses and hay that contain potential energy in the sugar units because their digestive systems can break down the fiber for usable energy.

● Fiber is only found in plant products and represents the structural material in plants that makes up the cell wall. Food sources of fiber include whole grains, vegetables, and seeds in their unprocessed states. There will be more about food sources in another section.

Glycogen

● This polysaccharide differs from starch and fiber because it is found in living humans and mammals in their muscles and liver. Like starch, glycogen is made of hundreds of glucose units. But glycogen's glucose is arranged in a highly branched chain (Figure 4.9).

● The unique design of glycogen allows for many exposed ends that can be clipped off, yielding many glucose units in times when energy is needed such as during exercise (muscle glycogen) or in maintaining blood sugar levels (liver glycogen). Compare glycogen to starch's structure. Plants do little running (none, actually) so the structure of starch is adequate for their need of glucose for fuel to support growth. However, for humans and other mammals, the design of glycogen allows for rapid release of glucose for fuel, which enables you to run or do another intense activity (more on this later).

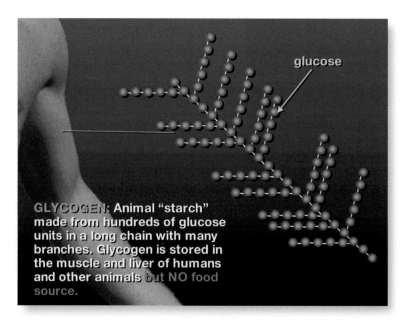

glucose

GLYCOGEN: Animal "starch" made from hundreds of glucose units in a long chain with many branches. Glycogen is stored in the muscle and liver of humans and other animals but NO food source.

FIGURE 4.9

- There are NO FOOD SOURCES of glycogen. Despite the fact that beef or other animal flesh may seem like a source, by the time we get it in the store, the glycogen has broken down and there is none present in the meat.

- Humans store about 1,600 calories worth of glycogen in the muscles (primarily) and the liver. This supply of carbohydrates as we will discuss in another section lasts about 24 to 36 hours in a person who is resting but not eating. This lasts only 2 to 3 hours if the person is rigorously exercising, such as in running a marathon.

CARBOHYDRATE DIGESTION

In this section we'll detail carbohydrate digestion by using a sample meal that you might eat—a glass of milk and a whole wheat bagel topped with jam (Figure 4.10).

This meal contains different carbohydrates:

- The milk contains lactose.
- The bagel contains starch and fiber.
- The jam contains sucrose. (Even though there is some fructose from the fruit, you will see this sugar requires no digestion.)

The two disaccharides (lactose and sucrose) are in fairly simple form, so for now we can ignore their digestion until they are farther down in the small intestine. At first, we'll track starch and fiber, the two polysaccharides, during digestion.

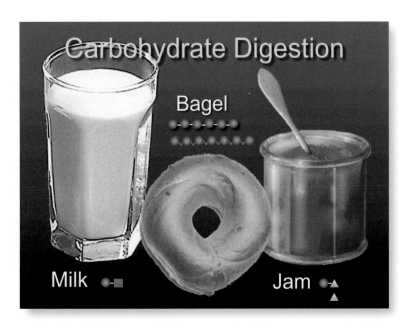

FIGURE 4.10

In the mouth: Saliva contains an enzyme called "salivary amylase," made by the salivary glands, that starts the process of chemical digestion of starch. (See Figure 4.11.) (The bonds that connect the glucose units in fiber, however, are left untouched.) Amylase works to break off smaller chains of starch. This chemical digestion of starch was most likely important in prehistoric times when some of the plant foods consumed took time to digest. But now, we could skip this step all together—you could swallow your bite of bagel without chewing (though a bit uncomfortable) and digestion would not be compromised. However, if you were to chew the bite of bagel long enough, it would start to taste mildly sweet as the maltose is released into your mouth.

In the stomach: Here, the chemical phase of digestion for starch stops because the acid in the stomach "kills" the enzyme. (Remember that enzymes are protein and proteins denature and become inactive in the stomach.) Although chemical digestion comes to a halt, physical digestion goes into full swing when the stomach makes a "smoothie" of the bagel-milk-jam meal. (See Figure 4.12.)

In the small intestine: The "smoothie" moves into the small intestine where the pancreas squirts in an enzyme called "pancreatic amylase" (the same enzyme as before, just from a different source). Chemical digestion restarts and the starch is broken down completely to maltose. As in the mouth, the bonds in fiber are not digestible so the fiber passes through untouched. (See Figure 4.13.)

At this point, our meal has been processed into three disaccharides: maltose (from the bagel), lactose (from the milk), and sucrose (from the jam). These disaccharides, however, are still too big to be absorbed through the wall of the small intestine, therefore, more chemical digestion must occur.

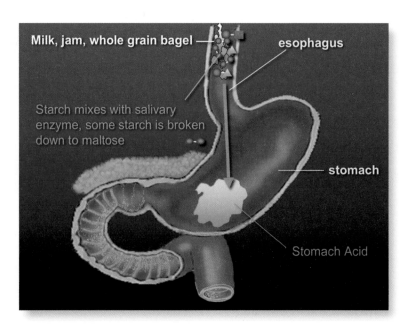

FIGURE 4.11

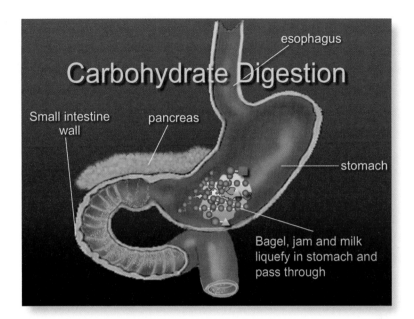

FIGURE 4.12

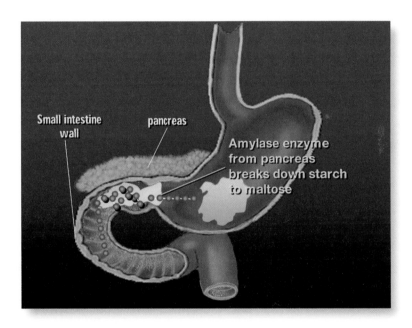

FIGURE 4.13

On the surface of the small intestine specific enzymes are made that break apart the specific disaccharide. As shown in Figure 4.14, each disaccharide is broken down into two monosaccharides.

Maltase is the enzyme that breaks apart maltose, **sucrase** breaks apart sucrose, and **lactase** splits lactose. In the next section we'll cover issues with lactose digestion.

As noted below, the end product of carbohydrate digestion is monosaccharides. Notice that the fiber is passing through undigested and unabsorbed. (See Figure 4.15.)

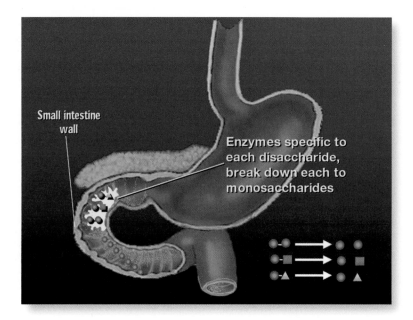

FIGURE 4.14

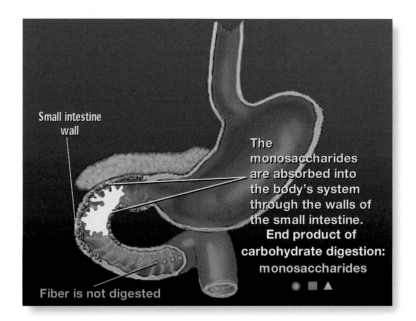

FIGURE 4.15

Lactose Intolerance

You may be or know one of the majority of people worldwide who has a limited ability to digest the milk sugar lactose. Most of these people either lack the enzyme lactase or have very little, so when a cup of milk is consumed, there is not enough lactase available to digest the milk sugar.

Trouble develops when lactose is not digested as shown in Figure 4.16. Since lactose is too big for absorption, it moves on down "the line" into

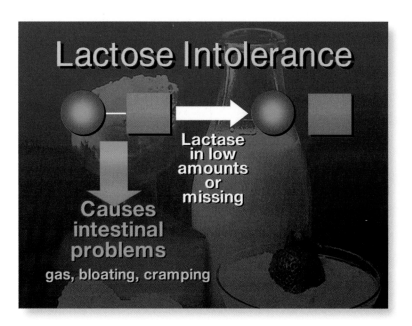

FIGURE 4.16

the large intestine (colon). There the bacteria go to work and start digesting it and their digestion products draw water into the area. This causes bloating. Also, gas forms. Get the picture? Lots of discomfort, even diarrhea may occur.

Note that lactose intolerance is NOT an allergy to milk but rather an inability to digest milk sugar.

Lactose intolerance is not uncommon. About 70% of the world's population is lactose intolerant. The ability to digest lactose decreases with age in most mammals. For example, dogs can drink milk when they are puppies, but as adults a bowl of milk can create discomfort. Since most mammals get their nutrition as babies from mother's milk, it makes sense to have lactase. And when weaning occurs, the amount of lactase declines. This doesn't appear to happen in humans as we retain some lactase activity. People of specific ethnic backgrounds seem to have retained the lactase enzyme. Those people who have maintained dairy herds as part of their culture, such as peoples from Northern Europe, tend to have more lactase activity as adults than those who traditionally did not, such as most Asian, African, and Native American peoples.

UNDERSTANDING THE POWER OF FIBER

No doubt you have heard before to get more fiber in your diet because it is good for your health. Studies show that people who eat ample fiber in their diet have lower risk for certain cancers and heart disease, and can assist weight loss than people who eat a low-fiber diet. But you have also learned that fiber is not digestible. So technically, fiber does not get into your circulation. How could it be that an indigestible substance can have such powerful health benefits?

Let's take a look at fiber: what it is, fiber types, and its health benefits.

What Is Fiber?

- Fiber is only in plants.

- Fiber is the structural material in plants such as the cell wall.

- Fiber is not digestible by human enzymes.

- Fiber does contain potential energy, but this energy is NOT available to us.

There are two fiber types with distinct properties in the intestinal tract that relate directly to their health benefits.

1. Water-Insoluble Fiber

- In technical terms this fiber type is called cellulose and hemi-cellulose. (Both are much like wood sawdust or the stringy material from celery and other vegetables.)

- Food sources of water-insoluble fiber include the outer husk or shell of wheat grain kernels (bran layers) and vegetables (especially the skins and peels).

- When water-insoluble fiber comes in contact with water (such as in your intestinal tract which is a very watery environment), it swells up. Think about a bowl of bran cereal—pour milk on it and the cereal swells as the little pieces of cereal absorb and hold water rather than dissolving.

- This "water holding" characteristic of water-insoluble fiber is key in your intestinal tract. As it moves through your intestines, it holds water and bulks up. This larger bulk swells, pushing against the intestinal wall, causing the muscle of the colon to "push back." (Just think of yourself in a line for a concert and someone pushes on you as the crowd swells; you push back and hold your ground, right? Well, so does your intestinal tract.)

- This pushing helps speed the passage of waste through the intestinal tract, which, in effect, tones or "workouts" the muscles of the intestinal tract. As the waste moves through, it does so with ease and exits the body easily as soft, bulky stool. Ultimately, this process avoids constipation, or the straining of a bowel movement.

● From this action comes several health benefits. Let's take a look at what happens if you eat a low-fiber diet and its consequence to understand the benefits of an ample fiber intake.

Figure 4.17 shows a comparison of a large intestine while on a low-fiber diet and a large intestine on an ample fiber intake.

Low-Fiber Diet

● With a low-fiber intake, there is not much mass of waste material to move through. This smaller amount of waste moves through the intestinal tract slowly, allowing more time for the body to pull water out, making it even smaller, harder, and drier.

● This hard, compact dry stool is difficult to move or evacuate. Thus, it will take some "effort" to expel this waste. If you have to strain or apply effort to have a bowel movement, you are constipated. Constipation is NOT about the number of times you have a bowel movement—once a day, or once every other day. Constipation is about having to "work" at it.

● If constipation is a regular occurrence, this frequent straining can put pressure on the blood vessels that are at the anus (the opening) and ultimately leads to the formation of **hemorrhoids**—varicose veins (bulging, swollen vessels) that become very painful.

● In addition, when this hard, dry, and slow-moving material sits in the intestines, it can lead to other health problems such as

FIGURE 4.17

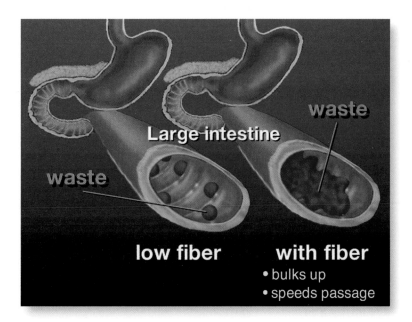

diverticulitis—when the lining of the intestinal wall becomes inflamed and forms small pouches as shown in Figure 4.18. It is possible that these small out-pockets may burst and infiltrate the intestinal cavity with waste material, which can lead to acute medical problems. (See Figure 4.19.)

- Another problem with a low-fiber diet is that this waste material most likely contains cancer-causing agents (often referred to as

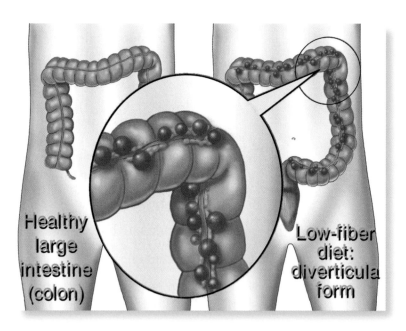

FIGURE 4.18

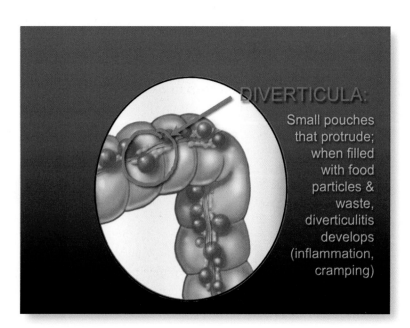

FIGURE 4.19

carcinogens). Increasing exposure time of the large intestinal wall to these harmful substances may lead to cancer of the large intestine (cancer of the colon) years down the road—a serious form of cancer that is linked to a low-fiber diet.

High-Fiber Diet

Take a look at the low- versus high-fiber diagram in Figure 4.18 again, and let's see what health benefits stem from getting ample fiber in your diet.

- The mass of waste material is larger and softer in the higher fiber situation. As a result, this mass moves through faster and you don't have to strain to have a bowel movement.

- Bottom line, you have a reduced chance of becoming constipated.

- This in turn means lower risk of developing hemorrhoids and diverticulitis.

- Since material doesn't sit for long, any potential carcinogens have little time for contact with the intestinal wall, and the potentially harmful substances are effectively diluted with the larger mass of waste material. This results in a lower risk of cancer of the large intestine with a high-fiber diet.

2. Water-Soluble Fiber

- This fiber type is called gums and pectins in technical terms. (You may notice gums and pectins on the ingredient list for some foods such as jams.)

- Food sources of water-soluble fiber include fruits, beans (kidney, black, pinto, and other beans), and oats.

- When water-soluble fiber comes in contact with water or other liquids such as milk (or your intestinal juices), it forms a gel. (Think of a bowl of oatmeal that has sat for awhile; it becomes gel-like and holds a shape.)

- In your intestinal tract this gel property helps to slow the emptying of your stomach content into the small intestines. This slowing may help you feel full longer (reduce your hunger levels) and studies show this fiber type may help with weight loss.

- Water-soluble fiber's gel-like quality also works to lower circulating cholesterol (a fatty, waxy substance covered in the next chapter) absorption in the body. This fiber "traps" cholesterol from your food or cholesterol by-products that are recycled in the intestinal tract. More on this will be covered in Chapter 6 when heart disease is covered.

- Once bound to the fiber, cholesterol is no longer available for absorption and it leaves the body in the stool with the fiber. This action effectively lowers your circulating level of cholesterol. As covered in Chapter 6, high blood cholesterol is a risk factor for heart disease.

The health benefits of water-soluble fiber are:

- Helps to reduce appetite and control the feeling of hunger after a meal
- Lowers blood cholesterol level
- Lowers heart disease risk

HERE'S THE FIBER CONTENT OF VARIOUS FOODS:

FOOD, SERVING SIZE	GRAMS FIBER / SERVING
Rice Krispies	0
White bread, 1 slice	1
100% wheat bread, 1 slice	2
Broccoli, 1 cup	2
Carrot, 7″	2
Prunes, 5 each	3
3 Oatmeal, plain, cooked, 1 packet	3
Banana, 1 large, 9″ long	4
Raisin bran cereal, 1 cup	4
Apple, 1 large, 4″ diameter	6
Bagel, whole grain	6
Artichoke	7
Lentil soup, 1 cup	7
Kidney beans, 1 cup	8
Soy burger on whole wheat bun, 1 each	8
Chilli-Vegtable, 1 cup	13
Fiber One Cereal—½ cup	14
Fast-Food • McDonald's Quarter Pounder • Taco Bell bean burrito, 1	 2 13

How Much Fiber Do You Need?

For starters, you need both types of fiber in your diet. Although some food sources of fiber may have more of one fiber type than another, wheat bran (water insoluble) and oat bran (water soluble) for example, most unrefined fruits, vegetables, beans, and grains supply both fiber types.

The Recommended Dietary Allowance (RDA) for fiber has been established for men and women:

38 grams / day for men

25 grams / day for women

This amount of fiber should be averaged over several days and include a mix of fibers from a variety fruits, vegetables, beans, and whole grains. The less processed the food, the greater the fiber content as milling grains along with various cooking techniques can reduce the fiber content.

Fiber on Food Labels

The Food and Drug Administration has established a Daily Value for fiber based on the typical consumer eating 2,000 calories per day.

Daily Value = 25 grams fiber/day from a mix of fibers

Listed on the food label, as shown in Figure 4.20, is the amount of fiber in a serving of the specific food and the percent Daily Value (DV) that this represents.

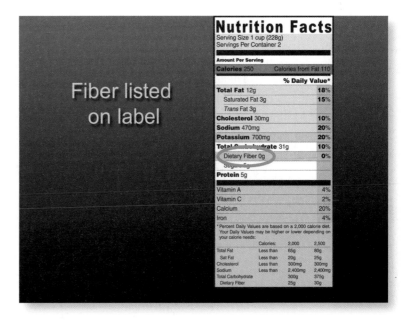

FIGURE 4.20

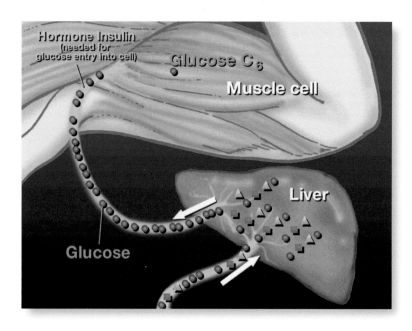

FIGURE 4.21

You calculate the percent DV for a high fiber breakfast cereal. Is your calculated value listed the same as the label?

$$\frac{10 \text{ grams fiber}}{25 \text{ grams fiber}} \times 100 = 40\% \text{ DV}$$

CARBOHYDRATE ENERGY METABOLISM

Recall when we first introduced the primary function of carbohydrate as an energy nutrient. Refer back to Figure 4.10 and our meal of milk, a whole wheat bagel, and jam to see what happens to the carbohydrate in these foods. After digestion, the end products were the individual monosaccharides—glucose, galactose, and fructose. We'll now track how these monosaccharides, once absorbed into the body, are used for energy.

As shown in Figure 4.21, the various monosaccharides make a brief stop at the liver, where they are all converted into glucose. Glucose is the basic "currency" of energy in the body. When someone says "my blood sugar" is low, glucose is the "sugar" they are talking about. The glucose then travels through the circulation for uptake into cells such as those in the muscle, which will then either use this monosaccharide for fuel or store it for later use.

However, the glucose must "get permission" to enter the cell. Glucose entry into most cells requires the hormone **insulin** made by the pancreas. Insulin is much like a monitor in a school that "knocks" on the "door" (cell receptor) of a cell for the door to open up and let glucose in as shown in Figure 4.22.

Once the cell recognizes that glucose is seeking entry, the "door" opens up and glucose marches inside for the cell to use. (See Figure 4.23.)

This process of glucose entry into cells does not occur that smoothly in some individuals. Unfortunately some people do not make insulin; they are Type 1 diabetics and must take a replacement of insulin via an

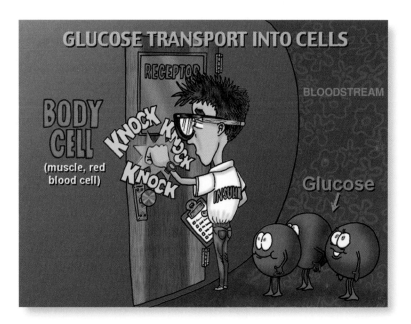

FIGURE 4.22

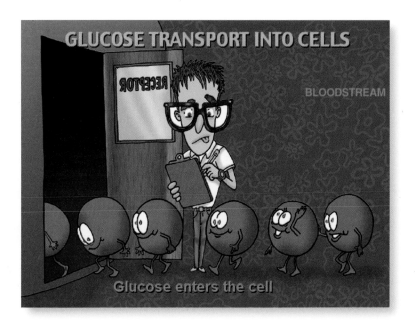

FIGURE 4.23

injection (or use of a pump) that puts insulin directly into the circulation. If insulin is lacking, the glucose accumulates in the bloodstream as shown in Figure 4.24. This pileup of glucose wreaks havoc on the body by damaging blood vessel walls, which leads to poor circulation, heart disease, and loss of eyesight (see Figure 4.25).

There is another form of diabetes, which actually represents about 90% of the diabetes in the United States. Called Type 2 diabetes, this condition is hallmarked by insulin that does not work very effectively; that is, the cell does not "hear" the insulin "knocking," as shown in Figure 4.26. In

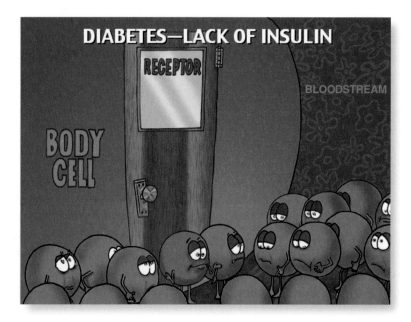

FIGURE 4.24

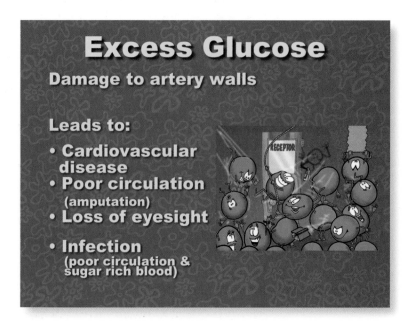

FIGURE 4.25

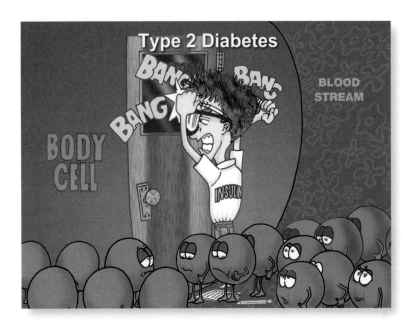

FIGURE 4.26

response, the pancreas secretes more insulin so that glucose may enter the cell. But in the meantime, the glucose accumulates and causes the same devastation on the body as Type 1 diabetes. Millions of Americans suffer from Type 2 diabetes, primarily due to a lack of exercise and obesity. In fact, the American Diabetes Association estimates 14.6 million Americans have been diagnosed with diabetes. Unfortunately, 6.2 million people are unaware that they have the disease.

Once glucose does enter the cell, it has an opportunity (depending upon the body's need for immediate energy) to be used as fuel or to be stored as a large "block" of carbohydrate.

Let's take a look at carbohydrate storage first. As shown in Figure 4.27, glucose enters a muscle cell. (Recall that glucose has six carbons—C_6—which becomes an important detail for later when we look at glucose's use as an energy source.) Hundreds of glucose units can be strung in branched chains called **glycogen,** which is **the body's storage form of carbohydrate.** We learned about glycogen in our discussion of carbohydrate structure.

Most of the body's glycogen is stored in the muscles. Some glycogen is also stored in the liver, which is a vital source of glucose for the bloodstream when you haven't eaten for a while. Recall that your brain relies on glucose for fuel.

The glycogen in the muscle serves that specific muscle as glucose storage. All told, the body can store about 1,600 calories of glycogen in the muscles. You can tuck away even more if you are physically fit and have been doing some endurance training such as running. As we'll see, storing more glucose energy makes sense because it is used during exercise. A fit person can store a few hundred extra calories worth of glucose as glycogen (a loaf of bread's worth of carbohydrate all together).

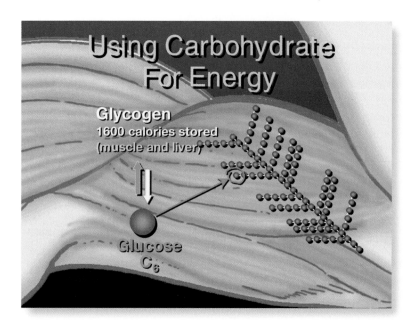

FIGURE 4.27

Now let's take a look at glucose being used as fuel by the muscle. (See Figure 4.28.) Glycogen can be broken back down into glucose or, the glucose enters the cell and is immediately used as a fuel source.

Glucose is a six-carbon molecule and in this first step, glucose is broken in half to release the potential energy out of these chemical bonds and give two three carbon units—C_3. (While it is shown in Figure 4.29 as one step, it actually takes a series of reactions to yield these three carbon units.)

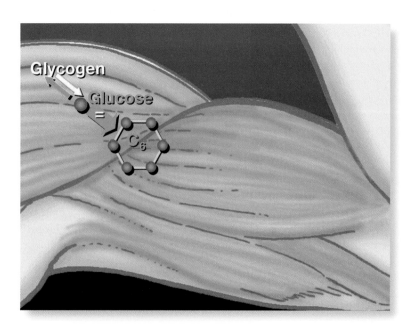

FIGURE 4.28

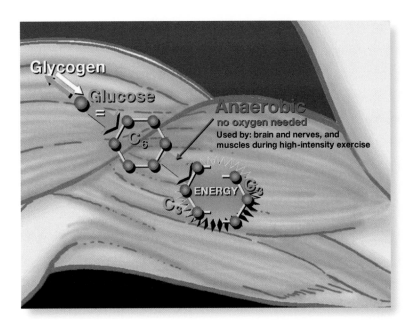

FIGURE 4.29

There is something very special about this breakdown of glucose (C_6) to C_3 units for energy. Unlike the breakdown of fat and protein for fuel, glucose can be broken down for fuel WITHOUT oxygen (you'll learn about this in the next chapter). This type of energy metabolism is called **anaerobic,** which means "without oxygen."

- The brain and central nervous system uses glucose for fuel anaerobically.

- There are also times when your body needs energy but little if any oxygen is present. During intense exercise for example, this breakdown of glucose for fuel provides immediate energy for hardworking muscles. The muscles, however, can only sustain this anaerobic energy metabolism for a short period of time—less than a few minutes—due to the accumulation of substances that hamper muscle contraction. The body must then slow down and take in oxygen for the further breakdown of glucose.

There is still more potential energy in the three carbon—C_3—units that can be released. These next steps however require the presence of oxygen. This process is called **aerobic** energy metabolism. As shown in Figure 4.30, oxygen is used when C_3 units are broken down to C_2 units and their carbon (C) is released as carbon dioxide—CO_2 and exhaled from the lungs. Since chemical bonds are broken, energy is released, which is used by the cells such as the muscle to drive contraction or carry out another metabolic processes such as build new protein.

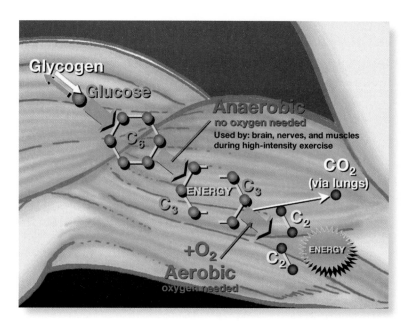

FIGURE 4.30

- An important side note: The step of $C_3 \rightarrow C_2$ is a one-way process (as noted by the one-way bold arrow). This means that once C_2 is made, the reverse process cannot occur. This fact becomes important when we discuss how the body resorts to making glucose when stores have run out.

There is still potential energy left in the C_2 units—right? (This means a chemical bond at least connecting the two carbons.) The body recognizes this and would not let this potential energy go to waste. Aerobic energy metabolism continues as shown in Figure 4.31 and the C_2 units are completely broken down for fuel and the carbon is released as CO_2. This, as in the previous step, is blow-off via the lungs. In addition to CO_2, water is made during the aerobic energy metabolism when the C_2 units completely break apart and energy is released. This process of breaking down C_2 units for energy, while shown here as "one" step is actually several biochemical reactions and is collectively called the Tri-Carboxcylic Acid (TCA) cycle. (You may learn about this energy metabolism cycle in another class.) As you will see in the next chapter, this cycle is the same cycle for the energy metabolism of fats and protein.

Now carbohydrate energy metabolism is complete.

- The end products of carbohydrate energy metabolism are:

Energy (4 calories/gram of carbohydrate) + CO_2 + H_2O

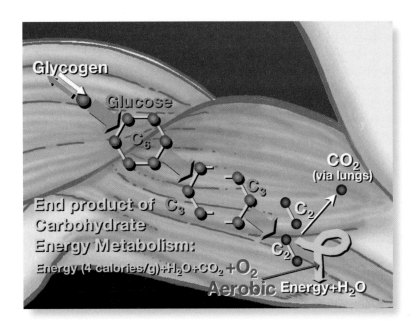

FIGURE 4.31

Carbohydrate Excess

During anaerobic and aerobic carbohydrate energy metabolism, energy is released for the cells to use. But what if you ate more carbohydrate than what your body needed for fuel at the time? Let's say you overate at your bagel meal and had a few bagels with lots of jam or a couple glasses of milk. If the body didn't need the fuel and glycogen stores are filled, what would happen to this potential energy?

Various metabolic signals go into place to tell the liver that excess carbohydrate energy is present. The liver takes the C_2 units and strings them together to build a fat (technically called a fatty acid) as shown in Figure 4.32.

The potential energy that was in the C_2 units has now been transformed into another molecule that contains potential energy—fat. This fat is packaged up into a carrier and then sent off into the circulation for eventual storage into fat cells. (This will be covered in detail in the next chapter.)

- So in the end, **carbohydrate eaten in excess of energy needs is converted to and stored as fat.**

Carbohydrate "Deficiency"

Up to this point, we have discussed the use of carbohydrate for fuel. What if carbohydrate is lacking in the diet, or at least inside the cell? What does the body do in this case since carbohydrate fuel is specifically necessary for the brain and central nervous system to function? Also, muscles rely

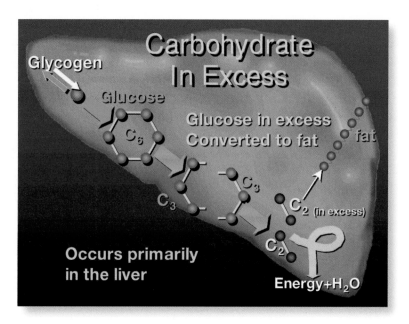

FIGURE 4.32

on glucose during high-intensity exercise. Additionally, other cells in the body use only glucose for fuel, such as red blood cells, so there is a specific reliance on carbohydrate in the body.

The following are situations when a "deficiency" of carbohydrate may occur:

- During a fast, when a person has not been eating anything for 24–36 hours or more

- During a very low carbohydrate diet such as popular weight-loss diets (Atkin's diet) that emphasize protein comsumption

- When insulin is lacking so that glucose does not get into cells (the cell is essentially "starving" for glucose fuel despite the fact there is plenty in the bloodstream), which may occur in a diabetic who is not taking replacement insulin!

The first action taken by the body is to break down any stored glycogen for glucose fuel. The glycogen in the muscle serves that specific muscle. The glycogen in the liver supplies the blood with glucose, which is in turn where the brain gets this sugar.

But stores of glycogen run out in about 24 to 36 hours. Usually liver glycogen runs out in less than 24 hours. If you are exercising, the use of glucose is greater so the glycogen stores may run out in two to four hours.

With stores of glucose depleted, the body must resort to making its own glucose because the brain MUST have glucose for fuel. As shown in Figure 4.33, the process of making glucose occurs in the liver and involves breaking down protein for conversion into glucose.

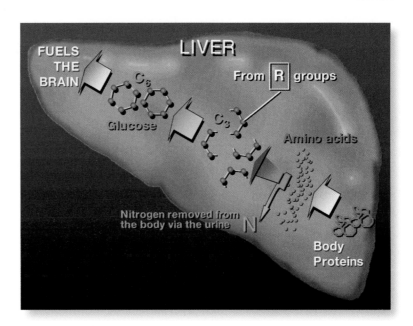

FIGURE 4.33

Hormonal signals that alert the body to this "no glucose" situation stimulate body proteins, such as those in muscle and elsewhere, to break down into individual amino acids and then get shuttled to the liver. As you may recall from Chapter 2, each of the 20 amino acids has a unique R group, and it's this R group that comes to the rescue. The nitrogen is pulled off each of the amino acids and excreted in the urine as urea. The remaining carbon skeletons, which contains the R groups, have the option of being converted into glucose.

Here's How It Works

- If the R group chemically "looks" enough like C_3 it gets converted into a C_3unit.

- This C_3 unit combines with another C_3 unit to make a glucose.

- This glucose then gets shuttled out into the bloodstream and can fuel the "hungry" brain.

- This process, called gluconeogenesis, is very costly to the body because vital proteins are used at the expense of making glucose. But this must happen since the brain needs carbohydrates for fuel.

- Also, this process of making glucose can only supply enough glucose fuel for the brain's central nervous systems and red blood cell's energy use, but not enough to restock glycogen stores so that a person can go run a marathon or do an extended session of exercise.

- If the R group is not chemically similar to C_3, it is converted to C_2 units and used for fuel in the TCA cycle (not pictured). This means that not all the amino acids get converted to glucose, which is another reason why this process of converting protein to glucose is so costly—you lose 2 grams of amino acids for every gram of glucose you make.

Need for Carbohydrate

So during a fast, high-protein/low-carb diet, or without insulin if you are diabetic, your body loses functional protein tissue (muscle, enzymes, and other body proteins).

- To prevent this protein breakdown, some carbohydrate is needed in the diet—about 130 grams of carbohydrate is necessary each day (though the daily value of 300 grams is recommended).

HERE IS THE CARBOHYDRATE CONTENT OF COMMON FOODS

FOOD, SERVING SIZE	GRAMS OF CARBOHYDRATE / SERVING
Low-fat milk, 1 cup	13
Sports drink, 1 cup	15
Peach, 1 medium	17
Crackers, Triscuit (7 ea)	21
Cereal, cornflakes, 1 cup	24
Apple, 1 large	32
Banana, 1 large	36
Pasta, 1 cup	40
Energy bar (Cliff)	42
Rice, white long grain, 1 cup	45
Baked potato, 1 medium	51
Beans, barbeque, 1 cup	64
Fast-Food • McDonald's french fries • Pizza Hut, pepperoni, medium 12″, 1 slice	57 21

- For optimal health, the Food and Nutrition Board suggests between 45 to 65 percent of calories come from a variety of carbohydrates (whole grains, vegetables and fruit). The Food and Drug Administration (the arm of the government in charge of food labels) has set the Daily Value for carbohydrate at 300 grams. This amounts to 55% of the calories for a typical consumer eating 2,000 calories per day.

Key Points about Carbohydrate Energy Metabolism

Let's review carbohydrate energy metabolism because grasping this will assist you in the next chapter when energy metabolism of carbohydrates, protein, and fats is integrated.

- Glucose (from a meal) can be stored as glycogen in the muscles and liver. (See Figure 4.34.) Glycogen lasts about 24 to 36 hours if you are at rest, or about 2 to 3 hours if you are exercising.

- Glucose can be broken down as an energy source in the absence of oxygen (anaerobically). (See Figure 4.35.) This process is especially important for the brain and central nervous system. Also, during intense exercise, anaerobic carbohydrate energy metabolism is vital. Fat and protein cannot be utilized this way.

- In the presence of oxygen, glucose can be broken down completely to release 4 calories per gram of energy, water is made and CO_2 is released. (See Figure 4.36.) If carbohydrates are eaten in excess, glucose is broken down to C_2 units and converted to and stored as fat.

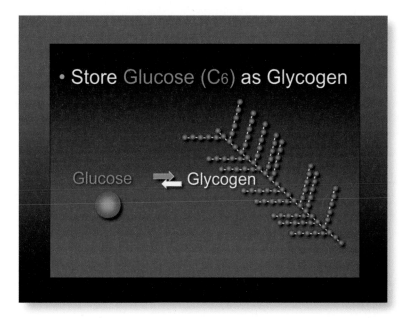

FIGURE 4.34

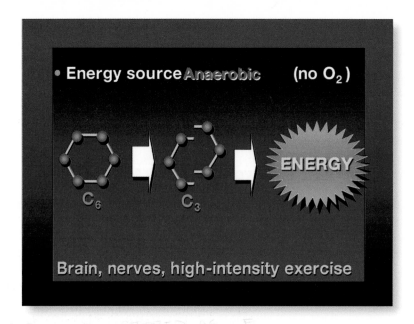

FIGURE 4.35

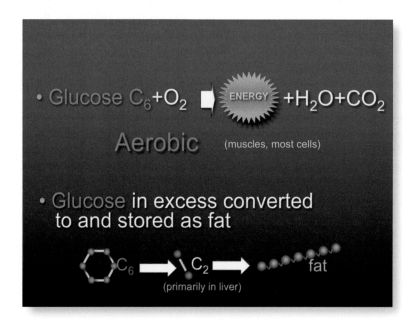

FIGURE 4.36

In the absence of dietary carbohydrate (or when insulin is lacking as in Type 1 diabetes), glycogen stores are depleted; thus, glucose must be made so that the brain can function. Glucose is made from protein, which is broken down into amino acids, which in turn are converted to glucose. (The nitrogen is excreted in the urine.) Making glucose from protein means a loss of functional tissue. (See Figure 4.37.)

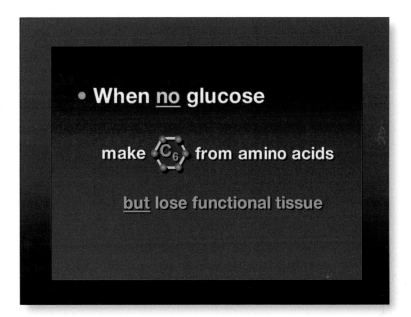

FIGURE 4.37

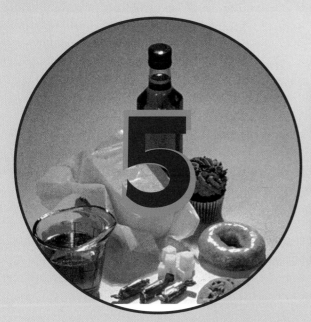

5 Fat—The Misunderstood Nutrient

No doubt you have thoughts about "fat" already. Most likely you have contemplated cutting back on fat in your diet, or perhaps you view fats as "bad" in general. In this chapter, your perspective on fat may change. Fats are not created equal when it comes to your health. This nutrient *is* vital in your diet. Certain types of fats have a negative impact on your health, while other fat types are essential for a variety of roles.

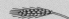

In this chapter, we will cover:

▶ The function of fat

▶ Fat types and food sources

▶ Essential fats and their role in health

▶ Fat in foods: processing and fat replacements (fat-free foods)

▶ Fat digestion and transport

▶ Fat energy metabolism

▶ Bringing it all together—energy metabolism (protein, carbohydrate, and fat)

▶ Cholesterol—its vital roles and transport in the body

THE FUNCTION OF FAT

Like protein and carbohydrate, fat performs all three basic functions of nutrients.

1. **Energy:** Fat supplies 9 calories/gram and is an excellent energy source. Most Americans eat about a third of their calories from fat—this translates to over 270,000 calories in fat per year or 6,000 teaspoons of fat! As we will discuss in future chapters, high-fat diets are linked with chronic diseases such as heart disease and cancer.

2. **Regulation:** Fat performs numerous regulatory roles in the body mediating a number of processes. An example is hormones. Some hormones, notably the sex hormones testosterone and estrogen, are made from fat and cholesterol.

3. **Structure:** Fat serves the body a number of ways in structure. Fat surrounding organs, such as the kidneys, help protect and cushion them from shock. Fat is also a very important component in the structure of cell membranes. As we will discuss in a later section, certain fats make up cell membranes and give the membrane its fluid characteristic and ability to serve as a selective barrier. This presence of fat in every single cell of your body means that you could never get rid of all your body fat even if you tried extreme dieting and exercising—about 3 to 4 percent of your body weight is fat in this capacity.

FAT TYPES AND FOOD SOURCES

Let's examine fat's chemical structure in food fat such as butter or a vegetable oil, as well as fat from a person (let's say it's been "sucked" out and is in a bowl). The chemical structure is the same in all three examples. All three fat examples consist of **triglycerides.**

The triglyceride shown in Figure 5.1 consists of **fatty acids** on a three-carbon backbone (called glycerol). For now, we are going to "pluck" off the fatty acids, from the glycerol, and take a look at these to understand their structure and characteristics.

Fatty Acids

There are two categories of fatty acids—saturated and unsaturated. It is the difference between these two categories that explains why butter is solid and olive oil is liquid at room temperature. Fatty acids are long chains of carbon that are typically even in number and range from about

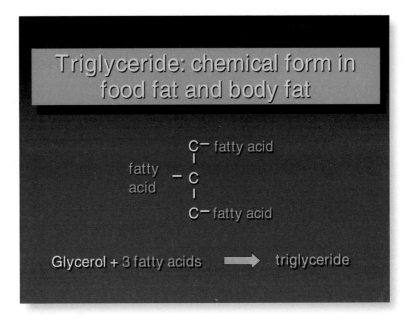

FIGURE 5.1

4 carbons to 26 carbons long (with 16 and 18 carbons in length being the most common fatty acid length in foods).

1. **Saturated Fatty Acids**

   ● "Saturated" means that each carbon is fully saturated with hydrogen atoms (recall that each carbon must bond four times to a neighboring element). The particular fatty acid in Figure 5.2 has 16 carbons and is called palmitic acid. Palm oil, a type of tropical fat from palm kernels and used in snack foods and cookies, consists of triglycerides with many of their fatty acids as palmitic acid.

   ● Notice below the C–H structure of palmitic acid in Figure 5.2 is a simplified drawing of this fatty acid that reflects the characteristic of this fatty acid—straight and stiff like a piece of wood. Thus, on the triglycerides, the saturated fatty acids tend to align themselves and stack up to form a solid fat at room temperature. If a food fat (triglycerides) has predominately saturated fatty acids, then it is **SOLID** at room temperature.

   ● Saturated fatty acids have an even number of carbons such as 6, 12, and up to 26 carbons.

   ● The most common saturated fatty acids are palmitic acid (16C), and stearic acid (18C). (*Note:* The number indicates the number of carbon atoms.)

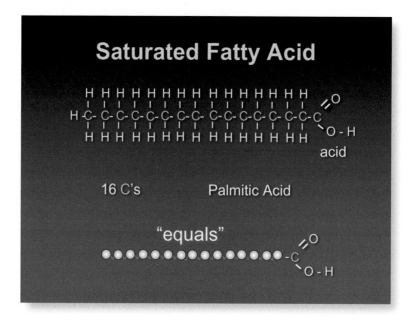

FIGURE 5.2

2. Unsaturated Fatty Acids

● Notice in Figure 5.3 that compared to the saturated fatty acid, two hydrogens are missing. Thus, the fatty acid is not fully "saturated" with hydrogen, or **unsaturated.** These carbons still must maintain the four-bond rule, so they end up bonding twice with each other. The chemical bond between the two carbons is called a **carbon-carbon double bond (C = C)**, which characterizes the unsaturated fatty acid. The fatty acid in Figure 5.3 is called oleic acid and is the predominate fatty acid found on the triglyceride from olive oil.

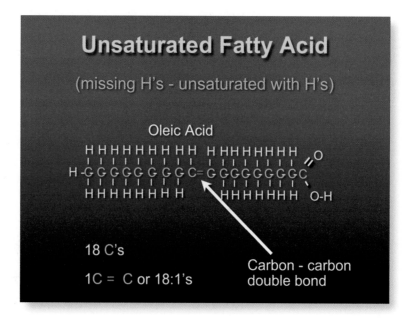

FIGURE 5.3

- Another way to represent this fatty acid is "18:1," which reflects the number of C atoms: number of C = C bonds. "18:1 fatty acid has 18 carbon atoms and one C = C bond and is called a monounsaturated fatty acid ("mono" means one).

- Let's take a look at how this double bond changes the property of the fatty acid. As shown in Figure 5.4 in the simplified drawing of the fatty acid, the double bond puts a bend or crimp in the strand of carbons. This changes everything. Now the triglycerides with these unsaturated fatty acids do not stack up neatly and increases movement which causes the fatty acids to be **LIQUID** at room temperature.

- Unsaturated fatty acids with more than one C = C bond are called polyunsaturated fatty acids. (Generally, fatty acids have no more than six C = C bonds.) (See Figure 5.5.)

- The placement of the C = C bond is very important. In oleic acid the C = C bond is in the "9" position; that is, it is 9 carbons in from the left. Your body, primarily in the liver, makes fatty acids and can make oleic acid if it wants. But the placement of C = C bonds in the "3" and "6" position the body cannot make. However, these resulting fatty acids have vital roles in the body, which makes them **essential fatty acids;** that is, you must eat a dietary source of these fats.

Figure 5.6 illustrates the common unsaturated fats and lists their food sources.

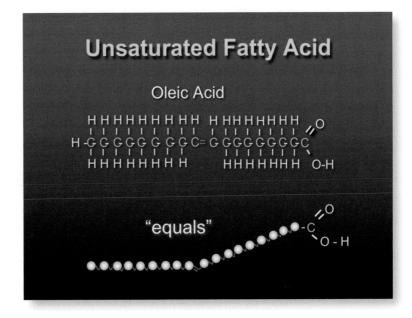

FIGURE 5.4

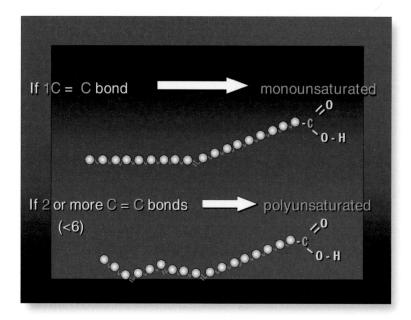

FIGURE 5.5

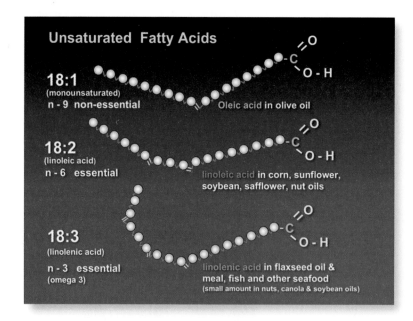

FIGURE 5.6

Notice that the two essential fats—18:2 linoleic (18 C's and 2 C = C bonds) and 18:3 linolenic (18 C's and 3 C = C bonds)—have an even more crimped structure. This imparts an even more "liquid" nature to these fats. Linolenic (18:3) is an essential fat found in fish, especially cold-water fish. This fatty acid is also called omega-3 fat. With the extra C = C bond, this fatty acid is very liquid at room temperature, and in cold seawater it doesn't solidify. (Just think, if fish did have monounsaturated or saturated fatty acids as part of their bodies, the fish would be "stiff as a board".)

ESSENTIAL FATS AND THEIR ROLE IN HEALTH

These vital fats are needed for important roles in the body—cell membrane structure and prostaglandin formation.

1. **Cell membrane structure**

   As shown in Figure 5.7, the cell membrane is made up of two layers of fatty acids (referred to as a "lipid bilayer"). Essential fats are components of this layer and allow the cell membrane to have a very fluid character while at the same time serving as a barrier.

2. **Prostaglandin formation**

   Essential fats are converted to a series of substances called prostaglandins, which act much like hormones in specific locations in

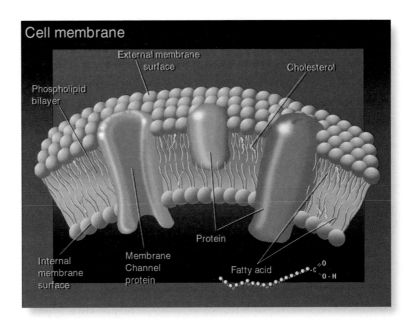

FIGURE 5.7

the body such as in blood vessels and in the uterus, mediating blood clot formation and uterine contractions (during menstrual bleeding). Prostaglandins also mediate the inflammatory response such as with swelling from an injury. The aspirin that you might take to ease the pain actually works against certain prostaglandins to lessen the inflammation, which will ease the pain.

How Much Essential Fatty Acid Do You Need?

- **Linoleic 18:2**—We need 12 to 17 grams or 5 to 10 percent of our total calories from this fat or about three teaspoons of corn oil daily. Most Americans easily get this amount from a variety of foods that contain vegetable oils.

- **Linolenic 18:3**—We need 1.1 to 1.6 grams or about 1 percent of our total calories as omega-3 fat daily. This would mean eating fish a few times per week; something most Americans don't do. Researchers feel that we fall short on our intake of this essential fatty acid. In fact, we have an imbalance of 18:2 to 18:3 fats, which may contribute to the development of age-related diseases such as heart disease and certain cancers. The theory is that the imbalance of essential fats creates changes in the cell membrane and prostaglandin profile in the body that promotes these chronic diseases.

What Happens if You Have a Deficiency of Essential Fatty Acids?

Essential fat deficiency is quite rare. Since our need is very little (about a teaspoon of oil daily) and we get plenty of vegetable oils in our diet, falling short on 18:2 (or linoleic acid) is not a risk. However, we tend not to get enough of 18:3 (or omega-3 fats). Even though this does not present an immediate problem, long-term imbalance, as mentioned above, may lead to age-related ailments. In rare situations, an essential fat deficiency may develop; for example, in a person with stomach or bowel disease typically on tube feeding (getting all their nutrients through liquid fed via a tube) in which too little or none of the essential fats were added to the mixture. In this case, growth failure results and dry flaky skin.

Nutrition Bite

Aspirin or other nonsteroidal anti-inflammatories work to help fight pain by blocking the action of certain prostaglandins, thereby reducing pain.

Fat in Food—Processing and Fat Replacements (Fat-Free Foods)

Let's go back to our original look at fat's chemical structure—the triglyceride. Fatty acids are attached as part of the triglyceride structure and don't exist in foods "unattached." (See Figure 5.8.)

As eluded to earlier, not all the fatty acids on a triglyceride are identical.

- A food fat is called a "saturated fat" if a majority (not all) of its fatty acids are saturated.

- Similarly, a food fat is called "unsaturated fat" if most (not all) of its fatty acids are unsaturated.

Let's look at a comparison of food fat from animal and vegetable sources. (*Note:* By "vegetable" what is meant are plant sources typically from a plant seed such as a sunflower seed, which is rich in fat, not a "vegetable" such as a carrot or lettuce.) (See Figure 5.9.)

Know your food sources of saturated and unsaturated fats. Figures 5.10, 5.11, and 5.12 show some examples.

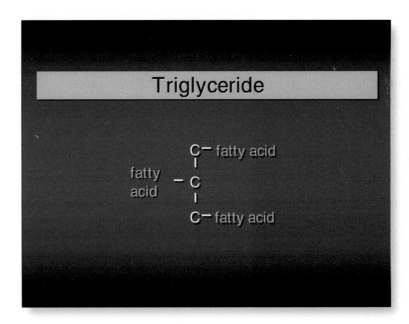

FIGURE 5.8

Fats and Food Processing

You may have been wondering up to this point why certain food fats, such as margarine and vegetable shortening, have not been mentioned. These fats are "manufactured" by processing natural food fats to change their properties, and hence, texture in foods. Margarine and vegetable shortening were developed decades ago (around the time of World War II) because

FOOD FAT	
ANIMAL	**VEGETABLE**
• Saturated fat	• Unsaturated fat
• Low 18:2 (linoleic) 18:3 (linolenic)	• High 18:2 • (very small amount of 18:3)
• Solid	• Liquid
Exceptions: Fish (18:3), chicken, egg	*Exceptions:* Coconut, palm oil

FIGURE 5.9

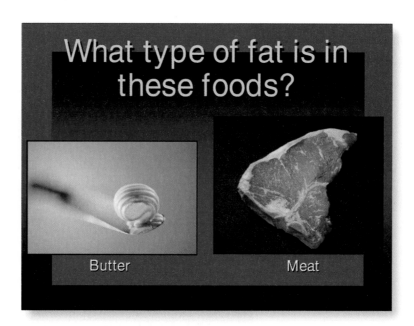

FIGURE 5.10

butter was in short supply and inexpensive vegetable oils were plentiful. But the C = C bond in unsaturated fats presented a challenge. This bond is very fragile. Exposing an unsaturated fat to oxygen in the air will cause the bond to "come undone" or, in scientific terms, oxidize and form free radicals as shown in Figure 5.13.

When a food fat is allowed to sit, let's say in a bowl or open bottle, exposed to the air, the free radicals that form can change the taste and appearance of the food. This off-taste is called **rancidity.** Obviously, food manufacturers don't want their food to become rancid, but they still want

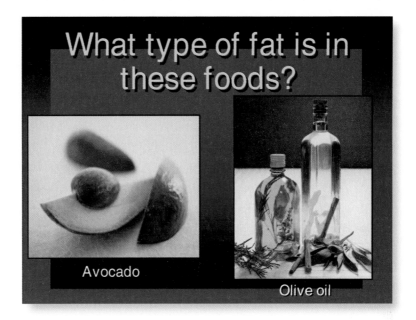

FIGURE 5.11

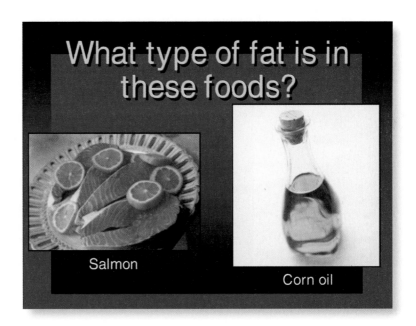

FIGURE 5.12

the ability to use these inexpensive vegetable oils. So the process of **hydrogenation** was "invented" as a way to stabilize the unsaturated fats by changing their chemical configuration about the C = C bond making the fat saturated, as shown in Figure 5.14.

Hydrogenation converts an unsaturated fatty acid to a saturated one. Hydrogen gas is bubbled into a vat of vegetable oil, such as corn oil or

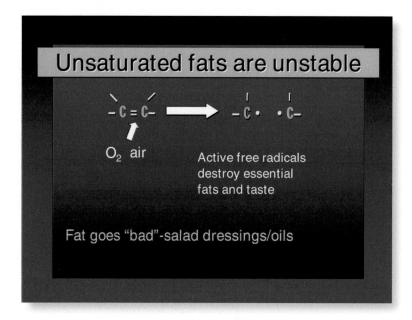

FIGURE 5.13

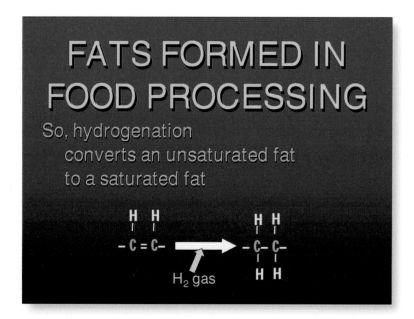

FIGURE 5.14

cottonseed oil, in the presence of a catalyst to start the reaction of "undoing" the C = C bond. Hydrogen is added to the C = C bond making the oil a saturated fat, thus changing a liquid fat to a solid fat. You may see the term "partially hydrogenated" on an ingredient list of a food. This simply means that the vegetable was "partially" hydrogenated; thus, most of its fatty acids were converted to saturated fats.

Hydrogenation results in several important changes to the original vegetable oil:

- The fat is now more stable having a longer shelf-life and it now can be stored at room temperature.
- The fat has changed from a liquid to a solid at room temperature.
- Unsaturated fatty acids become saturated.
- By removing the C = C bonds, the fatty acids that were once 18:2 linoleic or 18:3 linolenic (small amount in vegetable oils) NO longer possess double bonds. That is, hydrogenated vegetable oils are NOT a good source of the essential fats.
- The process of hydrogenation also forms a new type of fatty acid called "*trans*" fatty acids.

Let's take a closer look at *trans* fatty acids because scientific research shows that foods with these types of fatty acids on the triglycerides have health implications, specifically increasing the risk for heart disease.

Trans Fatty Acids

To compare how trans fat may impact health, let's remind ourselves how saturated and unsaturated fatty acids look. In these next few illustrations, we'll look at the simplified drawings of saturated and unsaturated fatty acids that reflect their straight and bent nature, respectively.

In Figure 5.15, the chain of carbon atoms in a saturated fatty acid is straight and stiff, allowing them to stack easily (as part of the triglyceride structure). This characteristic makes saturated fats solid at room temperature.

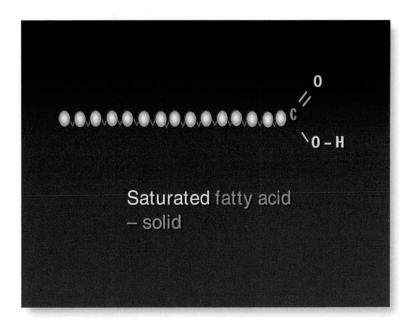

FIGURE 5.15

Now let's look at an unsaturated fatty acid and compare this to a saturated fatty acid. See Figure 5.16. The double bond causes a "kink" in the carbon chain that doesn't allow the fatty acids (while part of the triglyceride structure) to stack nicely. This is what keeps unsaturated fat liquid at room temperature. This particular type of "kink" caused by the arrangement of the C = C bond is called a "*cis*" configuration. (In the world of chemistry, this has to do with how the chain of carbons is oriented about the C = C bond.) The *cis* configuration is the way unsaturated fatty acids exist in nature.

Now let's take a look at what happens to some of the fatty acids during hydrogenation or partial hydrogenation. See Figure 5.17. During the hydrogenation process, many but not all of the fatty acids are converted into saturated fatty acids. Some of the unsaturated (*cis*) fatty acids are tweaked a bit—the double bond comes "undone" but does not get filled with hydrogen atoms but rather goes back to a double bond with a different configuration. This new arrangement about the C = C bond is called "**trans**" and as pictured, the chain of carbons is straight just like a saturated fatty acid despite its C = C bond. Thus, a trans fat is straight and stiff, solid at room temperature. This helps give margarine and other foods made with hydrogenated vegetable oil their texture.

Health Concerns about Trans Fats

Perhaps you've heard about the dangers of trans fat in the news, or seen products such as margarines that state "trans fat-free" on the label. All the fuss about trans fats has to do with how they behave like saturated fats,

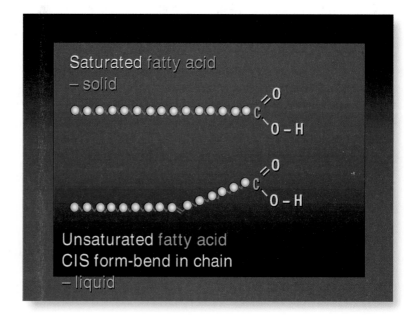

FIGURE 5.16

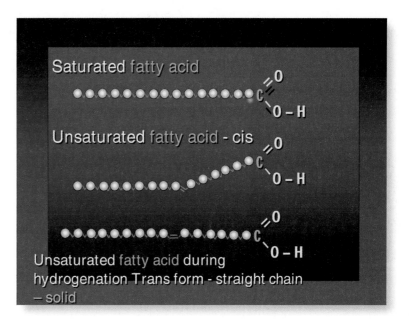

FIGURE 5.17

not only in food, but also in your body. As we'll discuss in our next chapter on heart disease, saturated fats increase your risk for this ailment by indirectly boosting your blood cholesterol levels. Unfortunately, trans fats do the same thing. Research shows that diets with high amounts of trans fat from margarine, snack foods, and cookies all made with hydrogenated or partially hydrogenated vegetable oils increase risk for heart disease. Therefore, the Food and Drug Administration has required that amounts of trans fat in food be listed on the Nutrition Facts food label. This will allow consumers to see how much trans fat is in a food, although a Daily Value (or suggested limit) for trans fat intake has not been determined (see Figure 5.18).

Fat Replacements

Fat is very important for the taste and texture of food. Just do a side-by-side comparison of full-fat ice cream (such as a premium brand) and a reduced-fat ice cream. No doubt you'll find the premium-brand ice cream full flavored and creamier than the low-fat version. However, even though fat may taste great, it also carries with it 9 calories for every gram. Thus, many high-fat foods are also packed with calories. In an effort to cut back on fat, both to reduce calorie intake and to lower fat intake for health benefits, many consumers have turned to reduced-fat or fat-free foods. Food manufacturers have worked hard to develop various fat replacements, some using standard food components such as protein and fiber. There is also a synthetic fat replacement being used in some foods.

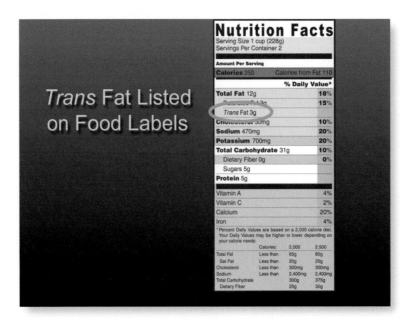

FIGURE 5.18

The following are fat replacements that are normal food constituents:

- **Protein:** Certain proteins can be "whipped" to form micro-particles that feel like fat in your mouth. (Just think how whipped egg whites look and feel like whipped cream.) This type of fat replacement can only be used in noncooked foods such as ice cream since cooking would denature the protein and alter the texture. This protein replacement has 4 calories per gram versus fat's 9 calories per gram.

- **Corn starch, fruit purees and oat fiber:** These are added to foods such as baked goods—muffins and pastries, for example—and gives these foods a texture much like that of fat. The oat fiber even adds fiber to the food. The energy content of these fat replacers is about 2 to 4 kcal per gram.

- **Fat as mono- and di-glycerides:** Sounds funny, but fat can substitute for fat. Small amounts of these modified triglycerides are added to salad dressing to help thicken (emulsify) and give the dressing a creamy texture. Because such small amounts are used, the food can be called "fat-free" and very few calories are added this way as well.

- **Water:** Water can be used to replace some of the fat in foods such as diet margarine or fat-free cream cheese. But don't try to cook with these foods because the water quickly evaporates and changes the texture of the food.

Synthetic Fat Replacement

Over 10 years ago, the Food and Drug Administration approved for the first time a synthetic fat replacement for use in snack foods. Olestra (trade name of Olean®) is the synthetic fat replacement used in potato chips and a few other snack foods. According to taste tests, olestra tastes like the real thing—it is oil and can be used just like vegetable oils for cooking and frying. Here is a look at olestra.

Olestra's size and structure make it indigestible—there are no "olestra" digestive enzymes. (See Figure 5.19.) So if olestra is not digested and absorbed, where does it go? It goes into the stool and with olestra go some fat-soluble nutrients.

In the intestinal tract as pictured in Figure 5.20, olestra attracts other dietary substances that are also soluble in fat—things like the fat-soluble vitamins A, D, E, and K (we'll learn about these in Chapter 11) and a family of substances known as carotenoids. These substances give vegetables and fruit their color, and studies show that carotenoids may help reduce the risk of certain age-related diseases such as cancer.

As shown in Figure 5.21, as olestra passes through the digestive tract unabsorbed, it takes these fat-soluble nutrients with it into the stool. This loss of nutrients is compensated by the fortification with the fat-soluble vitamins (but not carotenoids) in foods made with olestra. Additionally, consuming large amounts of foods made with olestra may present some gastrointestinal problems, as the olestra passes through it, resulting in cramping, bloating, and diarrhea. However, eating moderate amounts (a few servings) of chips or other snack foods made with this fat replacement should be well tolerated by most people.

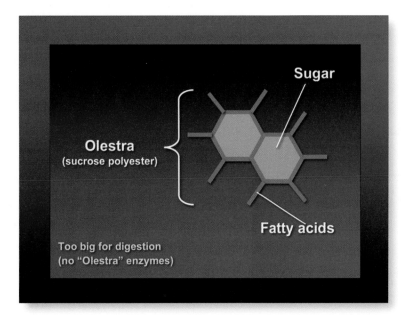

FIGURE 5.19

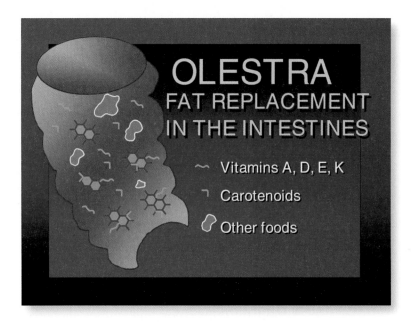

FIGURE 5.20

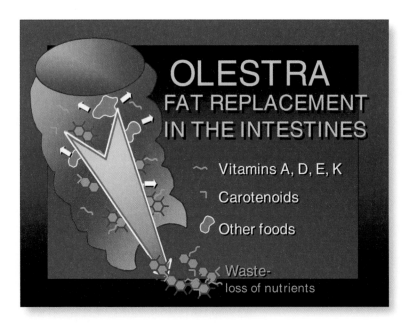

FIGURE 5.21

FAT DIGESTION, ABSORPTION, AND TRANSPORT

Fat is tricky stuff when it comes to its digestion, absorption, and transport in the body. Think about trying to dissolve a stick of butter in a pitcher of water versus dissolving a cup of sugar. There is no problem stirring the sugar into the water and watching it dissolve, but try as you may, the butter is not going to dissolve in the water. Fat and water don't mix, and this is the challenge the body is faced with since the body is over one-half water. The blood, for example, is mostly water. Fat must be made soluble every step of the way—during digestion, absorption, and transport. Emulsification is the process of making fat soluble in water. During fat digestion, absorption, and transport, emulsification on some level takes place for the fat to be "accepted" by the body.

Fat Digestion

Unlike protein and carbohydrate, there is no digestion of fat in the mouth or stomach. Digestion takes place in the small intestine as fat is made soluble in the watery environment and then fat can be chemically digested.

In the small intestine, as shown in Figure 5.22, triglyceride from a meal such as a bagel with cream cheese (which is about 90 percent fat, by the way) mixes with a substance called **bile.** Much like soap that you would put on a shirt or other fabric to wash away grease, bile acts to emulsify triglycerides and "wash" them into the digestive juices. Bile is made in the liver from cholesterol (more on this in another section) and is stored in the gallbladder. When you eat a meal, the gallbladder dispenses bile much like a pump dispenser of soap alongside a sink.

Once the triglyceride has been emulsified into solution, the enzyme **lipase** ("lip" = lipid or fat; "ase" = enzyme) secreted from the pancreas starts to chemically digest triglycerides. Lipase breaks off fatty acids from the triglycerides leaving monoglycerides (single fatty acid attached to the glycerol) and free fatty acids. As shown in Figure 5.23, fat droplets form a droplet called **micelles,** which contain a combination of fatty acids and monoglycerides. These small micelles are much like the tiny droplets of oil you see when you shake a bottle of oil and vinegar salad dressing.

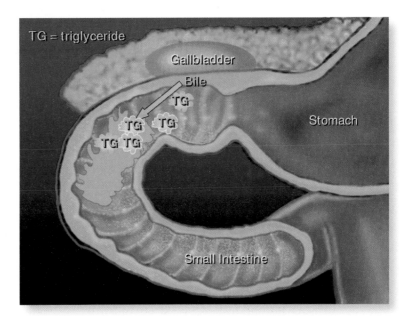

FIGURE 5.22

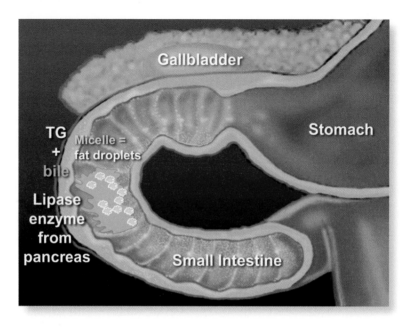

Gallbladder

Stomach

TG + bile

Micelle = fat droplets

Lipase enzyme from pancreas

Small Intestine

FIGURE 5.23

Fat Absorption

Once the micelles have formed, they migrate to the surface of the small intestine where they are absorbed. In the interior of the small intestine wall (before passing into the circulation) the triglycerides reform (fatty acids and monoglycerides rejoin). But before the triglyceride can move into the blood, as shown in Figure 5.23, the fat must be made soluble again.

A protein "coating" is put on the outside of the triglycerides to make the fat "acceptable" to travel in the blood since protein is soluble in water (and the blood is mostly water). This new fat + protein combination is called a **chylomicron.** (See FIgure 5.24.) As we are about to see, chylomicrons venture out into the circulation as a transport vehicle for triglyceride to cells. Chylomicrons are one of several types of **lipoproteins,** which are **the transport form of fat in the circulation,** as described in the next section.

Fat Transport

Chylomicrons migrate from the small intestine wall into the circulation to deliver triglyceride to the cells of the body. As mentioned, chylomicrons are a type of lipoprotein—fat + protein coating—that transports fat through the circulation.

To help visualize a chylomicron (as well as other lipoproteins that we will be introduced to), think of them as a special kind of bus. The outer shell of the bus is made of proteins (the advertisements represent different proteins), and the passengers inside (that we have met so far) are triglycerides.

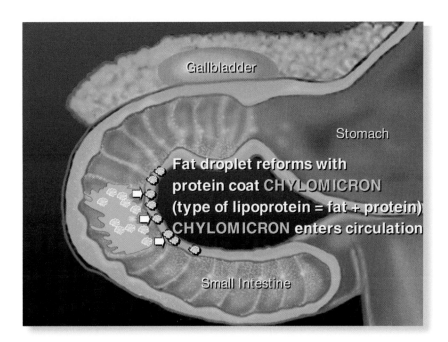

FIGURE 5.24

This bus (chylomicron) travels around the body; stops at muscle and fat cells, as pictured in Figure 5.25, opens its doors; and drops off its passenger—triglyceride. Most of the triglyceride "passengers" get off the bus and enter these cells, but not all. Which cell type—muscle or fat cell—depends upon your energy balance. If you're exercising and fit, the chylomicron likes to stop off at muscle cells so the triglyceride can be used immediately as fuel; but if you're sedentary, most likely this lipoprotein

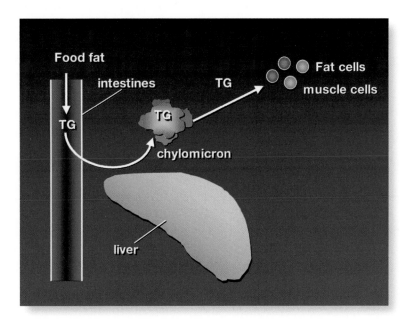

FIGURE 5.25

will stop at fat cells to put triglyceride away in storage for a rainy day when you do need the fat as fuel.

After a while, the chylomicron "fatigues" with delivering triglyceride to cells and heads to the liver. (See Figure 5.26.) Much like a bus depot or headquarters, the liver repackages the remaining triglyceride along with any new fat that has been made from excess protein or carbohydrate. This regrouped triglyceride now gets on a new "bus" and is shipped out of the liver. This new lipoprotein is called **VLDL** (short for **V**ery **L**ow **D**ensity **L**ipoprotein). The term *density* relates to the amount of triglyceride in the lipoprotein and its density in water—the more fat, the less dense or the more it floats in water.

VLDL is another lipoprotein—fat with a protein coat—and it also transports triglyceride to cells. Just like the chylomicron, VLDL "opens" its doors and drops off triglyceride to fat and muscle cells depending upon the need for energy. VLDL is a more compact or smaller version of a chylomicron with different proteins (different outside advertisements on the outside of the "bus").

This complex scheme of fat transport via the lipoproteins (chylomicrons, and VLDL) results from fat's insolubility in water (the blood). There's more to the fat transportation story—other lipoproteins and one more passenger in the lipoproteins, namely cholesterol, will be discussed in the last section of this chapter.

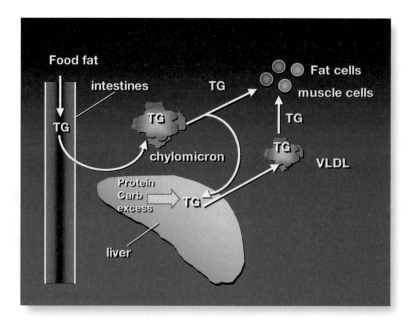

FIGURE 5.26

FAT ENERGY METABOLISM

Once the chylomicrons and/or the VLDLs have delivered triglyceride to cells, what happens to this fat? If put away in fat cells, the triglyceride waits until it is called upon to come out of storage for use as fuel by other cells. This would occur when a person has not eaten for several hours or when calorie intake falls below calorie expenditure for the day. More on this will be covered in Chapter 7 when we discuss obesity and weight loss.

If delivered to muscle cells, the triglyceride is used as fuel. Recall from Chapter 3 that fat contains 9 calories per gram, so it has potential energy in its carbon bonds.

Inside of a muscle cell, triglyceride is broken apart to release the fatty acids. (For sake of simplicity, we'll ignore the glycerol backbone and what happens to it.) These fatty acids contain potential energy and are broken down into C_2 units. (See Figure 5.27.) Energy is released and oxygen is used. This process is aerobic—with the presence of oxygen.

These C_2 units are just like the C_2 units from when carbohydrate was broken down aerobically. There is more potential energy in these two-carbon units, and they are sent through the TCA cycle to release more energy—all told, 9 calories per gram. At the same time CO_2 is released and water is made.

The end products of fat energy metabolism are energy (9 calories/gram) + CO_2 + H_2O.

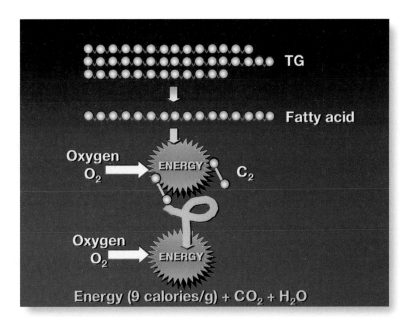

FIGURE 5.27

Now that we know the end products of fat and carbohydrate aerobic energy metabolism are the same, when does the cell decide to burn fat or carbohydrate as a fuel source? Well, BOTH are used simultaneously. In fact, both carbohydrate and fat must be burned together for operations in the C_2-burning (TCA) cycle to work best. When you are sedentary or not very active (such as walking), the body burns about 60 percent fat and 40 percent carbohydrate. However, as you step up the intensity of your activity, the muscle cell shifts to using more carbohydrate and less fat. So during a run (good effort) you are burning about 70 percent carbohydrate and 30 percent fat for fuel.

BRINGING IT ALL TOGETHER—ENERGY METABOLISM (PROTEIN, CARBOHYDRATE, AND FAT)

Let's integrate now what we know about how protein, carbohydrate, and fat are used for energy in the body. Energy metabolism is the collective term used to describe the body's use of fuel depending upon its status or state of energy balance. What the body uses for fuel, or what the body may decide to store for later use as fuel, depends upon different situations.

Let's take a look at three different energy metabolism "conditions" that your body may be routinely faced with and how energy metabolism works in each of these three situations.

1. After you eat a meal.

2. Several hours without eating, such as when you first wake up in the morning.

3. Without food for at least 24 hours—you are fasting.

For each of these three situations, we will look at Figure 5.28, which tracks each of the energy nutrients—carbohydrate, fat and protein. Then we'll summarize energy metabolism for each situation in a table.

Figure 5.28 shows the possibilities for each of the energy nutrients, such as carbohydrate (glucose), which can be stored as glycogen, used anaerobically and aerobically for energy, and in excess can be stored and converted to fat. Which the body chooses to do depends upon the current energy metabolism situation (situation 1, 2, or 3 listed above).

1. After Eating a Meal

When you eat a meal, it is similar to taking a trip to the grocery store and coming back to your apartment. What do you typically do with the bags of groceries? You put them away—in the refrigerator, freezer, and pantry. Your body does the same thing with energy nutrients. **Following a meal, energy nutrients are put away into storage.** Follow along

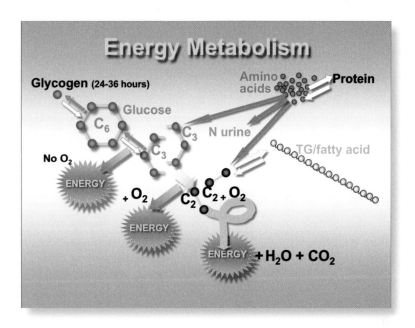

FIGURE 5.28

with each of the energy nutrients as they are put away in storage by following Figure 5.28.

Carbohydrate (Glucose)

After you eat a meal containing carbohydrate, it is digested, absorbed and transported to body cells as glucose. Glucose then enters the cell and can be used if needed for energy ($C_6 \rightarrow C_3 \rightarrow C_2 \rightarrow CO_2 + H_2O +$ energy).

Chances are, you've eaten a bit more than you need at the time for fuel so that you restock glycogen stores. Once these are filled in the muscles and liver, the excess glucose is converted to fat (in the liver), shipped out into the circulation via a VLDL and sent to fat cells.

Fat

Fat from your meal is already fat, and if you don't need it immediately for a fuel source in the muscle (that is, you're lounging around after your big meal), food fat is readily stored as body fat. Via a trip in a chylomicron, this excess fat from a meal makes a journey to fat cells for storage.

Figure 5.29 is a simplified diagram that shows the storage of energy nutrients following a meal.

Protein

Protein from your meal is broken down to amino acids and used for protein replacement needs (replenish or make any new proteins). If you've consumed more protein than what your body needs, the excess amino

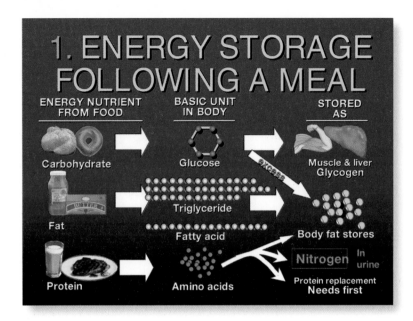

FIGURE 5.29

acids are stripped of their nitrogen (goes into the urine) and the leftover carbon skeleton is converted to fat (via conversion of C_2 units). Like carbohydrates, this is done in the liver and the fat is shipped out (via the VLDL) and sent to fat cells for storage.

2. Several Hours after Eating

When you first wake in the morning, it's been several hours since you have last eaten—dinner the evening before or perhaps a late night snack (overnight "fast"). This energy metabolism situation is much like you going into your kitchen when you are hungry and looking for something to eat but there's nothing out on the counter for munching. So what do you do? You open the cupboards or refrigerator and bring food "out of storage." This is exactly what your body does when you haven't eaten for a while. **Energy nutrients are brought out of storage when you haven't eaten for several hours.** Follow along using the integrated energy metabolism diagram in Figure 5.28 on page 127.

Carbohydrate (Glycogen)

Your brain and other parts of your body still need carbohydrate as fuel and even though you haven't eaten anything in the past few hours, there are readily available stores of carbohydrate for use—glycogen. This storage form of carbohydrate in the muscles and liver provides the body with carbohydrate fuel. Glycogen in a muscle is used by that specific muscle for fuel. (The right biceps muscle glycogen store, for example, is for that muscle, not some other part of the body.) Liver glycogen on the other hand, is used primarily for the brain and nervous system. (Glycogen breaks down to glucose and this moves out into the circulation to fuel the brain.)

Fat

Body fat stores are signaled that fuel is needed and triglycerides are brought out of storage. These are first broken down to C_2 units (aerobically) and then all the way to energy—9 calories/gram + CO_2 + H_2O.

Figure 5.30 is a simplified diagram that illustrates energy nutrients being brought out of storage after several hours without eating.

Protein

At this point, the protein in your body (which is all functional tissue—no "storage") is not touched since you have plenty of carbohydrate fuel. In other words, there's no reason to break protein down to make glucose since you have a supply of glycogen to last you about a day.

3. Fasting—without Food for at Least 24 to 36 Hours

This final energy metabolism situation is much like when you walk into your kitchen to get something to eat because you are famished, but unlike the previous situation, there's not much left in the cupboard or refrigerator. In fact, you're out of ready-to-eat food like breakfast cereal so you have to scrounge to find something edible. In your body, when you have gone without eating for 24 hours or more, and your store of carbohydrate—glycogen—is out, so you have to make your own source of glucose.

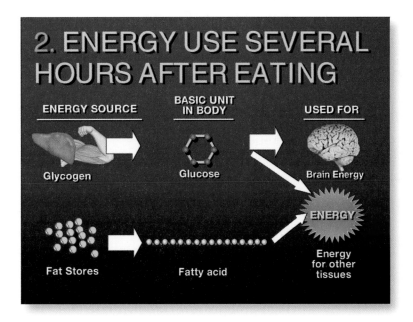

FIGURE 5.30

So the primary difference with the previous situation is that **with fasting, glycogen stores in both the liver and muscle have run out.** Follow along using the energy metabolism diagram in Figure 5.28 (page 127) to track how the body converts protein to glucose as well as using fat as fuel during a fast.

Glucose (Carbohydrate)

The stores of glycogen in muscle last approximately one day with fasting. These stores of glucose can run out sooner if you exercise, lasting about 2 to 4 hours of continuous exercise. Liver glycogen stores also run out in about a day's time.

Protein

With glycogen stores gone, and the brain and other cells in the body such as nervous tissue and red blood cells needing glucose, the body sends a signal to make carbohydrate from protein. Functional protein tissue such as muscle proteins, enzymes, and organ proteins are broken down into the amino acid building blocks. Recall from Chapter 4 that this occurs in the liver where the amino acids are stripped of their nitrogen, which gets excreted by the kidneys into the urine. The remaining carbon skeletons are converted to C_3 or C_2 units (depending upon the R groups). The C_3 units are "glued" together to form glucose (in the liver), which is then sent out into the circulation to fuel the brain and other needy tissues. This process is limited in that you can't make enough glucose to load up muscles with glycogen. In fact, you'll feel pretty weak during a fast, or even light-headed as glucose needs are barely met. The remaining C_2 units are used as fuel by the body.

Fat

At the same time protein is being broken down, hormones signal fat stores to initiate triglyceride break down to fatty acids, which are in turn broken down to C_2 units, and finally CO_2 + H_2O + energy. *Note:* Fatty acids are NOT converted to C_3 units; thus, they *cannot* be used to make glucose. This is why protein is lost—functional tissue—during a fast, in addition to body fat.

Another consequence occurs during a fast—the formation of **ketones,** which are a by-product of fat metabolism, are formed from C_2 units. Ketones form as C_2 units build up in part because carbohydrates are lacking to turn the cycle efficiently (you'll recall that CHO and fats work together in the TCA cycle to generate energy). This formation of ketones gives a person who is fasting a characteristic breath odor of acetone (a type of ketone). This metabolic state is called **ketosis.** It occurs in people who have fasted for a few days or more or following for several days a high-protein/low-carbohydrate diet, or untreated diabetes. During the

Nutrition Bite

If you ever fast for an extended period of time, you need to know the dangers associated with reintroducing food. When fasting for several weeks, such as hunger strike participants or victims of concentrations camps from World War II, the body is geared up for breaking down proteins. That is, the enzymes responsible for breaking down proteins to amino acids and then taking the nitrogen off are going full throttle. Thus, if a big steak meal—lots of protein—is given to a fasted person, this may present a life-threatening situation. With a big dose of protein, these enzymes go to work and break apart the protein and release the nitrogen, which then spikes in the blood. High blood nitrogen can be toxic; in fact, it may lead to instant death. Unfortunately, victims from concentration camps were given hearty meals upon their release and some died from this nitrogen poisoning. In addition, the intestinal tract becomes weakened with fasting, so food must be introduced slowly as the intestinal tract surface rebuilds to handle digestion and absorption of nutrients.

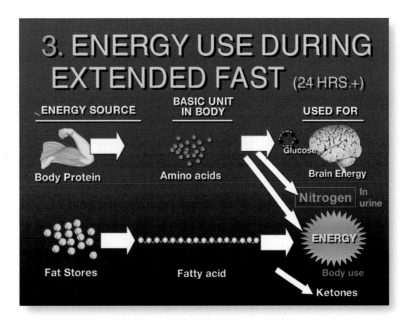

FIGURE 5.31

first few days, a "quick" five pounds of weight is lost. This occurs due to water loss as the glycogen stores run out. Water that is normally "packed" around glycogen is also lost. This rapid weight loss gives people the impression that fasting is a great way to lose weight or that a high-protein diet is a very effective way to lose weight quickly. Actually, the rate of weight loss slows down as the body adapts by slowing energy expenditure and lowering the Basal Metabolic Rate. In addition, the state of ketosis can be dangerous for people with kidney trouble because this puts a strain on kidneys to excrete these extra products.

This shift in energy metabolism during a fast can be simplified using the diagram in Figure 5.31. The key thing to remember is that glycogen stores have run out and the body must make its own glucose from body or food protein.

Cholesterol—Its Vital Roles and Transport in the Body

Let's finish our discussion about fat and its transport through the circulation. We need to meet one more member of the fat family—cholesterol.

Cholesterol is a fatty, waxy-like substance in the body and is handled like fat. Its chemical structure—shown in Figure 5.32—looks a bit like cyclone fence wire and belongs to the chemical family called sterols. Cholesterol performs several essential regulatory functions in the body, but cholesterol is NOT broken down to C_3 or C_2 and therefore provides no energy.

Cholesterol's functions include the following:

1. **Precursor to bile:** Recall that bile is just like a "soap" that the liver makes to emulsify fats in our small intestines so that fat can be digested and absorbed.

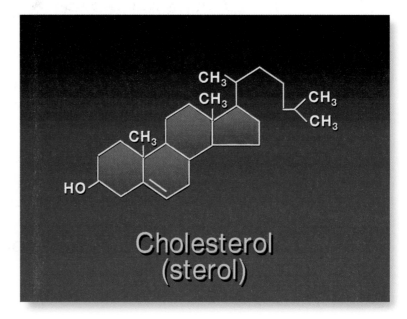

Cholesterol
(sterol)

FIGURE 5.32

2. **Precursor to sex hormones:** The sex hormones testosterone and estrogen are also made from cholesterol. (In fact, their chemical structures look very similar to cholesterol and are considered in the "sterol" family based upon their carbon-ring structure.)

3. **Precursor to vitamin D:** Cholesterol goes through a series of modifications in our body for eventual conversion to vitamin D. One of the first steps is the "activation" of cholesterol in the skin by ultraviolet light from the sun. We'll cover this in greater detail when we discuss vitamin D in Chapter 9.

4. **Component of cell membrane structure:** As shown in Figure 5.33, cholesterol sits in the cell membrane as the vital component giving the membrane its ability, in part, to control what goes in and gets out of the cell. Thus, cholesterol is a normal part of every cell in our body, and all mammals. (Remember this when we think about food sources of cholesterol.)

Even though cholesterol has all these vital roles in the body, it is not an essential nutrient. This must mean that the body can make cholesterol and make enough to meet its needs. Cholesterol is made in the liver of all mammals—you included. As shown in Figure 5.34, cholesterol is made from C_2 units that result from the breakdown of fats, protein, or carbohydrate.

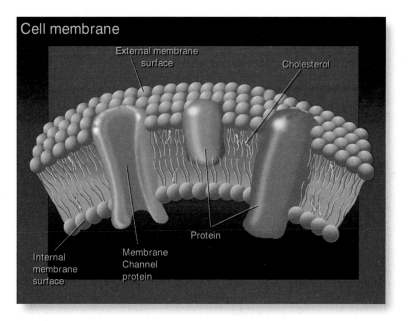

FIGURE 5.33

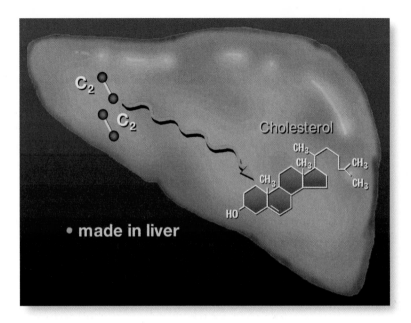

FIGURE 5.34

Sources of Cholesterol in the Body

- Each day the body manufactures about 1000 to 1500 milligrams of cholesterol.

- Each day you take in about 200 to 400 milligrams—this depends upon your diet (specifically how much you eat in the way of animal products—meats, milk, eggs, fish).

Food Sources of Cholesterol

Think about where cholesterol is made and then translate this to possible food sources. Any food that comes from something with a liver—in other words, any animal product—contains cholesterol.

Examples of foods that contain cholesterol: beef, chicken, seafood, eggs, milk (even skim milk), and, of course, liver and other organ meats.

How about avocado? Or what about olives or margarine? Even though these foods are high in fat, they are plant products and therefore contain NO cholesterol. Cholesterol is a type of fat, but that does not mean that only high-fat foods contain cholesterol. In Chapter 6 we'll discuss how high intakes of saturated fat and trans fats can indirectly elevate circulating levels of cholesterol and ultimately increase the risk for heart disease.

This brings up how cholesterol moves through the body via the circulation.

Cholesterol Transport

Let's go back to our discussion about lipoproteins and the transport of fat. We now have a new "passenger"—cholesterol. Since cholesterol is a type of fat, it is not soluble in water (hence, the blood), thus, it needs a ride in a lipoprotein as a means of transport through the body so cholesterol ultimately gets to cells and carries out its duties.

When you eat a food that contains cholesterol, it is absorbed along with fat in the micelle in the small intestinal wall, and then moves through the circulation as a "passenger" in chylomicrons, as shown in Figure 5.35. **Chylomicron, a type of lipoprotein, is made up of three items— triglyceride, cholesterol, and a protein coat.** As we'll see, **all lipoproteins are made of the same items,** just in different proportions.

As the chylomicron delivers triglyceride to fat and muscle cells, the cholesterol stays on board the "bus" and after several hours ends up at the liver. Here the cholesterol is repackaged with triglyceride (both cholesterol left over from the chylomicron along with new triglyceride made from excess carbohydrate and protein) and sent out in the **VLDL—Very Low Density Lipoprotein.** VLDL is also made of triglyceride, cholesterol, and a protein coat.

Recall that the VLDL's job was to drop off triglyceride at fat and muscle cells, and while it does this, cholesterol stays on board. As this happens, the VLDL transforms—it becomes smaller and becomes proportionately richer in cholesterol (although it still has triglyceride on board). This is now a new lipoprotein—**LDL** or **Low Density Lipoprotein.**

LDL, which is made of the three same items (triglyceride, cholesterol, and a protein coat—just different proportions compared to chylomicrons

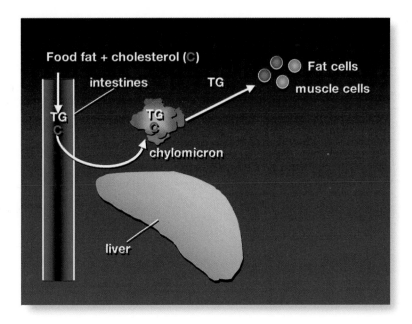

FIGURE 5.35

and VLDLs), now travels through the circulation with a job to do that is different from the chylomicron and VLDL. LDL delivers cholesterol to cells, as shown in Figure 5.36. LDL looks for cell receptors (similar to a bus stop sign) on the surface of cells to know if the LDL should make a stop there and deliver cholesterol. Every cell needs cholesterol for normal functioning. You may have heard about LDL as the "bad" cholesterol. In Chapter 6 we'll see how LDL cholesterol transport can go awry and lead to heart disease.

There's one more lipoprotein to this fat and cholesterol transport story. **HDL** or **High Density Lipoprotein** is also made up of triglyceride, cholesterol, and protein coat. But this lipoprotein is proportionately richer in protein so it's "heavier." HDL originates from the liver and has a very specific job—it acts like a scavenger. HDL picks up loose cholesterol that has fallen from lipoproteins or from dying cells. Once on board, the HDL travels to the liver where the cholesterol can get off and have the opportunity to become bile and leave the body or be recycled back on board a VLDL (as shown in the completed cholesterol and fat diagram in Figure 5.37).

HDL is frequently referred to as the "good" cholesterol since high levels of HDL is associated with a reduced risk for heart disease—more on this in Chapter 6. But we'll leave this discussion by noting that HDL levels can be boosted with exercise. It seems that with regular exercise, such as running, levels of HDL are increased due to a shift in lipoprotein transport, helping to explain why exercise lowers risk for heart disease.

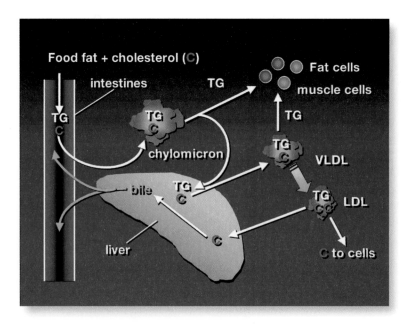

FIGURE 5.36

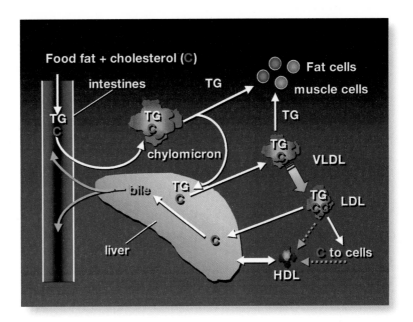

FIGURE 5.37

Also women tend to have higher levels of HDL compared to men. This is related to their greater estrogen levels. However, once a woman goes through menopause (estrogen levels fall), levels of HDL decline as this hormone plays a role in the formation of HDL, and heart disease risk subsequently goes up.

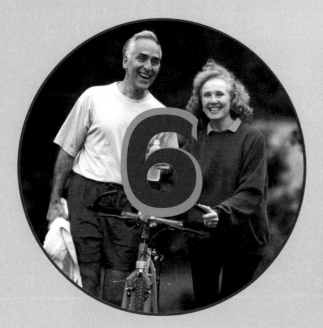

Keep Your Heart Healthy with the Right Foods

Congratulations, you just increased your knowledge about fats and cholesterol and their transport through the body as part of lipoproteins. Now we can move into unraveling heart disease, the leading cause of death in the United States for both men and women. The chance that, years from now, you may suffer from this age-related disease, or at least have a family member or close friend who suffers may not quite move you today. But perhaps knowing that the process of vascular damage—the buildup of cholesterol in your arteries—has most likely already started in your body may prompt you to sit up and take notice.

In this chapter we will cover:

▶ Lipoproteins and their implications heart disease

▶ Heart disease risk factors

▶ Diet and heart disease connection

▶ Dietary recommendations to reduce your risk for heart disease

THE LIPOPROTEIN STORY AND HEART DISEASE

Let's take a look at what vascular disease is and how it gets started.

Figure 6.1 shows a cross section of a normal artery leading to a muscle such as your heart (which pumps blood and, like other muscles in

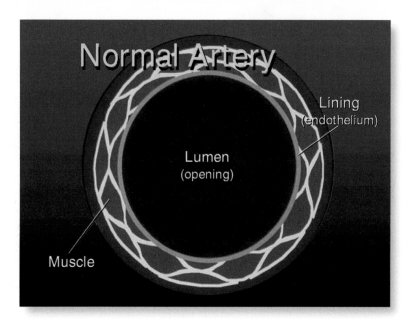

FIGURE 6.1

your body, it needs oxygen). The cross section is clear and unobstructed, meaning that there are no cholesterol deposits resulting from oxidized LDL particles infiltrating the lining of your artery wall. Your arteries looked like this when you were a newborn and perhaps the first few years of life. Probably by age 10 or even sooner, LDL particles have started "crashing" into your artery walls. White blood cells, platelets and immune cells, then attack the area to fight off what they see as invaders. Cholesterol which spills out is deposited and hardens, making "plaque" (a different plaque than on your teeth). Over time this process continues, and the plaque gets larger and harder, compromising the opening through which the blood has to travel. (See Figure 6.2.)

As the opening for blood flow narrows, danger of a heart attack or stroke lurks. When you exercise or climb a flight of stairs, your heart demands more oxygen. With limited blood flow, or even blockage when plaque breaks off and lodges in a narrowed artery, you feel chest pain and radiating discomfort down your left arm (or even flu-like symptoms). Your heart muscle is starved for oxygen, and you suffer a heart attack. If this same process happens in your brain, you suffer from a stroke when a portion of the brain is also starved for oxygen. This is usually the first sign of vascular disease. Unfortunately, the disease is quite progressed at this point because it has been developing for decades.

In Chapter 5 we referred to lipoproteins and their transport much like buses traveling through freeways and roads transporting the passengers, triglycerides and cholesterol. Using a cartoon analogy can help you understand this process of vascular disease, which in turn may assist you in making dietary and other lifestyle changes to decrease your risk for heart disease. (See Figure 6.3.)

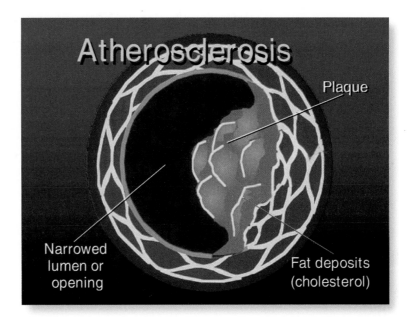

FIGURE 6.2

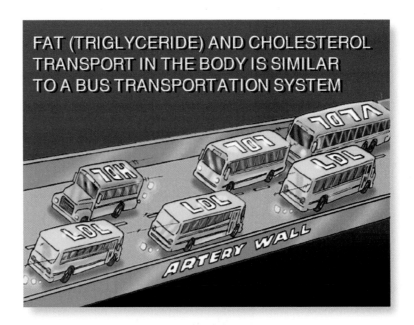

FIGURE 6.3

Remember that lipoproteins are made up of the same three components—triglyceride, cholesterol, and a protein coat—each lipoprotein with a different job to do "delivering" its passengers. (See Figure 6.4.)

Figures 6.5, 6.6, and 6.7 show Very Low Density Lipoprotein's (VLDL), Low Density Lipoprotein's (LDL) and High Density Lipoprotein's (HDL) transportation roles.

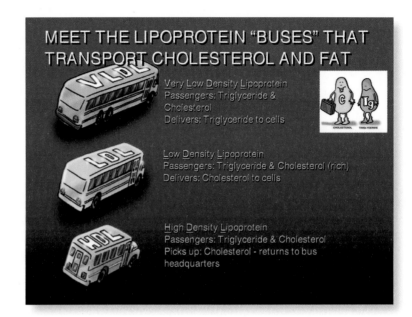

FIGURE 6.4

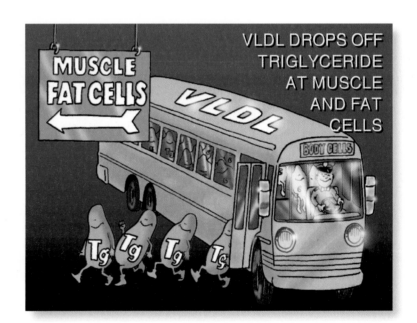

FIGURE 6.5

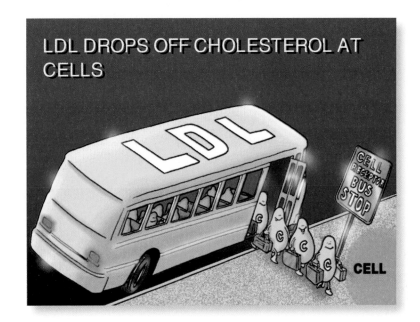

FIGURE 6.6

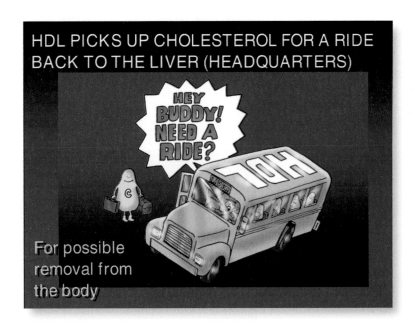

FIGURE 6.7

As the LDL travels through your roadways (arteries), transportation of cholesterol can go awry. The LDL can become damaged (referred to as oxidation) and drive out of control. (See Figure 6.8.)

Much like a real crash scene, debris litters the roadway. In your body, the cholesterol spills out, infiltrates the arteries and builds up into plaque. (See Figure 6.9.)

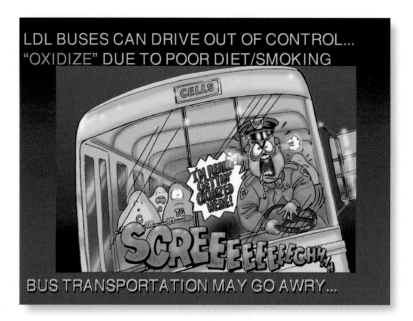

FIGURE 6.8

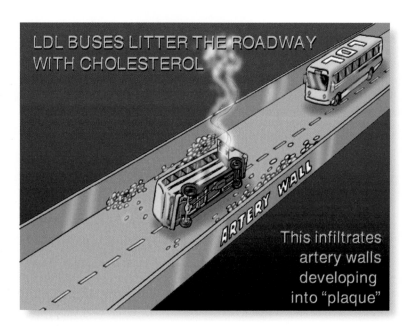

FIGURE 6.9

And like a real accident scene that draws the attention of rubber-neckers, your body sends platelets to the scene, which gather around the "injury," forming a blood clot. (See Figure 6.10.)

This process of "crashing" LDL buses continues over time and vascular disease develops, leading to a heart attack or stroke. (See Figure 6.11.)

FIGURE 6.10

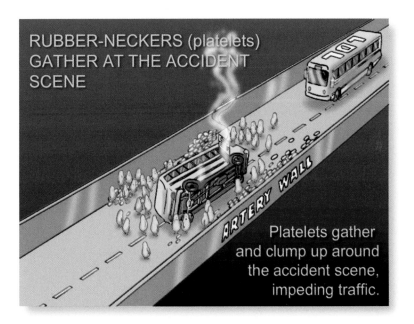

FIGURE 6.11

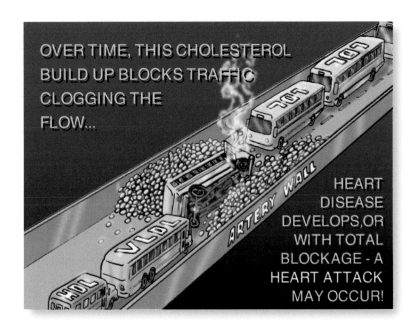

Vascular disease (heart attack or stroke) is a very frightening disease when it strikes you or someone you love. You can take charge of your health and your risk of developing vascular disease by altering your lifestyle and reducing your risk.

HEART DISEASE RISK FACTORS—ARE YOU AT RISK?

Let's take a look at the risk factors that predispose a person to increased chances of suffering a heart attack or stroke. These are characteristics—some are lifestyle related, such as smoking, and some you can't do anything about, such as genetics and gender—that influence your risk of heart disease (often referred to as coronary artery disease).

Coronary Artery Disease Risk Factors

- Cigarette smoking
- Hypertension*
- Hypercholesterolemia (low HDL, high LDL)*
- Diabetes*
- Heredity

- Increasing Age
- Obesity (abdominal body fat)*
- Male sex
- Inactivity
- Dietary factors*

*Indicates risk factors that are responsive to dietary intervention.

Nutrition Bite

Although men are generally at greater risk for developing heart disease, it is still the leading cause of death among women.

Some professional health organizations such as the National Cholesterol Education Program (NCEP) consider a cluster of certain coronary artery disease risk factors a set condition called **metabolic syndrome.** This syndrome, characterized by three or more of the following factors, is thought to pose a greater threat to heart health in combination than each factor poses individually.

- A waist circumference > 35 inches for women or > 40 inches for men (indicating abdominal obesity)
- A high fasting blood triglyceride level
- A low HDL level

- Elevated blood pressure (hypertension)
- High fasting blood glucose

Let's focus on high blood cholesterol as a risk factor as well as levels of LDL and HDL cholesterol. When scientists look at population data to determine what level of cholesterol presents a risk for heart health, the information looks like the graph in Figure 6.12.

Circulating cholesterol levels below 200 mg/dL are considered healthy and levels above this value are risky. The specific numbers and associated risks look like the following:

< 200mg/dL	desirable blood cholesterol level
200–239 mg/dL	borderline high blood cholesterol
> 240 mg/dL	high blood cholesterol

Recall that not all the lipoproteins are damaging to artery walls, so it is helpful to tease out LDL cholesterol levels (which can be measured with a lipoprotein screen). Here are LDL levels that are considered optimal to high risk:

< 100 mg/dL	optimal
100–129 mg/dL	above optimal
130–159 mg/dL	borderline high risk
160–189 mg/dL	high risk

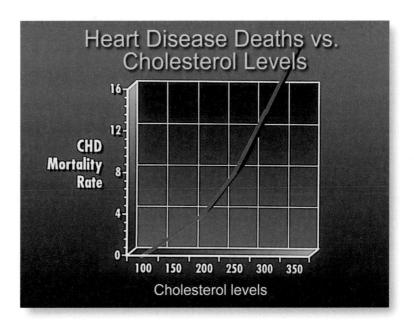

FIGURE 6.12

For HDL, the scavenger or "good" cholesterol carrier, levels that are risky are low and high levels are good:

< 35 mg/dL   low (high risk)

> 60 mg/dL   high (great!)

With all these numbers, let's not lose sight of what's important. You can look at overall blood cholesterol levels and get a good idea of a person's risk; 200 mg/dL and above is risky. Combined with other risk factors such as smoking and high blood pressure, elevated blood cholesterol levels can make matters worse, accelerating the progression of heart disease.

THE ROLE OF DIET—FAT, CHOLESTEROL, FIBER, AND MORE

The connection between diet and heart disease risk is very strong. You can modify several risk factors, such as high blood cholesterol and high blood pressure, by making changes in your diet along with exercise. Here are several of the major dietary factors, many of which we're going to discuss.

Diet and Heart Disease Connection

- Total dietary fat
- Type of dietary fat (saturated, trans, unsaturated)
- Cholesterol intake
- Protein intake
- Fiber intake
- Other dietary components
  fish oil (omega-3)
  garlic
  coffee
  wine

Total Fat Intake

Your total fat intake, typically expressed as a percentage of calories, has an impact on blood cholesterol levels and heart disease risk. Many studies that examine fat intake in different countries have shown a positive correlation between fat intake and heart disease risk. (See Figure 6.13.)

In countries such as the United States and England where fat intake is approximately one-third of the calories, risk for heart disease is high. In countries with low fat intakes such as Korea and Egypt, heart disease risk is significantly lower.

Two major exceptions to these observations are certain populations—native Eskimos and East African tribes. Native Eskimos, for example, consume nearly 60 percent of their calories in the form of fat (whale blubber and fatty fish), yet they have very low rates of heart disease. Tribes in Africa eat only animal products—meat, milk, and blood—yet their risk for heart disease is also very low. Researchers attribute this to their genetics and very active lifestyle.

FAT CONSUMPTION AND HEART DISEASE RISK

COUNTRY	% FAT CALORIE INTAKE	
USA	34%	
England	38%	high risk
Germany	38%	
Egypt	15%	
China	18%	low risk
Korea	10%	

*Exception: East African tribes, Eskimos
High fat/cholesterol diet → low risk

FIGURE 6.13

Type of Fat

Saturated Fat: (for example, butter, lard, margarine, meats, and full-fat dairy products) When saturated fats are the major source of fat in the diet, lipoprotein transport is effected, which in turn leads to elevated circulating cholesterol levels. This is NOT saying that saturated fat is cholesterol but instead that it indirectly impacts cholesterol levels (synthesis or formation).

- High saturated fat intake elevates LDL levels.
- This, in turn, increases heart disease risk.
- Trans fats also raise LDL levels and lower HDL and therefore heart disease risk.

ADVICE: Reduce intake of saturated fat and trans fats combined to less than 10 percent of total calories.

Monounsaturated Fat: (for example, olive oil, avocado, peanut oil, and canola oil) When monounsaturated fats are a major source of fat in the diet, lipoprotein transport is positively affected.

- Monounsaturated fats can lower total cholesterol levels (when substituted for saturated fats).
- Monounsaturated fats can lower LDL levels.
- Monounsaturated fats are neutral to HDL levels. (This is good news because these are the scavenger lipoproteins that help to lower heart disease risk.)

ADVICE: Consume about 10 percent or more of your calories as monounsaturated fats, but no more than 20 percent.

Polyunsaturated Fat: (for example, sunflower, soybean, safflower, and corn oils and nuts and nut oils) When polyunsaturated fats are a major source of fat in the diet, lipoprotein transport is affected both positively and negatively.

- Polyunsaturated fats can lower total cholesterol when substituted for other fats in the diet.
- Polyunsaturated fats can lower LDL levels.
- Polyunsaturated fats can also lower HDL levels.

ADVICE: Because polyunsaturated fats have a dual effect, it's best to limit intake to no more than 10 percent of total calories.

Cholesterol Intake

We learned from Chapter 5 that cholesterol has a variety of crucial roles in the body (sex hormone precursor, for example), but that cholesterol is NOT an essential nutrient because we can make it (in the liver) and make enough to meet our needs. Cholesterol is found in animal products such as eggs, cheese, meats, milk, fish, and other meats.

But does eating cholesterol mean that blood cholesterol levels are impacted? For most of the population, about 80 percent, homeostasis is in effect. That is, when we take in dietary cholesterol, our livers make less to keep things in balance. However for about 20 percent of the population, due to genetics or other lifestyle factors, the liver keeps pumping out cholesterol despite high levels in the diet. The end result is increased levels of total cholesterol and, particularly, high levels of LDL.

Thus, overall, the advice for the population is to moderate cholesterol intake because many foods rich in cholesterol may also be high in total fat and saturated fats.

ADVICE: Consume less than 300 milligrams of cholesterol per day; one egg per day is OK.

Dietary Fiber Intake

You also learned in Chapter 3 that fiber, specifically water-soluble fiber, helps to lower heart disease risk. Now it's time to take a closer look. Water-soluble fiber can lower blood cholesterol levels by binding bile (made from cholesterol and involved in fat digestion) and cholesterol (from food) in the intestinal tract, and therefore block cholesterol absorption and even effectively "drains" some of the cholesterol from the body. Here's how water-soluble fiber works. When you eat a meal with cholesterol along with a water-soluble food source (beans, fruit, and oats), the fiber attracts cholesterol, blocking its absorption (as noted by the dashed arrow from the intestines), taking the cholesterol into the stool. (See Figure 6.14.)

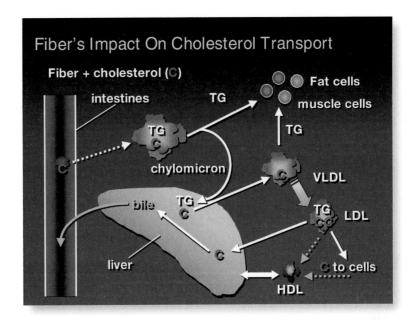

FIGURE 6.14

Nutrition Bite

Beans such as black, navy, and pinto beans are a great source of water-soluble fiber. Studies show including a daily serving of beans helps to lower blood cholesterol levels.

Water-soluble fiber also attracts bile, which ultimately comes from the liver (made from cholesterol). (See Figure 6.15.) The bile-fiber combo heads to the stool (as noted by the dashed arrow in the intestines), effectively taking away some of the body's cholesterol. The end result is lowering of blood cholesterol levels. In fact, eating more foods rich in water-soluble fiber is a very effective way to lower moderately elevated levels of blood cholesterol (200–250 mg/dL range).

ADVICE: Eat adequate fiber (both types) by meeting the Daily Value of 25 grams.

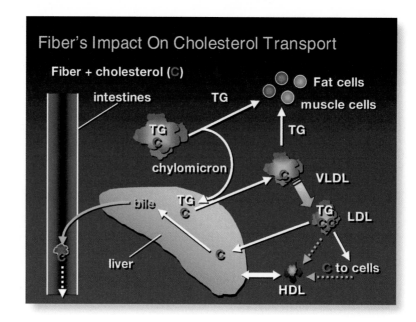

FIGURE 6.15

DIETARY RECOMMENDATIONS TO REDUCE YOUR RISK FOR HEART DISEASE

Now let's put all this advice together in the "Dietary Guidelines for Prevention and Treatment of Heart Disease" from the American Heart Association.

These guidelines are for all people over the age of 2.

- Total dietary intake fat should be less than 30 percent of total calories.

- Saturated fat intake should be less than 10 percent of total calories (trans fat included).

- Dietary cholesterol intake should be less than 300 milligrams per day.

- Meet the Daily Value for fiber of 25 grams per day.

- Salt intake should be less than 6 grams per day (2,400 milligrams of sodium—this will be discussed in Chapter 8).

- Limit alcohol intake.

- Achieve a healthy weight.

- Physical activity—30 minutes or more most days a week.

When you complete your Diet Project, you will compare your intake of calories from total fat and saturated fat and see where you stand. Also, you will make comparisons with the Daily Value for fiber and cholesterol (300 milligrams).

Computing Recommended Intake of Fat and Saturated Fat

From these guidelines, you can determine your recommended fat and saturated fat intake (or figure out anyone's) in grams per day based on your calorie intake.

Expect this type of calculation on the exam. Being knowledgeable about this may help you advise your folks or other friends about limiting their fat intake for better heart health.

> **Example:** A friend interested in reducing his risk for heart disease eats 2500 calories per day. What is his recommended fat and saturated fat intake?
>
> less than 30 percent calories as fat
> less than 10 percent calories as saturated fat

To calculate **total fat intake,** multiply the 30 percent recommendation by the total number of calories in your friend's diet:

$$2500 \text{ calories} \times 0.3 = 750 \text{ calories}$$

Convert this number to grams of fat by dividing this number by the physiological fuel value for fat:

$$750 \text{ calories divided by } 9 \text{ calories/gram} = 83 \text{ grams}$$

**Your friend should eat less than 83 grams of fat per day
for better heart health.**

To calculate **saturated fat intake,** multiply the 10 percent recommendation by the total number of calories in your friend's diet:

$$2500 \text{ calories} \times 0.1 = 250 \text{ calories}$$

Convert this number to grams of saturated fat by dividing this number by the physiological fuel value for fat:

$$250 \text{ calories divided by } 9 \text{ calories/gram} = 28 \text{ grams}$$

**Your friend should eat less than 28 grams of saturated fat per day
for better heart health.**

DAILY VALUE FOR FAT AND SATURATED FAT AND USING FOOD LABELS

The Daily Value for fat and saturated fat used on the Nutrition Facts food label are based on the dietary recommendations to reduce heart disease risk. Since the Daily Values are based on a 2,000-calorie diet, the same calculations from above can be applied. This is just what the Food and Drug Administration did in establishing the Daily Value for fat and saturated fat. (See Figure 6.16.)

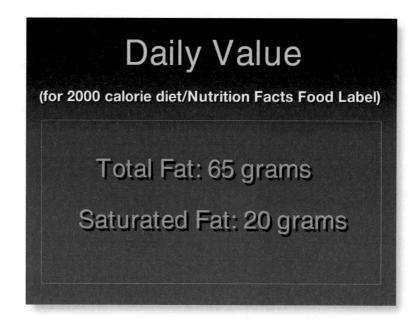

FIGURE 6.16

You should commit these numbers to memory for the exam but also for future reference so that you can quickly compute what percent of the Daily Value a food provides for fat or saturated fat. This way you can decide whether that food makes good sense in relation to the rest of your daily intake.

Let's put these Daily Values to work and interpret a food label.

Compute the percent Daily Value for fat and saturated fat using information from a food label (grams of total fat and saturated fat per serving). (See Figures 6.17 and 6.18.)

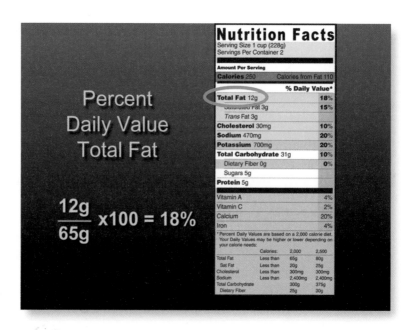

FIGURE 6.17

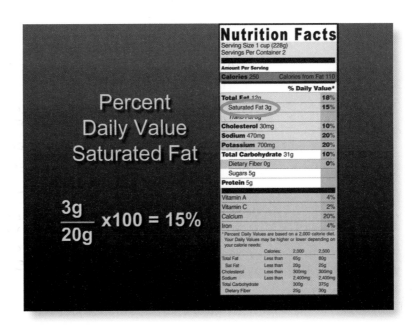

FIGURE 6.18

With knowledge about heart disease under your belt, you should feel confident about the dietary recommendations to reduce risk and why. Additionally, recognizing a person's risk factors should also become second nature: for example, high blood cholesterol level, inactive, smoker, and so on. Finally, make sure you feel comfortable about computing recommended fat and saturated fat intake (or budget) for a person given their calorie intake.

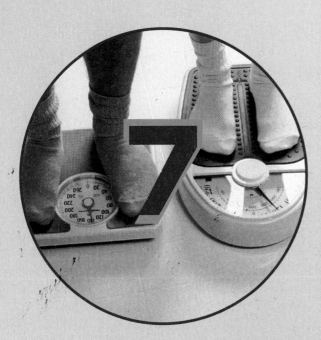

Obesity, Weight Control, and Eating Disorders— The Facts

Although heart disease is referred to as the single leading cause of death in the United States, another ailment is plaguing our nation—obesity. In this chapter we discuss the issue of energy imbalance, along with another related issue—eating disorders. At the onset, many of you may already have some views on obesity—its causes and the best ways to lose weight. We also have prejudices regarding obesity such as beliefs that obese people are "lazy" and that excess weight is an issue of overeating. I urge you to read this chapter and engage in the course material with an open mind. Obesity is a complex condition, with no simple solutions. Additionally, obesity prevention is paramount because much of our nation is either obese or overweight and this negatively impacts our nation with rising health-care costs due to obesity-related health problems.

In this chapter we will cover the following:

▶ A healthy weight for you

▶ Body fat distribution and fat cell development

▶ Control of food intake—the body's defense against weight loss

▶ Obesity causes—why energy balance becomes skewed

▶ Weight loss—the options: what works and what to avoid

▶ Eating disorders—prevalence and health risks

Obesity Statistics

Before we can discuss what is a healthy weight, let's take a look at the current numbers for obesity.

- Approximately 65 percent of the adult population is obese or overweight. (These terms will be defined in the next section.)
- About 20 percent of teenage boys and girls are obese.
- About 15 percent of children are obese.

These numbers represent a dramatic increase over the past few decades. According to the U.S. Surgeon General's office rising obesity rates have profound implications on health-care costs and about $120 billion a year is spent on obesity-related health problems, and an estimated 300,000 people die each year due to obesity-related health issues such as heart disease and diabetes.

HEALTHY BODY WEIGHT—IS YOURS?

Your body fat stores reflect your energy balance, that is, your calorie intake balanced with your energy output (BMR, TEF, activity), as shown in Figure 7.1.

Over time, if calorie intake equals output, then fat stores (just like your savings account in the bank) remains constant.

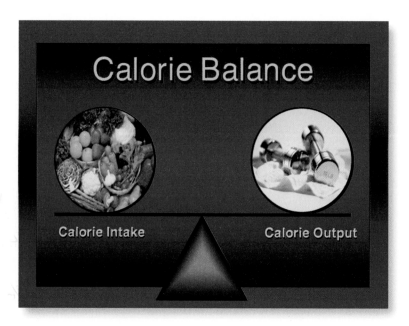

FIGURE 7.1

An increase in energy or fat stores occurs over time when energy balance is skewed: intake exceeds output. (See Figure 7.2.) This occurs several ways:

- when calorie intake increases and exceeds current caloric expenditure;
- when caloric intake is constant but caloric output decreases; or
- when both occur—caloric intake increases and caloric output decreases.

The end result is that these excess calories are stored as fat.

Our task now is to define how much fat, or using another measure such as body weight, is too much and presents health problems.

Defining Obesity

Obesity is defined as excess body fat that contributes to adverse health effects. There are several methods used for obesity classification.

Body Weight

Obesity is a body weight more than 20 percent above "desirable" body weight.

Desirable body weight is based upon a height-weight table that gives ranges for a healthy body weight for a given height. These values are derived from data that relate body weight to the risk of death. Both excess body weight and low body weight are associated with an increase risk for

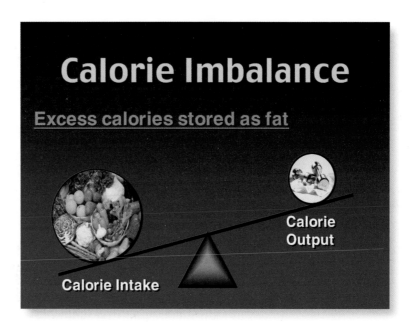

FIGURE 7.2

health problems. Desirable body weight is the weight at which there is the lowest risk of health problems.

- This method is great for assessing a large group of people because only two simple measurements are needed—weight and height.

- This method, however, can be inaccurate for people who have a large muscle mass but low body fat (i.e., weigh more than expected but are not obese, as seen in body builders).

Body Fat

> *Obese:* more than 20–25 percent body fat for men
> more than 30 percent body fat for women

Using these criteria, about 70 to 80 percent of the adult population would be defined as obese. The percent of body weight that is fat can be determined by several ways:

- Skin-fold thickness uses calipers to measure body fat through measurement of subcutaneous (underneath the skin) fat. This technique requires the individual to be skilled in using the calipers. Repeat measurements should be taken by the same technician to avoid error.

- Underwater-weighing or the hydrostatic technique measures body weight based upon the principle that fat floats (weighs less than water). The greater the difference between what you weigh in water compared to what you weigh out of water, the greater the body fat content.

- Bioelectrical impedance technique involves passing a very small electrical current through the body, with body fat determined based on transmission of the electrical current. Fat conducts electricity poorly due to its low water content while muscle transmits the current well.

All of these, as well as other techniques, involve measurement error so that the value determined is an approximation.

Body Mass Index (BMI)

> Obesity is a BMI equal to or more than 30. *Note:* BMI is not a percent but a ratio defined on the next page.

This technique involves computing a ratio of body weight to height, as shown in Figure 7.3. Note that height is measured in meters and is then squared.

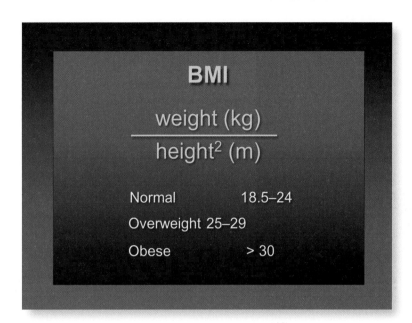

FIGURE 7.3

According to multiple research studies, this ratio is a good predictor that increasing BMI is associated with health problems and from this, cutoffs for overweight and obesity have been determined. A person who is overweight experiences a much greater risk for becoming obese than a healthy weight individual. Normal, overweight, and obese BMIs are given above.

What Is Your BMI?

Use the chart in Figure 7.4 to determine where your current body weight falls.

OVERWEIGHT AND OBESE CUT OFF POINTS

HEIGHT	BMI OF 25 OVERWEIGHT	BMI OF 30 OBESE
Inches	Pounds	Pounds
58	119	147
60	128	153
62	136	164
64	145	174
66	155	186
68	164	197
70	174	207
72	184	221
74	194	233
76	205	246

FIGURE 7.4

You can also use the graph in Figure 7.5 and plot what weight range is healthy for your height. Note there is no gender differentiation. Women, though, should be at the lower range of the healthy weight range for height and men toward the upper healthy weight range for height. (See Figure 7.5.)

While the BMI is fairly consistent in predicting obesity, the BMI may erroneously determine obesity for individuals who have large amounts of muscle mass as shown in the chart in Figure 7.6 that depicts BMI for several athletes and celebrities.

As you can see from our discussion, defining obesity is not quite black and white. There is "gray" around the definition and all individuals should be assessed separately.

BODY FAT DISTRIBUTION AND FAT CELL DEVELOPMENT

Determining if a person is overweight or obese represents part of the story. It is also important to determine where excess fat is located because certain profiles of body fat distribution present greater health risks than others. Additionally, understanding the nature of a fat cell is also important in deciphering obesity issues.

Both men and women have gender specific sites for fat storage, as shown in Figure 7.7.

These fat depot sites most likely have their origins from early humans when women stored body fat in thighs, hips, and buttocks to ensure reproduction and men stored fat in locations such as the trunk region, which allowed for greater mobility.

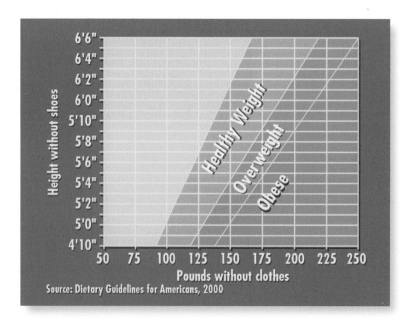

FIGURE 7.5

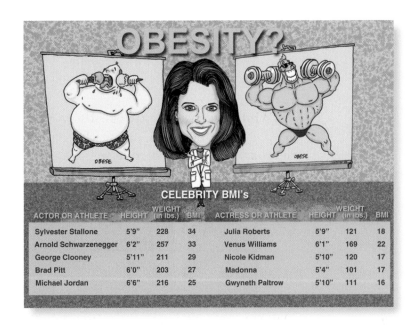

FIGURE 7.6

ACTOR OR ATHLETE	HEIGHT	WEIGHT (in lbs.)	BMI	ACTRESS OR ATHLETE	HEIGHT	WEIGHT (in lbs.)	BMI
Sylvester Stallone	5'9"	228	34	Julia Roberts	5'9"	121	18
Arnold Schwarzenegger	6'2"	257	33	Venus Williams	6'1"	169	22
George Clooney	5'11"	211	29	Nicole Kidman	5'10"	120	17
Brad Pitt	6'0"	203	27	Madonna	5'4"	101	17
Michael Jordan	6'6"	216	25	Gwyneth Paltrow	5'10"	111	16

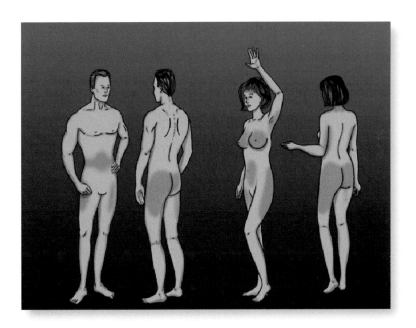

FIGURE 7.7

Lower- and Upper-Body Obesity

With these gender-specific fat depot sites in mind, now let's look at excess fat in these regions and their subsequent health risks. There are two general types of body fat distribution seen in people, and more dramatically in obese people: lower- and upper-body obesity. (See Figure 7.8.)

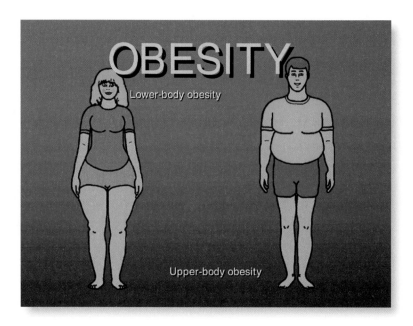

FIGURE 7.8

Lower-Body Obesity

- This type is sometimes called "pear-shaped" or "gynoid" obesity.

- Excess fat is stored in the hip and thigh region.

- This fat distribution is more common in women (based on gender-specific fat depot sites).

- Research suggests that fat in this region is more resistant to weight loss, perhaps a throwback to early human times when women needed to maintain fat stores for pregnancy and breast-feeding.

- This type of fat distribution, by itself and in the absence of other health factors such as high blood pressure, blood cholesterol, or waist measurement, does not pose a significant health risk.

Upper-Body Obesity

- This type is sometimes called "apple-shaped" or "android" obesity.

- Excess fat is stored in the abdominal/trunk area sometimes referred to as a "beer belly".

- This fat distribution is more common in men (based on gender-specific fat depot sites).

- This type of fat distribution is associated with a greater risk of health problems such as cardiovascular disease, diabetes, high blood pressure, and certain types of cancer. As shown in Figure 7.9, the location of this body fat—**visceral** fat—that is underneath the abdominal muscle wall, is near organs such as the liver and heart.

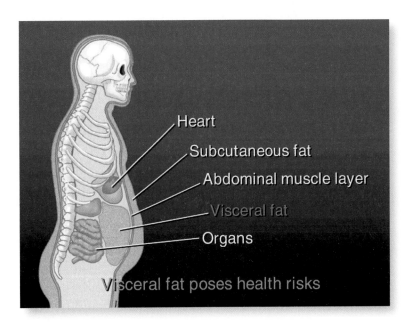

FIGURE 7.9

Heart
Subcutaneous fat
Abdominal muscle layer
Visceral fat
Organs

Visceral fat poses health risks

Determining Upper-Body Obesity

A simple measurement of the waist and hip is taken to compute a ratio, which determines upper-body obesity.

- Using a tape measure that is flexible, measure your waist at the belly button and at your hips at their widest point.

- Compute a waist-to-hip ratio:

   Upper body obesity is defined with a ratio more than 0.95 in men and more than 0.8 in women. For example, a man with a waist of 39 and hips of 38 equates to:

$$\text{Waist/hip} = 1.05 = >0.95 = \text{upper-body obesity}$$

Another way to assess upper-body obesity is simply use the waist measurement. If the waist exceeds 40 inches for men and 35 inches for women, this is defined as upper-body obesity.

Health Risks Associated with Obesity

Our discussion of body fat distribution brings us to summarize health problems associated with obesity in general. Obese individuals tend to be at greater risk for a variety of health problems including:

- Cardiovascular disease (heart disease)

- High blood cholesterol (this is particularly the case for younger obese men)

- Hypertension (high blood pressure)

- Diabetes (specifically type 2, which does not require insulin therapy)

- Certain types of cancer (uterine, breast, colon, and prostate)

- Osteoarthritis (joint trouble due to the excess body weight)

- Emotional disturbances (many obese individuals experience discrimination, issues of low self-esteem, and subsequent feelings of depression)

Fat Cells and Their Development

Fat is stored as triglyceride in cells called **adipose cells.** As shown in Figure 7.10, an adipose cell has a fat storage compartment, which can expand to hold more triglyceride or contract as triglyceride comes out of storage for energy use. Thus, when energy intake exceeds expenditure, triglyceride storage increases and fat cells expand. As you'll learn in the next section, the number of adipose cells may increase if more storage sites are needed.

Enzymes that sit at the surface of the adipose cell are involved in the storage and release of triglyceride inside fat cells. An enzyme vital to the storage of triglyceride is called **lipoprotein lipase** or **LPL** for short. This enzyme's activity is influenced by several factors, which in turn means that adipose cells have varying capacity to store fat (an important issue when understanding obesity).

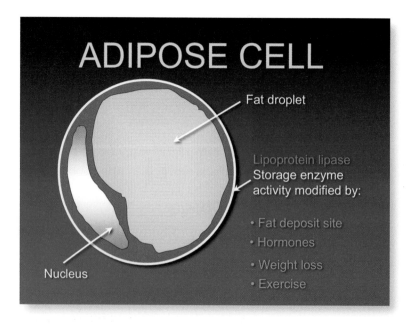

ADIPOSE CELL

Fat droplet

Lipoprotein lipase
Storage enzyme
activity modified by:

- Fat deposit site
- Hormones
- Weight loss
- Exercise

Nucleus

FIGURE 7.10

- Research studies show that LPL is more active at certain **fat depot sites** than others. Adipose cells in the hip and thigh region appear to have more active LPL than elsewhere in the body for women, but LPL activity is greater in the abdomen region for men. This is in keeping with how women and men differ in fat storage sites.

- **Hormone** changes, such as during pregnancy, also influence the activity of LPL. When a woman becomes pregnant, LPL activity goes up in the breasts and other sites in order to store more fat, which ensures energy stores for the developing baby and breast-feeding. This response makes sense, especially thinking back to our early ancestors who often went without food during scarce times.

- Following **weight loss,** LPL activity goes up, which means the adipose cell WANTS to store fat, filling the fat cell back up despite your efforts and desires for lasting weight loss. This may seem contrary to what you want, but again think back to what makes sense in terms of our early ancestors. Someone who lost weight would need to restock energy stores so that they could survive another situation of low energy intake such as a famine. So upping LPL activity with weight loss ensures a return of adequate fat reserves.

- **Exercise** also impacts LPL levels. When a person is physically active, their muscles need the triglycerides for fuel and their fat cells can do without. Thus, LPL activity at fat cells decline while this same enzyme that exists at muscle cells increases to meet energy demands at the muscle. This helps to explain why people who exercise routinely have less body fat (smaller fat cells) than folks who don't exercise.

Fat Cell Development

Understanding when and under what circumstances fat cells are made and altered helps us to understand the development of obesity. The number of adipose cells *normally* increases during periods of growth. There are believed to be two periods of cell number increase, which are sometimes termed "critical periods."

1. **The third trimester of pregnancy (the last three months of fetal development) is when energy stores in the fetus are increased.** Research studies in laboratory animals show that overfeeding during this time causes excess fat cell numbers and obesity develops. In humans, however, it is not clear whether a "big" baby necessarily means an obese teenager or adult.

2. **During the adolescent growth spurt, approximately ages 12 to 14.** At this point, adipose cell number increases and is believed to reach the adult fat cell number of approximately 25 billion in a

healthy weight individual. Excess weight gain during these ages DOES correlate to obesity later in life. Considering that these fat cells "want" to be filled with triglyceride for energy reserves, more fat cells translate to greater body fat levels. Excess body fat, defined as obesity during teen years, runs the risk of about 70 to 80 percent chance of being obese as an adult. Thus, prevention of excessive weight gain during teen years is encouraged considering the current trend in obesity rates among youth.

Although the fat cell number is considered to be stable during adulthood, evidence from research shows that the adipose number may increase when weight gain stimulus is sufficient, such as during pregnancy when desirable weight gain of 22 to 27 pounds is exceeded, such as 50 pounds, the fat cell number may increase. Also, during a period of extreme inactivity such as an injury, when a large amount of weight gain can occur, the fat cell number may increase. The significance of this is that **once a fat cell is made, it does not go away.** Considering that fat cells "want" to be filled with triglyceride for energy reserves, the more adipose cells a person has, most likely the more body fat they have. **With weight loss, fat cells shrink but they do not go away.**

Adipose development is summarized in Figure 7.11.

It is important to emphasize that, with weight loss, fat cell number does not change, and with excess weight gain earlier in life, adipose cell number is most likely increased and these cells are there to stay. (See Figure 7.12.)

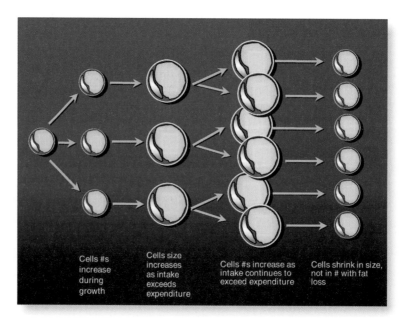

Cells #s increase during growth

Cells size increases as intake exceeds expenditure

Cells #s increase as intake continues to exceed expenditure

Cells shrink in size, not in # with fat loss

FIGURE 7.11

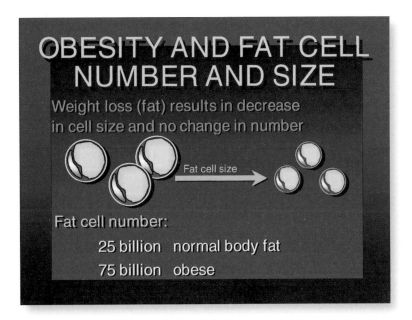

FIGURE 7.12

Nutrition Bite

Is there a way to get "rid" of adipose cells? A surgical procedure called liposuction removes fat (adipose cells) from specific areas. While this is not specifically a treatment for obesity, it has become a popular way to "sculpt" the body and lessen fat in certain areas such as the thighs (bulges around the hips) or the tummy. This procedure is costly and is wrought with side effects such as scaring and risks of blood clot.

FOOD INTAKE CONTROL

Before we can better understand the complexities of obesity, we need to discuss the basics about why we eat—termed **food intake control.** We initiate the action of eating and cessation of eating for a variety of internal and external reasons or factors. Consider that each of us on average eats about 900,000 to over 1 million calories per year. This intake of calories, if you recall, is balanced with calorie output, as shown in Figure 7.13.

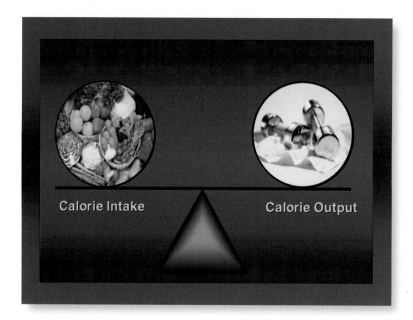

FIGURE 7.13

In energy balance, or weight maintenance, intake is balanced with output. This is actually quite an accomplishment considering being off by 50 or so calories per day (that is, intake greater than output of about half a small cookie each day) translates to about a one or two pound weight gain per year. Thus, small errors in energy balance can spell weight gain over time and the development of obesity.

People who keep their weight steady are in energy homeostasis. However, most Americans, according to statistics, are gaining weight and not balancing energy intake with output. So let's take a look at why some people balance energy intake with energy output, while others do not. What follows are the many factors—both internal and external—that influence our food intake control.

Internal Factors

Many factors that are internal, that is, within the body, impact food intake control. Internal factors include brain centers, blood metabolites, and other signals that stimulate the body to eat, feelings of **hunger,** or that signal the body to not eat, feelings of **satiety.** These signals may stimulate food intake or satiety over the short term—within hours or minutes— or may signal eating or not eating over the long term—days or weeks.

There is a general theme around the control of food intake that has profound implications in relation to obesity. **The body is designed to defend against weight loss.** That is, rather than "being satisfied" at a lower weight or body fat level, signals designed for survival kick in and prompt eating over the short and long term to ensure adequate energy stores. Here are several internal factors that influence food intake control.

Central Nervous System

Brain centers—There are several regions in the brain that respond to signals such as small proteins or hormones. One brain center called the **hypothalamus** responds to signals such as blood metabolites and hormones that stimulate or suppress eating.

Brain chemicals—Serotonin, a chemical produced in the brain that exerts feeling of calmness, has been shown to influence eating.

Peripheral Factors

Hormones—Insulin, sex hormones, and others impact food intake control. For example, in the brain, insulin signals the brain and food intake is increased.

Fat mass and fat cell size—A hormone released by fat cells called **leptin** signals the brain (as shown in Figure 7.14) that fat stores are adequate and this modulates (lessens) eating and stimulates metabolism. If fat cells have shrunk due to weight loss, leptin levels decrease and food intake increases so as to fill fat stores back up.

Stomach signals—The stomach sends out its own signals such as the small protein hormone called ghrelin. This hormone is thought to stimulate eating since levels of ghrelin rise immediately prior to eating. Also, the intestinal tract releases its own signals, one called CCK, and tells the brain in response to eating that you're full or satiated (satisfied).

Exercise—While this may at first appear as an external factor, exercise initiates a series of internal changes that impact food intake. On a short-term basis, an exercise session (particularly an intense one) inhibits food intake most likely because of a brief rise in body temperature. Over

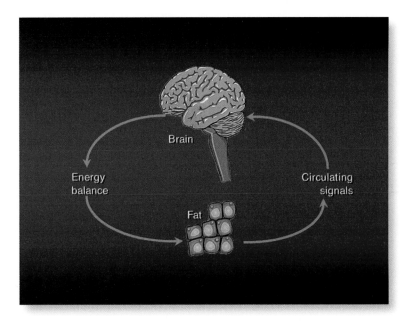

FIGURE 7.14

the long term, food intake increases with regular exercise but a person typically has less body fat, smaller fat cells, and the body has the ability to burn fat at muscle cells more effectively compared to a sedentary state.

Conditions or Diseases That May Alter Food Intake

Pregnancy and breast-feeding—Eating changes with pregnancy; hunger levels may fluctuate due to hormones and generally fat gain occurs to serve as reserves for pregnancy and breast-feeding. The hormones produced to maintain lactation (breast-feeding) stimulate food intake so that a woman has significant energy intake to contribute to breast milk production.

Obesity—The condition of obesity itself is known to impact food intake regulation, perhaps because of altered leptin levels, other blood signals to the brain, and the brains' ability to respond to these signals. This altered response may be a consequence of obesity or a genetic predisposition.

Eating disorders—Discussed in a later section of this chapter, eating disorders anorexia and bulimia are characterized by abnormal eating patterns and behaviors. This is believed to be both behaviorally and genetically rooted.

Cancer—With certain types of cancer, such as stomach or intestinal cancers, eating declines as the disease spreads. Additionally, cancer treatments are notorious for suppressing the appetite.

Psychological disturbances—Clinical depression and other psychological disturbances are often accompanied by changes in food intake. These are believed to have biological origins such as alterations in brain chemical levels.

External Factors

Various factors in our environment also impact our feelings of hunger and satiety. With external factors, our own personal experiences come into play as we respond based on childhood experiences, for example, in making decisions to eat certain foods. Here are a few external factors.

Time of day—Often we eat based on the "clock"—that is, when it is noon, we often decide it is time for lunch rather than basing the decision to eat on true feelings of hunger.

Temperature—the external temperature may stimulate hunger as with cold temperatures. This is believed to help build fat reserves in preparation for winter when food was scarce in early human evolution. Warmer temperatures suppress feelings of hunger (think of a very hot day and how you don't really feel like eating, especially a large meal).

Eating cues—We each respond to eating cues or visual signs of food such as all-you-can-eat buffets, food courts, and other eateries. Studies show that when people are given a variety of foods to choose from, such as with a buffet, that they eat more compared to offerings of a few foods. Also, the larger the portion size we are served, generally the more we eat.

Both of these have throwbacks to early human times when variety was important to ensure a good nutrient intake and that eating more when more food was available helped boost fat reserves for leaner times.

Food intake control is summarized in Figure 7.15.

OBESITY CAUSES—WHY ENERGY BALANCE BECOMES SKEWED

With your understanding of food intake control and the basic premise that the body is designed to defend against weight loss, let's now take a look into the many causes of obesity. Perhaps at the start of this chapter you had in mind a single "reason" for obesity—eating too much? Being lazy? By now though, you understand the complexities of how the body is designed to preserve fat stores, build up energy reserves to survive periods of famine or low energy intake, and ultimately, put fat "away for a rainy day."

When energy balance is skewed and the body puts excessive fat away (although contrary for optimal health), obesity develops. There are many reasons or causes behind why obesity develops in a given individual. Here are several proposed causes or theories behind obesity development.

Calorie imbalance: This may sound simple, but eating excess calories when calorie output is constant, means excess is converted to and stored as fat. An energy gap of approximately 50 to 100 calories daily can lead to a one to two pounds of weight gain per year and over 20 years, 10 to 20 pounds, and ultimately obesity develops. This increase in calorie intake may be very subtle, such as a change in jobs where food is available at break time, or a change in work or sleeping habits that means more time exposed to your kitchen or another eating environment.

FIGURE 7.15

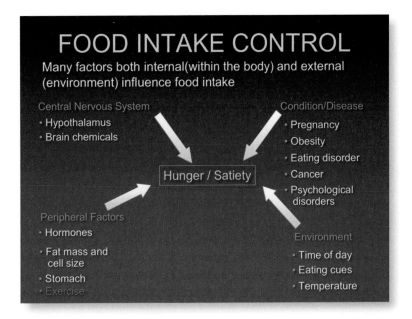

Inactivity: Expending fewer calories due to a decline of physical activity while caloric intake stays constant results in excess calories converted to and stored as fat. As with calorie imbalance above, an energy gap of about 100 calories daily results in a few pound weight gain per year, and over time obesity develops. This decline in physical activity and subsequent reduction in calories burned may be very subtle, such as in the greater use of labor-saving devices—washing machine, power lawn mower, and the like. A falloff in physical activity may also occur with a change in lifestyle—new job, starting a family, or even forced inactivity due to an injury. Inactivity can explain much of the rise in obesity in children, teens, and adults over the past few decades.

Genetic influence: A genetic predisposition to put away fat more efficiently or to burn fewer calories (BMR or TEF) while not adjusting caloric intake results in excess calories that are converted to fat and stored. Obesity develops over time, and perhaps may be more likely to occur during childhood and teen years. Some examples of genetic influence include a form of leptin that does not "connect" well with the brain, thus eating behavior is not well regulated in relation to fat stores, as shown in Figures 7.16 and 7.17. Another example may be that a person has a lower than expected TEF (energy needed to digest and assimilate food) thus fewer calories are burned and without caloric intake compensation, excess fat storage occurs and obesity develops over time.

Set point: This theory of obesity centers on the number of adipose cells a particular individual possesses and the average size of these cells. Consider a person who has 40 billion adipose cells, perhaps due to weight gain during teen years. Since fat cells prefer to be filled to a certain size (recall that fat cells are designed to serve as energy reserves and not

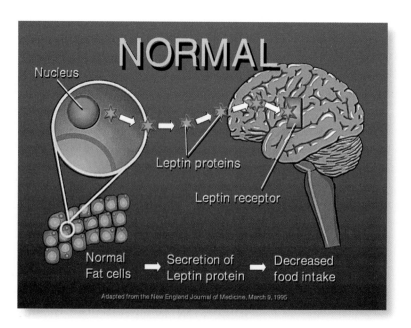

FIGURE 7.16

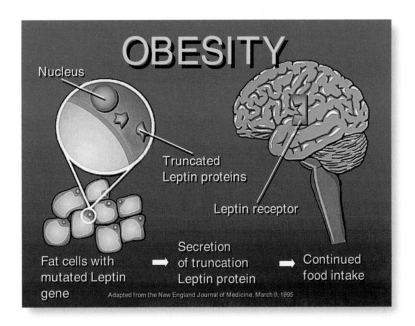

FIGURE 7.17

shrink away to nothing), this person would have more body fat (obesity) compared to a person with 25 billion adipose cells. This suggests that a person with a high adipose cell number is "doomed" to be obese. As will be discussed in the next section, exercise can overcome this by encouraging fat cells to "accept" being smaller.

"Thrifty" metabolism: Along the lines of genetic influence, a "thrifty" metabolism or a lower than expected BMR would mean that person conserves or uses less energy than another person of equal body size. Thus, without reducing caloric intake, excess calories would accumulate (converted to fat) fat stores would increase and obesity would develop over time.

Diet composition: The composition of a person's diet over the long run may have an impact on obesity development. Studies show that eating a high-fat diet, compared to an equal calorie diet with a greater carbohydrate content, can lead to excess weight gain. How can this be if calorie intake is the same? When excess calories are consumed as fat, this is efficiently stored as body fat (not much to do in taking food fat and storing it in fat cells). But for excess calories eaten as protein or carbohydrate, there must first be a conversion to triglyceride in the liver and this must then be shipped to fat cells via lipoproteins. This metabolic work costs some calories so carbohydrate and protein are stored less efficiently as body fat compared to dietary fat's conversion.

Meal patterns: Some research suggests that the pattern of eating, specifically skipping meals, may have an influence in the development of obesity. Skipping meals, such as breakfast and lunch, may lead to overeating at the next meal. This, of course, would then lead to excess calories stored as fat. In an effort to lose weight, some people skip meals, inadvertently ending up eating more because they become ravenous. It's important to point out that eating in the evening does not necessarily lead to weight gain and obesity. If you balance calories in against calories out, then your weight stays steady even if you eat late into the evening. If you overeat, more calories in than calories out, then weight gain occurs, regardless of when you take in the excess calories.

Nutrition Bite

Sumo wrestlers of Japan practice a specific eating pattern of large meals a few times a day to induce weight gain. Many sumo wrestlers are very obese with BMIs over 35.

WEIGHT LOSS OPTIONS—WHAT WORKS, WHAT TO AVOID

At this point in our obesity discussion, you undoubtedly see the complexities to this condition. This carries over to the treatment of obesity. Perhaps through your own personal experience, you recognize the difficulty in losing weight and then maintaining it. We are a nation obsessed with weight loss, despite the fact that over 60 percent of the population is obese or overweight, suggesting we are not successful with our efforts. According to statistics, about 44 percent of women and 29 percent of men are actively trying to lose weight on any given day and another 35 percent of both women and men are trying to maintain their weight.

Why is it that weight loss efforts by most people using diet plans, such as the low-carb/high-protein diets, weight loss supplements such as appetite suppressants, and other gimmicks such as skin patches that claim to help boost calorie burning, don't work? An estimated 85 percent of those who try these types of obesity treatment regain their lost weight and often then some. In this section we take a look at obesity treatment—what works and what to avoid. Much can be learned from individuals who have lost weight *and* kept this weight off for extended periods of time—several years or more. Bluntly put, it's relatively easy to lose weight; the trick is keeping it off and this requires lifestyle changes. So let's take a look at what works—a successful obesity treatment program.

The three key components to a successful program:

1. **Reduced energy diet**

2. **Behavior modification**

3. **Physical activity or exercise**

Research studies with people who have kept lost weight off reveal that they exercise on a regular basis, practice behavior modification strategies, and make efforts to control calorie intake to maintain weight loss. Let's take a look at each of these components in more detail.

1. Reduced Energy Diet

Calorie intake must be less than calorie output for weight loss to occur. An energy deficit forces fat out of storage for fuel use, and in turn, body fat decreases. Creating this calorie deficit involves:

- **Consuming a diet that meets nutrient needs (protein, fiber, vitamins, and minerals) except for energy.** Excluding food groups such as fruits, and grains to avoid carbs (high-protein diets) means missing out on fiber and other essential nutrients (such as vitamins).

- **Meeting individual tastes and habits.** Setting up a diet plan that meets the person's individual food preferences is important for compliance during the weight loss phase and important in the long term for weight maintenance. Forbidding certain foods such as sweets or making a person eat foods that they don't care for often results in failure when the individual reverts to overeating their favorite foods and excluding "good-for-you" foods that they didn't care for.

- **Designing a plan that minimizes fatigue and hunger.** Creating a large energy deficit can leave a person feeling weak and very hungry. Not only does this hamper a person's ability to function, but can easily lead to diet failure when they find it difficult to fight ravenous hunger pangs. Additionally, severe calorie restriction leads to a loss of muscle mass as well as body fat since the body is forced to make carbohydrate out of protein tissue to fuel the brain. Instead of rapid weight loss, losing about a half pound to no more than two pounds per week can avoid this problem. This translates to a calorie gap of about 250 to 1000 calories per day. (This energy gap can also be created by exercise as well as cutting back on calorie intake, or a combination of the two.)

2. Behavior Modification

Changing current eating behavior leads to decreased calorie intake and the establishment of new eating behavior conducive to weight loss and maintenance.

- **Changing eating behavior.** This involves tracking current eating habits through the use of a detailed food diary. In this log a person writes down not only what they eat and the amount, but also the time it took to eat the meal or snack, associated activities such as watching TV, mood, and hunger level. Through the assistance of a professional skilled in behavior modification, the diary is then evaluated for patterns such as rapid eating pace or munching mindlessly on snacks while watching TV.

- **Understanding response to environmental cues.** Also through the diary, a person can track which environmental cues trigger eating, such as being alone or TV viewing. Understanding response to these environmental triggers helps a person see what aspects of their environment should be changed to assist in weight loss and maintenance.

- **Cognitive restructuring.** Step-by-step behavior is modified such as techniques to slow eating pace, finding alternative activities to TV viewing, or moving the TV from the eating area. Each of these steps is unique for each individual based on their own eating behaviors.

  Behavior modification works well for mildly overweight individuals. Once weight is lost, returning to the food diary every so often helps keep a person on track with their new habits.

3. Physical Activity

Increasing caloric expenditure through purposeful physical activity while keeping caloric intake the same (or decreasing it) creates an energy deficit that leads to fat loss. Beyond this benefit, there are many other health benefits attributable to increasing physical exercise.

- **Food intake control.** Perhaps the most important outcome of regular physical activity is better food intake control. This means that the body is better able to balance intake with output. Studies show that people who exercise regularly eat more than people who don't but that exercisers have less body fat. Thus, exercise must allow the body to better balance in and out. On a short-term basis, exercise (especially intense forms such as an interval running workout) blunts appetite, thus decreasing calorie intake soon after exercise.

- **Body weight, fat loss, and lean tissue preservation.** Exercise specifically helps with fat loss. Triglycerides are pulled out of fat cells for use as fuel by the muscles. Also, exercise stimulates lean tissue or muscle to develop—tone and increase in size. This means a person can lose fat but preserve lean mass and get a sleeker look which cutting calories alone won't do. Also, an increase in muscle or lean tissue increases the number of calories burned at rest since this tissue costs more for the body to maintain than fat tissue.

- **Increased metabolism.** Exercise boosts the BMR so that a person is burning more calories at rest (see Chapter 3). This may be an extra 50 calories per day or perhaps more. In the long run, this means burning more calories compared to when your "body" was sedentary.

- **Weight maintenance.** Studies show that people who exercise keep lost weight off better than people who just diet or restrict calories. Much of what we have discussed thus far suggests that our bodies were designed to be physically active.

- **Improved sense of well-being.** Exercise has been shown to improve mood and sense of self. Often people who are overweight or obese have low self-esteem. With the addition of physical activity, self-esteem improves. Dieting alone as a way to lose weight does not have this benefit.

- **Chronic disease prevention.** Regular exercise has a variety of health benefits including lowering risk for heart disease, certain forms of cancer, improving blood sugar control and symptoms of diabetes, lowering high blood pressure, and boosting bone mineral density, which protects against osteoporosis. All these benefits are something that dieting alone can't do!

Combined, these three key components—reduced energy diet, behavior modification, and exercise—are essential in successful weight loss and maintenance. (See Figure 7.18.)

Obesity Treatments with Poor Outcomes

Many different weight loss options are available—diet books, supplements, even surgery. While some people find success with a particular program, most attempt and fail. Here's a rundown on a few options with words of caution.

Very low-calorie diets. Often administered through a physician or another type of medically supervised facility, very low-calorie diets

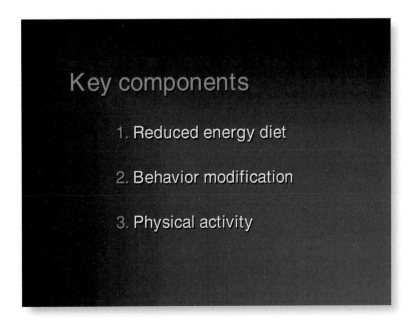

FIGURE 7.18

Key components

1. Reduced energy diet

2. Behavior modification

3. Physical activity

restrict energy intake to about 300 to 800 calories daily. Obese individuals with health problems should be medically supervised and monitored to prevent heart or kidney trouble. Also, participants should be counseled to make lifestyle changes in activity and eating habits to avoid regaining lost weight. These programs may be successful if well supervised, but often people don't stick with the program because these diets are very restrictive (usually liquid formulas) and monotanous.

Special formulas or products. These types of weight loss programs are centered on a product (or product line) that replaces real food. As with low-calorie diets, these are very restrictive and limit a person's ability to eat in "real" situations such as with family and at social outings.

Extremes in macronutrient restriction. Weight loss programs that omit carbohydrate or fat generally don't work in the long run because they are very restrictive and people find them difficult to stick with in the long term. While people may find short-term success, long-term weight maintenance is poor with these diets. Additionally, they often lack in meeting essential nutrient needs, which is problematic in the long run.

Surgery. Several surgical procedures are used in treating severe obesity. Physicians may opt to recommend surgery for a person whose immediate health is greatly compromised by their excess weight. Gastric bypass, as shown in Figure 7.19, involves bypassing most of the stomach and the top portion of the small intestines and reconnecting the intestines to the top part of the stomach. This prevents foods from being digested and absorbed, which means most calories (along with nutrients) don't enter the body. Dramatic amount of weight is lost but there are potentially severe health problems and these patients must be monitored closely.

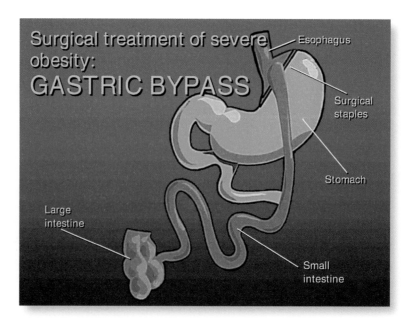

FIGURE 7.19

Another procedure called gastric band essentially limits the size of the stomach so very little food can fit. The band, as shown in Figure 7.20, can be tightened to make the stomach capacity smaller. Eating too much food creates discomfort so the person eats less and loses weight. These and other surgical procedures are expensive and typically not covered by medical insurance. While some people do find success with obesity surgery, it requires changes in lifestyle as well as including the incorporation of exercise.

Drug therapy. Several drugs have been used in the treatment of obesity, but unfortunately, not with much success. Altering a level of a brain chemical through drug treatment may change eating behavior, but as we have learned, it is not the only factor in controlling calorie intake and obesity development. One drug currently used, called Orlistat, blocks fat absorption. As a result, a low-fat diet must be eaten in conjunction with drug therapy to avoid intestinal trouble. For the most part, drugs have a very modest effect and must be used in conjunction with lifestyle changes, including the addition of increased physical activity.

Nutrition Bite

Dietary supplements such as those purchased on the Internet promoted as weight loss aids are not clinically tested—that is, unlike prescription obesity drugs, dietary supplements sold as weight loss aids are not proven nor is their safety guaranteed.

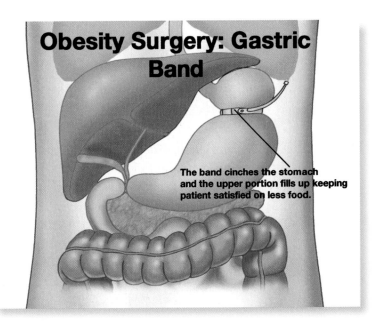

Obesity Surgery: Gastric Band

The band cinches the stomach and the upper portion fills up keeping patient satisfied on less food.

FIGURE 7.20

EATING DISORDERS—PREVALENCE AND PROBLEMS

Beyond obesity, there are other situations where energy balance is skewed—eating disorders. Some 2 million people in the United States, mostly young and primarily women suffer from the two eating disorders, **anorexia nervosa** and **bulimia.** These serious conditions are believed to have their origins in dieting, or restrictive eating, combined with environmental issues such as family life and participation in weight-conscience sports. In this section we discuss these two conditions and their related nutritional problems.

Anorexia Nervosa

This eating disorder is characterized by self-induced starvation and typically afflicts young women—mostly teenagers. About 5 to 10 percent of anorectics are male, though these numbers appear to be on the rise as more boys and men become overly concerned about their body images. Another characteristic of an anorectic is that she often comes from an affluent family and exhibits signs of perfectionism. Other criteria for those suffering from anorexia:

- Below or less than 85 percent of expected healthy body weight.
- Intense fear of becoming fat even though she is underweight for her age and height.
- Distortion of body image (unable to determine rationally that she is underweight). (See Figure 7.21.)
- Loss of a regular menstrual cycle—amenorrhea—for at least three months.

Anorexia sufferers deny their hunger and it is not clear if regulatory mechanisms for food intake control become "damaged" with starvation or that a person may be susceptible to anorexia since this eating disorder appears to run in certain families.

Bulimia

This eating disorder is characterized by recurrent episodes of binge eating and purging, or other methods to rid the excess calories. Bulimia is believed to afflict approximately 5 to 25 percent of college-aged females. Males also suffer from bulimia, especially men involved in weight-restrictive sports such as wrestling and crew, even though cases appear to be underreported. Bulimia most likely gets its start when a person diets or restricts eating in an effort to lose weight. She often forbids herself to eat certain foods, lasting several days and then "giving in" and overeating on that food such as

FIGURE 7.21

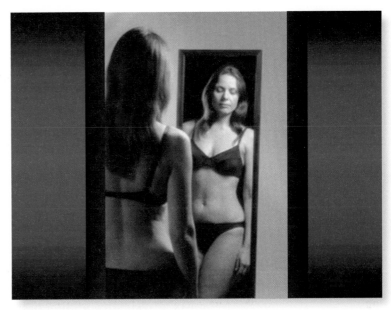

Suze Scalora/Getty Images

cookies or ice cream. Extreme guilt follows and she restricts again, only to succumb later. A cycle begins of restricting, binging, and soon she tries methods such as vomiting or the use of laxatives to rid her body of the excess. Here are some specific characteristics of a person with bulimia.

- Eating large amounts of food in a short or discrete period of time. Binges may be 1,000 to over 10,000 calories of food—usually sweets. Binges are often planned and carried out in privacy.

- A feeling of no control during the binge, which is followed by feelings of extreme guilt.

- Purging type of behavior follows the binge, such as vomiting (self-induced with use of fingers or medication that induces vomiting), use of laxatives or diuretics (cause increase in urine output to reduce bloated feelings), periods of fasting and/or excessive exercise.

- This behavior occurs twice a week for at least three months for bulimia to be diagnosed. (But as you might imagine, a person doesn't "wake up" one day and become bulimic. Instead this disorder develops over time as a person continues the dieting and binging cycle.)

Nutritional Problems Associated with Eating Disorders

Anorexia—Since this is basically malnutrition brought on by starvation, many of the same symptoms are seen as in a person who is malnourished from a poor country.

- Protein deficiency and related problems (see Chapter 2)

- Calcium deficiency and related bone problems (stress fractures and early osteoporosis—covered in Chapter 8)

- Zinc and iron deficiency (anemia and poor immune health are often seen in anorexia sufferers)

- Vitamin deficiencies (with little food being eaten, various vitamin needs are not met and related symptoms are seen)

- Fine hair covers body—lanugo or peach fuzz like hair grows on the back, face, and arms as the body tries to stay warm (with starvation, the BMR drops so heat production is reduced and a person is often chilled or cold much of the time, dressing in layers of warm clothing)

Treatment for anorexia involves a team approach with psychiatrists, family therapists, physicians, and dieticians. The longer a person suffers from this eating disorder the harder it is to treat. Anorexia suffers have a high rate of suicide deaths and death from organ failure.

Bulimia—With intermittent caloric restriction and overeating, the nutritional problems are generally less severe compared with anorexia.

- Loss of potassium due to heavy vomiting (in extreme cases, this may result in heart failure)

- Loss of fat-soluble vitamins when laxatives are abused (this decreases their absorption)

- Erosion of teeth enamel due to acid in vomit

Bulimics are treated with much more success when structured eating is implemented to avoid swings (dieting and binging). Also, therapy with antidepressant medication may be helpful to many sufferers because this eating disorder may have origins in altered levels of brain chemicals.

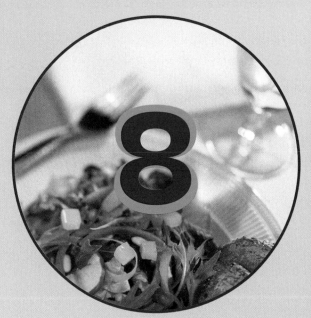

Minerals— From Bones to Hormones— The Work Hard Nutrients

Now that we've covered the first three classes of nutrients, actually the *macro*nutrients protein, carbohydrate, and fat, it's time for the *micro*nutrients. First up: minerals. This class of nutrient is the simplest. Minerals are elemental substances such as iron, calcium, and sodium. While they may be simple elements, the roles of minerals are far reaching, as we will see—from bone structure to the delicate workings of hormones.

This chapter will cover several important minerals; however, not all of them will be covered because there are some 20 of nutritional significance. For each mineral, the following will be covered:

▶ The mineral's function

▶ Consequence of the mineral's deficiency (specifically related to its function)

▶ Issues of the mineral's bioavailability (described in the next section)

▶ Food sources of the mineral

▶ Relationship of the mineral to specific health issues such as bone health or heart disease

MINERALS—THEIR ORIGIN AND PATH THROUGH THE FOOD CHAIN

Let's define minerals as a nutrient category:

● Minerals are elemental substances other than carbon, hydrogen, oxygen, and nitrogen. Thus, they are inorganic. (In chemistry terminology this means without carbon. For example, water is inorganic, but carbohydrate is organic.)

- Minerals represent about 5 to 6 percent of your total body weight. Mineral content of the body varies with gender and race. Males generally have a greater mineral content (due to a greater skeletal mass). For people of Asian descent, mineral composition is just below 5 percent of body weight, while those of African descent or blacks have a great mineral content of about 6 percent (primarily due to greater bone/skeletal mass).

- Minerals are essential nutrients and the body is unable to make them; thus, food (and water) is the only source.

- Minerals function in a regulatory and/or structural role, but minerals do not provide energy. (What nutrients do provide energy?)

- Minerals originate from rocks and make their way into water, soil, and eventually plants, animals, and then us.

Here Is the Path of Minerals through the Food Chain

An estimated 4 billion years ago when the earth formed, minerals were integrated into the earth's crust. Over time, they have made their way into water, as water trickles over and through layers of rock in the earth. Rocks and water become part of soil; then plants take up water and use minerals from the soil for their needs. Animals then eat the plants and drink the water. Finally, we drink the water, eat plants, and also eat animal products such as meat and milk. Thus, we get the minerals "directly" from the earth as shown in Figure 8.1.

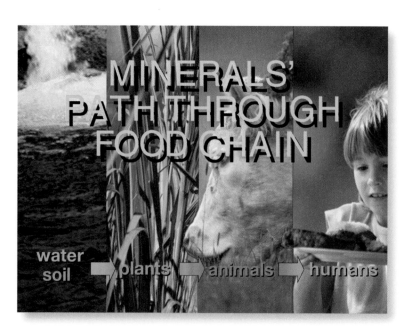

FIGURE 8.1

With this in mind, you can see that a particular plant growing on mineral-deficient soil (such as the mineral iodine) would then lead to deficient intake of this mineral for the animals and people of this land. This is particularly true for people living in isolated areas such as parts of Africa and Asia who eat only locally grown vegetables, fruits, grain, and animals existing in mineral-deficient soils. It is not necessary for us, however, to worry whether our neighborhood soil is mineral deficient or replete since we eat foods grown all over the United States and other countries.

There are two major classifications of minerals, which are based upon their presence in the body (as a percentage of body weight) and the amount required in our diets.

Major (Major) Minerals

- present in the body at levels greater than 0.01 percent of the body weight
- required in amounts greater than 100 milligrams per day
- function in both structural and regulatory roles

Some of the major minerals include calcium, phosphorous, sodium, potassium, magnesium, and chloride. In this course, we cover in detail calcium, sodium, and potassium. Although the others are just as vital in the diet, these three have particular health significance to you.

Trace (Micro) Minerals

- present in the body at levels less than 0.01 percent of the body weight (all the trace minerals added together would fit into a soup spoon!)
- required in amounts less than 50 milligrams per day
- function primarily in regulatory roles since their presence in the body is in such small amounts

Some of the trace minerals present in you and food include iron, zinc, copper, selenium, fluoride, iodine, and manganese. In this course, we cover zinc, iodine, and fluoride. As with the major minerals, these select trace minerals have a particular relevance to you.

BIOAVAILABILITY

The concept of bioavailability is important in the discussion of minerals. Bioavailability the amount or proportion (percentage) of a nutrient and, in our case mineral that is available for absorption. Recall from earlier chapters that when we eat protein, carbohydrate, or fat, we are able to absorb about 90 to 95 percent of the nutrient (Chapter 3). The remaining 5 to 10 percent is undigested and unabsorbed, ending up in the stool. Thus, the bioavailability for protein, carbs, and fat is about 90 to 95 percent. For minerals, however, the numbers are quite different. Most minerals range in bioavailability from under 5 percent in the case of iron from foods like spinach, to over 60 percent for sodium from foods like snack crackers.

Several factors can increase or decrease a mineral's bioavailability. Throughout our discussion of minerals, take note of these factors and their significance for that particular mineral. Many of these bioavailability factors may have personal significance and may contribute to poor mineral status for you.

How Is Bioavailability Taken into Account in Setting Nutrient Requirements?

Knowing that iron bioavailability from spinach is low, does this mean that we need to eat 10 to 20 times that amount to meet our needs? Look back to the notes on the RDA in Chapter 1. Several factors were mentioned that went into determining the RDAs for the nutrients. For example, issues of gender, physiological state (lactation, for example), and age are taken into account when setting nutrient requirements. The nutrient's bioavailability is also taken into account. Thus, for iron, the RDA is set knowing that about 10 percent of this mineral is absorbed on average from most foods. The RDA for various minerals, both major and trace, are set with issues of bioavailability in mind. As we cover each mineral, you will see that for some minerals, bioavailability factors can be significant.

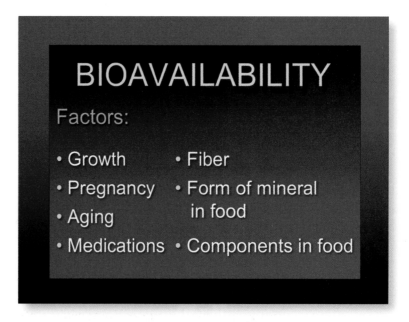

FIGURE 8.2

MAJOR MINERALS

As each of these minerals are covered, keep in mind the function and how its deficiency relates to the mineral's role. Also, consider bioavailability factors, and how this may influence the requirement for the specific mineral. While memorizing the specific RDA is not necessary, you should recognize differences in need based on prominent factors such as age, and, of course, learn about some good food sources.

Calcium

Perhaps the most famous of minerals, calcium plays both structural and regulatory roles. This mineral accounts for about 2% of your body weight or roughly 3 pounds.

Function

- **Structure:** Approximately 99 percent of the body's calcium is found in your teeth and bones. Bone formation starts with a protein latticework of collagen fibers (much like a trellis that roses climb upon), which is then overlaid with a calcium-phosphorous salt called hydroxyapatite. Your bones undergo constant remodeling by two types of cells called osteoblasts (building or construction cells) and osteoclasts (the breakdown or demolition cells). These two bone cell types work together over time to determine bone growth and bone changes. You can build bone mineral content or density (calcium) during your younger years until about ages 25 to 30. Typically after this time, calcium is lost from the bones and as we'll see with calcium deficiency, this speeds up with a calcium-deficient diet and other lifestyle factors such as inactivity and smoking.

- **Regulatory:** The remaining 1 percent of calcium is found in body tissues performing roles such as in blood clot formation and in muscle and nerve cell impulse transmission. For example, the heart muscle must have the proper levels of calcium for normal heart function. Another regulatory role of this mineral is as part of the calcium-binding protein called calmodulin. This protein mediates many cellular processes such as cell division and cell secretions.

Deficiency

Can you imagine the possibility of your heart stopping or your blood not clotting after a shaving nick if there was insufficient calcium in your system? These horrific consequences will not happen because maintenance of these regulatory roles is so vital to life. Remember the concept of homeostasis? Well, calcium homeostasis is a perfect example of many systems coming into play to maintain constant internal conditions (tissue levels of calcium). Essentially, your body "robs" your bones of calcium to maintain regulatory roles. Here's how it works. Visualize your bones as a "bank" of calcium just like your savings account that you use to make such purchases as college tuition and a car. Your tissue levels of calcium represent the ready cash you have on hand. If you're low on cash, you take cash out of your savings to make purchases. Your body works the same way. If tissue levels dip slightly due to a low intake from the diet, then the body responds by withdrawing calcium from your bones through the osteoclasts (much like an ATM machine that allows you to withdraw cash). In addition to this, other systems work to boost tissue levels back to normal. (See Figure 8.3.)

Calcium homeostasis is achieved three ways:

1. The bioavailability of calcium goes up in times of need (when tissue levels take a dip). A signal is sent to the intestines—vitamin D, which is needed to make a protein carrier for calcium absorption to help boost bioavailability.

2. Hormones (released from the parathyroid gland) work on the excretion end and tell the kidneys not to excrete as much of this mineral in urine. The kidneys play a major role in the homeostasis of most major minerals (particularly sodium and potassium) in addition to calcium.

3. The osteoclast cells in the bone are stimulated by hormones to release calcium into the bloodstream.

Net result: Blood/tissue levels of calcium return to normal and vital calcium regulatory roles continue. But there is a price to pay. Over time, continued withdrawal of calcium from the bone without return "deposits"

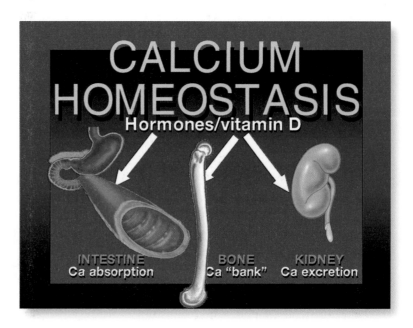

FIGURE 8.3

results in loss of bone mineral or calcium content. The results in children and adults differ.

Children: Calcium deficiency results in poor growth and bone mineralization. Mineral content of bone is low, and as a result, bones are soft and bow with the weight. This condition is called rickets, which we will discuss in more detail with vitamin D deficiency in Chapter 9.

Adults: Osteoporosis develops. This literally means "porous" bones and is characterized by weak bones with low mineral content. As shown in Figure 8.4, the cross section of a normal healthy bone looks like a sponge (with holes that allow for interchange with the circulation) but the osteoporotic bone looks lacy in appearance, much like a loofah pad with bigger holes and weak mineral structure.

Osteoporotic bones break easily, especially the bones in the spine, hip, and wrist. The spine or vertebral bones actually become so weak and fragile that they crush onto themselves, causing the person to shrink in size (lose height) and become slumped over. (See Figure 8.5.) This also causes great pain and severely limits motion and activity. Hip fractures and fractures of other bones due to osteoporosis put many older people in the hospital costing millions of dollars and severely limiting their mobility and often leading to secondary problems such as pneumonia and possible death.

The risk of developing osteoporosis is very high for women—about one in three will develop age-related mineral loss from bones and related fractures. Men also are at great risk later in life. Even though poor calcium intake is an important factor, there are several other factors including lifestyle issues that impact bone density and bone health. Are you at risk for osteoporosis?

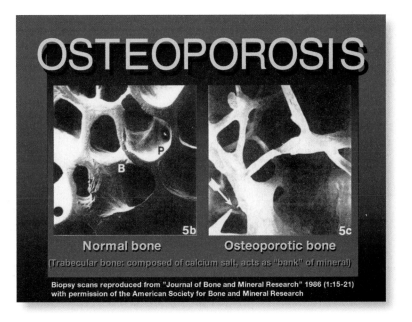

FIGURE 8.4

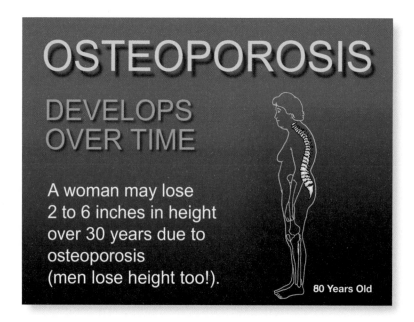

FIGURE 8.5

- **Risk increases with age.** The older a person is, the more they are at risk when calcium loss from the bone exceeds "deposits" in our later years.

- **Risk increases with long-term low-calcium intake.** If calcium intake is low during your formative (growth) years or during young adulthood, you have less calcium in your bone "bank" or in reserve to cover losses.

- **Risk is greater for women than men.** Men generally have greater bone mineral density (content of calcium), thus a bigger savings account. Women tend to live longer than men, thus signs of calcium loss from the bone eventually show up in these later years. After menopause, when a woman's body ceases to make estrogen, bone loss is accelerated. This hormone helps maintain bone density, thus many women opt for estrogen replacement therapy post-menopause to help slow this loss.

- **Risk is greater in inactive people.** Physical activity, especially weight-bearing exercises such as weight lifting and brisk walking help build denser bones.

- **Smoking and heavy alcohol consumption speed mineral loss from the bone.**

- **There is also evidence that a high intake of sodium from processed foods and possibly coffee may accelerate bone mineral loss in some people.**

So ask yourself again—are you at risk for developing osteoporosis? Check your calcium intake on your Diet Project to see how your intake ranks with requirement.

Bioavailability Issues

Calcium bioavailability is about 30 percent for adults. However, during times of greater needs such as pregnancy (forming skeletal mass of a newborn and building reserves for lactation) bioavailability boosts to about 50 percent. During teen years and other times of rapid growth, bioavailability also goes up to about 50 percent. Vitamin D is also needed for calcium absorption, thus factors that alter status of this vitamin may impair calcium bioavailability (more in Chapter 9). Bioavailability of calcium is decreased in the presence of particular food factors—phytate (phytic acid) found in whole grains and oxalate (oxalic acid) found in leafy green vegetables—they bind to calcium in the stomach and small intestine, and decrease calcium's absorption.

Requirement

Calcium requirements are listed in Figure 8.6 for various age groups. While we often refer to the requirement as the RDA, it is actually the Adequate Intake or AI because insufficient data exists to accurately determine the RDA for calcium. Note that the requirement for a woman who is pregnant or lactating is not greater. Since bioavailability goes up for this mineral in these conditions, this required level is considered sufficient.

Food Sources

A variety of food sources are listed in Figure 8.7. Calories for calorie, non-fat dairy products, such as non-fat yogurt, are the best sources of this mineral. There are many calcium-fortified foods including orange

CALCIUM REQUIREMENTS		
INDIVIDUAL		**AI**
Child	1–3 years	500 mg
	4–8 years	800 mg
Child/teen	9–18 years	1300 mg
Adult	19–50 years	1000 mg
	51 + years	1200 mg
(pregnancy, lactation—same as age group)		

FIGURE 8.6

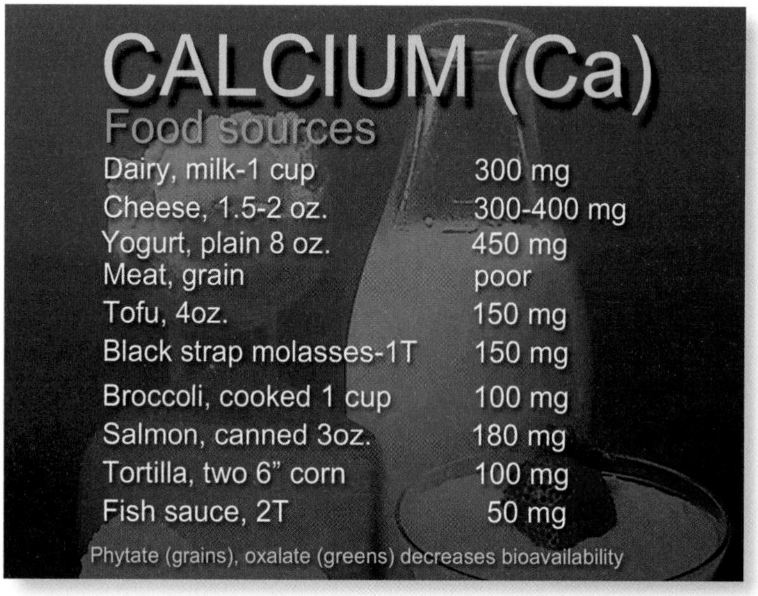

FIGURE 8.7

juice and other fruit juices, breakfast cereals, and even milk boosted with extra calcium.

Issues of Calcium Supplementation and Excess

The real threat of developing osteoporosis has many people, particularly women, selecting calcium-fortified foods and taking calcium supplements. Supplements of this mineral may be a wise decision for many people who do not eat dairy products or eat other good sources of calcium. If you are considering a calcium supplement, keep a single dose to no more than 500 milligrams and take it with food. To ensure maximum calcium absorption, take it with a meal that is not rich in calcium. There is no need to purchase fancy supplements—calcium carbonate is effective and inexpensive. Avoid supplements of bone meal or oyster shell because these may have small amounts of heavy metals such as mercury, which may present toxicity problems over the long term.

Should you be concerned about taking too much calcium? It's best to avoid excessive calcium supplementation because this can hamper the absorption of another mineral, iron. The Safe Tolerable Upper Limit (UL) for calcium is 2,500 milligrams per day. As shown in Figure 8.8, you can come close to this amount in just one meal if you go overboard taking supplements and eating calcium-fortified and calcium-rich foods.

Sodium and Potassium

These two major minerals are covered together because they work closely together in regulating fluid balance and other roles. Sodium (better known

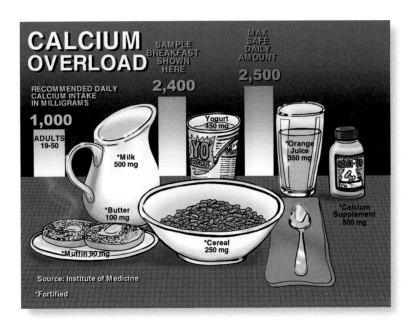

CALCIUM OVERLOAD

SAMPLE BREAKFAST SHOWN HERE

MAX SAFE DAILY AMOUNT 2,500

2,400

RECOMMENDED DAILY CALCIUM INTAKE IN MILLIGRAMS

1,000

ADULTS 19-50

*Milk 500 mg

*Butter 100 mg

*Muffin 90 mg

Yogurt 450 mg

*Cereal 250 mg

*Orange Juice 350 mg

*Calcium Supplement 500 mg

Source: Institute of Medicine

*Fortified

FIGURE 8.8

as a component of table salt) is a notorious culprit in high blood pressure. However, both of these minerals play a role in healthy blood pressure regulation.

Function

Both sodium and potassium are called electrolytes, simply a term used to describe minerals which dissolve in water and can form or carry an electrical charge.

- **Both minerals are crucial in the regulation of fluid homeostasis.** The distribution of sodium and potassium differs in and outside the cell as shown in Figure 8.9. A majority of the sodium (chemically abbreviated Na^+) is located outside the cell, called extracellular; potassium is located intracellular or inside the cell (chemically abbreviated K^+). Recall from Chapter 1 that two-thirds of the body water is intracellular and one-third is extracellular. This set distribution must be maintained for proper cellular function and metabolic reaction, and it is the division of sodium outside the cell and potassium inside the cell that ensures this fluid balance. These two minerals work in concert not only to aid in fluid balance but also maintenance of healthy blood pressure (blood is mostly water).

- **Both minerals serve in the transmission of nerve impulses.** It is again their distribution in and outside the cell that allows for nerve function.

Minerals—From Bones to Hormones—The Work Hard Nutrients | 201

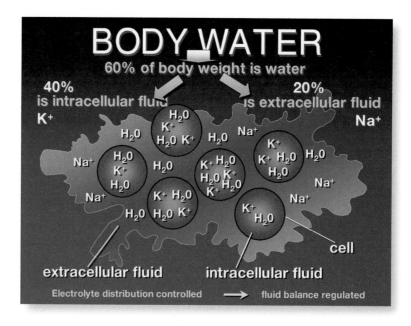

FIGURE 8.9

As with calcium, the kidneys along with several hormones maintain the homeostasis of both sodium and potassium. For example, excess sodium intake would result in hormonal signals to the kidneys to rid the excess in the urine.

Deficiency

Lack of these minerals would rarely occur as a result of poor dietary intake since both are very plentiful in our diets. (However, a low potassium intake relative to sodium intake may be an issue for some people and contribute to the development of high blood pressure—discussed later.)

The more likely possibility of a deficiency of either mineral results from a sudden loss of body fluids. This may occur with heavy sweating (primarily a loss of extracellular fluid, thus sodium—taste your sweat next time you're finished with a tough workout). Also, bouts of vomiting and diarrhea, which occur with food poisoning, the flu, or with an eating disorder, cause the loss of both potassium and sodium.

Symptoms of sodium or potassium deficiency include a drop in blood pressure, which gives you a light-headed, dizzy feeling. Also, muscle weakness and cramping along with nausea occur. During long bouts of exercise such as running a marathon and drinking copious amounts of plain water can lead to a dilution of sodium in the circulation called hyponatremia. This condition can be life-threatening and requires medical attention. As a result, slower runners who most likely are sweating less are cautioned not to over-hydrate so as to avoid hyponatremia.

Bioavailability Issues

Both minerals are very bioavailable in the diet—over 60 to 80 percent. Excess intake and regulation of levels in the body occurs through the monitoring of fluid levels by a series of hormones and the action of the kidneys to excrete excess or hold on to either mineral if needed.

Requirement

There is an Adequate Intake (AI) established for both minerals:

- Sodium: 1,500 milligrams daily
- Potassium: 4,700 milligrams daily

Note that potassium intake should be about three times that of sodium. However, due to our intake of sodium from processed foods (added salt and other forms of sodium), our intake of sodium easily reaches 3,000 to over 5,000 milligrams daily. This coupled with the fact that processed foods are very low in potassium and that our intake of potassium-rich foods—fruits, vegetables, and juices—is low, our intake of potassium is overshadowed by sodium. Health professionals and researchers note that this disparity contributes to the development of high blood pressure, a major risk factor for heart disease.

As a result of this relationship between these minerals to heart health, the Food and Drug Administration has set Daily Values on food labels for both minerals.

- Sodium: 2,400 milligrams (a value not to exceed)
- Potassium: 3,500 milligrams (a value to try and achieve, if not go beyond)

Food Sources

As a general rule, processed foods are loaded with sodium and fresh, unprocessed foods are loaded with potassium. This makes sense because potassium is found inside of cells (fruit and vegetables cells included). When you cut or process fruits and vegetables, you break open cells and potassium is lost in the rinsing and preparation of the foods. Typically, salt or other forms of sodium are added in the processing for taste and preservation of the foods. This explains why a fresh tomato has virtually no sodium and a few hundred milligrams of potassium. When you make that tomato into tomato sauce or ketchup, virtually all the potassium is lost during the processing while oodles of sodium is added. It's no wonder Americans consume so much unnecessary sodium, which may be contributing to health problems, while at the same time getting little potassium, which also is contributing to the same health ailments.

Figure 8.10 shows how processed and fresh foods compare on sodium and potassium.

TRACE MINERALS

As a reminder, these minerals are called "trace" because they are present in the body in such small amounts and their requirements are also quite small—less than 50 milligrams daily. The trace minerals function primarily in regulation rather than structure as the major minerals do. Again, bioavailability issues reign supreme for trace minerals. This issue may be of significance for you personally because your iron or zinc status and intake may be compromised by bioavailability factors.

Iron

Although one of the most abundant minerals in the earth's rocks and soils, iron deficiency ironically is the most common nutrient deficiency worldwide.

Function

- **As a regulatory mineral, iron is most noted for its ability to carry oxygen.** In the red blood cell iron is part of an oxygen-carrying protein called hemoglobin. As the blood cell moves to the lungs, it picks up oxygen as you breathe and this gas binds to iron (abbreviated by Fe in Figure 8.11). The blood cell then travels through your body and delivers the oxygen to cells for its use in

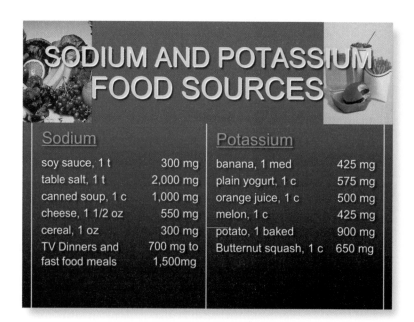

FIGURE 8.10

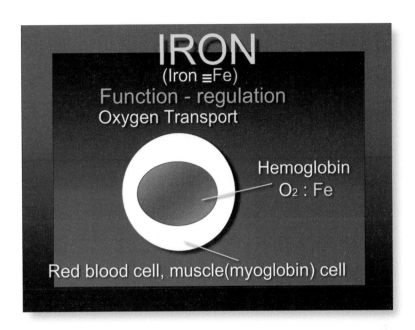

FIGURE 8.11

energy metabolism. (Recall that fats and carbohydrates are broken down aerobically to release energy.) In the muscle cell, another oxygen-carrying protein called myoglobin, which also contains iron, actually picks up the oxygen from the blood cell to transfer it inside the cell for energy metabolism.

Nutrition Bite

Muscle cells that get a lot of "action" such as leg muscles have more myoglobin, hence more iron. This is why dark meat poultry (leg meat) contains more iron and is darker in color than white meat poultry (chest from the bird).

- **Iron also serves as a cofactor in several enzyme reactions involved in energy metabolism.** Iron plays a vital role in the actual release of energy from carbohydrates, fats, and protein.

Deficiency

Before we get into problems with inadequate iron (diet or losses from the body), there are a few things to establish about iron. The body treats this mineral much like a precious gem. Once inside the body, it tries hard not to lose it.

- The body does this by not losing much iron (if any) in the urine and other excretions.

- Blood cell iron is recycled; that is, when a blood cell dies (1 percent do every day), the iron is plucked out and reused.

- Additionally, the body has the ability to change iron absorption in the small intestine. Thus, bioavailability changes as a reflection of need (more on this later).

- The body has the ability to store extra iron in storage proteins called ferritin and hemosiderin.

Iron deficiency can result from poor diet or from losses of iron from the body such as blood losses. Iron deficiency results in low iron stores and low levels of hemoglobin. This is called iron-deficiency anemia. Anemia means "sick blood" and as you will see with other nutrient deficiencies, anemia may result. It is important to note that iron-deficiency anemia has specific characteristics. The blood has poor oxygen-carrying capacity, thus a person feels tired and very fatigued with exertion such as exercise. Other symptoms include a smooth tongue (cells on the surface are unable to regrow properly), and in some cases spooned finger nails, as shown in Figure 8.12.

Nutrition Bite

While spooned fingernails may be a sign of iron deficiency anemia, alterations to fingernail growth and appearance are an unlikely consequence of diet problems. Some Internet sites offer fingernail analysis. Beware not to fall prey to such an inaccurate assessment of your diet adequacy. Fingernails may become ridged, split, and flake as a result of detergents and exposure to other environmental factors. Your fingernails' composition and appearance is not a window to your diet adequacy. Instead, take a good look at your Diet Project assignment and see how you faired with your intake of protein, vitamins, and minerals.

Those at risk for iron deficiency include those who are rapidly growing such as infants and children. Also, women who are in their childbearing years are at risk because of the amount of blood (iron) that is lost due to menstruation.

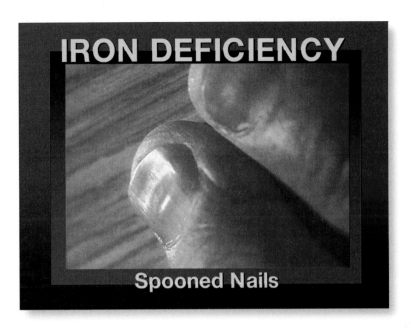

FIGURE 8.12

Bioavailability

Several factors can alter the bioavailability of iron, including (a) your iron status, (b) the form of iron in the food, and (c) meal composition or food factors.

a. Iron status—How great is your need for iron?

Iron entry into the body through absorption via the small intestine is controlled. (Compare this to calcium, sodium, and other major minerals where excretion through the kidneys is mechanism for major mineral homeostasis.)

- *Poor iron status:* Sites for absorption are empty, which signifies that iron stores are on the low side. Many women and children are in this situation. End result: Iron absorption or bioavailability gets a boost, hence more iron is absorbed from food.

- *Good iron status:* Sites for absorption are mostly full, which signifies good iron stores. Most men are in this situation. End result: Iron absorption is reduced.

Figure 8.13 illustrates how need for iron affects bioavailability.

b. Form of iron in food—meat versus nonmeat foods

There are two forms of iron related to the particular state of the iron—heme and non-heme iron.

- Heme iron is the form of iron found only in meats (red meat, poultry, fish) and blood (clotted blood is eaten in some Asian

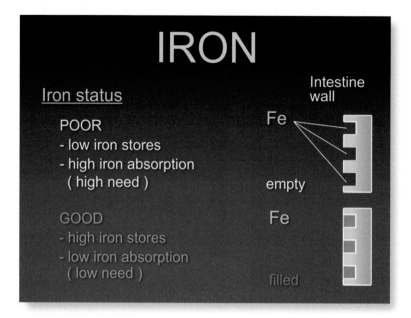

FIGURE 8.13

cultures). The iron is bound to hemoglobin and myoglobin. This form of iron has good bioavailability—about 20 to 30 percent is available for absorption.

- Non-heme iron is found in plants such as beans, grains, and green leafy vegetables. About 40 to 60 percent of the iron in meat is non-heme iron as well (this simply means iron is not bound to hemoglobin). The bioavailability of this iron form is much lower—less than 5 percent up to about 10 percent.

c. Meal composition or food factors

A variety of factors in foods can either increase or decrease the bioavailability of non-heme iron. Numbers given here are for non-heme iron in a breakfast cereal.

- Vitamin C (from berries, oranges, peppers, or a supplement) increases the bioavailability from 10 percent to about 20 percent.

- A protein factor exists in meat that increases the bioavailability of non-heme iron eaten at the same meal (e.g., the non-heme iron both in the meat and in other foods such as beans at that same meal).

- Oxalate (found in greens such as spinach and Swiss chard) and phytates (in whole grains) reduce iron bioavailability by binding with the iron in the intestine and preventing its absorption. This can greatly impact iron status for a person who avoids meats and relies on greens as their major source of iron.

- Extreme intakes of fiber about 50 grams or more (remember that the Daily Value for fiber is 25 grams) can decrease iron bioavailability by binding with the iron at that meal.

- Tannins, which are compounds found in coffee, tea, and red wines, decrease iron bioavailability.

Requirement

The requirement for iron, shown in Figure 8.14, illustrates that women have a greater need due to higher losses of this mineral with regular menstruation.

Remember that iron's low bioavailability is taken into account in establishing the RDA for this mineral. The RDA for pregnant women is so high that a supplement is required to meet this need. Also note that the typical American diet supplies about 6 milligrams of iron for every 1000 calories. Thus, women often don't meet their need for iron with their calorie intake that usually falls below 2000 calories daily.

Food Sources

Iron in foods exists as either heme or non-heme. Recall that flesh and blood are heme iron sources (but not milk, even though it is an animal product). Whether you choose to eat meat or not, non-heme iron is your major source of iron in your diet. If you eat breakfast cereals regularly, your iron intake is most likely more than adequate since most cereals are iron-fortified. (See Figure 8.15.)

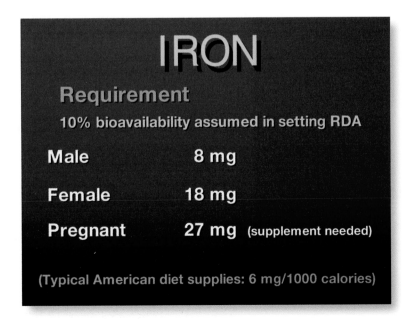

FIGURE 8.14

IRON

Requirement

10% bioavailability assumed in setting RDA

Male	**8 mg**
Female	**18 mg**
Pregnant	**27 mg** (supplement needed)

(Typical American diet supplies: 6 mg/1000 calories)

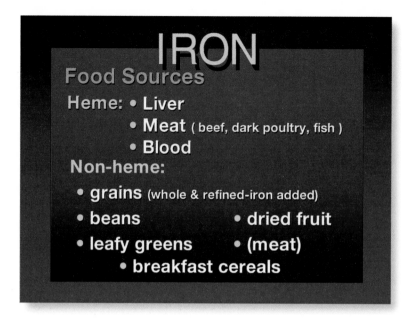

FIGURE 8.15

Toxicity

Getting too much iron in your body can spell trouble, because your body has no active way to expel it—iron is stored, recycled, and little is lost from the body (compare this with sodium, for example, which excess is promptly excreted in the urine). Iron is a potent oxidant, which means it can cause some cellular damage. Therefore, excess iron should be avoided. There is a somewhat rare genetic defect (one in 250 people carry the gene) where iron absorption is not controlled, which leads to iron overload called **hemochromatosis.** This condition can cause serious damage to the liver, because excess iron is stored there, causing damage to tissue. Over time, iron builds up elsewhere and leads to liver cancer or failure. A person with this condition must avoid iron-fortified foods such as breakfast cereal and must go in for blood-lettings (taking blood out) as a way to lower body iron stores.

Acute iron poisoning is a very serious problem in young children. A toddler who ingests vitamin or iron supplements can easily die of acute iron poisoning when the excess iron overwhelms the intestinal tract and enters the body and wreaks havoc. Remember to keep your vitamin supplements and other possible sources of iron in childproof containers and out of the reach of kids.

Finally, even if you think you are anemic due to poor iron intake, don't just take an iron supplement without the advice of a physician. Iron supplements can hamper the absorption of other minerals such as zinc.

Zinc

Touted as the "male mineral," you'll find zinc added to supplements that claim to enhance sexual performance and fertility. Although zinc is involved in sperm production, among other things, claims about sexual performance have yet to be proven.

Function

This mineral operates as a regulatory nutrient and as an enzyme assistant or cofactor in many different enzyme-controlled reactions. A majority of these enzymes are involved in cell replication, or the making of new cells. Thus, during periods of growth and development (pregnancy, childhood, puberty), zinc status is important. (See Figure 8.16.)

Deficiency

In the early 1960s, researchers in the Middle East discovered that men did not develop normally in terms of sexual maturation. Growth during puberty was hampered; secondary sexual characteristics such as emergence of pubic hair and testicle enlargement did not occur. The diet of these men (women as well) was deficient in zinc because of a mostly vegetarian fare and a diet high in phytates (found in whole grains) since unleavened bread was a dietary staple.

Primary symptoms of zinc deficiency include:

● delayed sexual development—young adults appear to be in their childhood years

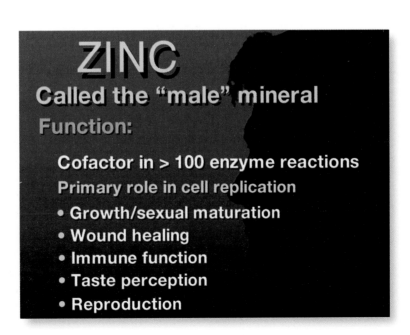

FIGURE 8.16

- impaired immune function (increased susceptibility to colds and flu)

- decreased taste perception (particularly seen in the elderly)

- reduced sperm count (although this has been produced experimentally, few cases of male infertility are due to poor zinc intake)

Bioavailability

As the researchers in the Middle East noted during the 1960s, zinc deficiency resulted from a low bioavailability of this mineral from unleavened bread. Unleavened bread is high in phytates because it is made from whole grains without leavening agents (yeast) so the phytate remains intact. Since 70 percent of the daily calories typically came from unleavened bread, zinc status was impacted as phytate reduces zinc's bioavailability.

In your diet, eating whole grains does not appreciably alter zinc bioavailability since you don't consume a majority of your calories from these foods. Most whole grain breads are made with yeast, which "deactivates" phytate and allows greater zinc bioavailability from whole grain breads.

Requirement

The RDA for zinc is shown in Figure 8.17. As for iron, zinc is not plentiful in the typical diets eaten by Americans (6 milligrams for every 1000 calories). Zinc status may be marginal in the diets of people who take in few calories such as inactive women and the elderly.

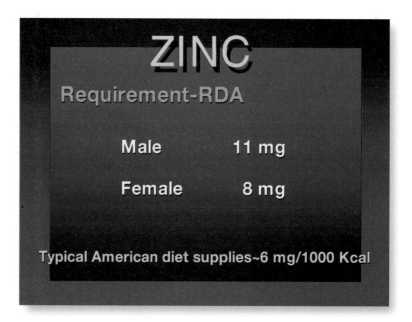

FIGURE 8.17

Food Sources

Meats provide a very good and bioavailable (absorbable) source of zinc. Figure 8.18 shows several good food sources of zinc.

Iodine

Iodine is an excellent example of a mineral whose deficiency is linked to geographical location; that is, in areas where the soil is deficient in this mineral, and where people only eat locally grown food (plant and animal), iodine deficiency results.

Function

Iodine is incorporated into the hormones made by the thyroid gland. This gland is located at the base of your neck and often during physical exams, your physician will ask you to swallow to perform a quick check on the size of your thyroid, which may reflect iodine deficiency as well as other diseases of the thyroid.

The thyroid hormones direct oxygen use by each and every cell in the body. Big job! Thus, thyroid hormones are vital in setting the energy use of the body. More specifically:

- energy use or Basal Metabolic Rate
- reproductive function
- growth

FIGURE 8.18

Food for Boosting Zinc Intake

Food	mg Zinc
Oysters (Eastern), 6 medium	77
Fortified Breakfast Cereal, 1 oz.	5–15
Beef, 3 oz. roasted	6.1
Turkey, dark 3 oz. roasted	3.8
Wheat germ, 2T	2.3
Garbanzo beans, 1/2 cup	1.3
Milk, 1 cup	1.0
Kidney beans, 1/2 cup	0.9

Deficiency

Inadequate intake of iodine comes from eating foods (both plant and animal products) that were grown or raised on iodine-deficient soils. Since in many poor, under-developed communities, people consume only food grown locally, iodine deficiency can readily develop. Iodine-deficient soil occurs in areas where there is lots of erosion such as in the mountains of Peru, or here in the United States within the Great Lakes region (northern Mideast.) Worldwide, iodine deficiency afflicts about 200 million people.

Iodine deficiency leads to the following:

- Inadequate intake of this mineral results in low levels of the iodine-containing thyroid hormones.

- The body senses this imbalance (remember homeostasis?) and sends a signal from the pituitary gland to make more thyroid hormone.

- In an effort to boost thyroid hormone production, the thyroid gland actually grows larger in size to trap more iodine from the blood.

- This enlarged gland is called **goiter.** Goiter is shown in Figure 8.19. The Vietnamese woman on the right subsists on low-iodine intake from her locally grown foods.

- People with goiter also become sluggish and gain weight because their BMR has been lowered. In a small community, sluggish people can in turn impact the productivity of the community at large.

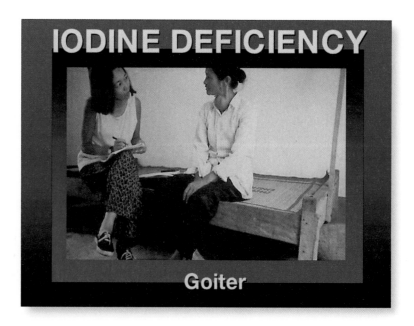

FIGURE 8.19

- A pregnant woman who becomes iodine deficient gives birth to an infant with **cretinism,** which is a permanent defect characterized by mental retardation, deafness, and blindness. This tragic outcome of pregnancy can also have an impact on the entire community suffering from iodine deficiency as an individual with cretinism requires care and resources, and thus, is not able to effectively contribute to the community in return.

In the United States, iodine deficiency was determined to be the cause for goiter and the government implemented the first food fortification program with iodine fortification of table salt.

Requirement

The RDA for iodine is 150 micrograms, which is very easy to meet with a varied diet (i.e., food that is from various geographical locations—different parts of the United States and the world).

Food Sources

Iodine is present in most foods (dependent on soil and water content). In general, food grown closer to the ocean (coastal communities) have great iodine content because this mineral is in sea water and sea water's evaporation and eventual depositing as rain along the coast contributes to the iodine in the soil and water supply. Iodine also makes its ways into our food supply through the use of iodine-containing disinfectants used to clean machinery at restaurants, particularly fast-food eateries.

Fluoride

Chances are that you grew up using fluoridated toothpaste or perhaps you were given fluoride pills to boost your intake in an effort to protect your teeth from tooth decay.

Function

- Fluoride is incorporated into bone and teeth structure through your system when this mineral is taken in drinking water or in pill form. This is particularly important for young children because it becomes a part of the tooth structure as it develops.

- When applied to the teeth topically as with toothpaste, mouthwashes, and even drinking water (which may contain fluoride) or during a fluoride treatment at the dentist's office, this mineral actually interchanges with tooth minerals and becomes incorporated into the enamel structure.

- Once part of the tooth structure, the fluoride helps the tooth become more resistant to decay that causes dental carries or cavities. Dental carries are caused by the action of bacteria-fermenting carbohydrate into acids that etch away at the enamel forming holes and divots that lead eventually to rotting of the teeth. Fluoride actually fights the action of the acid, thereby protecting the teeth.

Deficiency

- Some areas where there is naturally a low level of fluoride in the water supply (less than 1 part per million [ppm] or 1 milligram per liter of drinking water), there is a greater rate of dental carries.

- In those areas where the fluoride in the water supply is greater than 1 ppm, there is a lower rate of dental carries. (Water is the best way to get fluoride because food contains very little of this mineral.)

- Why is fighting tooth decay of such importance? Teeth that are riddled with cavities need dental care that many people cannot afford. Additionally, with many fillings as a result of cavities, these teeth are prone to other problems such as needing crowns or root canal work. This eventually may lead to missing teeth and denture work. Eventually with age the dentures don't fit and the person has a difficult time eating. This in turn may lead to life-threatening nutritional deficiencies. Bottom line: Get adequate fluoride when you are young and use fluoridated toothpaste all through your life to maintain healthy teeth.

Toxicity

For fluoride, getting too much does present a problem, even though only a cosmetic one. In areas where the fluoride is over several ppm, the condition fluorosis develops. This is characterized by chalky or mottled appearance to the enamel. In extreme cases, the teeth appear stained with mottled brown swirls. In this state, the teeth are very resistant to dental carries, but there are no health problems associated with fluorosis.

Children run the risk of mild fluorosis if they are given fluoride supplements and brush with fluoridated toothpaste (particularly if they don't rinse their mouth out and swallow the toothpaste). So it's important for caregivers to monitor a child's brushing activities.

Requirement

The Adequate Intake (AI) for fluoride is 4 milligrams daily.

Food Sources

Water can contain fluoride if the geographical location is such that it gets into the water supply from surrounding rocks; toothpaste and mouthwash contain fluoride if it has been added. Some drinking waters are fluoridated; that is, this mineral is added to the water supply to help the entire local community ward off dental carries. This costs about $1 per person per year and is a great way to protect against tooth decay. Not all local water supplies opt for this measure because some people express fear of adding a "chemical" to the water supply. Now that you know fluoride is an essential mineral that helps keep your teeth healthy for a lifetime, what do you think?

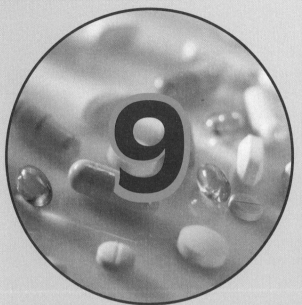

9 Vitamins— The Wondrous Regulatory Nutrients

With minerals under our belts, let's move on to the next group of micronutrients—vitamins. No doubt you have heard about vitamins. Frequent news stories expound on the health benefits of vitamins; the Internet is loaded with websites selling various vitamin supplements; and perhaps you take a vitamin supplement. This intriguing class of nutrient captures the interest of many such as health seekers, high-performance athletes, and those looking to defy aging. Vitamins work in the body as regulators that influence virtually everything from skin and bone health to the workings of energy metabolism and the immune system. In this chapter we cover the wondrous work of vitamins and the truth behind some of the claims made about their "powers."

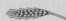

This chapter will cover many, but not all, of the 13 different vitamins. Specifically, we cover:

▶ Roles and classification of vitamins
  ● Water-soluble vitamins
  ● Fat-soluble vitamins
▶ Do you need a vitamin supplement?
▶ Dietary supplements—regulation and safety

ROLES AND CLASSIFICATION OF VITAMINS

- As a class of nutrients, vitamins are organic substances. This means they contain the element carbon (unlike minerals that are inorganic).

- In the body, vitamins function as regulators. Vitamins DO NOT provide energy nor do they provide the body with structure.

- Each vitamin has a unique structure. That is, unlike protein or carbohydrates, vitamins do not have a common unit of structure such as an amino acid. We will cover 11 of the 13 vitamins.

- Vitamins needs differ among different species. For example, humans and other primates require vitamin C but dogs and cats do not.

- Overall, vitamin requirements are small in the milligram or microgram quantity.

- Vitamins function in virtually all body cells, but they don't work together as a "complex" (this is despite what you may see on a bottle of vitamin supplements that reads "B complex").

There are two classifications of vitamins based on their solubility in water. Due to a vitamin's particular chemical structure, it may "like" water and dissolve in it versus "dislike" water and prefer to be around fat (recall from Chapter 5 that fat and water don't mix). The two classifications of vitamins are water-soluble and fat-soluble.

Water-Soluble Vitamins

Characteristics of water-soluble vitamin category (compare and contrast these with fat-soluble vitamins):

- Water-soluble vitamins are found in the watery parts of the cell (inside compartments such as the mitochondria responsible for oxidation of carbohydrates and fats for energy).

- Turnover from the body is rapid, about 48 hours or so. Therefore, your need for water-soluble vitamins is on a frequent basis.

- When consumed in excess, either from the diet or supplement, the body will maintain homeostasis and excrete the extra (either "whole" or in a broken-down form) in urine.

- Excess of water-soluble vitamins is not likely to be toxic.

- Water-soluble vitamins function as coenzymes, which means they facilitate enzyme action. Each water-soluble vitamin functions with one or more enzymes that allows a chemical reaction to occur.

The water-soluble vitamins covered in this chapter are listed in Figure 9.1.

WATER-SOLUBLE	
B VITAMINS	**VITAMIN C**
Thiamin (B_1)	Ascorbic acid
Riboflavin (B_2)	
Niacin (B_3)	
Pyrodoxine (B_6)	
Folate (folic acid)	
Vitamin B_{12}	

FIGURE 9.1

Fat-Soluble Vitamins

- Since these vitamins are NOT soluble in water, they are found in the fatty parts of the body and cells such as adipose tissue and cell membranes.

- Turnover within the body is very slow—months. Therefore, the need is less frequent compared to water-soluble vitamins. (This difference becomes important when discussing deficiency of a vitamin—water-soluble deficiency can occur in several weeks on a poor diet, but it may take years to become deficient in some of the fat-soluble vitamins.)

- Excess of fat-soluble vitamins, whether from diet or a supplement, will stay in the body and be stored (in extreme cases of overdoing with a particular fat-soluble vitamin, the excess is deposited in fatty tissue). Thus, excess is NOT excreted in the urine.

- As a result, excess can be toxic and some fat-soluble vitamins such as vitamin A can even be fatal.

- Fat-soluble vitamins function in more general roles than the water-soluble vitamins. (They are not coenzymes.) The fat-soluble vitamins tend to "oversee" a system such as vitamin D, which is involved in the homeostasis of calcium and bone health.

The fat-soluble vitamins covered in this chapter are listed in the Figure 9.2.

Vitamins and the RDA

Throughout this book we have referred to the RDA (Recommended Dietary Allowances) and factors taken into account when establishing the RDA for a given nutrient. (See Chapter 2; for example, the quality of dietary proteins was taken into account in establishing the RDA for protein.)

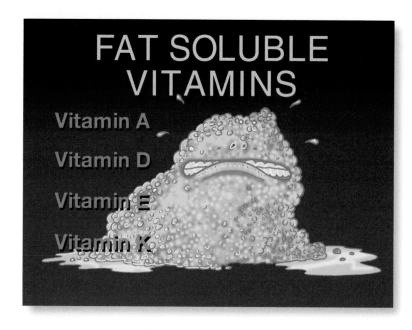

FIGURE 9.2

As a reminder, the RDA represents the recommended intake for many essential nutrients such as protein, fiber, vitamins, and minerals meant to meet the needs of nearly all healthy people in the population. The RDA is not a minimum value, nor is it an average but rather a safe and adequate intake that is meant to be averaged over several days.

Factors taken into account in establishing a given RDA include different age groups, pregnancy, and lactation. For minerals, issues of bioavailability are also considered. (Recall for the iron RDA, for example, that a 10 percent bioavailability from the diet is assumed.)

For vitamins, other considerations are factored in when establishing the RDAs. Many of the vitamins have chemical structures that make them unstable when exposed to heat, light, and even air. Thus, the RDA for many of the vitamins account for this issue of instability and the RDA reflects a greater value in accordance with this.

WATER-SOLUBLE VITAMINS

Before we get into each individual vitamin, let's take a look at the progression of water-soluble vitamin deficiency. You may have thought that you could develop deficiency problems within days of eating a vitamin-poor diet, when actually it takes several weeks.

Here's the progression of a water-soluble vitamin deficiency in a person who previously had been eating a diet with ample amounts of this particular vitamin.

Tissue saturation of the vitamin (which means the body fluids have an ample amount of the vitamin from diet)

Vitamin-deficient diet ↓

Tissue levels of vitamin decline steadily

About 3 to 4 weeks ↓

Biochemical lesion (enzyme activity decreases)

About 6 to 8 weeks ↓

Clinical lesion (outward sign of deficiency — skin, tongue, etc.)

Following three to four weeks of a vitamin-deficient diet (very low amounts relative to requirement), you won't look any different and chances are you won't feel different (except perhaps some general fatigue). However, your cells will "look" different. A laboratory test could detect low activity of the enzyme that needs the particular vitamin which is deficient.

By six weeks or so, you will have an outward sign of deficiency. For water-soluble vitamins, common signs are:

- Skin disorders (dermatitis) such as cracking in the corner of the mouth, granular skin, darkening and peeling of the skin

- Intestinal tract trouble since these cells are high turnover cells (smooth tongue, diarrhea)

- Muscle fatigue because the enzymes needed for energy metabolism become less effective (or not effective at all) in the absence of their vitamin helpers (coenzymes)

Nutrition Bite

Vitamins were discovered around the beginning of the 1900s and got their name from "vital amine" (or vitamin) because nitrogen was associated with, what scientists thought at the time, a single vital substance that was not protein, carbohydrate, fat, or mineral. As each of these different compounds was discovered, they received names in the order of the alphabet. B vitamin was determined to be several different vitamins so they earned a numbering system that is still partially used today (e.g., vitamin B_6 and B_{12}).

For each of the water-soluble vitamins, we will cover:

1. Function
2. Deficiency problems (related to the vitamin's function)
3. Requirement
4. Food sources

Where Do the B Vitamins Work?

Most of the B vitamins are coenzymes in energy metabolism—the breakdown of carbohydrates, fats, and protein for fuel and in the manufacturing of glycogen, fat, and protein. Figure 9.3, as you may recall from Chapter 5, summarizes energy metabolism and indicates where some of the B vitamins operate. Seeing this may help you visualize how vital these B vitamins are for every cell's functioning.

Thiamin (Also Referred to as Vitamin B₁)

1. **Function:** Thiamin's basic function is regulatory and specifically works as a coenzyme in carbohydrate energy metabolism, as shown in Figure 9.4.

2. **Deficiency:** Thiamin deficiency appeared in populations that relied on grains, especially rice, for the bulk of their calories. In the 1800s, the process for refining grains—removing the coarse outer fiber and vitamin-rich hull—became widespread. The poorer people who had traditionally eaten brown rice (with the outer hull)

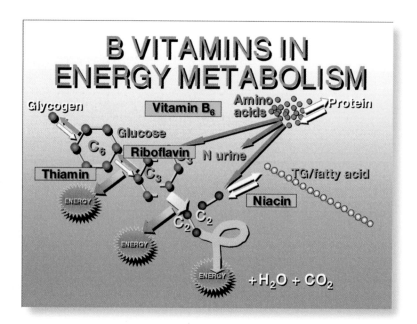

FIGURE 9.3

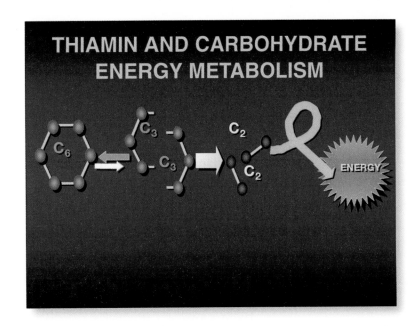

FIGURE 9.4

began to eat white or "polished" rice as this was desirable since the more well-to-do people had long eaten hand-milled grains. But the wealthy also ate a varied diet and didn't rely on rice for a majority of their calories. (See Figure 9.5.) Since the poorer people ate about 80 percent of their calories as "polished" rice, thiamin deficiency developed, called **beriberi** (which means "I cannot, I cannot"). Beriberi is characterized by muscle fatigue and nervous system dysfunction (these cells use carbohydrate for energy)—the people

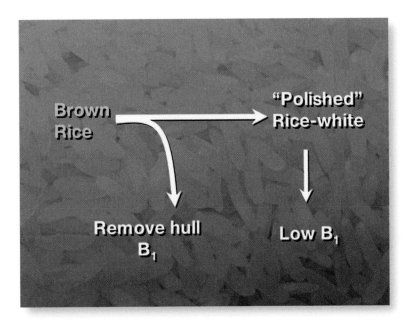

FIGURE 9.5

had trouble standing up and balancing (hence "I cannot get up"). Beriberi is also fatal and can result in heart failure.

Because beriberi was a problem, along with a few other B vitamin deficiencies, the government implemented a grain enrichment program in the 1930s and 1940s to combat these problems. Now, by law, refined grain products have thiamin added back to whole grain levels (more on this in another section).

3. **Requirement:** Listed in Figure 9.6 is the RDA for thiamin. While memorizing the numbers is not important, notice the milligram units and that women have greater needs when pregnant and lactating. The need for thiamin is based upon energy and carbohydrate intake—thus, a very active person who exercises quite a bit would take in more carbohydrate and therefore need more thiamin (but this increase in need can easily be met by food and does not require the use of supplements).

4. **Food sources:** Thiamin is found in many foods—meat, whole grains, beans, and liver being good sources. Pork is very high in thiamin. Food sources of thiamin are listed in Figure 9.7.

Riboflavin (Also Referred to as Vitamin B₂)

1. **Function:** Riboflavin's basic function is regulatory and it specifically serves as a coenzyme in carbohydrate energy metabolism. (See Figure 9.8.)

2. **Deficiency:** Riboflavin deficiency often occurs with other B vitamin deficiencies and similar symptoms develop. The condition is called **ariboflavonosis** and is characterized by a smooth tongue, cracking at the corners of the mouth, and general fatigue.

3. **Requirement:** The requirement for riboflavin is listed in Figure 9.9.

RDA FOR THIAMIN (B₁)	
19+ years male	1.2 mg/day
19+ years female	1.1 mg/day
Pregnancy	1.4 mg/day
Lactation	1.4 mg/day

FIGURE 9.6

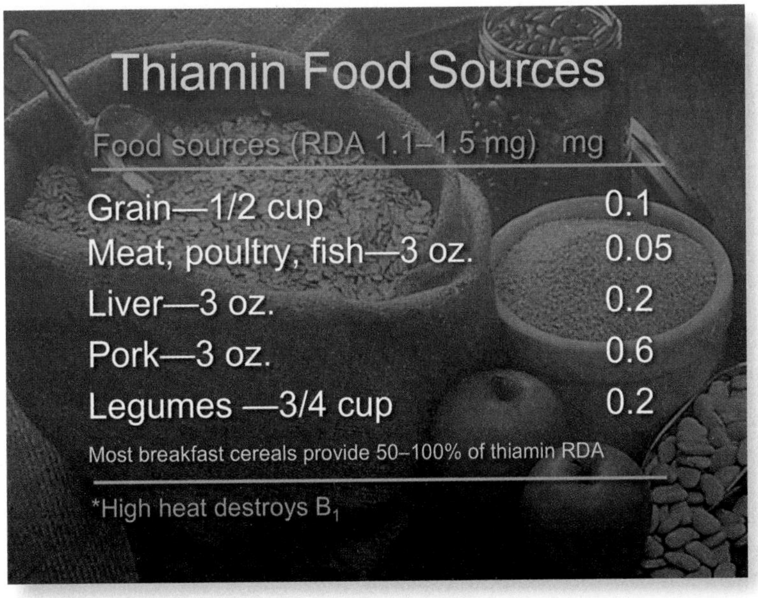

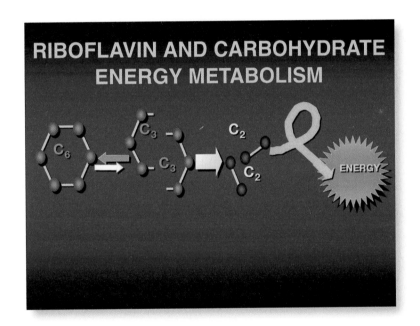

FIGURE 9.7

FIGURE 9.8

4. **Food sources:** As shown in Figure 9.10, dairy products are a good source of riboflavin and for milk drinkers this is the source of about half of the dietary riboflavin. Many foods such as breakfast cereals, breads, and soymilk are either fortified (amounts added that are greater than what occurs in the food) or enriched (added back to original quantities) with riboflavin. Riboflavin is another B vitamin added back to refined grain products.

RDA FOR RIBOFLAVIN (B_2)	
19+ years male	1.3 mg/day
19+ years female	1.1 mg/day
Pregnancy	1.4 mg/day
Lactation	1.6 mg/day

FIGURE 9.9

RIBOFLAVIN (B_2) FOOD SOURCES	
FOOD SOURCES	**mg**
Milk – 1 cup	0.4
Soy milk	1.2
Meat – 3 oz.	0.15
Egg – 1	0.15
Dark green veggies	0.25
Whole grain	0.05/slice
Enriched grains	0.05/slice
1/2 intake from dairy products	
*UV light destroys B_2	

FIGURE 9.10

Niacin (Also Referred to as Vitamin B_3)

1. **Function:** Niacin's basic function is regulatory. Specifically it works as a coenzyme in several reactions involved in the oxidation of carbohydrates, fats, and protein for fuel. Niacin also is a coenzyme in the building or making of fat. (See Figure 9.11.) Interestingly, our bodies can make some niacin from the amino acid tryptophan.

2. **Deficiency:** In the early 1900s, niacin deficiency was a killer disease in the southern United States. The diets of many poor people in this region consisted of just a few foods: refined corn grits, black-eyed peas, and salt pork (fatty pork with not much meat). This monotonous fare led to a serious disorder called **pellagra,** which was characterized by a dermatitis ("blackening" of skin exposed to

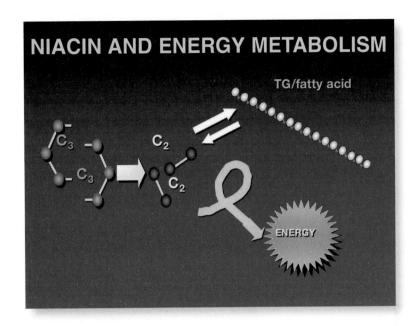

FIGURE 9.11

light), diarrhea, dementia (severe mood swings and derangement), and then death. Notice that the symptoms are characteristic of water-soluble vitamin deficiency described earlier.

Nutrition Bite

The mental disorder characteristic of pellagra was widespread and many mental institutions were built to handle the many thousands who suffered. At the time, the medical community did not realize that this disorder was caused by a lack of a nutrient in the diet. A physician Dr. Goldberg worked to show that pellagra was caused by the people's traditional diet and a dietary cure was soon developed.

The traditional diet led to the niacin deficiency in three ways:

- The diet was very low in niacin.
- The niacin in corn is not very available for absorption (low bioavailability).
- The black-eyed peas are an incomplete protein and salt pork is low in protein. This presents a problem since the essential amino acid tryptophan can be converted to niacin in the body. It takes about 60 milligrams of tryptophan to make one milligram of niacin. Therefore, niacin is an essential nutrient that can be made by the body but not in sufficient amounts to meet needs.

Vitamins—The Wondrous Regulatory Nutrients | 231

Bottom line, these people were not getting enough or making enough niacin to meet their needs, and so pellagra developed. In the 1930s and 40s the government implemented the enrichment program for refined grains; niacin is another one of the B vitamins added back to grains after milling.

3. **Requirement:** The need for niacin, like thiamin, is based on energy needs. The requirement is listed in Figure 9.12.

4. **Food sources:** Niacin needs are easily met with a variety of foods. Good sources of niacin are listed in Figure 9.13.

FIGURE 9.12

RDA for Niacin (B₃)

19+ years male	16 mg/day
19+ years female	14 mg/day
Pregnancy	18 mg/day
Lactation	17 mg/day

FIGURE 9.13

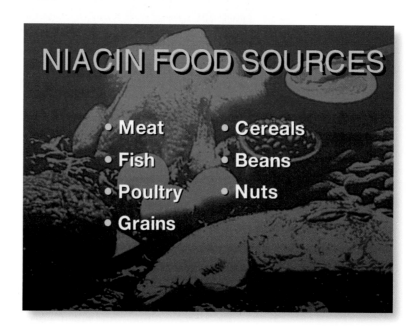

NIACIN FOOD SOURCES

- Meat
- Fish
- Poultry
- Grains
- Cereals
- Beans
- Nuts

Vitamin B$_6$ (Also Referred to as Pyridoxine)

1. **Function:** Vitamin B$_6$'s basic function is regulatory. Specifically it acts as a coenzyme in protein metabolism assisting the transfer of nitrogen from one amino acid to another. B$_6$ is also involved in the breakdown of glycogen to glucose. (See Figure 9.14.)

2. **Deficiency:** Lack of B$_6$ causes similar water-soluble deficiency signs already discussed—diarrhea, skin changes, muscle fatigue. Anemia results because B$_6$ is also needed for the making of the hemoglobin protein found in red blood cells.

3. **Requirement:** The need for B$_6$ is related to protein requirement and intake. The RDA has been set at a level adequate for typical protein intakes of about 50 to 100 grams. The RDA for B$_6$ is listed in Figure 9.15. Notice that it increases in older people due to increased losses and turnover with aging combined with a poor intake.

4. **Food sources:** Food sources are listed in Figure 9.16. Whole grains are a good source but not refined grains, because vitamin B$_6$ is not added back during the enrichment process.

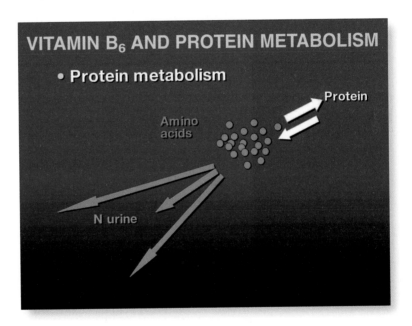

FIGURE 9.14

Vitamin B$_{12}$ and Folate (Also Called Folic Acid—The Chemical Form Used in Enrichment, Fortification, and Supplements)

These two B vitamins are discussed together since their roles are similar and they actually work together.

1. **Function:** These vitamins function as regulators and specifically work in the replication of genetic material (DNA and RNA) inside

RDA FOR VITAMIN B$_6$		
19–50 years Male/female		1.3 mg/day
50+ years	female	1.5 mg/day
	male	1.7 mg/day
Pregnancy		1.9 mg/day
Lactation		2.0 mg/day

FIGURE 9.15

VITAMIN B$_6$ FOOD SOURCES	
FOOD SOURCES	**mg**
Meat, 3 oz.	0.1–0.9
Legumes, 1 cup	0.4
Banana, 1 medium	0.4
Green veggies, 1 cup	0.15
Whole grain breads	0.05/slice
Yeast, 1T	0.2

FIGURE 9.16

cells. Thus, they both play a crucial role in the growth and turnover of new cells. Vitamin B$_{12}$ also functions in the manufacturing of the nerve covering called the myelin sheath.

2. **Deficiency:** Cells that turnover frequently in the body will be quickly affected by a deficiency of B$_{12}$ or folate. This includes red blood cells, which turnover or die at a rate of 1 percent each day so they need to be replaced often.

   Anemia (sick blood) develops with deficiency of B$_{12}$ or folate. This form of anemia (different than iron-deficiency anemia) is characterized by large, immature blood cells. If a person is deficient in B$_{12}$, the nerves may also be damaged due to problems with myelin sheath formation and result in paralysis. This makes it imperative to determine the cause of anemia—B$_{12}$ or folate deficiency. Taking folate can mask a B$_{12}$ deficiency, which may ultimately lead to serious and permanent nerve damage.

Lack of folate pre-conception or during the first several weeks of pregnancy may lead to serious birth defects when cells are rapidly growing in the fetus. Studies show that taking folate before becoming pregnant and during pregnancy itself helps reduce the incidence of neural tube defects (a type of birth defect that involves the spinal cord and is often characterized by paralysis). For this reason, the government has added folate to the list of B vitamins added to refined grain products to improve intake in the general population. This will ensure that women will get adequate folate even if they are not planning a pregnancy. (About 50 percent of all pregnancies are unplanned and many women do not even know they are pregnant until a few weeks into the pregnancy when the spinal cord has developed.) Studies show that this fortification of grain products has helped significantly reduce the incidence of neural tube defects in the United States.

3. **Requirement:** The RDA for both B_{12} and folate are in the microgram quantity as shown in Figure 9.17. Notice the increased need for pregnant and lactating women. The need for B_{12} may increase with aging as the ability to absorb this vitamin declines due to a reduction in acid production.

4. **Food sources:** Good food sources of folate include: liver, citrus fruits such as oranges and orange juice, and green leafy vegetables such as spinach and asparagus. Grain products and breakfast cereals are fortified with folate (in the form of folic acid).

   Good sources of vitamin B_{12} include most animal products—meats, fish, poultry, dairy, and B_{12} fortified soymilk, soy products, and some breakfast cereals.

Special Considerations for Vitamin B_{12}:

This vitamin is unlike other water-soluble vitamins in several ways.

- Since B_{12} is a very large and fragile molecule, it needs some special care in the intestinal track. The acid in the stomach can

RDA FOR VITAMIN B_{12} + FOLATE		
	B_{12}	FOLATE
19+ years Male/female	2.4 µg/day	400 µg/day
Pregnancy	2.6 µg/day	600 µg/day
Lactation	2.8 µg/day	500 µg/day

FIGURE 9.17

damage B_{12}. So to protect B_{12}, a special factor, called **intrinsic factor,** is manufactured by the stomach to bind with B_{12} and serve as protection and transport. This allows for absorption in the small intestine. A small group of people may genetically lack the ability to make this factor, and therefore need B_{12} injections on a regular basis since they cannot absorb the vitamin.

- The mineral cobalt is part of vitamin B_{12} structure, unlike other vitamins that don't have minerals as part of their chemical makeup.

- Vitamin B_{12} is stored in the liver. If you eat a diet with sufficient amounts of this vitamin, you have about a year's supply stored. Recall that the other water-soluble vitamins are not stored.

- The distribution of B_{12} in foods is unique—it is only found in animal products (meat, dairy, eggs, fish, etc.) and fermented foods. Fermented foods with bacteria such as miso (fermented soy) generally are not adequate in B_{12} content to meet needs.

Whole Grains, Refined Grains and Enrichment

Throughout our discussion of B vitamins, reference has been made to refined grains and the depletion or loss of nutrients. Let's take a look at the nutritional difference of whole grains compared to refined grains and how *some* of this disparity has been corrected.

Figure 9.18 shows a whole grain kernel, actually a seed of a plant such as wheat or barley, which would grow into a new plant if allowed to sprout. So it makes sense that this whole kernel is rich in a variety of nutrients.

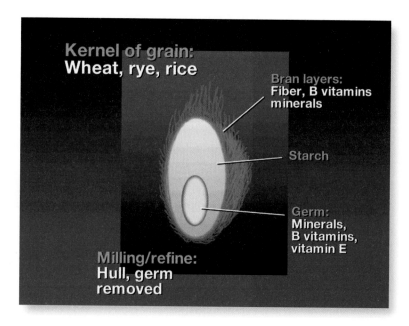

**Kernel of grain:
Wheat, rye, rice**

**Bran layers:
Fiber, B vitamins
minerals**

Starch

**Germ:
Minerals,
B vitamins,
vitamin E**

**Milling/refine:
Hull, germ
removed**

FIGURE 9.18

The outer layer—the bran layers or hull—contains water-insoluble fiber, B vitamins, and some minerals. The bulk of the kernel—what we eat and what feeds the developing plant—is starch (complex carbohydrate). The part that actually sprouts into a new plant is called the germ (rich in minerals and vitamins B and E). The germ also has a very small amount of polyunsaturated fats, which is why the vitamin E is there to protect these fats from oxidative damage due to sunlight or air.

If the germ is left with the grain during milling and made into flour or another grain item, the small amount of polyunsaturated fat may go "bad" or rancid due to its oxidation. This is the main reason why the germ is removed during processing to improve the shelf life of the grain product. In addition to shelf life, many people don't like the texture or taste of whole grain breads and other such products. Also, this dislike for whole grains is a bit of a throwback to when the peasants ate whole grain while the wealthy ate the refined grains.

As mentioned earlier in this chapter, during the 1800s, grain processors developed a way to refine grain—remove the coarse outer layers and the germ, leaving just the starch as shown in Figure 9.19. This starch could then be milled into flour and stored for long periods of time without going bad, which the public preferred. The down side—the whole grain had been stripped of many nutrients—fiber, B vitamins, vitamin E, and minerals such as iron, zinc, and magnesium. As a result, many people by the late 1800s and 1900s had developed vitamin and mineral deficiencies such as pellagra, beriberi, and iron-deficiency anemia.

To combat these nutrient deficiencies, the government instituted the grain enrichment program. Under law, grain manufacturers are required to add thiamin (B_1), riboflavin (B_2), niacin (B_3), and iron at levels comparable

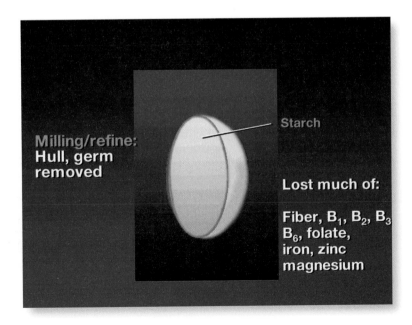

FIGURE 9.19

to the unrefined whole grain. In 1998, folate was added to the list of enrichment nutrients. However, as shown in Figure 9.20 enriched refined grain products are not nutritionally comparable to whole grains because several nutrients are still lacking, including fiber, zinc, and other minerals and several vitamins. Additionally, unrefined grains also supply a wealth of protective compounds referred to generally as phytochemicals. Discussed in the next chapter, these compounds protect against cancer and other age-related diseases.

When you make grain choices in your diet, keep in mind that whole grain provides better nutrition than refined grain. So make an effort to use 100 percent whole wheat bread, brown rice, whole barley, and oats over their refined counterparts. The 2005 Dietary Guidelines (Chapter 12) recommend at least three whole grain servings daily.

Vitamin C (Also Referred to as Ascorbic Acid)

1. **Function:** Vitamin C's basic function is regulatory. Specifically it works in a chemical reaction to make the protein collagen. Recall from Chapter 2 that this protein has structural duties—collagen is the "glue" that holds your bones, connective tissue, lung tissue, blood vessels, and teeth together. Of the thousands of different proteins in your body (about 10,000 different ones), collagen makes up about 25 percent of your total body protein. (As you might guess, deficiency of vitamin C must have devastating consequences and it does.)

Vitamin C also aids in iron absorption. Recall from Chapter 8 that iron's bioavailability is improved by the presence of vitamin C.

Vitamin C also functions as an **antioxidant** in protecting fats—the liquid polyunsaturated fats—against oxidation (much like a fire

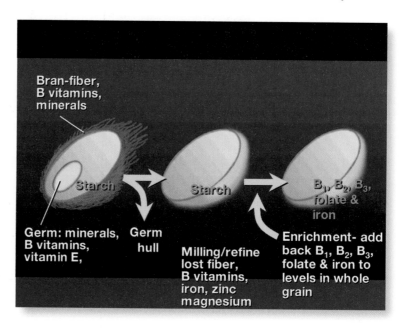

Bran-fiber, B vitamins, minerals

Starch

Germ: minerals, B vitamins, vitamin E,

Germ hull

Starch

Milling/refine lost fiber, B vitamins, iron, zinc magnesium

B$_1$, B$_2$, B$_3$, folate & iron

Enrichment- add back B$_1$, B$_2$, B$_3$, folate & iron to levels in whole grain

FIGURE 9.20

extinguisher that puts out small kitchen fires). Research shows that ample vitamin C intake over many years may lead to a lower risk of developing age-related diseases such as cataracts that are linked to oxidation of fats and other substances within the eye.

2. **Deficiency:** The deficiency of vitamin C actually impacted the exploration of the New World and the slave trade hundreds of years ago. The deficiency disease called **scurvy** was rampant among sailors on long voyages—many (about two-thirds) would die a hideous death of teeth falling out, hemorrhages under the skin, and painful joints and bones. Africans taken from their villages were brought on slave boats across the Atlantic Ocean and a good three-fourths would die from scurvy. This disease was not known on land because people ate fruits and vegetables that provided vitamin C. Scurvy is characterized by the following:

   ● Painful, swollen and bleeding gums result because the collagen is not being remade (remember protein turnover).

   ● Teeth become loose and fall out.

   ● Joints become painful and sore.

   ● Bones become fragile. (Collagen is part of the bone matrix.)

   ● Small hemorrhages form under the skin when blood leaks from the weakened blood vessels.

   ● Eventually scurvy is fatal.

3. **Requirement:** Vitamin C is a good example of a vitamin NOT required by all species. In fact, only humans, other primates, guinea pigs, fruit-eating bats, and trout are among the few mammals that require vitamin C. The reason is that we lack the enzyme to make vitamin C from glucose (a very simple chemical reaction that we and the few other species cannot perform). Therefore, vitamin C is required in the diet.

   The RDA for vitamin C is listed in Figure 9.21. Notice that there is an additional 35 milligrams needed by people who smoke because this increases the breakdown of vitamin C in your system and the oxidative stress.

   There is a safe upper limit of 2000 milligrams daily established for vitamin C, which is commonly taken in supplement form. Above this level there may be adverse effects. Even though vitamin C is water-soluble, such large amounts may be detrimental. For example, at this level, the vitamin C interferes with urine tests for diabetes and may cause gastro-intestinal trouble, reduction in iron absorption and an increased risk for the formation of kidney stones.

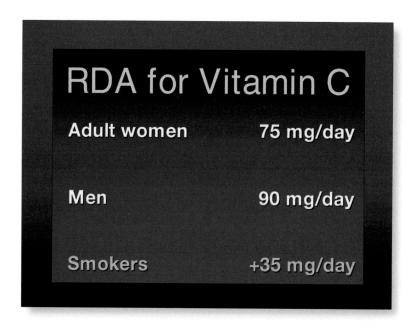

FIGURE 9.21

VITAMIN C FOOD SOURCES	
FOOD SOURCES	**mg**
Milk, meat	0
Fresh fruit: kiwi, orange, strawberry, cantaloupe (1 cup)	40–100 +
Orange juice, 6 oz.	90
Tomato, broccoli (1 cup)	40
Pepper (green, red, hot) (½ cup)	30–60 +

FIGURE 9.22

4. **Food sources:** Vitamin C is easily obtained from food. Many fruits, particularly citrus (oranges, grapefruit, tangerines) are excellent sources of this vitamin. Vegetables such as peppers, tomatoes, and broccoli are also very good sources as shown in Figure 9.22.

What about Vitamin C Supplements?

Many people opt to take vitamin C supplements in amounts well over the RDA such as 500 or 1000 milligram tablets in an effort to ward off diseases such as cancer or to fend off the common cold. Research does suggest that getting ample vitamin C from the foods you eat may help lower your risk for age-related diseases. The scientific evidence for supplements, however, is not as compelling. This brings up the possibilities that the vitamin may interact with other substances such as phytochemicals in food to provide the health benefit rather than the vitamin C supplement alone. As for preventing or curing the common cold, research does not support that taking vitamin C on a regular basis prevents the cold virus. If, however, you have a low vitamin C intake, this may weaken your immune system and make you more susceptible to getting a cold. Instead, taking vitamin C at the onset of a cold may help lessen the symptoms.

FAT-SOLUBLE VITAMINS

As described in the first section, fat-soluble vitamins are chemically different from water-soluble. This in turn influences fat-soluable vitamin turnover and storage in the body, and subsequently the need and possible toxicity issues for these vitamins. As we cover the four fat-soluble vitamins, issues of storage and toxicity will be covered, which was not done for water-soluble vitamins. Also note the functions of fat-soluble vitamins do not involve a specific coenzyme duty but rather function in a more general manner. Deficiency of fat-soluble vitamins progresses at a much different rate than water-soluble due to the storage and relatively slow turnover of fat-soluble vitamins. Consequently, it may take years to become deficient, for example, in vitamin E.

Vitamin A

1. **Function:** Vitamin A's basic function is regulatory and specifically plays a role in several areas:

   - Vitamin A plays a role in the vision cycle—the ability to perceive light during low-light situations such as dusk and dawn, or a dimly lit room. In the back of the eye, there are specialized cells that contain vitamin A, which is chemically modified when light comes in contact with these cells. This chemical modification in turn signals the brain of the presence of light.

   - Most of the body's vitamin A is involved in the maintenance of **epithelial** cells, which is the covering tissue in the body—skin, lining of the lungs, intestines, sinus cavities, urinary tract, and reproductive system. When totaled, epithelial cells account for a large surface area of the body.

   - Vitamin A is also involved in the growth of new bones, which occurs primarily at the ends where remodeling of the bones allows growth in length—a vital role for this vitamin during childhood and adolescence.

2. **Deficiency:** Several deficiency problems arise in response and may take months or years to develop depending upon the person's status (storage) of vitamin A prior to the inadequate diet.

- **Night blindness** (related to the vision cycle), which is the inability to see in low-light situations (trouble driving at night, etc.)

- **Xeropthalmia**—the surface of the eye or cornea sloughs off (the surface and inner eyelid are epithelial surfaces) and blindness occurs. In poor underdeveloped countries and communities, about 500,000 children go blind every year as a result of vitamin A deficiency.

- Infection of the lungs, skin, urinary tract, and other epithelial surfaces occurs when these surfaces are no longer maintained with a vitamin A deficiency. Bacteria and other pathogens invade the body and often a person dies from infection due to vitamin A deficiency.

- Bone growth is halted with vitamin A deficiency and this leads to stunting of growth in children.

3. **Requirement:** Figure 9.23 illustrates vitamin A's structure as it is found in animal products such as liver and milk. It is a ring structure with a long fatty-acid like chain attached. (This is why vitamin A is fat soluble.)

   In plants, there are pigment substances that give plants a yellow, orange, or red color called carotenes. There are some 400 different carotenes, and a few have what is called "vitamin A activity." As shown in Figure 9.24, carotenes look like two vitamin A units

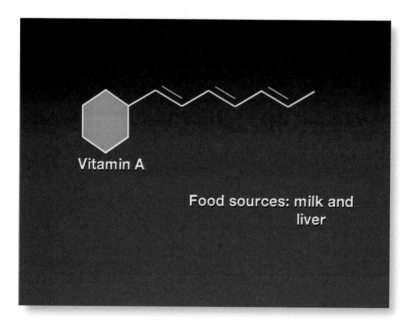

Vitamin A

Food sources: milk and liver

FIGURE 9.23

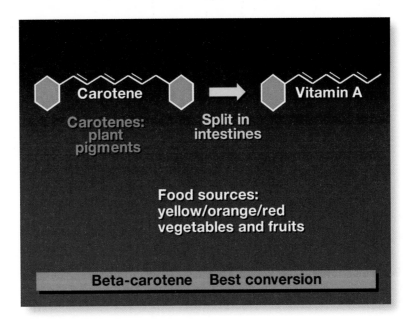

FIGURE 9.24

joined together. In fact, when you eat them, enzymes in the intestinal wall break carotene apart and vitamin A is formed. Not all carotenes are converted to vitamin A, and not all at the same efficiency. Beta-carotene (found in carrots, cantaloupe, and papaya) is converted the best.

Plant food sources contain carotenes and animal sources contain vitamin A. In order to have a common "currency" when talking about vitamin A and its precursors like beta-carotene, we use a measurement called Retinal Activity Equivalent or RAE. Although these numbers are not to be memorized, 1 RAE = 1 microgram of retinol (animal vitamin A), 2 micrograms of beta-carotene from a supplement (converted more efficiently than from food), 12 micrograms of beta-carotene from food, and 24 micrograms of carotenes (other than beta-carotene).

With all of this said about vitamin A in animal products and carotenes in food, the requirement for vitamin A is expressed in RAE because you can meet your need from animal sources or plant sources, or both. The RDA for vitamin A is listed in Figure 9.25.

4. **Food sources:** Typically, about half of your vitamin A comes from animal sources (especially if you eat dairy products, which come fortified with vitamin A). Liver is an extraordinary source of vitamin A, as shown in Figure 9.26, because this organ is a site of storage for this vitamin.

5. **Toxicity and supplementation:** As a fat-soluble vitamin, vitamin A has some major toxicity concerns since excess from food or supplements stays in the body, which is either stored in the liver

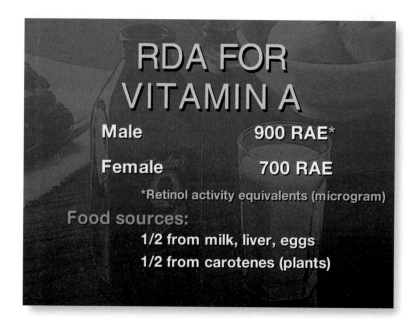

FIGURE 9.25

VITAMIN A FOOD SOURCES	
FOOD SOURCES	**RAE**
Liver (3 oz.)	9000
Egg (1)	84
Milk (1 cup)	100
Orange–yellow fruit: Cantaloupe, apricot, papaya (1 cup)	100 +
Orange–yellow vegetables: Carrot, butternut squash, pumpkin (1 cup)	300–1000 +

FIGURE 9.26

or tucked away in fatty tissue. Taken during pregnancy in large amounts (25 times the RDA), it can cause serious birth defects. At this level of intake, liver damage occurs along with swollen and painful gums.

For beta-carotene and other carotenes, there is no toxicity concerns (in terms of health) other than pigmentation of the skin, primarily an orange tinge to the palms and soles of the feet. This pigmentation develops when a person drinks copious amounts of carrot juice or takes beta-carotene supplements.

As a side note, derivatives of vitamin A (Retin-A and Accutane) are used in the treatment of acne as well as the treatment of fine wrinkles (skin aging process). These vitamin A analogs cause the skin to slough off rapidly, revealing "fresh" skin. There is a danger in taking oral vitamin A analogs (Accutane) for acne treatment because these can also cause severe birth defects. A woman using this medication should be on birth control to prevent pregnancy.

Vitamin D

1. **Function:** The basic function of this vitamin is regulatory and it oversees the homeostasis of calcium metabolism:

   - Regulates calcium absorption in the intestinal tract through a protein carrier.

   - Directs the bones to mineralize (calcium-phosphorous salt called hydroxyapatite).

   - Regulates blood levels of calcium by directing the amount of calcium the kidneys excrete or retain.

2. **Deficiency:** Severe bone maladies were noted in children at the turn of the century in urban London, England. The city used coal for heat and fuel. This produced smoke, which clouded the sky and blocked UV light from the sun. The children, who also spent much of their time indoors, suffered from soft bones that bent under their bodyweight—a condition called **rickets.**

   Why might rickets—vitamin D deficiency—be tied into sunlight exposure? Vitamin D is actually much like a hormone. Your body can make this vitamin, and make enough to meet your needs given sufficient exposure to sunlight—about 30 minutes to hands and face per day for fair skin people and up to two hours for darker skin. Cholesterol is the building block for vitamin D and after a few chemical modifications, the first of which involves UV light, it becomes the vitamin as shown in Figure 9.27. Rickets is characterized by:

- Soft bones that bow out or in (the long bones of the legs being most affected)

- Cartilage overgrows to compensate for lack of mineralized bone.

- The head of a young child becomes enlarged because the skull plates do not mineralize properly and migrate apart with cartilage filling in the gaps.

In adults, a type of rickets forms where the bones become soft. Elderly who do not get enough sunlight exposure and inadequate vitamin D in their diet are likely to suffer. Additionally, their kidney and liver function may be compromised because of aging and medication use further aggravating the problem.

3. **Requirement:** Since exposure to sunlight varies, and many people also have dark skin, which in effect hampers the manufacturing of vitamin D (as does sun block), this vitamin is deemed essential. But the need for vitamin D is quite small. Instead of an RDA being set for vitamin D, an Adequate Intake or AI has been determined as listed in Figure 9.28. (Recall from Chapter 1 that AI reflects a value established on the best available evidence but it is not as precise as RDA, typically set for gender and age differences.) Note that need increases with age since the body's ability to manufacture this vitamin declines with age.

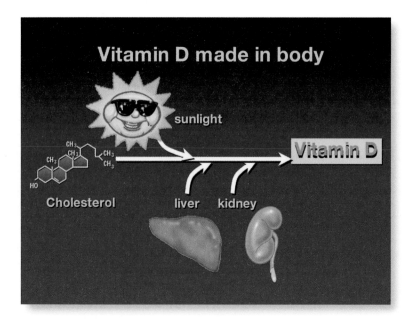

FIGURE 9.27

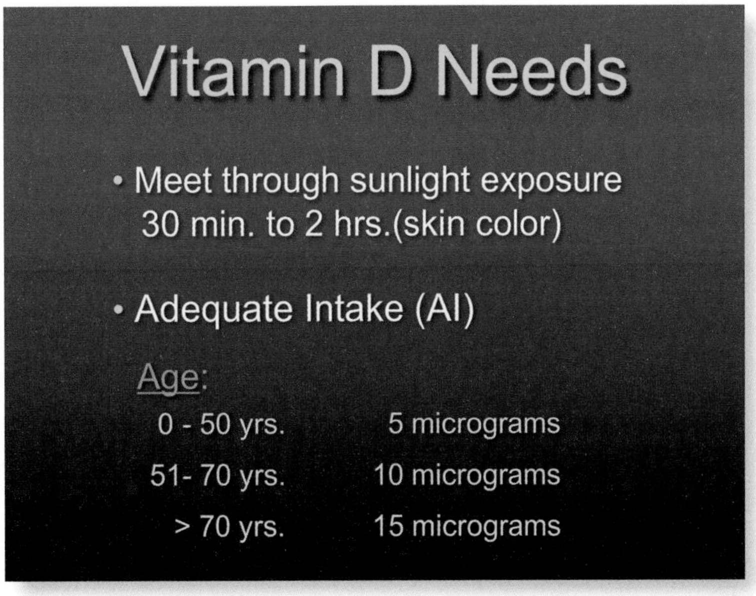

FIGURE 9.28

Vitamin D Needs

- Meet through sunlight exposure 30 min. to 2 hrs.(skin color)

- Adequate Intake (AI)

  Age:

0 - 50 yrs.	5 micrograms
51- 70 yrs.	10 micrograms
> 70 yrs.	15 micrograms

4. **Food sources:** Few foods are good sources of vitamin D. Primarily fatty fish such as salmon and mackerel are the best sources of vitamin D. (In the early 1900s, cod liver oil was used as a treatment for rickets and was later found to contain vitamin D.) Also liver and eggs contain vitamin D. In the United States, milk is fortified with vitamin D as are some breakfast cereals.

5. **Toxicity:** At intake about three times the AI, vitamin D can be toxic in children since their bones are rapidly growing. Calcium levels in the blood increase and calcium is then deposited in soft tissue such as organs. Overgrowth of bones in the face may occur, causing gross malformations.

Vitamin E

1. **Function:** The basic function of this vitamin is regulatory and specifically it acts as an antioxidant (like vitamin C and beta-carotene) protecting fatty acids with double bonds from oxidation. These fats reside in the cell membrane. So consider those cells exposed to oxygen (which can easily cause oxidative damage or rancidity of the fatty acid)—lungs, red blood cells, etc. Vitamin E actually rests on the cell membrane to protect these fats from oxidative damage. (See Fiure 9.29.)

   This brings up the impact of exercise on oxidative damage and need for vitamin E. During exercise, more oxygen is taken in to support the energy demands of the workout. This means the possibility of increased oxidative damage to polyunsaturated fatty

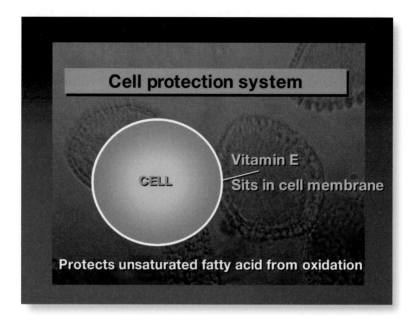

FIGURE 9.29

acids in the membranes of muscle cells. Studies show that this does in fact occur, and that people who exercise may benefit from a greater intake of dietary antioxidants such as vitamins E and C.

2. **Deficiency:** True vitamin E deficiency is rare and is believed to take at least five to seven years to develop because this vitamin turns over very slowly. The consequence of vitamin E deficiency is a type of anemia called **hemolytic anemia** where the red blood cells break open because the cell membranes have been weakened as shown in Figure 9.30.

   A lifetime marginal intake of vitamin E is believed linked to age-related ailments such as cancer, heart, and Alzheimer's diseases. For example, with weakened cell membranes, carcinogens may be able to damage DNA more readily, leading to cancer. Many people take supplements of vitamin E in an effort to ward of these conditions. Research is not clear as to whether food sources or supplements may be beneficial.

3. **Requirement:** The requirement for vitamin E is based upon polyunsaturated fat intake. If a person has a very high intake of these fats (vegetable oils), vitamin E needs would increase.

   ● The RDA for this vitamin is set at 15 milligrams daily for both men and women, and increases to 19 milligrams during lactation.

4. **Food sources:** Vitamin E comes from plant sources rich with polyunsaturated fats. (Recall that whole grains contain the germ

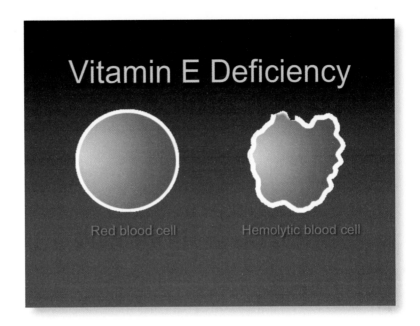

FIGURE 9.30

with small amounts of these fats that need protection from oxidation so the plant has ingeniously put vitamin E there for that very reason.) Food sources are listed in Figure 9.31.

5. **Toxicity:** Out of the four fat-soluble vitamins, vitamin E appears to be the least toxic. The Tolerable Upper Safe Limit (UL) is set at 1,000 milligrams daily. Risks associated with excess vitamin E include bleeding (the blood does not clot as well) and flu-like symptoms.

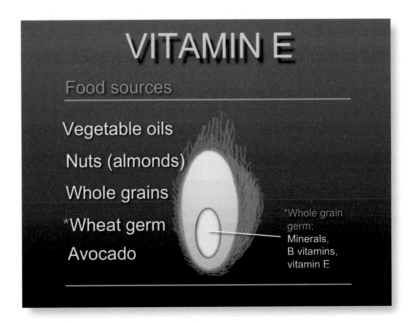

FIGURE 9.31

1. **Function:** This vitamin functions as a regulatory nutrient and specifically:

   - Plays a role in several steps of blood clot formation

   - Is involved in the mineralization of bone (specifically a modification of a bone protein)

2. **Deficiency:** Vitamin K deficiency is not common since some of our "intake" of this vitamin comes from the contribution of intestinal bacteria. These friendly microbes in our intestines make vitamin K, providing us a source of the vitamin even if our intake is low. Deficiency typically arises when a person has been taking antibiotics for an extended period of time (these medications kill infectious bacteria along with our beneficial intestinal bacteria).

   Also, certain people take anti-vitamin K drugs so that their blood will be less likely to clot. Can you guess whom? People with heart disease and narrowed arteries don't want their blood to clot in these clogged vessels so "thinner" blood is best.

3 and 4. Requirement and food sources: The requirement and basic food sources are listed in Figure 9.32.

At birth when you entered the world your intestines were sterile or free of friendly bacteria. During the first few days of life, you got by with an injection of vitamin K given to all newborns to avoid the risk of bleeding.

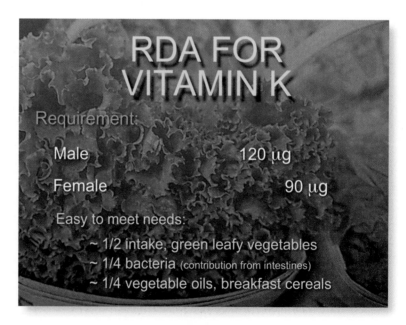

FIGURE 9.32

RDA FOR VITAMIN K

Requirement:

Male	120 µg
Female	90 µg

Easy to meet needs:

~ 1/2 intake, green leafy vegetables
~ 1/4 bacteria (contribution from intestines)
~ 1/4 vegetable oils, breakfast cereals

Do You Need a Vitamin-Mineral Supplement?

After our two chapter discussion of the micronutrients—minerals and vitamins—you may have the feeling that you might be in need of supplementation. Deficiency consequences sound devastating and you may realize by now that your diet is not optimal. From your Diet Project forms you can assess your typical intake and compare it to established requirements. This comparison may alert you to a less than adequate diet in one or more nutrients. Should you consider a supplement to boost your intake of the vitamins and minerals? As we will learn in Chapter 10, whole foods offer a wealth of phytochemicals in addition to vitamins and minerals that help protect our bodies from age-related diseases. This is one of the benefits of whole foods over supplements.

For the most part, our intake of many vitamins and minerals is more than adequate due to our consumption of vitamin- and mineral-fortified foods such as breakfast cereals, energy bars, and beverages. There are times, however, when you may want to consider a supplement. Here are several considerations for use of a general multivitamin and mineral supplement that contains no more than 100 percent of the RDA for the micronutrients.

If your calorie intake is less than 1,500 calories daily (especially if you are female or elderly). At low-calorie intakes, it is challenging to meet your need for all the micronutrients. You must choose fruits, vegetables, whole grains, beans, lean meats, etc. This leaves little if any room for empty calorie foods such as candy or soda.

If you consume alcohol regularly and in excessive amounts. As discussed in the next chapter, alcohol effects nutrient status several ways, essentially putting you at risk for vitamin and mineral deficiencies.

If you are pregnant, or planning on becoming pregnant. Nutrient needs change and having good folate status is important for the prevention of certain birth defects. Also, iron needs rise so dramatically during pregnancy that a supplement is necessary.

If your eating habits are irregular or if you habitually make poor food choices. This perhaps fits your eating habits and hopefully by this point in the course you are interested in improving your food choices. In the event you do continue to eat irregularly, a multivitamin and mineral supplement helps fill in the gaps on those days when you eat poorly.

When choosing a multivitamin and mineral supplement, there are many choices such as high-priced brands to generic or store-name brands. Generally these less expensive brands are made by some of the best supplement makers and are just as good as high-priced varieties. Unfortunately, as we will learn in the next section, the quality of supplements overall is poorly regulated so you can never be sure of what you are purchasing.

Dietary Supplements—Regulation and Safety

Vitamin pills, herbal preparation, and protein powders are just a few of the some 29,000 different dietary supplements sold in the United States. An estimated 40 percent of all Americans take one or more dietary supplements on a regular basis, leading to sales that exceeds $16 billion annually. What you may not be aware of are the laws that regulate the safety and efficacies of supplements are different than that that governs food. In fact, purchasing a dietary supplement is a "buyer beware" type of situation because the Food and Drug Administration does not strictly regulate this industry.

Let's first define a dietary supplement. (See Figure 9.33.)

The Food and Drug Administration, which is responsible for overseeing dietary supplements, states that they are intended to supplement the diets of some people, but not to replace the balance of the variety of foods important to a healthy diet.

The Dietary Supplement Health and Education Act (DSHEA) of 1994 has impacted the supplement industry and what manufacturers are able to state as claims on the label, in advertising and promotional materials including websites. In accordance with DSHEA, supplement labels may carry "statements of nutritional support," which describes the effect of the ingredient on the body. This is called a structure function claim. But label claims cannot make statements of drug-like effects. Examples of permissible and prohibited claims are shown in Figure 9.34.

Since the FDA has not evaluated manufacturers' claims, they must bear a disclaimer on the label as shown in Figure 9.35.

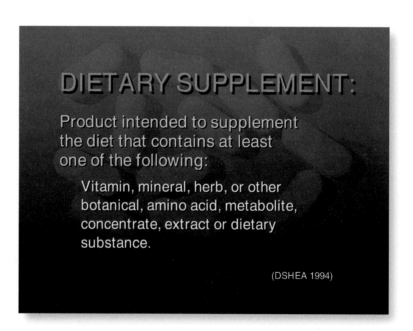

DIETARY SUPPLEMENT:

Product intended to supplement the diet that contains at least one of the following:

Vitamin, mineral, herb, or other botanical, amino acid, metabolite, concentrate, extract or dietary substance.

(DSHEA 1994)

FIGURE 9.33

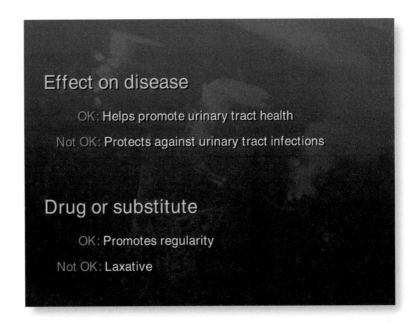

FIGURE 9.34

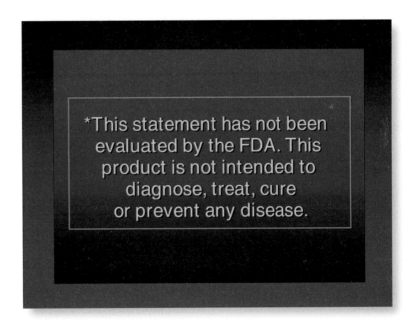

FIGURE 9.35

The manufacturer must be able to substantiate that structure/function statements are truthful, but they are NOT required to provide substantiation unless asked. So in other words, the FDA does NOT approve statements of nutritional support, but the FDA can object to them.

When considering a dietary supplement, there are some things you should consider such as how to spot a fraudulent product. The following are some bogus claims that should alert you that the claims are most likely "too good to be true."

- "break through"
- "magical"
- "miracle cure"
- "new discovery"

Here are several things to consider about supplements as it relates to potential health problems:

- Dietary supplements are NOT checked for quality and quantity of active ingredients. (This means you can't be sure what you are taking.)
- Some supplements may interact with prescriptions and over-the-counter medicines.
- Some supplements may increase complications during surgery (such as causing excessive bleeding).
- Many supplements have unsafe side effects. (Under the DSHEA of 1994 this is out of FDA's control.)

When you use the Internet for supplement information, here are some tips before you buy:

Look for sites operated by the government, health organizations, or universities (FDA, American Heart Association, or National Institute of Health).

Look for sites without advertisements (commercial sites promote their products).

Question the source of the information (referenced with scientific journals, qualified author).

Check this site for good info—*http://dietary-supplements.info.nih.gov.*

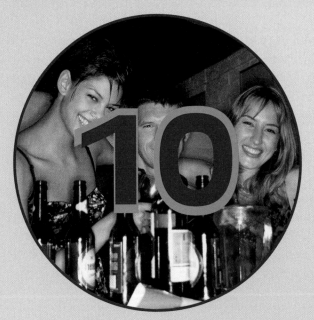

Special Topics That May Save Your Life!

We've covered all the nutrient classes and looked at the impact that some of these have on health and disease (fat and heart disease, for example). Now let's turn our attention to two special topics—alcohol and cancer. In the case of alcohol, consumption of this substance profoundly impacts a person's nutritional status. In our discussion, you will see how both in the short and long term, alcohol compromises health. Our discussion of cancer is an excellent way to tie in the various nutrients, their functions, and the role they may play in the prevention of this often age-related disease.

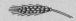

NUTRITIONAL IMPACT OF ALCOHOL

Our discussion of alcohol first focuses on its metabolism and then on how this substance impacts nutritional status.

Alcohol and Its Metabolism

● Alcohol is a two-carbon molecule that is made from the fermentation of carbohydrates. Hops and barley (complex carbohydrates), for example, are fermented to make beer (with the aid of organisms such as yeast), which breaks down the carbohydrate to a two-carbon unit (similar to how glucose and fatty acids are broken down during their aerobic energy metabolism—recall from Chapters 4 and 5). Fruit such as grapes are fermented to make wine. Even though alcohol comes from carbohydrate—it is NOT a carbohydrate. Contrary to what some people may think, alcohol is not a nutrient.

- Alcohol is small and a very simple molecule, thus it requires NO digestion. Unlike other substances we eat, alcohol can be absorbed through the stomach. If food is present, then the absorption through the stomach is slowed and the alcohol moves on to the small intestine for absorption (as shown in Figure 10.1). So, on an empty stomach, more alcohol enters your circulation, thereby impacting your brain and subsequently motor function, speech, and judgment compared to drinking alcohol with food.

- In the stomach lining, there is a small amount of an enzyme that can break down alcohol before it reaches the bloodstream. Men possess a bit more of this enzyme than women. Thus, at this first stage, less of the alcohol passes through into the circulation when a man has an alcoholic drink compared to a woman drinking the same amount of alcohol.

Nutrition Bite

Men and women also differ in their ability to handle alcohol because of body composition differences. Since alcohol is water soluble, it "dissolves" in the blood and body water. Men have more body water than women (greater lean mass, less body fat—see Chapter 1), which means that for a man and woman of equal body size, the man has a greater volume of body water (blood included) to "dissolve" the alcohol. This means that after drinking the same of amount of alcohol, a woman would have a greater blood alcohol level compared to an equal-sized man.

- The liver is the primary site for the metabolism or breakdown of alcohol, as shown in Figure 10.2. The enzyme, alcohol dehydrogenase, is responsible for converting alcohol (two-carbon unit) on to its way into the same two-carbon unit that is obtained from the breakdown of fats, carbs, and protein for fuel that then feeds into the TCA cycle (look back to Chapter 5). Taking it through this cycle would break chemical bonds and release energy.

  Alcohol yields 7 calories per gram. The other option for alcohol is that, once converted to C_2 units, several can be "glued' together and a fatty acid can be made (which in turn leads to the making of a triglyceride or fat). This fat can then be shipped out of the liver and stored as body fat.

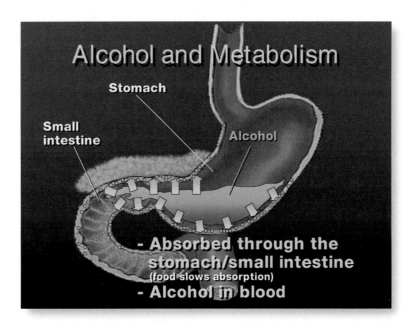

10.1

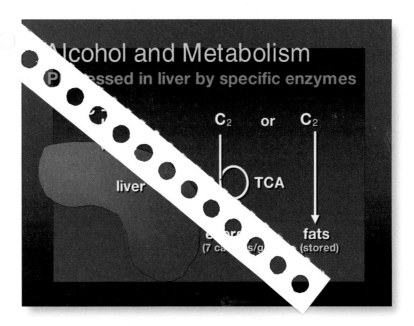

FIGURE 10.2

- Most livers (or people) have the ability to process 15 grams of alcohol per hour. This translates to one alcoholic drink per hour (12 ounces of beer, 5 ounces of wine, and 1.5 ounces of distilled spirits such as vodka). But this is just an estimate, because smaller people particularly women may not be able to process this much alcohol in one hour. Exceeding this intake would lead to elevated blood alcohol levels and the subsequent impact alcohol has on the brain (speech, inhibition level, coordination, etc.).

- Asians have a decreased ability to process alcohol due to lack of proper enzyme to deal with alcohol. This means Asians feel the effects of alcohol more readily and also have discomfort (facial redness) due to the buildup of an alcohol by-product that is not processed normally.

- Another set of enzymes also break down alcohol called the drug-metabolizing enzymes. These enzymes are also responsible for processing drugs such as painkillers and anesthesia. With chronic alcohol consumption (several drinks many days of the week), these enzymes adapt and can tolerate more alcohol and more drugs. This is why physicians ask about your alcohol use before going into surgery so as to know how much anesthesia to give. They don't want to under-dose and have you wake up on the operating table!

Impact of Alcohol on Liver Function

You can tell by this discussion that the liver is very busy processing alcohol each time a person takes a drink. But also recognize that the liver puts alcohol on the top of its priority list. This means the liver puts aside its regular duties such as building fluid balance proteins (Chapter 3) or the packaging of fat into lipoproteins (Chapter 5). The consequence on continued presence of alcohol can be devastating to liver function and overall body health.

- **The liver has a decreased ability to convert amino acids to glucose.** This means that during times without food, glucose levels will not be maintained well (part of the reason why some people feel hungry after a night of drinking). The brain, in turn, will not get the necessary carbohydrate (glucose) that it normally would have from the liver.

- **The liver's ability to produce proteins decreases.** The liver makes a host of regulatory proteins such as fluid balance proteins, coating proteins for lipoproteins, and transport proteins that move vitamins and other substances in the blood. The most important proteins affected are the lipoprotein "coats" that allow the lipoproteins to move through the watery environment of the blood. (Go back to Chapter 5 to get a feel for this again—recall that lipoproteins transport fat and cholesterol to cells.)

- **Fat accumulates in the liver and further disrupts liver function.** Without the protein coat, the fat and cholesterol droplets get "stuck" in the liver. This leads to fat accumulation in the liver, and eventually fatty liver and liver disease results, ultimately leading to death in many alcoholics.

ALCOHOL'S INFLUENCE ON NUTRITIONAL STATUS

Beyond alcohol's interference with liver function, this beverage also impacts nutritional status. Alcohol does this four ways:

1. **Ingestion:** When you drink alcohol, you most likely are not eating what you would have otherwise. This means you are "drinking" your calories rather than sitting down to a healthful meal. Also, alcohol can reduce your appetite. Thus, you may eat less food, particularly nutritious foods such as fruits and vegetables.

   Most nutrients are impacted by reduced ingestion—protein, vitamins, and minerals.

2. **Absorption:** In the intestinal tract, alcohol reduces or impairs the absorption of many micronutrients. Those most impacted include thiamin, folate (alcohol interferes with the conversion of folate to folic acid—the form the body uses), iron, and vitamin B_{12}. (The formation of Intrinsic Factor—made in the stomach—is interfered with by alcohol.)

3. **Metabolism:** Alcohol can actually alter the way a specific nutrient is handled or metabolized by the body. Several nutrients are "mishandled" because of alcohol, including vitamins D and A. (A healthy liver is needed for the proper metabolism of these vitamins.)

4. **Excretion:** Alcohol acts as a diuretic, which means it increases urine production. As a result, the kidneys are compromised in doing their job of filtering the blood. The result is an increased excretion of minerals zinc, potassium, calcium, and magnesium, along with folic acid.

EMPTY CALORIES AND YOUR DIET

It's a great time to bring up the concepts of **empty calorie foods** and **nutrient dense foods.** Alcohol provides 7 calories per gram and no essential nutrients. These calories then are "empty" in terms of overall contribution to your diet (see Figure 10.3 for calorie content of alcoholic beverages).

Empty Calorie Food: This food (or beverage) provides little or nothing in the way of essential nutrients relative to the number of calories per serving.

Examples of empty calorie foods include candy, chips, soda, and alcohol. Think back to your Diet Project and what you ate—what are a few empty calorie foods in your diet? Consider the amount of empty calorie foods you eat and what room is left for meeting your need for

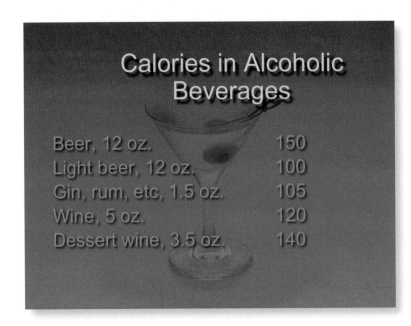

FIGURE 10.3

protein, fiber, and other essential nutrients. Figure 10.4 shows what most Americans consume in the way of empty calories.

Eating fewer empty calorie foods and replacing them with foods and beverages that have more to offer in the way of essential nutrients may make sense for you.

Nutrient Dense Foods: These foods or beverages provide a good amount of one or more essential nutrients relative to the number of calories per serving.

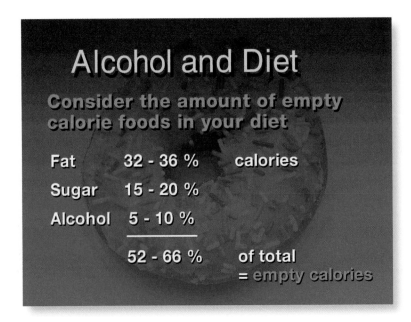

FIGURE 10.4

Examples of nutrient dense foods include low-fat or non-fat dairy products, fruits, vegetables, and lean meats. Think about what nutrient dense foods you already eat and what nutrient dense foods that you could substitute for empty calorie foods you are currently eating such as an apple for candy.

CHRONIC DISEASE—CANCER

In Chapter 6 we discussed the leading cause of death in the United States—heart disease. Cancer, another chronic, age-related disease, is number two on the list. Similar to heart disease, diet plays a major role in cancer risk (both increased and decreased). To get an understanding of cancer, let's take a look at its development on a cellular level. We'll use the development and progression of stomach cancer as our example.

- Cells in various organs and other tissues such as the stomach are constantly being replaced. A glitch can occur at some point when the genetic material called the DNA, which rests inside the nucleus of the cell, becomes altered or damaged. Referred to as **initiation** (shown in Figure 10.5), this alteration is caused by carcinogens (cancer-causing agents). Carcinogens can have dietary origins such as substances that form in food due to broiling or high-heat cooking. The cell now has a different or "bad" set of DNA, making it an altered cell.

- Given the right environment, this altered cell can grow (multiply) rapidly (shown in Figure 10.6)—referred to as **promotion,** this

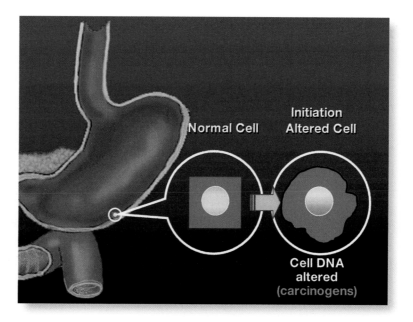

FIGURE 10.5

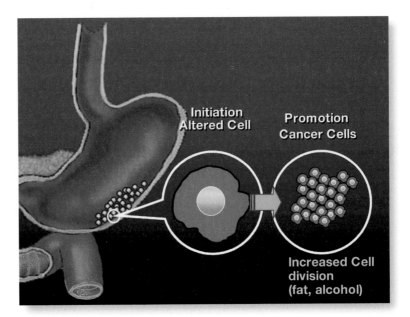

FIGURE 10.6

phase allows altered cells to quickly grow in numbers into cancer cells. High-fat diets and chronic alcohol consumption both act as cancer promoters to stomach cells.

- Once cancerous cells gain momentum, they take over an organ such as the stomach by taking nutrients away from healthy cells, compromising that organ's ability to function normally. Additionally, the cancer cells can migrate through the circulation and spread to other parts of the body. (See Figure 10.7.)

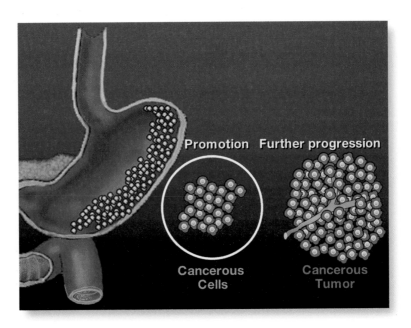

FIGURE 10.7

ROLE OF DIET—FOODS THAT WARD OFF CANCER OR THAT INCREASE YOUR RISK

The dietary link to cancer is very strong—research suggests that 30 to 60 percent of all cancers are preventable through diet modification. This diet-cancer prevention connection was demonstrated in a population research looking at prostate cancer risk in men from Japan and the United States. Prostate cancer risk is very low in Japan and researchers associate this with a traditional Eastern diet that includes several servings of soy foods weekly. When Japanese men move to the United States and adopt a Western diet (low soy food content, high in fat, low in fruits and vegetables), prostate cancer risk goes up and is comparable to American men of non-Japanese heritage. This suggests diet as a major factor rather than genetics.

Let's now take a look at specific factors in the diet that either increase or decrease cancer risk.

1. **Fat: ↑ risk**

   High-fat diets are linked to an increased risk of various cancers such as cancer of the large intestine (colon), breast cancer, and prostate cancer. Fat acts as a promoter.

2. **Fiber: ↓ risk**

   A diet that is ample in whole grains such as barley, whole wheat, and brown rice, along with fruits and vegetables, supplies plenty of fiber and is associated with a reduction of cancer risk, particularly of the large intestine. Fiber (recall from Chapter 4) helps speed the passage of waste and this would in turn reduce the exposure time to potential carcinogens. Also, fiber bulks up the mass of material and dilutes carcinogens in the large intestine.

3. **Antioxidants (Vitamins C and E and beta-carotene): ↓ risk**

   A diet rich in these antioxidants found in fruits, vegetables (especially yellow-orange and green leafy types), and whole grains (source of vitamin E) have been linked to a reduced cancer risk. These antioxidants are believed to protect cell membranes and cell nuclei from oxidative damage (caused by air pollution, cigarette smoke, etc.). This antioxidant protection helps ward off carcinogens and possible cancer initiation.

4. **Salt-cured, char-broiled, pickled, or smoked foods: ↑ risk**

   A diet that supplies these foods on a very regular basis (such as frequent or daily eating of barbeque meats, deli meats, and pickled foods) has been linked to increased cancer risk. These foods contain carcinogens. Char-broiled meats, for example, contain a carcinogen called heterocyclic amines or HAA for short (HAAs form when the protein in meat is burnt or cooked at high heat). You needn't worry though, if these foods are not a large part of your diet.

5. Protective factors in food called phytochemicals: ↓ risk

Plants—like fruits, vegetables, and whole grains—contain an array of substances that protect the plant (a tomato growing on a vine, for example) from its environment—UV light, air pollution, and parasites. These protective substances are called **phytochemicals** and when you eat a tomato, these substances go to work in you. Some phytochemicals actually block tumor growth; others halt or interfere with the initiation phase. Many of these phytochemicals have become popular for people to take as supplements. Isoflavones in soy foods, for example, are sold as supplements and people take them in hopes of reducing breast or prostate cancer risk. It's important to point out that research supports foods (soy foods) that supply isoflavones as cancer protection and not supplements. Researchers feel that isoflavones may interact with other items in food such as fiber or other nutrients to give the cancer protection benefit. Taking a supplement of isoflavones only gives you the one phytochemical, not the phytochemical in context with the whole food where the protection lies.

6. Alcohol: ↑ risk

Studies show that drinking more than two alcoholic drinks per day increases cancer risk. Alcohol is a promoter and makes the environment more conducive for cancer cells to thrive. Adding smoking cigarettes to the "mix" with alcohol increases the risk for cancer exponentially. Smoke and substances in cigarettes are carcinogens. When combined, the two (cigarette smoking and drinking) become more dangerous than when alone.

7. Mutagens: ↑ risk

Mutagens are substances that cause cells to mutate and more likely to turn into cancer cells. Some foods contain mutagens that are naturally present. Celery and mushrooms, for example, contain mutagens. However, these vegetables also supply protection against cancer with their phytochemical content. The cancer risk of naturally occurring mutagens is very low unless a person goes overboard and eats an excessive amount of a particular food (eating celery morning, noon, and night and drinking celery juice).

8. Additives and pesticides: ↑ risk

Some additives in foods do have carcinogenic potential, if consumed in large enough amounts. But the Food and Drug Administration strictly controls the use of additives and prohibits the use of those that represent a true cancer threat. Eating a varied diet helps lower even further this low risk from additives.

The same goes for pesticides that are used in traditional growing methods of fruits, vegetables, and whole grains. But this risk is very low. Since fruits, vegetables, and grains offer cancer-protection benefit, researchers feel that this very small risk is not worth worrying about.

DIETARY RECOMMENDATIONS TO REDUCE CANCER RISK

After discussing these various factors that increase and decrease cancer risk, specific dietary recommendations can be made. These dietary recommendations are listed in Figure 10.8 and incorporate the major dietary components such as fat, fiber, fruits, vegetables, and other sources of protective factors that modify cancer risk.

After reviewing these, you should be prepared to tell a friend who is interested in lowering cancer risk what dietary modifications to make and why.

FIGURE 10.8

RECOMMENDATIONS TO REDUCE CANCER RISK

- Control weight/obesity prevention
- Eat <30% of calories as fat
- Eat 25–35 grams of fiber daily
- Include a variety of fruits and vegetables (orange-yellow and leafy types, cruciferous)
- Consume salt-cured, smoked and char-broiled foods in moderation
- Consume alcoholic beverages in moderation

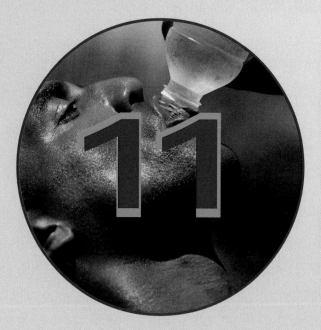

11 Nutrition and Athletic Performance

As we wrap up our overview of introductory nutrition in these final chapters, applying what we've learned to certain groups of individuals helps solidify our new understanding of nutrition. In this chapter, we integrate and apply what we've learned about nutrition and its role in physical activity and performance. A person who participates in regular physical activity, which I refer to as an *athlete* (you don't have to compete to be an athlete!), has specific nutritional concerns. Undoubtedly, you've seen ads on the Internet or in magazines about special sports-related drinks, powders, and pills that claim to enhance athletic performance. Although many of these ads may be enticing, true nutritional issues for athletes focus more on the macronutrient needs (protein, carbohydrate, and fat) rather than special substances said to enhance performance. Certainly sport drinks and energy bars have their place in an athlete's diet, but a grasp of the basics goes a long way when setting up an eating plan for active people.

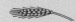

In this chapter, you will be pulling information from previous chapters and applying it to nutrition issues for athletes. We will cover:

▶ Energy use during exercise—role of carbs and fat

▶ Importance of carbohydrates for performance and recovery

▶ Water and sport drinks—what's best to drink and how much

▶ Performance boosting aids—what works and what to avoid

From this we develop practical recommendations about energy, carbohydrate, and protein needs, along with vitamins and minerals. Additionally, we also include issues regarding competition such as what to eat before exercise and how best to stay hydrated. With these topics and the additional sports nutrition articles in the Appendix, you may well find some practical dietary advice that will assist you in your efforts to stay healthy and fit.

ENERGY USE DURING EXERCISE—ROLE OF CARBOHYDRATE AND FAT

Determining an athlete's nutritional need involves revisiting energy metabolism. In Chapter 5, we integrated energy metabolism of carbohydrate, protein, and fat. In this chapter, we'll take another look at energy metabolism but in relationship to the impact of exercise. Think of the different types of physical activity you engage in—running, weight lifting, walking, bike riding, and kick boxing, to name a few. These activities require differing efforts on your part and, in turn, require different proportions of carbohydrate and fat as fuel. Let's take a look at the energy expenditure for different types of exercise and then the types of fuel used during these activities.

Taking a look at the chart in Figure 11.1, you can see why an athlete requires more energy or calories per day than a person who is sedentary. Competitive athletes may need anywhere from 3,000 to over 5,000 calories daily compared to a typical inactive person who needs about 1,800 to 2,200 calories. Also notice that the weight-bearing exercises such as running burn more calories per hour than a non-weight-bearing activity. Moving your body against gravity requires more effort. In addition, men burn more calories than women for the same activity because they have more muscle mass and require more energy to support and move muscle than women who have more "inexpensive" fat tissue.

Energy expenditure during exercise (calories/hour)

	Male 170 lbs	Female 130 lbs
Bicycling (15 mph)	800	600
Running (8.5 min/mile)	925	700
Stair Climbing (machine med. effort)	485	370
Swimming (freestyle, moderate)	645	490
Walking (4 mph)	320	245

FIGURE 11.1

Fuel Sources

What are fuel sources in the body to support this activity? Recall from previous chapters that the energy nutrients are protein, carbohydrate, and fat. In your body, you can store both fat and carbohydrate but protein is not stored. Instead, body protein is functional tissue—serving a purpose. As review:

- **Carbohydrate:** Stored in the body as glycogen in the muscle and liver in limited quantities.

- **Fat:** Stored in virtually unlimited quantities throughout the body.

- **Protein:** Not stored in the body but is functional tissue such as muscles, organ protein or enzymes (little of your energy needs come from protein—about 5 to 10 percent).

Inside a typical athlete, how much does all this represent in the way of calories? Since protein is not stored as energy and little is used as fuel, let's just look at stored carbohydrate and fat. Figure 11.2 shows the energy store of a fit, 70 kg (155 pound) man who has about 10 percent body fat. (Recall that 15 percent body fat is average or normal for a college-aged male.)

Fuel Use during Exercise

Let's go back to the integration of carbohydrate, fat, and protein energy metabolism to understand what fuel sources, and in what proportion they are used during various exercises. The diagram in Figure 11.3 (from Chapter 5) summarizes carbohydrate, fat, and protein energy metabolism. Since protein use for fuel is small, we'll ignore this for now. (However,

Body energy stores in 70 kg male (10% body fat)

Body Fuel	Weight (kg)	Calories
Fat	7	63,000
Glycogen		
Liver	0.08-0.1	300-400
Muscle	0.3-0.4	1,200-1,600
Blood glucose	0.03	100

FIGURE 11.2

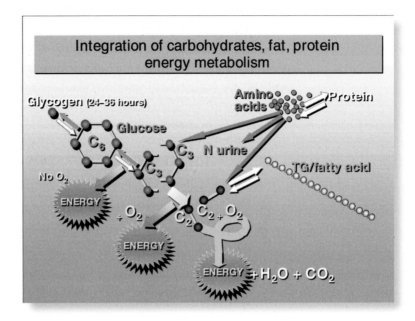

FIGURE 11.3

protein fuel use can be an issue if glycogen stores have been depleted and no incoming carbohydrates are available—glucose must be made from protein to supply fuel for the brain.) This can occur during endurance exercise lasting more than a few hours.

What fuel sources are used during exercise, and under what conditions are certain fuels (specifically carbohydrate versus fat) preferred by the working muscles?

High-Intensity, Sprint Types of Activity

All muscle activity or work is driven or powered by a high-energy molecule called ATP. You have enough ATP in your muscles to last a few seconds for a burst of activity and then the ATP must be regenerated with the help of phosphocreatine. (More on creatine as a supplement to boost performance will be presented later in this chapter.) Even with this regeneration, you have less than 30 seconds worth of ATP. Your body then kicks into using glucose or C_6 anaerobically for fuel. Breaking down glucose without the presence of oxygen releases ATP (fuel) quickly and gives C_3 (see Figure 11.3).

Another name for this C_3 unit is lactic acid and if the amount of lactic acid produced exceeds what can be cleared by the muscle (and sent to the liver), the lactic acid accumulates. This along with an increasing acidity in the muscle contributes to fatigue during intense exercise (you know that "lead-like" feeling you may get as you do very intense exercise). This exclusive anaerobic use of glucose lasts up to about two minutes at which point the body can't keep up with the ATP demands and the lactic acid accumulation and must slow down to now use glucose and fat aerobically to regenerate ATP. (See Figure 11.4.)

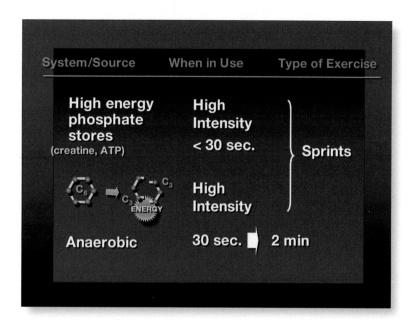

System/Source	When in Use	Type of Exercise

High energy phosphate stores (creatine, ATP) — High Intensity < 30 sec.

Anaerobic — High Intensity 30 sec. ▸ 2 min

Sprints

FIGURE 11.4

Continuous, Endurance Types of Activity

For exercises lasting more than two minutes, aerobic use of *both* carbohydrate and fat occur. Glucose (C_6) is broken down completely to CO_2, H_2O, and energy (ATP) and fat is also broken down to these same end products. The amount or proportion of carbohydrate and fat used during exercise is dependent upon the intensity of that activity. The more intense exercise, such as hard running or an intense game of soccer, uses more energy per minute and a greater proportion of that energy is supplied by carbohydrate compared to less-intense exercises, such as walking or moderate cycling. During lower intensity exercises, less energy per minute is spent and a greater proportion of that fuel comes from fat. (See Figures 11.5 and 11.6.)

Figure 11.7 shows the use and site of fat and carbohydrate fuel stores. Fat (triglyceride) comes out of the fat cells as well as some triglyceride that is stored as small droplets in the muscle. Glycogen, which is stored in muscles, is used by that muscle for carbohydrate fuel.

What about "Fat-Burning" Exercises?

Perhaps you heard from a friend or read in a popular magazine that certain exercises "burn" more body fat than others, so you'll lose more weight. Before you decide to buy into this idea, first let's go back—how is body fat lost? Recall from Chapter 7 on obesity and weight loss that calorie intake must be less than calorie output to lose body fat. You can do this by reducing the number of calories going in (what you eat), increasing the number going out (your activity), or a combination of both.

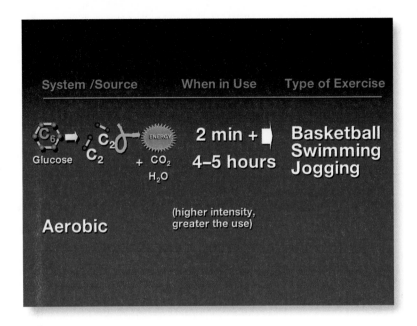

FIGURE 11.5

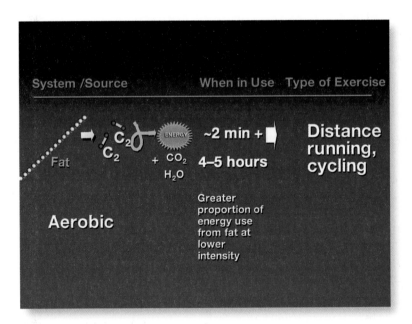

FIGURE 11.6

If you choose to boost your activity to lose weight, it actually makes no difference what you do in the way of activity—just do it! Burning calories by walking slowly or running fast both expend calories and ultimately you will lose body fat if you end the day in a calorie deficit. Even though walking may burn proportionately more fat while fast running burns mostly carbohydrate and little fat, you readjust fuel burning during the rest of the day. Ultimately, creating a calorie deficit leads to fat loss as long as you don't compensate by filling in the energy gap by eating more food.

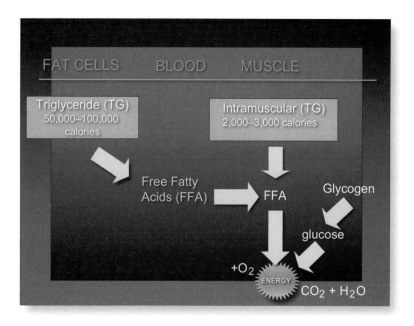

FIGURE 11.7

IMPORTANCE OF CARBOHYDRATES FOR PERFORMANCE AND RECOVERY

Now that we know the importance of both fat and carbohydrate as fuel sources during exercise, let's take a look at carbohydrates specifically since they are stored in limited amounts. As described above, a typical athlete stores approximately 2,000 calories of carbohydrate as glycogen in the muscles and liver. But fat is stored in a virtually "unlimited" supply. So as you might expect, during continuous exercise such as cycling or running (or a long game of soccer) glycogen stores are depleted, specifically in the muscles that do most of the work. This depletion of glycogen stores is illustrated in Figure 11.8.

Research studies have shown repeatedly that boosting glycogen stores through increasing dietary carbohydrate intake in turn raises glycogen stores and prolongs endurance. In short, if you increase the amount of carbs in your diet, you can run, cycle, swim, etc. farther and longer. Figure 11.9 illustrates results of scientific research and the relationship of dietary carbohydrate intake, muscle glycogen stores, and endurance performance.

Researchers put a set of highly trained cyclists on a low-carbohydrate diet of about 40 percent carbohydrate calories (certainly not as low as an Atkin's type diet). The cyclists ate this diet for several days and then showed up to the laboratory for testing. Their muscle glycogen levels (in calf muscle) were measured and then they were asked to pedal at a set workload for as long as they could. The researchers noted that the cyclists could only pedal for 50 minutes. **Low carbs in the diet meant low glycogen levels and, in turn, poor endurance.**

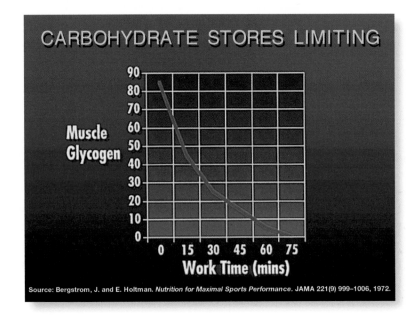

FIGURE 11.8

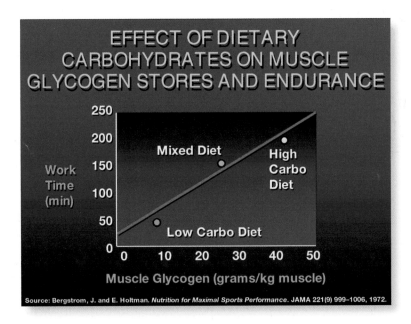

FIGURE 11.9

The same cyclists were then put on another diet—about 55 percent of calories as carbohydrate for several days. The same muscle glycogen and endurance tests were performed. This time the cyclists had more glycogen in their calf muscles and could pedal 150 minutes at that same workload. **So more dietary carbohydrate and greater muscle glycogen stores meant better endurance.**

For a third time the same cyclists were put through the test following a high-carbohydrate diet of 70 percent of the calories. Muscle glycogen stores were greater (but note not as dramatic an increase from the low to the medium carb diet, suggesting a limit to glycogen storage). The cyclists' endurance also improved, but as with muscle glycogen, not as dramatic an increase compared to the previous diet. But still, the relationship of increasing dietary carbohydrate, which increases muscle glycogen, and in turn endurance remains true.

From this research, others are able to make recommendations regarding carbohydrate intake for athletes (particularly endurance types). The Daily Value for carbohydrate is 300 grams (for a person eating a 2,000 calorie diet) and for athletes, 450 to 600 grams daily or about 60 to 65 percent of calories as carbohydrate is suggested. An athlete can also base his or her carbohydrate intake relative to body weight. Most athletes are recommended to consume between 6–10 g per kg body weight. This amount ensures recovery of glycogen stores following workouts so that another workout can be performed the next day.

Figure 11.10 summarizes the benefits of boosting carbohydrate intake for athletes.

So *Where Does Protein and Fat Fit in the Diets of Athletes?*

Recall from Chapter 2 that protein needs increase with exercise. This occurs for two reasons: (1) small amounts of protein are needed to repair damaged muscle proteins as a result of exercise (bumps and bruises along with tissue rebuilding following strength training exercise); and (2) the small amount of protein that is used as fuel during exercise can add up for an endurance-type athlete who is working out for a couple of hours or more daily. The amount of increase above the RDA of 0.8 grams/kg body per day is about 50 percent (or about 1.2 to 1.6 g/kg body weight daily).

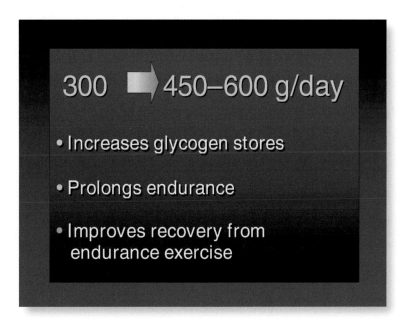

FIGURE 11.10

But this amount can easily be met through diet. Taking in about 15 percent of the total calories from protein from foods such as soy, fish, poultry, lean meats, low-fat dairy, and bean-grain combinations is recommended for athletes.

Fat is an important source of calories in an athlete's diet. Especially for those expending over 4,000 to 5,000 plus calories daily, a source of calorie-dense fat helps keep energy intake up because the sheer volume of food eaten becomes a challenge for some athletes. Healthful fats such as olive oil (in cooking or salads), avocados, nuts, and fish are good choices.

Figure 11.11 puts this all together in a recommended distribution of calories for athletes.

WATER AND SPORT DRINKS—WHAT'S BEST TO DRINK AND HOW MUCH

As you probably know from personal experience, your fluid needs increase with exercise. How you meet that need, through drinking plain water, sport drinks, or other beverages such as soda, fruit juice, or fitness water, is often hotly debated. Let's first look at why fluid needs increase and then how best to meet that need.

Water is an absolutely essential nutrient and even more so for athletes:

- As you exercise, your muscles generate heat—recall that you burn some 100 calories for every mile of running—and this heat must be dissipated or you would literally "cook" your muscles and other proteins in the body. The body rids itself of this heat by releasing water onto the surface of the skin as sweat. As this sweat evaporates, the

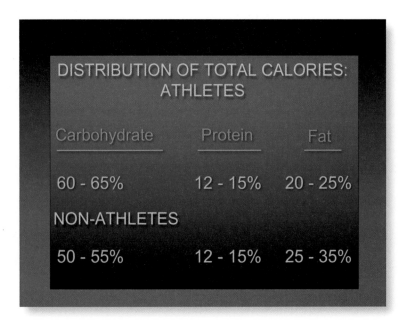

FIGURE 11.11

heat is "taken away." On average, you lose about a liter of water as sweat for every hour of continuous exercise. Evaporation of this liter takes away about 600 calories of heat.

- Water is also the medium that makes up the blood, which transports oxygen, carbohydrates, and other nutrients to hard-working muscles.

- With exercise, waste products are produced that must be transported out of cells via the circulation and excreted through the lungs (CO_2) or urine (metabolic waste). Again, we rely on body water to carry out this process.

Nutrition Bite

Sweat rates are greater in endurance-trained athletes—marathon runners have been known to lose over 2 ½ liters of sweat per hour!

As the body loses water due to sweating, several changes take place:

- A reduction of cardiac output (volume the heart pumps) as blood volume drops
- Drop in blood flow to the muscles and skin surface
- Reduction in sweat rate

With this loss of body water and compromise to several body systems comes symptoms and consequences of **dehydration,** the loss of body fluids.

Some signs and consequences of dehydration due to sweating are heat accumulation in the body—you feel nauseous, fatigued, and experience loss of appetite; with declining cardiac function and increasing body temperature, performance is decreased; and you may feel flushed, lightheaded, and suffer from muscle cramps.

Fluid replacement is key before, during, and after exercise to avoid dehydration and its consequences. Here are some fluid replacement guidelines:

- Drink about 2 cups of fluid prior to exercise
- Drink ½ cup to 1 cup every 20 minutes during exercise. You may need less if you are exercising in a cooler climate or have a low sweat rate.

What's Best to Drink?

Water? Sport drink? Or what about the new fitness waters? Athletes must consider the amount of time they are working out and the intensity of that exercise to make a decision about what's best to drink. Carbohydrate stores become limiting after about 90 minutes to over two hours of continuous exercise. Low blood sugar levels, which result when liver glycogen stores run low, also become a limitation to performance. As just described, dehydration limits performance as well. Thus, during continuous exercise lasting about 90 minutes or more, taking in a source of *both* carbohydrate and water makes sense.

Research shows that sport drinks help replenish lost fluids and provide carbohydrate to prolong endurance. Most sport drinks consist of a carbohydrate source such as sucrose, glucose, or maltodextrin (a small complex carbohydrate) dissolved in water at the concentration of about 6 to 9 percent by weight (carbohydrate). This amount of carbohydrate allows for fluid absorption in the intestine while at the same time providing energy for exercising muscles. A higher concentration of carbohydrate would slow fluid absorption (as in fruit juices, energy drinks, fruit drinks, and sodas) and may cause sloshing in the stomach or even nausea if consumed during exercise. Most sport drinks also supply small amounts of minerals (electrolytes) that help replenish what's lost in sweat and encourage further drinking. Figure 11.12 lists some popular sport drinks. (See Appendix p. 480 for more on sport drinks and uses.)

During exercise, aim for replenishing lost fluids and carbohydrates by:

- Drinking ¼ to ½ cup every 15 to 20 minutes

COMPARING SPORTS DRINKS
(per 8-ounce serving)

	Calories	Protein (g)	Carbohydrate (g)	Fat (g)
Accelerade	94	6.5	17	0
Cytomax	45	0	10	0
Gatorade	50	0	14	0
GU₂O	50	0	14	0
Powerade	65	0	17	0

Sport drinks are solution of 6-9% carbohydrate (sucrose, maltodextrins)

FIGURE 11.12

- Consuming 30 to 60 grams of carbohydrate every hour of continuous exercise

- Besides sport drink, also eating solid carbohydrate sources such as fruit, dried fruit, carbohydrate gels (sold in sporting good stores), or energy bars (check the label for carbohydrate content) (See Appendix p. 475 and 482.)

- Avoiding food with fat and protein because these are slow to digest and may cause stomach upset (additionally, fat and protein are not fuel sources in limiting supply during exercise). Some sport drinks contain protein which a limited amount of research suggests certain amino acids may help delay fatigue during endurance exercises.

What to Eat Before Exercise?

- While we're discussing how best to keep your body hydrated, you also may be curious about what's best to eat before a workout. Many athletes skip eating before they head off to a long practice or run several miles. Not a good decision. Your muscles are in need of carbohydrate energy and your brain is also dependent upon glucose for fuel. Eating a few hours before you exercise helps to keep energy levels up and boosts your endurance. Here are some guidelines for pre-workout eating:

  - Eat two to fours hours before you work out or compete. (Especially after a night's sleep, your body needs fuel.)

  - Eat food high in carbohydrate—about 100 to 200 grams depending upon your body size and level of exercise.

  - Choose food with a moderate amount of protein and low in fat. (These slow digestion but some is OK)

Example meal: Two slices whole wheat bread spread with jam and peanut butter, one banana, and a cup of soymilk or low-fat milk.

You can read more about preparing yourself for a race such as a marathon in the Appendix (see p. 478).

PERFORMANCE BOOSTING AIDS—WHAT WORKS AND WHAT TO AVOID

Athletes strive for their best whether that's running fast, scoring goals, or making a quick tackle. Beyond staying hydrated, eating ample carbohydrates, and in general consuming a healthful diet, athletes often turn to supplements that claim to enhance performance. These aids, sometimes called ergogenic aids, which means work-enhancing aids, are available on the Internet, in grocery stores, and at sport shops. Recall from our discussion of dietary supplements in Chapter 9, the FDA regulation of these products are minimal and that claims made are for the most part, not sub-stantiated. Here's a brief list of a few ergogenic aids:

- Amino acids
- Baking soda
- Bee pollen
- Caffeine
- Carnitine
- Creatine
- Ginseng
- Inosine
- Phosphate
- RNA/DNA
- Spirulina

You now know that, just because a supplement is sold, doesn't mean that it works or comes through on its claims. Many of these fall short on their performance claims, but a few have been shown through well-controlled scientific research to enhance performance. So how are you to know when you come across a potential supplement whether or not it lives up to its claims?

Here are some guidelines when evaluating a supplement:

- **Does the performance claim make sense?** That is, would it make sense for your body to adjust itself based on taking this substance or mixture? Remember homeostasis and the body's drive to stay constant internally.

- **What is the supporting evidence for the performance claim?** What supports the performance claim? Is it testimonials from ath-letes or scientific studies?

- **What is the consequence of taking the performance aid?** Are there any safety issues or concerns about the substance's legality (caffeine and other stimulants for example are banned in college and international competition).

When evaluating information on the Internet or in printed literature, it's important to determine the credibility of the source. Often manufac-turers may give a "science-like" look to their product information when actually it is written by the supplement makers and is not supported by unbiased scientific research.

Check the Appendix p. 484 for information on a variety of perform-ance aids, including creatine, caffeine, and others.

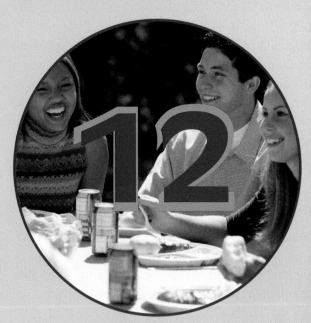

Pulling It All Together— Dietary Guidelines for Americans and Food Labeling

Take a moment and think about all that you have learned—from proteins, carbohydrates, and fats; to minerals, vitamins, and supplements; and obesity, cancer, and athletic performance. Immersing yourself in nutrition during this course has given you the knowledge to take charge of your health today and for a lifetime. In this chapter, you will pull together the concepts, principles, and facts from the previous eleven chapters and summarize them into guidelines for a healthy lifestyle. You can compare your food choices from the Diet Project you completed to the recommendations made here regarding optimal diet and health.

In this chapter we cover:

▶ Dietary guidelines—principles for healthy eating and physical activity

▶ Using food labels for choosing an optimal diet

As you read this last chapter think beyond the scope of this class and how the information you have learned can be incorporated into your daily life for better health.

DIETARY GUIDELINES—PRINCIPLES FOR HEALTHY EATING AND PHYSICAL ACTIVITY

The government, specifically the U.S. Department of Agriculture and Department of Health and Human Services, takes responsibility for making recommendations regarding diet and health. Every five years, these groups jointly issue a set of guidelines called the Dietary Guidelines for

Americans. Find in the Appendix on page 495 the actual booklet issued by the government, *Finding Your Way to a Healthier You* which we discuss here. Also, you can view this and more information about the Dietary Guidelines at www.healthierus.gov/dietaryguidelines.

The Dietary Guidelines for Americans are key recommendations that assist us in putting together a healthful lifestyle through an eating plan and recommendations for physical activity.

- This chapter covers the 41 key recommendations dealing with diet and exercise, divided into nine focus areas.

- Each focus area reflects the most current knowledge about diet, exercise and health. In January of 2010, the U.S. Department of Agriculture will issue a revision to these current Guidelines that will reflect new research and its implication to diet and exercise recommendations.

- The Dietary Guidelines are for use by everyone two years of age and older. There are specific recommendations for children, teens, and pregnant women. Refer to *www.healthierus.gov/dietaryguidelines* for more details on these and other detailed recommendations. (Figure 12.1)

- A Food Guide Pyramid developed from the Dietary Guidelines is available to assist in planning a healthy diet. This tool, explained later in this chapter, is an interactive and personalized guide that people can access via the Internet *www.mypryamid.gov*—and determine how their current diet and activity levels fit in with the current recommendations.

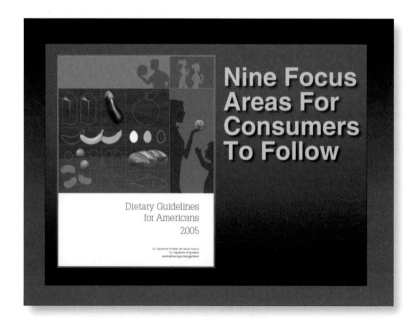

FIGURE 12.1

Focus Area #2

Weight Management: As discussed in Chapter 7, the prevalence of obesity in the US over the past 20 years has doubled—65% of the population is either overweight (BMI between 25 and 30) or obese (BMI > 30, 30% of the population). The number of children and teens that are overweight today also represents a doubling from 20 years ago. Excess body fat in both adults and youth represents a variety of health risks such as type 2 diabetes (insulin resistance), high blood cholesterol, high blood pressure, and heart disease. Maintaining a healthy weight will optimize health for adults and may reduce the likelihood that children will become overweight or obese as adults. As we discussed in Chapter 7, maintaining a healthy weight means achieving a balance with calorie intake and physical activity. Key recommendations made for this focus area include:

- To maintain body weight in a healthy range, balance calories from foods and beverages with calories expended.

- To prevent gradual weight gain over time, make small decreases in food and beverage calories and increase physical activity.

Promotion of general health: Managing your weight and keeping it in a healthy range (or making an effort to lose weight) boosts your health for today by enabling you to move freely and to reduce the likelihood of suffering from diabetes and other ailments that may hamper your daily living. See Figure 12.3 for determining your current BMI based upon your weight and height.

Prevention of chronic disease: By managing your weight, and keeping it in the healthy range for your height, you reduce your risk for a variety of ailments linked to excess body fat—heart disease, cancer, diabetes, high blood pressure, and more.

Focus Area #3

Physical Activity: Many Americans spend little time doing physical activities such as yard work, walking, or playing Frisbee, and spend too much time doing sedentary activities such as screen time in front of computers or TV. This lack of physical activity or sedentary lifestyle increases the risk of weight gain (overweight and obesity) and many chronic diseases such as heart disease, certain types of cancer, and osteoporosis. Incorporating daily physical activities can help lower risk for these and other diseases as well as help boost feelings of self-esteem and reduce feelings of anxiety. Key recommendations for physical activity include:

ADULT BMI CHART

Locate the height of interest in the left-most column and read across the row for the weight of interest. Follow the column of the weight up to the top row that lists the BMI. BMI of 19-24 is the health weight range, BMI 25–29 is the overweight range, and BMI of 30 and above is in the obese range.

BMI	19	20	21	22	23	24	25	26	27	28	29	30	31	32	33	34	35
Height	Weight in Pounds																
4'10"	91	96	100	105	110	115	119	124	129	134	138	143	148	153	158	162	167
4'11"	94	99	104	109	114	119	124	128	133	138	143	148	153	158	163	168	173
5'	97	102	107	112	118	123	128	133	138	143	148	153	158	163	158	174	197
5'1"	100	106	111	116	122	127	132	137	143	148	153	158	164	169	174	180	185
5'2"	104	109	115	120	126	131	136	142	147	153	158	164	169	175	180	186	191
5'3"	107	113	118	124	130	135	141	146	152	158	163	169	175	180	186	191	197
5'4"	110	116	122	128	134	140	145	151	157	163	169	174	180	186	192	197	204
5'5"	114	120	126	132	138	144	150	156	162	168	174	180	186	192	198	204	210
5'6"	118	124	130	136	142	148	155	161	167	173	179	186	192	198	204	210	216
5'7"	121	127	134	140	146	153	159	166	172	178	185	191	198	204	211	217	223
5'8"	125	131	138	144	151	158	164	171	177	184	190	197	203	210	216	223	230
5'9"	128	135	142	149	155	162	169	176	182	189	196	203	209	216	223	230	236
5'10"	132	139	146	153	160	167	174	181	188	195	202	209	216	222	229	236	243
5'11"	136	143	150	157	165	172	179	186	193	200	208	215	222	229	236	243	250
6'	140	147	150	162	169	177	184	191	199	206	213	221	228	235	242	250	258
6'1"	144	151	159	166	174	182	189	197	204	212	219	227	235	242	250	257	265
6'2"	148	155	163	171	179	186	194	22	210	218	225	233	241	249	256	264	272
6'3"	152	160	168	176	184	192	200	208	216	224	232	240	248	256	264	272	279
	Healthy Weight						Overweight					Obese					

Source: *Evidence Report of Clinical Guidelines of the Identification, and Treatment of Overweight and Obesity in Adults,* 1998. NIH/National Heart, Lung, and Blood Institute (NHLBI). Dietary Guidelines for Americans 2005.

FIGURE 12.3

- Engage in regular physical activity and reduce sedentary activities to promote health, psychological well-being, and healthy body weight.

- To reduce risk of chronic disease in adulthood: Engage in at least 30 minutes of moderate-intensity physical activity, above usual activity, at work or home on most days of the week.

- To help manage body weight and prevent the gain of gradual unhealthy body weight in adulthood: Engage in approximately 60 minutes of moderate– to vigorous-intensity activity on most days of the week while not exceeding caloric intake requirements.

- To sustain weight loss in adulthood: Participate in at least 60 to 90 minutes of daily moderate-intensity physical activity while not exceeding caloric intake requirements.

- Children and adolescents: Engage in at least 60 minutes of physical activity on most, preferably all, days of the week.

While these recommended amounts of physical activity may seem daunting for some of us, know that it is the accumulated total minutes each day for health and weight control effects. You can accumulate 60 minutes of activity for example through 6 bouts of 10 minutes of moderate to vigorous physical activity throughout the day (climbing the stairs, a quick walk to class, carrying groceries a few blocks home, and so forth).

See Figure 12.4 for a listing of moderate and vigorous physical activities and the approximate number of calories burned for a 154 pound person (70 kg.)

Promotion of general health: Being physically active on a daily basis builds endurance and strength and enhances well-being, making it possible for you to function better during your day. Daily physical activity also enhances your ability to perform daily tasks such as carrying groceries, climbing upstairs, and lifting boxes.

Prevention of chronic disease: Regular physical activity reduces your risk for developing many of the major chronic ailments Americans suffer—heart disease, certain cancers, diabetes, osteoporosis, high blood pressure, and others. And by helping you manage your weight, physical activity helps reduce the health risks brought on by excess body fat.

Focus Area #4

Food Groups to Encourage: No one food has it all—protein, fiber, essential fats, all the vitamins, minerals, and other micronutrients (phytochemicals) crucial for good health. Eating a variety of foods, from fruits,

CALORIES/HOUR EXPENDED IN COMMON PHYSICAL ACTIVITIES

Some examples of physical activities commonly engaged in and the average amount of calories a 154-pound individual will expend by engaging in each activity for 1 hour. The expenditure value encompasses both resting metabolic rate calories and activity expenditure. Some of the activities can constitute either moderate- or vigorous-intensity physical activity depending on the rate at which they are carried out (for walking and bicycling).

Moderate Physical Activity	Approx. Calories/Hr for a 154 lb Person[a]
Hiking	370
Light gardening/yard work	330
Dancing	330
Golf (walking and carrying clubs)	330
Bicycling (<10 mph)	290
Walking (3.5 mpg)	280
Weight lifting	220
Stretching	180

Vigorous Physical Activity	Approx. Calories/Hr for a 154 lb Person[a]
Running/jogging (5 mph)	590
Bicycling (>10 mph)	590
Swimming (slow freestyle laps)	510
Aerobics	480
Walking (4.5 mph)	460
Heavy yard work (chopping wood)	440
Weight lifting (vigorous effort)	440
Basketball (vigorous)	440

[a] Calories burned per hour will be higher for persons who weigh more then 154 lbs (70 kg) and lower for persons who weight less.

Source: Adapted from the *2005 DGAC Report/Dietary Guidelines for Americans,* 2005.

FIGURE 12.4

vegetables, whole grains, and low-fat or fat-free dairy will help ensure we get all the vital nutrients in the amounts needed. Research shows that people who eat a variety of fruits and vegetables have reduced risk for the chronic diseases such as heart disease and certain cancers. Consuming adequate calcium from dairy products for building healthy bones in young people and later in life is crucial for maintaining bone health. This focus area gives specific recommendations for intake of fruits, vegetables, whole grains, and dairy (or equivalent calcium rich foods/beverages). The Food Guide Pyramid (MyPyramid) incorporates these recommendations and bases them on caloric needs/intake. Key recommendations include the following food groups:

- Eat 2 cups of fruits and 2½ cups of vegetables per day for a reference 2,000 calorie intake with higher or lower amounts depending on the calorie level.

- Choose a variety of fruits and vegetables in each group. In particular, select from all five vegetable subgroups (dark green, orange, legumes, starchy vegetables, and other vegetables) several times a week. (See Figure 12.2 for specifics.)

- Consume 3 or more once-equivalents of whole grain products per day, with the rest of the recommended grains coming from enriched or wholegrain products. In general, at least half the grains should come from whole grains. (See Figure 12.5 for a listing of whole grains.)

- Consume 3 cups per day of fat-free or low-fat milk or equivalent milk products.

Promotion of general health: Selecting a variety of foods from the various food groups will ensure adequate intake of various essential nutrients needed for good health. **MyPyramid** in the next section outlines the food groups and recommended amounts based upon calorie needs.

Prevention of chronic disease: Eating a diet with ample amounts of fiber, vitamins, minerals, and phytochemicals from plant foods (vegetables, fruits, and whole grains) along with getting adequate calcium and protein will aid in lowering risk for chronic diseases such as certain forms of cancer, heart disease, diabetes, and more.

Focus Area #5

Fats: We learned in Chapters 5 and 6 that certain fats are essential, and that other fats—namely saturated and trans fats—when consumed in excess increase risk for heart disease. Fats are also an important source of fuel and are necessary for absorption of fat-soluble vitamins A, D, E, and K along with other fat-soluble micronutrients. Key recommendations for fat include:

- Consume less than 10 percent of calories from saturated fatty acids and less than 300 mg/day of cholesterol, and keep trans fatty acid consumption as low as possible.

WHOLE GRAINS AVAILABLE IN THE UNITED STATES

Whole grains that are consumed in the United States either as a single food (i.e., wild rice, popcorn) or as an ingredient in a multi ingredient food (i.e., in multi-grain breads).

Whole Wheat

Whole oats/oatmeal

Whole-grain corn

Popcorn

Brown rice

Whole rye

Whole-grain barley

Wild rice

Buckwheat

Bulgur (cracked wheat)

Millet

Quinoa

Sorghum

Source: *Agriculture Research Database CSFII 1994–1996/Dietary Guidelines for Americans, 2005.*

FIGURE 12.5

- Keep total fat intake between 20 to 35 percent of calories, with most fats coming from sources of polyunsaturated and monounsaturated fatty acids such as fish, nuts, and vegetable oils.

- When selecting and preparing meat, poultry, dry beans, and milk or milk products, make choices that are lean, low-fat, or fat-free. See Figure 12.6 for comparisons in saturated fat amounts in some common foods.

- Limit intake of fats and oils high in saturated and/or trans fatty acids, and choose products low in such fats and oils.

Promotion of general health: Limiting your intake of saturated and trans fat along with cholesterol helps make room for more fruits and vegetables (and of course, you take in more vitamins, minerals, and fiber

DIFFERENCES IN SATURATED FAT AND CALORIE CONTENT OF COMMONLY CONSUMED FOODS

This table shows a few practical examples of the differences in the saturated fat content of different forms of commonly consumed foods. Comparisons are made between foods in the same food group (i.e., regular cheese and low-fat cheddar cheese), illustrating that lower saturated fat choices can be made within the same food group.

Food Category	Portion	Saturated Fat Content (grams)	Calories
Cheese			
Regular cheddar cheese	1 oz	6.0	114
Low-fat cheddar cheese	1 oz	1.2	19
Ground beef			
Regular ground beef (25% fat)	3 oz (cooked)	6.1	236
Extra lean ground beef (5% fat)	3 oz (cooked)	2.6	148
Milk			
Whole milk (3.24% fat)	1 cup	4.6	146
Low-fat milk (1% fat)	1 cup	1.5	102
Breads			
Croissant (medium)	1 medium	6.6	231
Bagel, oat bran (4")	1 medium	0.2	227
Frozen desserts			
Regular ice cream	1/2 cup	4.9	145
Frozen yogurt, low-fat	1/2 cup	2.0	110
Table spreads			
Butter	1 tsp	2.4	34
Soft margarine with zero trans	1 tsp	0.7	25
Chicken			
Fried chicken (leg and skin)	3 oz (cooked)	3.3	212
Roasted chicken (breast, no skin)	3 oz (cooked)	0.9	140
Fish			
Fried Fish	3 oz	2.8	195
Baked Fish	3 oz	1.5	129

Source: ARS Nutrient Database for Standard Reference, Release 17. *Dietary Guidelines for Americans*, 2005.

FIGURE 12.6

while most likely eating fewer calories, as many fatty foods also pack in extra calories). This translates to better health.

Prevention of chronic disease: As described in Chapters 6 and 10, high-fat diets increase the risk for heart disease and cancer. Lowering saturated fat intake helps lower blood cholesterol levels (specifically LDL levels). And limiting trans fats also helps lower heart disease risk.

Focus Area #6

Carbohydrates: In Chapter 4 we learned the importance of carbohydrate as a fuel source, especially during exercise. Food sources of carbohydrate such as fruits and whole grains provide essential vitamins and minerals along with fiber crucial for intestinal tract health. Foods with added sugar (sweeteners such as sucrose and corn syrup) are often void in essential nutrients (candy, sodas, cookies, and cakes) and the more of these foods in the diet the more challenging it is for people to meet their need for the essential nutrients. Additionally, sugars as well as starches contribute to tooth decay. Choose carbohydrate-rich foods with thought as to how that food fits in the overall scheme of the diet in terms of providing essential nutrients. Key recommendations regarding carbohydrates include:

- Choose fiber-rich fruits, vegetables, and whole grains often.
- Choose and prepare foods and beverages with little added sugars or caloric sweeteners.
- Reduce incidence of dental caries by practicing good oral hygiene and consuming sugar- and starch-containing foods and beverages less frequently.

Promotion of general health: Limiting intake of foods with added sugar makes room for more nutrient-dense fruits, vegetables, and whole grains. The amount of added sugar in a person's diet depends upon the caloric intake (which is a function of age, gender, and activity level.) The amount is small for most people, ranging from 100 to 300 calories daily (termed **discretionary calories**—see next section.)

Prevention of chronic disease: Eating fewer foods with less added sugars and more nutrient-dense foods will help control calorie intake and prevent weight gain. Also, eating more fruits, vegetables, and whole grains provides additional nutrients that may help lower risk for several chronic diseases.

Focus Area #7

Sodium and Potassium: As covered in Chapter 8, the minerals sodium and potassium play a role in healthy blood pressure. A high intake of sodium (found in table salt and processed foods) links with high blood pressure, while ample potassium (found in fruits and vegetables) aids in maintaining healthy blood pressure. And high blood pressure is a major risk factor for heart disease as well as for kidney disease and stroke. Key recommendations for sodium and potassium include:

- Consume less than 2,300 mg (approximately 1 tsp. of salt) of sodium per day.
- Choose and prepare foods with little salt. At the same time, consume potassium-rich foods, such as fruits and vegetables.

Promotion of general health: By limiting sodium through decreasing your intake of processed foods, you make more room for fruits, vegetables, and whole grains. Figure 12.7 shows the major contribution that processed foods make to overall sodium intake in the typical American diet. As described in other focus areas, this boosts intake of fiber, vitamins, and minerals crucial for good health.

Prevention of chronic disease: Lowering sodium intake while increasing potassium intake will aid in maintaining healthy blood pressure. Additionally, the increase in intake of fruits, vegetables, and grains (potassium rich foods) will supply a wealth of disease-fighting phytochemicals that may aid in lowering the risk for certain cancers, heart disease, and other age-related conditions.

Focus Area #8

Alcoholic Beverages: In Chapter 10 we discussed that alcohol is a source of empty calories and that excess alcohol consumption negatively impacts nutrient status. Additionally, heavy alcohol consumption increases the risks for certain cancers, high blood pressure, liver disease, and accidental death. But moderate alcohol consumption may have beneficial effects on health. Moderate alcohol consumption defined as one to two drinks per day is associated with lower risk for heart disease. This risk reduction is evident in middle-aged and older adults while among young adults, moderate alcohol consumption provides minimal health benefits. Key recommendations for alcoholic beverages include:

- Those that choose to drink alcoholic beverages should do so sensibly and in moderation—defined as the consumption of up to one drink per day for women and up to two drinks per day for men.

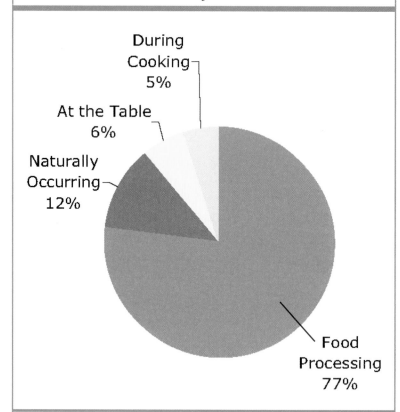

SOURCES OF DIETARY SODIUM

The relative amounts of dietary sodium in the American diet.

During Cooking 5%

At the Table 6%

Naturally Occurring 12%

Food Processing 77%

Source: Mattes RD, Donnelly D. Relative contributions of dietary sodium sources. *J AM Coll Nutr.* 1991, Aug;10(4): 383–393/Dietary Guidelines for Americans, 2005.

FIGURE 12.7

- Some individuals should not consume alcoholic beverages. This includes those who cannot restrict their alcohol intake, women of childbearing age who may become pregnant, and pregnant or lactating women.

Promotion of general health: Moderate alcohol intake promotes good health by lowering your risk for injury at work and while driving. Limiting alcohol also makes room for nutrient-dense foods such as fruits and vegetables, and helps control calorie intake to aid in weight control. See Figure 12.8 for calorie counts in alcoholic beverages. Avoiding heavy alcohol consumption will minimize the impact alcohol has on nutrient status (see Chapter 10.)

CALORIES IN SELECTED ALCOHOLIC BEVERAGES

This table is a guide to estimate the caloric intake from various alcoholic beverages. An example serving volume and the calories in that drink are shown for beer, wine and distilled spirits. Higher alcohol content (higher percent alcohol or higher proof) and mixing alcohol with other beverages, such as calorically sweetened soft drinks, tonic water, fruit juice, or ice cream, increases the amount of calories in the beverage. Alcoholic beverages supply calories but provide few essential nutrients.

Beverage	Approx. Calories Per 1 Fluid Oz[a]	Example Serving Volume	Approx. Total Calories[b]
Beer (regular)	12	12 oz	144
Beer (light)	9	12 oz	108
White wine	20	5 oz	100
Red wine	21	5 oz	105
Sweet dessert wine	47	3 oz	141
80 proof distilled spirits (gin, rum, vodka, whiskey)	64	1.5 oz	96

[a] **Source:** Agricultural Research Service (ARS) Nutrient Database for Standard Reference (SR), Release 17. (*www.nal.usda.gov/fnic/foodcomp/index.html*) Calories are calculated to the nearest whole number per 1 fluid oz.

[b] The total calories and alcohol content may vary depending on the brand. Moreover, adding mixers can contribute calories in addition to the calories from the alcohol itself.

Source: *Dietary Guidelines for Americans,* 2005.

FIGURE 12.8

Prevention of chronic disease: Excessive alcohol consumption links to stroke, cancer and other diseases. And while moderate alcohol consumption may confer health benefits in some, other individuals who have difficulty in restricting their intake may need to avoid alcohol altogether.

Focus Area #9

Food Safety: Eating foods that are free from harmful bacteria, parasites, and chemical contaminants is vital for good health. Thousands of people, primarily infants, children, and the elderly, die of food-borne illnesses every year. We can take simple steps in handling, preparing, and cooking foods to minimize our risk for food-borne illness. Key recommendations for food safety include:

● Clean hands, food contact surfaces, and fruits and vegetables. Do not wash or rinse meat and poultry.

- Separate raw, cooked, and ready-to-eat foods while shopping, preparing, or storing foods.

- Cook foods to a safe temperature to kill microorganisms. See Figure 12.9 for safe cooking temperatures for various foods.

- Chill perishable food promptly and defrost foods properly.

- Avoid raw (unpasteurized) milk or any products made from unpasteurized milk, raw or partially cooked eggs, or foods containing raw eggs, raw or undercooked meat and poultry, unpasteurized juices, and raw sprouts.

Promotion of general health: Preparing and eating safe foods allows a person to stay free of food-borne illnesses and other related problems, which clearly is essential for good health.

Prevention of chronic disease: Keeping foods safe to eat ensures you will take in a variety of foods—fruits, vegetables, protein sources, whole grains, and more—that together provide nutrients that help lower chronic disease risk.

MyPyramid

In conjunction with the Dietary Guidelines for 2005, the U.S. Department of Agriculture developed an interactive Internet based tool—MyPyramid—that illustrates and informs consumers in a personalized way about plan-

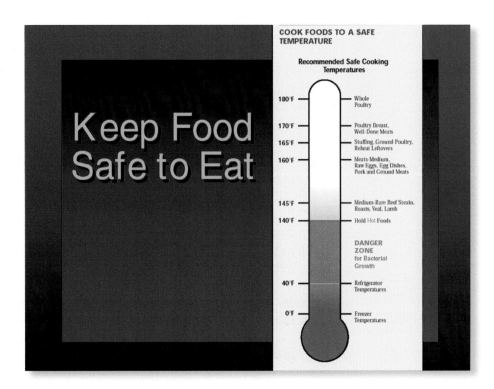

FIGURE 12.9

ning a healthy diet and physical activity. Consumers can log on to *www.mypyramid.gov* and assess their current food choices and get recommendations for types and amounts of foods based upon age, gender, and current activity level. The Food Guide Pyramid shown in Figure 12.10 illustrates several components and messages from the Dietary Guidelines.

- Activity: The steps and the person climbing signify the importance of daily exercise.

- Moderation: The colored bands widening at the base illustrate the fact that we should eat those foods with little or no added fats or added sugars more often than foods at the top of the pyramid with added sugars and fats.

- Personalization: The slogan "MyPyramid" and the Web site www.mypyramid.gov both show personalization for you can find a diet plan to fit your needs.

- Proportionality: This feature appears in the different widths of the colored bands, which show that we should eat food groups in differing amounts (for example, amount of grains versus fruits).

- Variety: Variety appears in the six colored bands representing the five food groups and oils. All food groups are necessary daily for good health.

- Gradual improvement: The slogan "Steps to a healthier you" shows that improvements toward good health occur gradually.

MyPyramid illustrates five food groups and oils [see Figure 12.10]. There is also an amount of discretionary calories for each calorie intake to "spend" on other foods as you desire, such as soda, cookies, or other foods from the pyramid groups.

Grains—Make half your grains whole: This group (orange band) provides B vitamins, iron, zinc, magnesium, protein, and fiber. The emphasis is to eat at least 3 oz equivalents of grains daily that are whole (brown rice, whole grain breakfast cereal, whole wheat pasta, and so forth).

Vegetables—Vary your veggies: The message illustrates (green band) the importance of eating a variety of vegetables each day. Listed in the green box of Figure 12.10 are the different vegetable categories, such as dark green and orange.

Fruits—Focus on fruits: The same variety message that accompanies the vegetable group holds for fruits as well (red band). Also, the MyPyramid emphasizes eating whole fruits and some fruit juice but not consuming all fruit as juice as valuable nutrients may be lost in making

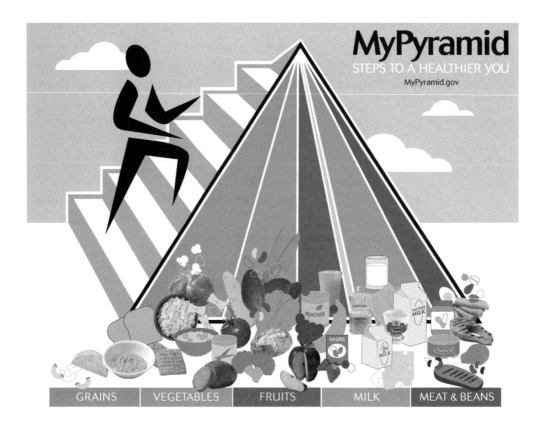

MyPyramid
STEPS TO A HEALTHIER YOU
MyPyramid.gov

| GRAINS | VEGETABLES | FRUITS | MILK | MEAT & BEANS |

GRAINS Make half your grains whole	VEGETABLES Vary your veggies	FRUITS Focus on fruits	MILK Get your calcium-rich foods	MEAT & BEANS Go lean with protein
Eat at least 3 oz. of whole-grain cereals, breads, crackers, rice, or pasta every day 1 oz. is about 1 slice of bread, about 1 cup of breakfast cereal, or ½ cup of cooked rice, cereal, or pasta	Eat more dark-green veggies like broccoli, spinach, and other dark leafy greens Eat more orange vegetables like carrots and sweetpotatoes Eat more dry beans and peas like pinto beans, kidney beans, and lentils	Eat a variety of fruit Choose fresh, frozen, canned, or dried fruit Go easy on fruit juices	Go low-fat or fat-free when you choose milk, yogurt, and other milk products If you don't or can't consume milk, choose lactose-free products or other calcium sources such as fortified foods and beverages	Choose low-fat or lean meats and poultry Bake it, broil it, or grill it Vary your protein routine — choose more fish, beans, peas, nuts, and seeds

For a 2,000-calorie diet, you need the amounts below from each food group. To find the amounts that are right for you, go to MyPyramid.gov.

| Eat 6 oz. every day | Eat 2½ cups every day | Eat 2 cups every day | Get 3 cups every day; for kids aged 2 to 8, it's 2 | Eat 5½ oz. every day |

Find your balance between food and physical activity
- Be sure to stay within your daily calorie needs.
- Be physically active for at least 30 minutes most days of the week.
- About 60 minutes a day of physical activity may be needed to prevent weight gain.
- For sustaining weight loss, at least 60 to 90 minutes a day of physical activity may be required.
- Children and teenagers should be physically active for 60 minutes every day, or most days.

Know the limits on fats, sugars, and salt (sodium)
- Make most of your fat sources from fish, nuts, and vegetable oils.
- Limit solid fats like butter, stick margarine, shortening, and lard, as well as foods that contain these.
- Check the Nutrition Facts label to keep saturated fats, *trans* fats, and sodium low.
- Choose food and beverages low in added sugars. Added sugars contribute calories with few, if any, nutrients.

MyPyramid.gov
STEPS TO A HEALTHIER YOU

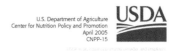

U.S. Department of Agriculture
Center for Nutrition Policy and Promotion
April 2005
CNPP-15

FIGURE 12.10

juice from whole fruit (particularly fiber.) The pyramid does not combine fruits and vegetables for although they provide many of the same nutrients (fiber, vitamins A and C, for example), they contain many different nutrients. Thus eating a variety of both vegetables and fruits helps ensure ample intake of key essential nutrients.

Oils—Know your limits: The message with oils (yellow band) is to select those that are healthy over those fats that increase risk for chronic diseases. The emphasis is to choose fats and oils found in fish, nuts, and vegetable oils over hard cheeses, lard, and fatty meats.

Milk—Get your calcium-rich foods: The emphasis in this group is to select low-fat or fat-free dairy foods (blue band). This group encourages those who cannot eat dairy products containing lactose to choose calcium-rich or fortified foods and beverages such as soy milk and calcium-fortified juices.

Meats and beans—Go lean on protein: This group (purple band) includes dry beans, eggs, and nuts along with lean meats, poultry, and fish. The emphasis is selecting a lean version prepared in lean fashion—baking, broiling, or grilling.

Discretionary calories: Once you've selected the recommended servings of whole grains, vegetables, fruits, healthy oils, milk and meat, and beans for your calorie needs (as outlined below), there are some calories left to use on "extra" foods if you desire. This represents your "discretionary calories," which are much like a bit of cash you can spend each day on frivolous items such as butter on your whole grain bread, a can of soda, or a few cookies. You could also choose to use these calories on more fruit or whole grain items or other foods from the food groups as you desire (and ranges from 100 to over 400 calories daily). The amount of discretionary calories depends upon your calorie intake. The more active you are, the greater the number of calories you need to support your active lifestyle. This translates to a great number of discretionary calories allotted to you.

Your Personal Food Guide Pyramid

When you log on to *www.mypyramid.gov,* you can get your own personalized eating plan. Simply enter your age, gender, and activity level, and you will be assigned one of 12 food plans or pyramids that range in calorie intake from 1000 to 3200 calories daily. Each pyramid plan designates the number of daily servings for each of the five food groups detailed above and the number of discretionary calories. Figure 12.11 illustrates the food guide for five different caloric intakes.

What are the serving sizes in each food group—for a whole grain or a vegetable for example? The serving sizes for each food group are listed in

MYPYRAMID FOOD GUIDE FOR FIVE DIFFERENT ENERGY INTAKES

Food Group	1200 calories/day	1600 calories/day	2000 calories/day	2400 calories/day	3000 calories/day
Grains	4 oz-equiv.	5 oz-equiv.	6 oz-equiv.	8 oz-equiv.	10 oz-equiv.
Vegetables	1.5 c	2 c	2.5 c	3 c	4 c
Fruits	1 c	1.5 c	2 c	2 c	2.5 c
Milk	2 c	3 c	3 c	3 c	3 c
Meat and Beans	3 oz-equiv.	5 oz-equiv.	5.5 oz-equiv.	6.5 oz-equiv.	7 oz-equiv.
Oils	3.5 tsp	4.5 tsp	5 tsp	6 tsp	9 tsp
Discretionary Calorie Allowance	171	132	267	362	512

FIGURE 12.11

Figure 12.12. An ounce-equivalent (oz-equivalent) is an amount of the food equal to one ounce (28 grams.) An important note about serving sizes: There is no standard definition for a serving size for a food group. You will find a serving size of grain listed in MyPyramid as an oz.-equivalent (1/2 cup of breakfast cereal), but this is different from a serving size listed on a box of whole grain breakfast cereal (1 cup of breakfast cereal or two oz-equivalents). As you select packaged foods, be sure to check the serving size listed on the package and compare it to your recommend food guide so as not to over-consume calories.

Figures 12.13 and 12.14 list the food guides for an active college-aged male and female. Note the different number of servings for various food groups such as grains and vegetables based upon calorie intake. Discretionary calories also differ for these two people to fit their calorie needs, emphasizing the goal of balancing calorie in with calories spent.

USING FOOD LABELS FOR HEALTHIER EATING

The primary goal behind the Nutrition Facts food label is to help you plan and choose foods that are part of a healthy diet based on the Dietary Guidelines for Americans and their principles of promoting general health and prevention of chronic disease. Now, at the end of the course we have a more complete "nutritional" view of food labels from when it was first brought up in Chapter 2.

MYPYRAMID FOOD GROUP SERVING SIZES

Food Group	Equivalent
Grains	1 oz-equivalent: 1 slice bread 1/2 c cooked pasta, rice 1 c ready-to-eat cereal 1 small muffin 1/2 burger roll
Vegetable	1 cup-equivalent: 1 c cooked broccoli, carrots, green beans 2 c leafy greens (romaine lettuce, raw spinach) 1 c vegetable juice
Fruit	1 cup-equivalent: 1 c sliced fruit (strawberries, melon) 1/2 grapefruit 1 medium apple, pear
Milk	1 cup-equivalent: 1 c milk 1 c yogurt 1 c ice cream 1 1/2 oz hard cheese
Meat and Beans	1 oz-equivalent: 1 oz beef, pork, fish, poultry 1/4 c cooked lentils, pinto and other beans 1/4 c tofu 1 egg 1 T peanut butter 1/2 oz nuts and seeds

FIGURE 12.12

The information on the Nutrition Facts food label is all about comparison—how does a serving of that specific food compare with reference intakes for total fat, saturated fat, protein, carbohydrate, fiber, and various vitamins and minerals. These reference intakes are the **Daily Values** that you have already learned about in previous chapters. The Daily Value is an intake that is recommended (and in some cases, such as fat, an intake not to exceed) based on a typical consumer eating a 2,000 calorie per day diet. Figure 12.15 shows the Daily Values used for comparison on food labels.

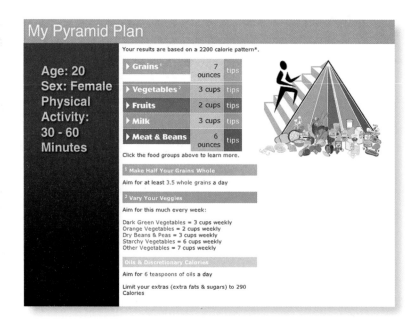

FIGURE 12.13

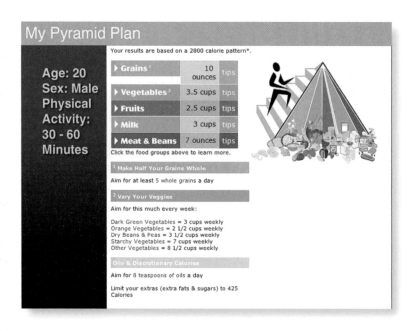

FIGURE 12.14

How to read a food label: Let's take a "walk" through a Nutrition Facts food label and point out many of the important features.

- At the top portion of the label is information on the serving size. (See Figure 12.16.) This is important to note because what you serve yourself may in fact be two or more servings, which of course impacts the amount of calories, fat, and so on that you take in from this food.

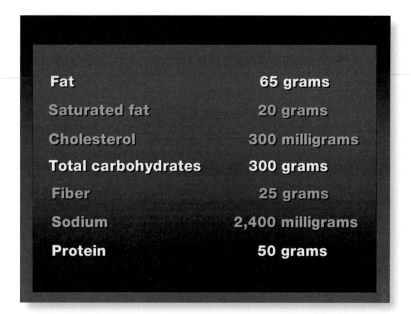

Fat	65 grams
Saturated fat	20 grams
Cholesterol	300 milligrams
Total carbohydrates	300 grams
Fiber	25 grams
Sodium	2,400 milligrams
Protein	50 grams

FIGURE 12.15

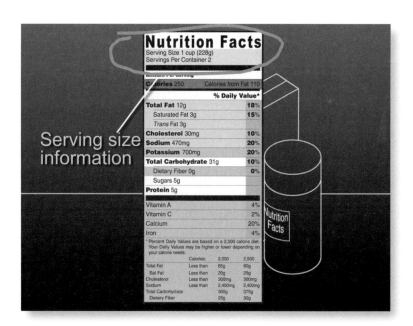

FIGURE 12.16

- The midsection of the label presents information on the number of calories per serving along with the number of fat calories. (See Figure 12.17.) This allows you a quick assessment of the food and a means of comparing this food to another.

- The amounts of fat, saturated fat, trans fat, cholesterol, and sodium per serving are listed and this value is compared with the Daily Value for that nutrient. (See Figure 12.18 and 12.19.) Remember

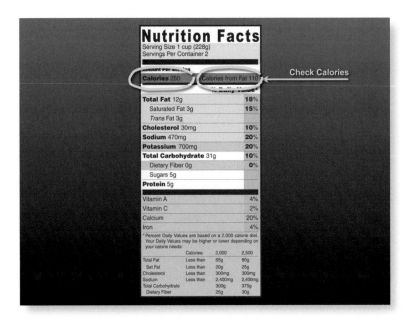

FIGURE 12.17

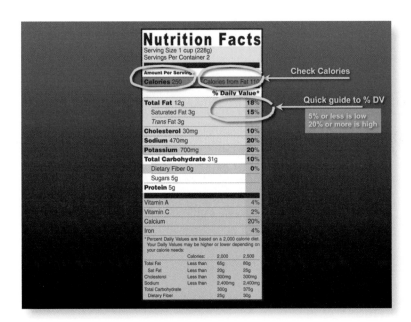

FIGURE 12.18

from the Dietary Guidelines that these items are to be limited in the diet because of their connection with chronic disease. When the Percent Daily Value is 5% or less this considered low and 20% or more is considered high.

- Amounts of carbohydrate, fiber, sugar (naturally occurring such as fruit sugar and lactose in milk, and added sugars such as in candy), and protein is presented. (See Figure 12.20.) These are compared to the Daily Value but note only for carbohydrate and fiber. The

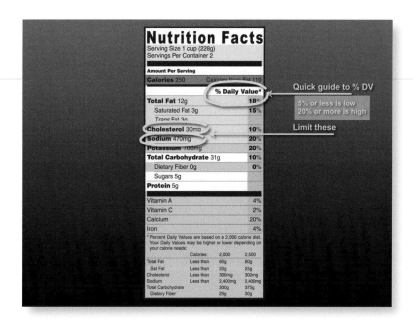

FIGURE 12.19

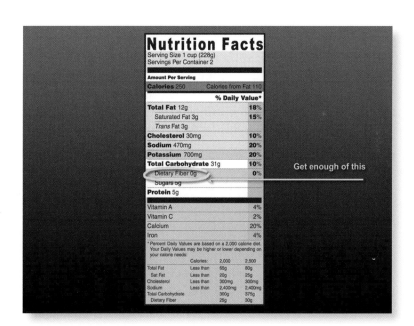

FIGURE 12.20

FDA does not require protein to be listed as a percent of Daily Value unless a claim is made on the package about the protein in the food. There is no Daily Value for sugar for comparison, but be aware that 4 grams of sugar is equivalent to a teaspoon.

● The FDA requires that four micronutrients—vitamins A and C and minerals calcium and iron—be listed on the label as a percent of the Daily Value. (See Figure 12.21.) If a food is fortified with other micronutrients, these too would be listed as percent Daily Value.

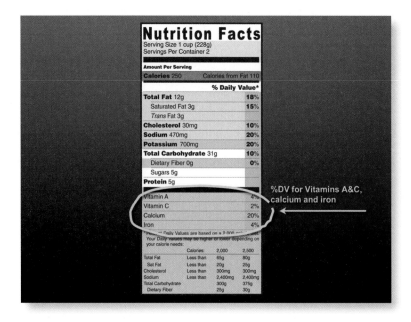

FIGURE 12.21

At the bottom of the label, room permitting, the Daily Values are listed along with adjusted amounts for a 2,500 calorie diet.

Putting the Dietary Guidelines for Americans, Food Guide Pyramid, and Nutrition Facts food label all together in this way has perhaps given you a different perspective on these tools in planning a healthful diet. (See Figure 12.22.)

Congratulate yourself—you now have a wealth of knowledge about your health and how diet plays a vital role for today and your future.

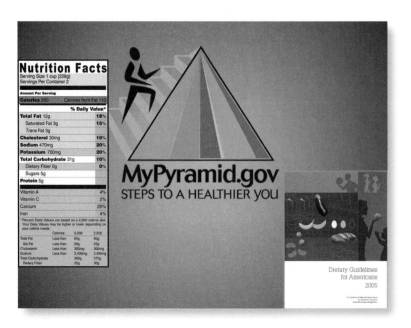

FIGURE 12.22

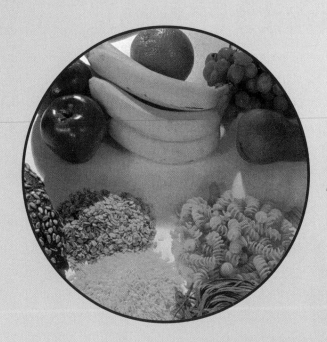

Appendix

Diet Project (with forms)

DIET PROJECT GUIDE

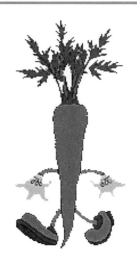 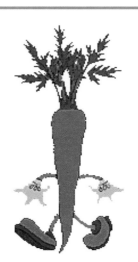 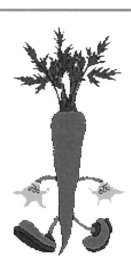

Important Dates to Remember:

* **Project Due Date** _____

   Late Due Date (for partial credit) _____

   Projects Returned _____

** **Re-Grade Submittal** _____

   *In class, or by 5 p.m. at 1334 Meyer (no other location accepted)

  **In class only! (no other location or time accepted)

Checklist for Turning In Your Diet Project:

- ☐ **Food Record Forms for Three Days**   (pp. 325–329)
- ☐ **Summary & Comparison Forms**   (p. 331)
- ☐ **Calculations Page**   (p. 333)
- ☐ **Unsealed Return Envelope**   (Distributed in Class on due date)
     with completed grade forms

How Does *Your* Diet Rate?

Diet Project Guide Contents

BACKGROUND / INTRODUCTION

As you'll learn in class, the Recommended Dietary Allowances are the suggested levels of intake for a variety of important nutrients. Because not everyone can possibly eat "perfectly" every day, they are meant to apply to the average of several days' intake. Think of them as intake goals that you should be aiming for.

In keeping with the purpose of this class—putting nutrition knowledge into the context of personal health—you will record your diet for three days and then average the nutrient content from those three days. You will then compare your actual three-day average with the RDA goals and other dietary guidelines. This comparison will give you a idea of how good a job you are doing in meeting your body's needs for today and preventing chronic disease in years to come. Later, when you learn more about the functions of these nutrients and good food sources for them, you will understand their importance and be able to make choices that can improve your diet.

- To complete this project, you will need the following tools:
  - Your completed Food Record Pages (instructions will follow)
  - Food Composition Tables (starting on page 340 of the Appendix)
  - A calculator

- To get full credit for your project, you must submit (in the *unsealed* envelope provided in class):
  - Completed Food Record Pages for three days (extra Food Record form if needed)
  - Completed Calculation Page
  - Completed Summary and Comparison Forms

If you have made several errors on your Diet Project, or you have omitted one or more of the required pages/forms, you will be given a "No Pass" grade. **IF** you correct these errors or omissions you get Dr. Applegate's or one of the Teaching Assistants' initials indicating corrections are correctly made, and **IF** you re-submit it by the deadline on the front page of this packet, you will still be able to get full credit. The TAs and Dr. Applegate are happy to look over your corrected Project to be sure you are on the right track—there is no reason not to get full credit, **if** you meet all the deadlines.

COMPLETING YOUR FOOD RECORD FORMS

STEP ONE: Record *everything* **that you eat or drink (except water) for three consecutive days.** You must choose either Sunday, Monday, and Tuesday, or Thursday, Friday, and Saturday. We all tend to eat differently on the weekends, so including at least one weekend day will give you a better representation of your typical eating patterns. And please try to continue to eat as you usually would; being overly "good" (however you might define that) will not give you an accurate picture of your diet.

- **Don't record any nutrient supplements you might be taking (even though these are listed in the food tables).** This Project is your tool for discovering how well your food choices deliver the nutrients you need. (You may though record protein powders, nutritional bars and other supplement products that provide calories.)

- Place each food item on its own line. If you eat more items in one day than there are lines on the form, use the extra Food Record Form on page 335.

- When you are recording your food items, take careful note of the measure—cups, ounces, tablespoons and teaspoons. Don't just write "bowlful" or "glassful" because not all bowls and glasses are the same size. It might be helpful to use kitchen measuring cups at first, until you can estimate with some accuracy. For items such as meat or cheese, remember that 3 oz of cooked meat is about the size of an ordinary playing card, that one oz of cheese is a cube about 1½ inches on a side, and that 4 oz of raw meat usually cooks down to 3 oz., a medium size piece of fruit is about the size of a tennis ball. Also note that for household measures: 2 cups = 1 pint; 1 cup = 16 T; 2 T = 1 ounce, 3 t = 1 T; 8 ounces = 1 cup.

- If you are eating most common frozen dinners or entrees or at a fast-food restaurant, write down the exact name of the item: *Healthy Choice* Chicken Chow Mein, *Taco Bell* Chicken Taco Supreme,

MacDonald's Big Mac, *Burger King* Whopper with cheese, etc. Enter drinks by the number of ounces they contain, not as "large" or "extra-large."

● Combination-type foods and drinks, such as casseroles or smoothies or mochas, present a challenge. Try to find out the types and amounts of ingredients that went into the casserole, and then estimate the share your serving represents (though many combination-type foods such as stews, soups and casseroles are listed in the food tables. For example, a casserole might be made from 12 oz. of penne pasta, 2 medium zucchini, a half-pound of ground turkey, and a 28-oz can of tomatoes. (Don't worry about entering spices or herbs.) If you ate one-fourth of this casserole, you would enter 3 oz. penne pasta, $\frac{1}{2}$ medium zucchini, ~2 oz of cooked ground turkey, and 7 oz. of canned tomatoes.

STEP TWO: Determine the nutrient values for each food item. Use the Food Composition Tables found in the Appendix of this Reader starting on page 337, which have listings for most commonly consumed foods listed alphabetically. There are many categories, so look through the entire set of tables to find each food item. Categories include beverages, fast food (listed by restaurant), fish, fruits, grains (breads, pasta, rice), breakfast cereal, meals and dishes (including frozen, canned, and pizza), meats (including meat substitutes), nuts (peanut butter), poultry, sauces, snack foods, soups, sports products (energy bars, supplements, and sport drinks), and vegetables (fresh, canned & frozen). Find the food item that most closely matches the one on your Food Record. In some cases if the food item you recorded is not listed you may need to substitute, that is, choose the food item that most closely resembles, in terms of nutrient profile, what you ate. *Using a ruler or straight edge* (to be sure you stay on the same line), record nutrient values for each item listed on the Food Record. Note that not all nutrient values listed in the tables will be recorded; phosphorus and potassium, for example.

● **DO NOT** use the Nutrition Facts Food Label from a food's packaging for nutrient information. While they are helpful in allowing consumers to compare food products, these labels don't serve our needs because they don't list all the nutrients we are interested in. Use the Food Composition Tables.

● Make careful note of the units and serving sizes. Don't write the food values for a loaf of bread when you only had two *slices!* What if the Table listing shows a serving of 1 cup of milk, but you actually consumed 2½ cups? You would then need to make the appropriate adjustment to all the food nutrient values given by multiplying them by 2.5.

- **If information is listed for an entire package or container, figure out what fraction of the container you ate and make appropriate adjustments such as, multiply by 0.25 if you ate ¼ of a whole pizza.**

- If a "—" is listed for the content of a particular nutrient, record it as "—" and assume a value of zero (0). The dash line means the information is not available.

- If you have eaten a food that is not in the Food Composition Tables (and you can't find an appropriate substitute), you can use one of the reference books on reserve at Shields Library. Start with Bowes & Church, *Food Values of Portions Commonly Used.* For more unusual foods, you may need to turn to the appropriate section of the *USDA Handbook 8,* which contains nearly every food item ever analyzed. You may also refer to the USDA web site www.nal.usda.gov/fnic/foodcomp/search and enter your food item to obtain the nutrient profile. (Make appropriate adjustments based on serving size listed compared to what you ate.)

- Some reference books will use the short names for some of the B vitamins. Remember that vitamin B_1 is thiamin, B_2 is riboflavin, and B_3 is niacin.

- Some reference books may list nutrients as " < 1". Please convert " < 1" to "0". **NOTE: You MUST SEE THE " < " SYMBOL FOR THIS TO APPLY.** In addition, values with a superscript (i.e., 8^5) are not to be multiplied. The superscript refers to a footnote.

STEP THREE: Total each column (except for the "serving size" column) on each of your three Food Record Forms, and place the totals in the appropriate boxes at the bottom of the Forms.

How to Fill Out Your Summary Form

STEP ONE: Transfer the Totals from each Food Record Form to the appropriate column. Be very careful to enter each item in its correct column.

STEP TWO: Total each column. Total the nutrient values from your three days.

STEP THREE: Find the average value. Divide the totals for each column by three to find your three-day average intake.

Completing Your Calculation Page

STEP ONE: Calculate your daily Energy and Protein Requirements.
Don't try to complete this portion of the page until we have covered these topics in class (see chapters 2 and 3). After that point, you will have all the information you need to complete Parts 1, 2, and 3.

STEP TWO: Calculate your Energy Intake Distribution. (Part 4)
Transfer the three-day average intakes for carbohydrate, protein, and fat from the last line of your Summary Page to the appropriate lines in Part 4 of the Calculation Page. Convert these intakes from grams to kcalories by using the appropriate physiological fuel value. Finally, total these kcalories to determine your total calculated energy.

STEP THREE: Calculate your % Energy Distribution. (Part 5) Using the kcalorie results that you calculated in Part 4, compute the relative percentages of your total calories coming from carbohydrate, protein, fat, and saturated fat.

How to Fill Out Your Comparison Form

STEP ONE: Transfer your three-day average intakes from the last line of the Summary Form to the first line of the Comparison Form—EXCEPT for fat and saturated fat. For these entries, use the "% kcal from fat" figure you computed in Part 5 and "% kcal from saturated fat" figure in Part 6 of the Calculation Page.

STEP TWO: Enter your daily Energy and Protein Requirements into the first two boxes of the "Standard" line of the Comparison Form.

STEP THREE: Enter the appropriate set of RDAs/DRIs in the remaining boxes of the "Standard" row of the Comparison Form.
The RDAs/DRIs are on pages 323–334. RDAs/DRIs are listed for males, females, and by age—be sure you choose the set appropriate for you. Notice that some boxes have already been filled for you. These represent dietary recommendations of the National Research Council for the prevention of chronic diseases. The values in this "Standard" row are the "goals" that you will make a comparison to your actual intake.

STEP FOUR: Calculate what percent (%) of the "Standard" you are consuming. To do this, you would divide your average intake by the Standard, and then multiply by 100 to get a percentage.

STEP FIVE: Circle all nutrients for which your average daily intake was less than 100% of the standard.

Turning In Your Diet Project

STEP ONE: Tear out (at perforations) Food Record forms (3 days), summary and comparison forms, and calculation page.

STEP TWO: Place the completed Diet Project pages into the manila envelope provided to you in class. Use the checklist of these instructions found on page 316 and be sure that you have recorded your name [LAST, FIRST] and ID number on the outside of the envelope and on both the pink and white grade sheets inside the envelope.

DO NOT SEAL THE ENVELOPE!

STEP THREE: Turn your Diet Project in on the date indicated on the cover of the Diet Project Guide. You can do so in class that day or later at the TA office. *NOTE:* No other location is acceptable for diet project submission other than in class or the TA office in 1334 Meyer. Projects turned in later than 5:00 P.M. that day will be considered late and will receive only half-credit.

Dietary Reference Intakes: RDA & AI for Vitamins

Life Stage Group	Vitamin A (µg/d)[a]	Vitamin D (µg/d) (AI)	Vitamin E (mg/d)[b]	Vitamin K (µg/d) (AI)	Vitamin C (mg/d)	Thiamin (mg/d)	Riboflavin (mg/d)	Niacin (mg/d)[c]	Biotin (AI)	Folate (µg/d)[d]	Vitamin B6	Vitamin B12 (µg/d)	Choline (mg/d) (AI)
Children													
1-3 y	300	5	6	30	15	0.5	0.5	6	8	150	0.5	0.9	200
4-8 y	400	5	7	55	25	0.6	0.6	8	12	200	0.6	1.2	250
Males													
9-13 y	600	5	11	60	45	0.9	0.9	12	20	300	1.0	1.8	375
14-18 y	900	5	15	70	70	1.2	1.3	16	25	400	1.3	2.4	550
19-30 y	900	5	15	120	90	1.2	1.3	16	30	400	1.3	2.4	550
31-50 y	900	5	15	120	90	1.2	1.3	16	30	400	1.3	2.4	550
51-70 y	900	10	15	120	90	1.2	1.3	16	30	400	1.7	2.4	550
> 70 y	900	15	15	120	90	1.2	1.3	16	30	400	1.7	2.4	550
Females													
9-13 y	600	5	11	60	45	0.9	0.9	12	20	300	1.0	1.8	375
14-18 y	700	5	15	75	65	1.0	1.0	14	25	400	1.2	2.4	400
19-30 y	700	5	15	90	75	1.1	1.1	14	30	400	1.3	2.4	425
31-50 y	700	5	15	90	75	1.1	1.1	14	30	400	1.3	2.4	425
51-70 y	700	10	15	90	75	1.1	1.1	14	30	400	1.5	2.4	425
> 70 y	700	15	15	90	75	1.1	1.1	14	30	400	1.5	2.4	425
Pregnancy													
≤ 18 y	750	5	15	75	80	1.4	1.4	18	30	600	1.9	2.6	450
19-30 y	770	5	15	90	85	1.4	1.4	18	30	600	1.9	2.6	450
31-50 y	770	5	15	90	85	1.4	1.4	18	30	600	1.9	2.6	450
Lactation													
≤ 18 y	1200	5	19	75	115	1.4	1.4	17	35	500	2.0	2.8	550
19-30 y	1300	5	19	90	120	1.4	1.4	17	35	500	2.0	2.8	550
31-50 y	1300	5	19	90	120	1.4	1.4	17	35	500	2.0	2.8	550

Note: These are from the DRI reports (see www.nap.edu). RDAs are set to meet the needs of almost all (97%-98%) individuals in a group. AI are more tentative values as insufficient research exists currently to set an RDA. Both RDAs and AIs may be used as goals for individuals.

[a] Given as a retinal activity equivalents (RAEs).

[b] Also known as a-tocopherol

[c] Given as niacin equivalents (NE)

[d] Given as dietary folate equivalents (DEF)

Sources: Adapted from the Dietary Reference Intakes series, National Academic Press. Copyright 1997, 1998, 2000, 2001, by the national Academy of Sciences. These reports maybe accessed via www.nap.edu. Courtesy of the National Academies Press, Washington, DC.

Dietary Reference Intakes: RDA & AI for Minerals

Life Stage Group	Calcium (mg/d) (AI)	Phosohorus (mg/d)	Magnesium (mg/d)	Iron (mg/d)	Zinc (mg/d)	Selenium (µg/d)	Iodine (µg/d)	Copper (µg/d)	Manganese (µg/d) (AI)	Fluoride (mg/d) (AI)	Chromium (µg/d) (AI)
Children											
1-3 y	500	460	80	7	3	20	90	340	1.2	0.7	11
4-8 y	800	500	130	10	5	30	90	440	1.5	1	15
Males											
9-13 y	1300	1250	240	8	8	40	120	700	1.9	2	25
14-18 y	1300	1250	410	11	11	55	150	890	2.2	3	35
19-30 y	1000	700	400	8	11	55	150	900	2.3	4	35
31-50 y	1000	700	420	8	11	55	150	900	2.3	4	35
51-70 y	1200	700	420	8	11	55	150	900	2.3	4	30
> 70 y	1200	700	420	8	11	55	150	900	2.3	4	30
Females											
9-13 y	1300	1250	240	8	8	40	120	700	1.6	2	21
14-18 y	1300	1250	360	15	9	55	150	890	1.6	3	24
19-30 y	1000	700	310	18	8	55	150	900	1.8	3	25
31-50 y	1000	700	320	18	8	55	150	900	1.8	3	25
51-70 y	1200	700	320	8	8	55	150	900	1.8	3	20
> 70 y	1200	700	320	8	8	55	150	900	1.8	3	20
Pregnancy											
≤ 18 y	1300	1250	400	27	12	60	220	1000	2.0	3	29
19-30 y	1000	700	350	27	11	60	220	1000	2.0	3	30
31-50 y	1000	700	360	27	11	60	220	1000	2.0	3	30
Lactation											
≤ 18 y	1300	1250	360	10	13	70	290	1300	2.6	3	44
19-30 y	1000	700	310	9	12	70	290	1300	2.6	3	45
31-50 y	1000	700	320	9	12	70	290	1300	2.6	3	45

Note: These are from the DRI reports (see www.nap.edu). RDAs are set to meet the needs of almost all (97%-98%) individuals in a group. AI are more tentative values as insufficient research exists currently to set an RDA. Both RDAs and used AIs may be as goals for individuals.

Sources: Adapted from the Dietary Reference Intakes series, National Academic Press. Copyright 1997, 1998, 2000, 2001, by the national Academy of Sciences. These reports maybe accessed via www.nap.edu. Courtesy of the National Academies Press, Washington, DC.

Table of Contents
for Food Composition Table

Food Composition Table

Food Name	Amount	Measure	Weight (g)	Calories	Protein (g)	Total Carb (g)	Dietary Fiber (g)	Total Fat (g)	Sat Fat (g)	Mono Fat (g)	Poly Fat (g)	Chol (mg)	Vit A (mcg RAE)	Vit D (mcg)
BEVERAGE AND BEVERAGE MIXES														
Carbonated Drinks														
Drink, lemonade, cnd, Country Time	1	Cup	247.20	90.00	0.00	23.00	0.00	0.00	0.00	0.00	0.00		0.00	
Soda, 7 Up	1	Cup	240.00	100.00	0.00	26.00	0.00	0.00	0.00	0.00	0.00	0.00	0.00	
Soda, club	1	Cup	236.80	0.00	0.00	0.00	0.00	0.00	0.00	0.00	0.00	0.00	0.00	
Soda, Coca Cola/Coke	1	Cup	246.00	102.67	0.00	26.67	0.00	0.00	0.00	0.00	0.00	0.00	0.00	0.00
Soda, Coca Cola/Coke, diet	1	Cup	239.50	1.00	0.00	0.08	0.00	0.00	0.00	0.00	0.00	0.00	0.00	0.00
Soda, cola	1	Cup	248.00	104.16	0.12	26.66	0.00	0.00	0.00	0.00	0.00	0.00	0.00	
Soda, cola Pepsi	1	Cup	240.00	100.00	0.00	27.33	0.00	0.00	0.00	0.00	0.00	0.00	0.00	
Soda, cola, diet Pepsi	1	Cup	240.00	0.00	0.00	0.00	0.00	0.00	0.00	0.00	0.00	0.00	0.00	
Soda, cola, diet, caff free Pepsi	1	Cup	240.00	0.00	0.00	0.00	0.00	0.00	0.00	0.00	0.00	0.00	0.00	
Soda, cola, diet, w/asp	1	Cup	236.80	2.37	0.24	0.24	0.00	0.00	0.00	0.00	0.00	0.00	0.00	
Soda, cream	1	Cup	247.20	126.07	0.00	32.88	0.00	0.00	0.00	0.00	0.00	0.00	0.00	
Soda, Dr Pepper	1	Cup	246.00	100.00	0.00	27.00	0.00	0.00	0.00	0.00	0.00		0.00	
Soda, ginger ale	1	Cup	244.00	82.96	0.00	21.40	0.00	0.00	0.00	0.00	0.00	0.00	0.00	
Soda, ginger ale, diet, Schweppes	1	Cup	246.70	0.00	0.00	0.00	0.00	0.00	0.00	0.00	0.00		0.00	
Soda, grape	1	Cup	248.00	106.64	0.00	27.78	0.00	0.00	0.00	0.00	0.00	0.00	0.00	
Soda, lemon lime	1	Cup	245.60	98.24	0.00	25.54	0.00	0.00	0.00	0.00	0.00	0.00	0.00	
Soda, lemon lime, dietSlice	1	Cup	240.00	2.67	0.00	0.67	0.00	0.00	0.00	0.00	0.00	0.00	0.00	
Soda, not cola/pepper, diet, w/sacc	1	Cup	236.80	0.00	0.00	0.24	0.00	0.00	0.00	0.00	0.00	0.00	0.00	0.00
Soda, orange	1	Cup	248.00	119.04	0.00	30.50	0.00	0.00	0.00	0.00	0.00	0.00	0.00	
Soda, pepper type, w/caff	1	Cup	245.60	100.70	0.00	25.54	0.00	0.25	0.17	0.00	0.00	0.00	0.00	
Soda, root beer	1	Cup	246.40	101.02	0.00	26.12	0.00	0.00	0.00	0.00	0.00	0.00	0.00	
Coffee and Substitutes														
Coffee, brewed, prep w/tap water	1	Cup	237.00	2.37	0.28	0.00	0.00	0.05	0.00	0.04	0.00	0.00	0.00	
Coffee, cappuccino, w/lowfat milk, double, tall Starbucks	1.5	Cup	244.00	110.00	8.00	11.00	0.00	3.50	2.50			15.00		
Coffee, cappuccino, w/whole milk, tall Starbucks	1.5	Cup	244.00	140.00	7.00	11.00	0.00	7.00	4.50			30.00		
Coffee, decaf, inst, prep w/water	1	Cup	179.00	3.58	0.21	0.77	0.00	0.00	0.00	0.00	0.00	0.00	0.00	
Coffee, espresso	1	Cup	240.00	21.60	0.02	3.67	0.00	0.43	0.22	0.00	0.22	0.00	0.00	0.00
Coffee, frappuccino, mocha, tall Starbucks	1.5	Cup	311.00	230.00	6.00	44.00	0.00	3.00	2.00			0.00		
Coffee, latte, iced, w/lowfat milk, double, tall Starbucks	1.5	Cup	392.00	90.00	7.00	10.00	0.00	3.00	2.00			15.00		
Coffee, latte, w/nonfat milk, double, tall Starbucks	1.5	Cup	367.00	120.00	12.00	17.00	0.00	0.50	0.00			5.00		
Coffee, latte, w/whole milk, double, tall Starbucks	1.5	Cup	366.00	210.00	11.00	17.00	0.00	11.00	7.00			45.00		
Coffee, mocha cappuccino, decaf, inst, dry pkt Maxwell House	1	Each	23.00	100.00	2.00	17.00	0.00	2.50	1.00			0.00	0.00	
Coffee, reg, inst, prep w/water	1	Cup	238.40	4.77	0.24	0.81	0.00	0.01	0.00	0.00	0.00	0.00	0.00	
Dairy Mixed Drinks and Mixes														
Drink, chocolate, dairy, rducd cal, w/asp, dry pkt, .75oz	1	Each	21.30	63.47	5.32	10.69	2.00	0.55	0.40	0.11	0.01	5.11	33.23	1.00
Drink, chocolate, dry mix	2.5	Teaspoon	21.60	75.38	0.71	19.50	0.95	0.67	0.40	0.22	0.02	0.00		
Drink, chocolate, prep f/dry mix w/milk	1	Cup	266.00	226.10	8.59	31.68	1.06	8.62	4.95	2.21	0.49	23.94	69.16	
Drink, strawberry, prep f/dry mix w/milk	1	Cup	266.00	234.08	7.98	32.72	0.00	8.25	5.08	2.36	0.30	31.92	69.16	2.66
Hot Cocoa, dry pkt Swiss Miss	1	Each	28.00	120.00	2.00	22.00	1.00	3.00	1.00			0.00	0.00	
Hot Cocoa, prep f/dry mix w/water	1	Cup	274.67	151.07	2.22	31.97	1.37	1.51	0.90	0.50	0.05	2.75		
Hot Cocoa, prep f/recipe w/milk	1	Cup	250.00	192.50	8.80	26.58	2.50	5.82	3.58	1.69	0.08	20.00	127.50	2.48
Hot Cocoa, rich chocolate, dry pkt Nestle	1	Each	28.00	112.00	1.30	24.24	0.67	1.11	0.29	0.35	0.27	1.68	0.00	1.96

Vit E (mg)	Vit C	Vit B$_1$-Thia (mg)	Vit B$_2$-Ribo (mg)	Vit B$_3$-Nia (mg)	Fol (mcg)	Vit B$_6$ (mg)	Vita B$_{12}$ (mcg)	Sodi (mg)	Pota (mg)	Cal (mg)	Phos (mg)	Magn (mg)	Iron (mg)	Zinc (mg)	Caff (mg)	Alco (g)	Sol Fiber (g)	Insol Fiber (g)
	0.00							90.00							0.00	0.00	0.00	0.00
	0.00						0.00	50.00			45.00				0.00	0.00	0.00	0.00
0.00	0.00	0.00	0.00	0.00	0.00	0.00	0.00	49.73	4.74	11.84	0.00	2.37	0.02	0.24	0.00	0.00	0.00	0.00
0.00	0.00	0.00	0.00	0.00	0.00	0.00	0.00	5.33	2.46	7.38	36.00	2.46	0.07	0.02	30.67	0.00	0.00	0.00
0.00	0.00							4.00	12.00		18.00				31.00	0.00	0.00	0.00
0.00	0.00	0.00	0.00	0.00	0.00	0.00	0.00	9.92	2.48	7.44	32.24	2.48	0.05	0.02	24.80	0.00	0.00	0.00
	0.00						0.00	23.33		0.00	35.33		0.00		24.67	0.00	0.00	0.00
	0.00						0.00	23.33	5.33	0.00	27.33		0.00		24.00	0.00	0.00	0.00
	0.00						0.00	23.33		0.00	27.33		0.00		0.00	0.00	0.00	0.00
0.00	0.00	0.01	0.05	0.00		0.00	0.00	11.84	14.21	7.11	26.05	2.37	0.07	0.00	33.15	0.00	0.00	0.00
0.00	0.00	0.00	0.00	0.00	0.00	0.00	0.00	29.66	2.47	12.36	0.00	2.47	0.12	0.17		0.00	0.00	0.00
	0.00							35.00							27.20	0.00	0.00	0.00
0.00	0.00	0.00	0.00					17.08	2.44	7.32	0.00	2.44	0.44	0.12	0.00	0.00	0.00	0.00
	0.00							60.00							0.00	0.00	0.00	0.00
0.00	0.00	0.00	0.00	0.00	0.00	0.00	0.00	37.20	2.48	7.44	0.00	2.48	0.20	0.17	0.00	0.00	0.00	0.00
0.00	0.00	0.00	0.00	0.04	0.00	0.00	0.00	27.02	2.46	4.91	0.00	2.46	0.17	0.12	0.00	0.00	0.00	0.00
	0.00						0.00	23.33		0.00	0.00		0.00		0.00	0.00	0.00	0.00
0.00	0.00	0.00	0.00	0.00	0.00	0.00	0.00	37.89	4.74	9.47	0.00	2.37	0.09	0.12	26.05	0.00	0.00	0.00
0.00	0.00	0.00	0.00	0.00	0.00	0.00	0.00	29.76	4.96	12.40	2.48	2.48	0.15	0.25	0.00	0.00	0.00	0.00
0.00	0.00	0.00	0.00	0.00	0.00	0.00	0.00	24.56	2.46	7.37	27.02	0.00	0.10	0.10	24.56	0.00	0.00	0.00
0.00	0.00	0.00	0.00	0.00	0.00	0.00	0.00	32.03	2.46	12.32	0.00	2.46	0.12	0.17	0.00	0.00	0.00	0.00
0.02	0.00	0.03	0.18	0.45	4.74	0.00	0.00	4.74	116.13	4.74	7.11	7.11	0.02	0.05	94.80	0.00	0.00	0.00
	2.40							110.00		250.00			0.00		180.00	0.00	0.00	0.00
	2.40							105.00		250.00			0.00		90.00	0.00	0.00	0.00
0.00	0.00	0.00	0.03	0.50	0.00	0.00	0.00	3.58	82.34	5.37	7.16	8.95	0.11	0.00	1.79	0.00	0.00	0.00
0.00	0.48	0.00	0.42	12.50	2.40	0.00	0.00	33.60	276.00	4.80	16.80	192.00	0.31	0.12	168.00	0.00	0.00	0.00
	0.00							180.00		100.00			0.00		130.00	0.00	0.00	0.00
	1.20							100.00		250.00			0.00		180.00	0.00	0.00	0.00
	3.60							170.00		400.00			0.00		180.00	0.00	0.00	0.00
	3.60							170.00		400.00			0.00		180.00	0.00	0.00	0.00
	0.00						0.00	70.00	150.00	60.00			0.00			0.00	Fiber	Fiber
0.00	0.00	0.00	0.00	0.56	0.00	0.00	0.00	4.77	71.52	9.54	7.15	7.15	0.10	0.02	61.98	0.00	0.00	0.00
0.00	1.19	0.02	0.41	0.27	7.03	0.02	0.51	140.37	477.12	300.76	190.21	44.73	1.64	0.77	3.83	0.00		
0.01	0.15	0.01	0.03	0.11	1.51	0.00	0.00	45.36	127.66	7.99	27.65	21.17	0.68	0.33	7.78	0.00		
0.16	0.27	0.11	0.48	0.38	13.30	0.09	1.06	154.28	457.52	252.70	234.08	47.88	0.80	1.28	7.98	0.00		
0.27	2.39	0.09	0.42	0.22	13.30	0.10	0.88	127.68	369.74	292.60	228.76	31.92	0.21	0.93	0.00	0.00	0.00	0.00
	0.00							130.00		40.00			1.08			0.00		
0.19	0.55	0.04	0.21	0.22	0.00	0.04	0.49	195.02	269.18	60.43	118.11	32.96	0.47	0.58	5.49	0.00		
0.08	0.50	0.10	0.45	0.33	12.50	0.10	1.05	110.00	492.50	262.50	262.50	57.50	1.20	1.58	5.00	0.00		
0.04	0.00	0.03	0.12	0.16	1.96	0.03	0.10	101.64	194.32	40.04	70.84	27.44	0.28	0.36	5.04	0.00		

Food Name	Amount	Measure	Weight (g)	Calories	Protein (g)	Total Carb (g)	Dietary Fiber (g)	Total Fat (g)	Sat Fat (g)	Mono Fat (g)	Poly Fat (g)	Chol (mg)	Vit A (mcg RAE)	Vit D (mcg)
Hot Cocoa, rich chocolate, w/o add sugar, dry pkt Nestle	1	Each	15.00	54.75	4.30	8.43	0.75	0.43	0.20	0.14	0.01	2.85	0.00	1.05
Hot Cocoa, w/asp add sod & vit A, prep f/dry w/water	1	Cup	256.00	74.24	3.23	13.93	1.28	0.59	0.01	0.19	0.02	0.00	35.84	
Hot Cocoa, w/marshmallows, dry pkt Nestle	1	Each	28.00	111.72	1.35	24.25	0.50	1.02	0.39	0.29	0.35	1.68	0.00	1.96
Instant Breakfast, chocolate malt, prep f/dry w/skm mlk Carnation	9	Fluid ounce	280.44	220.00	12.50	39.00	1.00	1.95	1.00			6.00		2.50
Instant Breakfast, milk chocolate, creamy, rtd, 10 fl oz can Carnation	10	Fluid ounce	314.00	220.00	12.00	37.00	2.00	2.50	1.00			10.00		2.51
Kefir, European	1	Cup	233.20	149.24	7.70	11.20	0.00	8.16						
Malt Beverage	1	Cup	236.80	87.62	0.50	19.06	0.00	0.28	0.06	0.04	0.13	0.00	0.24	
Malted Milk, chocolate, dry mix	3	Teaspoon	21.00	78.75	1.07	18.44	1.41	0.80	0.45	0.22	0.07	0.21	0.84	0.03
Malted Milk, chocolate, prep w/milk f/dry mix	1	Cup	265.00	225.25	8.93	29.68	1.33	8.72	4.99	2.19	0.55	26.50	68.90	
Malted Milk, chocolate, w/add nutrients, prep f/dry mix	1	Cup	265.00	222.60	8.90	28.94	1.06	8.64	4.95	2.17	0.54	26.50	903.65	
Malted Milk, natural, w/add nutrients, prep f/pwd w/milk	1	Cup	265.00	227.90	9.73	28.28	0.00	8.51	4.85	2.13	0.56	29.15	744.65	

Juice and Fruit Flavored Drinks

Food Name	Amount	Measure	Weight (g)	Calories	Protein (g)	Total Carb (g)	Dietary Fiber (g)	Total Fat (g)	Sat Fat (g)	Mono Fat (g)	Poly Fat (g)	Chol (mg)	Vit A (mcg RAE)	Vit D (mcg)
Drink, breakfast, orange, prep f/pwd	1	Cup	248.00	121.52	0.00	31.37	0.25	0.00	0.00	0.00	0.00	0.00	190.96	
Drink, cherry, sug free, prep f/dry mix, 1/8 pkg Kool-Aid	1	Cup	237.00	5.00	0.00	0.00	0.00	0.00	0.00	0.00	0.00	0.00	0.00	
Drink, cherry, sug free, w/asp & Vit C, dry pkg Kool-Aid	1	Each	9.60	27.84	0.59	8.15		0.03						
Drink, cherry, unswtnd, dry pkg Kool-Aid	0.125	Each	0.50	0.00	0.00	0.00	0.00	0.00	0.00	0.00	0.00	0.00	0.00	
Drink, diet, kiwi strawberry Snapple	1	Cup	251.70	20.00	0.00	5.00		0.00	0.00	0.00	0.00	0.00		
Drink, fruit punch, cnd	1	Cup	248.00	116.56	0.00	29.69	0.50	0.01	0.00	0.00	0.01	0.00	4.96	
Drink, fruit punch, dry mix Crystal Light	0.5	Teaspoon	1.20	5.00	0.00	0.00	0.00	0.00	0.00	0.00	0.00	0.00		
Drink, fruit punch, prep f/fzn conc w/water	1	Cup	247.20	113.71	0.15	28.82	0.25	0.01	0.00	0.00	0.00	0.00	1.36	
Drink, fruit punch, sug free, low cal, rtd Crystal Light	1	Cup	241.00	5.00	0.00	0.00	0.00	0.00	0.00	0.00	0.00	0.00	0.00	
Drink, fruit, low cal	1	Cup	240.00	43.20	0.00	11.28	0.00	0.00	0.00	0.00	0.00	0.00	1.20	0.00
Drink, Island Punch Snapple	1	Cup	251.70	110.00	0.00	27.00		0.00	0.00	0.00	0.00	0.00		
Drink, lemonade, low cal, w/asp, prep f/pwd w/water	1	Cup	236.80	4.74	0.05	1.23	0.00	0.00	0.00	0.00	0.00	0.00	0.00	
Drink, lemonade, prep f/pwd w/water	1	Cup	264.00	102.96	0.00	26.85	0.00	0.00	0.00	0.00	0.00	0.00	0.00	
Drink, lemonade, sug free, low cal, rtd Crystal Light	1	Cup	241.00	5.00	0.00	0.00	0.00	0.00	0.00	0.00	0.00	0.00	0.00	
Drink, orange, cnd	1	Cup	248.00	126.48	0.00	31.99	0.00	0.02	0.00	0.00	0.01	0.00	2.48	
Gelatin, drinking, orange, prep f/pwd pkt w/water	1	Cup	240.00	117.60	10.80	18.48	0.00	0.48	0.05	0.09	0.22	0.00	0.00	
Juice Drink, citrus fruit, prep f/fzn conc w/water	1	Cup	248.00	124.00	0.45	30.23	0.25	0.12	0.00	0.00	0.00	0.00	2.48	
Juice Drink, cranberry apple, 10% juice Everfresh	1	Cup	236.40	120.00	0.00	31.00	0.00	0.00	0.00	0.00	0.00	0.00	0.00	
Juice Drink, cranberry apple, btld	1	Cup	244.80	173.81	0.17	44.33	0.24	0.12	0.00	0.00	0.00	0.00	0.37	
Juice Drink, cranberry apple, w/vit, low cal	1	Cup	240.00	45.60	0.24	11.28	0.24	0.00	0.00	0.00	0.00	0.00	0.36	0.00
Juice Drink, cranberry raspberry Snapple	1	Cup	251.70	120.00	0.00	29.00		0.00	0.00	0.00	0.00	0.00		
Juice Drink, fruit punch, prep f/fzn conc w/water	1	Cup	248.00	124.00	0.25	30.26	0.25	0.50	0.06	0.06	0.12	0.00	0.74	0.00
Juice Drink, grape, cnd	1	Cup	250.40	125.20	0.25	32.00	0.00	0.00	0.00	0.00	0.00	0.00	0.25	
Juice Drink, kiwi strawberry, rtd Snapple	1	Cup	244.00	117.12	0.24	28.79	0.00	0.00	0.00	0.00	0.00	0.00	0.00	

Vit E (mg)	Vit C	Vit B₁-Thia (mg)	Vit B₂-Ribo (mg)	Vit B₃-Nia (mg)	Fol (mcg)	Vit B₆ (mg)	Vita B₁₂ (mcg)	Sodi (mg)	Pota (mg)	Cal (mg)	Phos (mg)	Magn (mg)	Iron (mg)	Zinc (mg)	Caff (mg)	Alco (g)	Sol Fiber (g)	Insol Fiber (g)
0.01	0.41	0.06	0.22	0.18	5.85	0.05	0.45	142.05	288.15	123.45	135.00	27.00	0.39	0.60	15.75	0.00		
0.08	0.26	0.05	0.28	0.22	2.56	0.06	0.33	227.84	540.16	120.32	179.20	43.52	1.00	0.69	2.56	0.00		
0.04	0.00	0.03	0.12	0.10	1.12	0.03	0.12	96.04	141.96	41.16	57.96	16.24	0.24	0.20	2.24	0.00		
6.82	30.00	0.38	0.43	5.00	100.00	0.50	1.50	264.00		500.00	250.00	100.00	4.50	3.75		0.00		
6.85	30.00	0.38	0.44	5.02	100.48	0.50	1.51	230.00	609.16	500.00	348.54	100.48	4.50	3.77		0.00		
								107.28	373.12		209.88	32.64	0.30		0.00	0.00	0.00	0.00
0.00	1.18	0.04	0.11	2.64	33.15	0.06	0.05	30.78	18.94	16.58	37.89	16.58	0.14	0.05	0.00	0.71	0.00	0.00
0.02	0.31	0.04	0.04	0.42	10.71	0.03	0.04	52.71	129.78	12.60	36.75	14.70	0.48	0.17	7.77	0.00		
0.16	0.27	0.14	0.49	0.69	23.85	0.12	1.11	159.00	455.80	259.70	241.15	39.75	0.56	1.09	7.95	0.00		
0.16	31.80	0.76	1.32	11.08	18.55	1.01	1.14	230.55	577.70	339.20	288.85	45.05	3.76	1.17	5.30	0.00		
0.32	27.56	0.73	1.21	10.58	15.90	0.86	1.06	190.80	530.00	325.95	283.55	39.75	3.60	1.09	0.00	0.00	0.00	0.00
0.00	73.16	0.00	0.22	2.54	0.00	0.25	0.00	9.92	59.52	126.48	47.12	2.48	0.02	0.02	0.00	0.00		
	6.00						0.00	5.00	0.00	0.00	0.00		0.00		0.00	0.00	0.00	0.00
	53.76						0.00	40.51	0.00	0.00			0.00		0.00	0.00		
	6.00						0.00	5.00	0.00	0.00			0.00		0.00	0.00	0.00	0.00
	0.00							10.00							0.00	0.00		
0.05	73.41	0.05	0.06	0.05	9.92	0.03	0.00	94.24	62.00	19.84	7.44	7.44	0.22	0.02	0.00	0.00		
	6.00						0.00	0.00	45.00	0.00					0.00	0.00	0.00	0.00
0.00	108.27	0.02	0.03	0.05	2.47	0.01	0.00	9.89	32.14	9.89	2.47	4.94	0.22	0.05	0.00	0.00		
	0.00							20.00	105.00	0.00	0.00		0.00		0.00	0.00	0.00	0.00
0.00	77.52	0.02	0.05	0.05	4.80	0.00	0.00	50.40	50.40	16.80	4.80	4.80	0.65	0.26	0.00	0.00	0.00	0.00
								10.00							0.00	0.00		
0.00	5.92	0.00	0.00	0.00	0.00	0.00	0.00	4.74	0.00	52.10	23.68	2.37	0.09	0.02	0.00	0.00	0.00	0.00
0.00	8.45	0.01	0.00	0.03	2.64	0.01	0.00	10.56	31.68	71.28	34.32	2.64	0.16	0.05	0.00	0.00	0.00	0.00
	0.00							20.00	160.00	0.00	0.00		0.00		0.00	0.00	0.00	0.00
0.05	84.57	0.01	0.01	0.08	9.92	0.02	0.00	39.68	44.64	14.88	2.48	4.96	0.69	0.22	0.00	0.00	0.00	0.00
0.00	89.04	0.00	0.00	0.00	0.00	0.00	0.00	57.60	4.80	4.80	0.00	2.40	0.00	0.05	0.00	0.00	0.00	0.00
0.05	36.21	0.04	0.02	0.15	7.44	0.04	0.00	4.96	121.52	12.40	9.92	9.92	0.12	0.05	0.00	0.00		
								0.00							0.00	0.00	0.00	0.00
0.00	78.34	0.01	0.05	0.15	0.00	0.05	0.00	17.14	68.54	12.24	4.90	4.90	0.29	0.44	0.00	0.00		
0.00	76.80	0.00	0.05	0.14	0.00	0.05	0.00	4.80	64.80	16.80	7.20	4.80	0.14	0.10	0.00	0.00		
	0.00							10.00							0.00	0.00		
0.00	13.89	0.00	0.16	0.15	0.00	0.03	0.00	12.40	190.96	17.36	0.00	9.92	0.57	0.55	0.00	0.00		
0.00	40.06	0.02	0.03	0.17	2.50	0.04	0.00	2.50	82.63	7.51	10.02	7.51	0.25	0.05	0.00	0.00	0.00	0.00
	0.00							7.32		0.00			0.37		0.00	0.00	0.00	0.00

Food Name	Amount	Measure	Weight (g)	Calories	Protein (g)	Total Carb (g)	Dietary Fiber (g)	Total Fat (g)	Sat Fat (g)	Mono Fat (g)	Poly Fat (g)	Chol (mg)	Vit A (mcg RAE)	Vit D (mcg)
BEVERAGE AND BEVERAGE MIXES *(continued)*														
Juice Drink, Mango Madness Snapple	1	Cup	251.70	110.00	0.00	29.00		0.00	0.00	0.00	0.00	0.00		
Juice Drink, pineapple grapefruit, cnd	1	Cup	250.40	117.69	0.50	29.05	0.25	0.25	0.02	0.03	0.07	0.00	0.13	
Juice Drink, pineapple orange, cnd	1	Cup	250.40	125.20	3.26	29.55	0.25	0.00	0.00	0.00	0.00	0.00	2.50	
Juice Drink, raspberry peach Snapple	1	Cup	251.70	120.00	0.00	29.00		0.00	0.00	0.00	0.00	0.00		
Juice, Snapple Farms, apple juice Snapple	1	Cup	251.68	120.00	0.00	29.33		0.00	0.00	0.00	0.00	0.00		
Lemonade, pink, prep f/fzn conc w/water	1	Cup	247.20	98.88	0.25	25.96	0.00	0.05	0.01	0.00	0.03	0.00	0.25	0.00
Lemonade, white, prep f/fzn conc w/water	1	Cup	248.00	131.44	0.22	34.05	0.25	0.15	0.02	0.00	0.04	0.00	0.25	
Limeade, prep f/fzn conc w/water	1	Cup	247.20	103.82	0.10	26.13	0.00	0.02	0.00	0.00	0.00	0.00	0.12	
Other Beverages														
Cocktail Mix, Bloody Mary, tabasco tomato, mild McIlhenny Company	8	Fluid ounce	242.00	55.66	2.18	11.86	0.97	0.00	0.00	0.00	0.00			
Drink, apple cider, spiced, inst, dry pkt Swiss Miss	1	Each	22.00	90.00	0.00	21.00	0.00	0.00	0.00	0.00	0.00	0.00	0.00	
Drink, energy, zesty flax, dry mix Natural Ovens	1	Tablespoon	10.00	40.00	2.00	5.00	3.00	2.00	0.50		1.00	0.00	0.00	
Teas														
Tea, brewed w/tap water	1	Cup	236.80	2.37	0.00	0.71	0.00	0.02	0.00	0.00	0.01	0.00	0.00	
Tea, chai, original, brewed w/water only Celestial Seasonings	1	Cup	236.80	0.00	0.00	0.00	0.00	0.00	0.00	0.00	0.00	0.00	0.00	
Tea, green Snapple	1	Cup	251.70	100.00	0.00	25.00		0.00	0.00	0.00	0.00	0.00		
Tea, herbal, not chamomile, brewed	1	Cup	236.80	2.37	0.00	0.47	0.00	0.02	0.00	0.00	0.01	0.00	0.00	
Tea, lemon flvr, diet, w/sacc, inst, prep f/pwd	1	Cup	236.80	4.74	0.05	1.04	0.00	0.00	0.00	0.00	0.00	0.00	0.00	
Tea, lemon flvr, unswtnd, inst, prep f/pwd	1	Cup	238.00	4.76	0.01	0.95	0.00	0.00	0.00	0.00	0.00	0.00	0.00	
Tea, lemon flvr, w/sug & vit C, inst, prep f/pwd	1	Cup	259.00	88.06	0.26	22.01	0.00	0.03	0.01	0.00	0.02	0.00	0.00	0.00
Tea, sweet, can Lipton Brisk	1	Cup	259.00	70.00	0.00	18.00	0.00	0.00	0.00	0.00	0.00	0.00	0.00	
Tea, unswtnd, inst, prep f/pwd	1	Cup	236.80	2.37	0.07	0.40	0.00	0.00	0.00	0.00	0.00	0.00	0.00	
Water														
Water, btld, Perrier	1	Cup	236.56	0.00	0.00	0.00	0.00	0.00	0.00	0.00	0.00	0.00	0.00	
Water, tonic	1	Cup	244.00	82.96	0.00	21.47	0.00	0.00	0.00	0.00	0.00	0.00	0.00	
BEVERAGES, ALCOHOLIC														
Aquavit, 80 proof	1	Fluid ounce	27.80	64.22	0.00	0.00	0.00	0.00	0.00	0.00	0.00	0.00	0.00	
Beer, can/btl, 12 fl oz	12	Fluid ounce	356.40	139.00	1.07	10.76	0.00	0.00	0.00	0.00	0.00	0.00	0.00	
Beer, golden draft, each Anheuser-Busch	12	Fluid ounce	356.00	149.91	1.59	12.81		0.00	0.00	0.00	0.00	0.00		
Beer, Light Coors	12	Fluid ounce	352.90	105.00	0.70	4.99	0.00	0.00	0.00	0.00	0.00	0.00	0.00	
Beer, light, can/btl, 12 fl oz	12	Fluid ounce	354.00	102.66	0.99	5.17	0.00	0.00	0.00	0.00	0.00	0.00	0.00	
Beer, Light, each Anheuser-Busch	12	Fluid ounce	356.00	110.00	1.20	6.60		0.00	0.00	0.00	0.00	0.00		
Beer, non alcoholic Coors	12	Fluid ounce	352.90	72.99	0.79	14.20	0.00	0.00	0.00	0.00	0.00	0.00		
Brandy, 80 proof	1	Fluid ounce	27.80	64.22	0.00	0.00	0.00	0.00	0.00	0.00	0.00	0.00	0.00	
Gin, 80 proof	1	Fluid ounce	27.80	64.22	0.00	0.00	0.00	0.00	0.00	0.00	0.00	0.00	0.00	
Liqueur, coffee, 53 proof	1	Fluid ounce	34.80	116.93	0.03	16.29	0.00	0.10	0.04	0.01	0.04	0.00	0.00	
Mixed Drink, daiquiri, 6.8 fl oz can	1	Each	207.40	259.25	0.00	32.56	0.00	0.00	0.00	0.00	0.00	0.00	0.21	0.00
Mixed Drink, martini, prep f/recipe	1	Fluid ounce	28.20	68.53	0.01	0.58	0.00	0.00	0.00	0.00	0.00	0.00	0.00	
Mixed Drink, pina colada, cnd, 6.8 fl oz	1	Each	221.68	525.38	1.33	61.18	0.22	16.85	14.57	0.98	0.30	0.00	2.22	
Mixed Drink, whiskey sour, 6.8 fl oz can	1	Each	209.44	249.23	0.00	28.06	0.21	0.00	0.00	0.00	0.00	0.00	2.09	
Tequila, 80 proof	1	Fluid ounce	27.80	64.22	0.00	0.00	0.00	0.00	0.00	0.00	0.00	0.00	0.00	
Vodka, 80 proof	1	Fluid ounce	27.80	64.22	0.00	0.00	0.00	0.00	0.00	0.00	0.00	0.00	0.00	
Wine, all table types	6	Fluid ounce	177.00	136.29	0.35	5.66	0.00	0.00	0.00	0.00	0.00	0.00	0.00	
Wine, cooler	1	Cup	226.67	113.02	0.26	13.45	0.07	0.05	0.01	0.00	0.01	0.00	0.16	0.00

Vit E (mg)	Vit C	Vit B₁-Thia (mg)	Vit B₂-Ribo (mg)	Vit B₃-Nia (mg)	Fol (mcg)	Vit B₆ (mg)	Vita B₁₂ (mcg)	Sodi (mg)	Pota (mg)	Cal (mg)	Phos (mg)	Magn (mg)	Iron (mg)	Zinc (mg)	Caff (mg)	Alco (g)	Sol Fiber (g)	Insol Fiber (g)
	0.00							10.00							0.00	0.00		
0.03	115.18	0.08	0.04	0.67	22.54	0.11	0.00	35.06	152.74	17.53	15.02	15.02	0.78	0.15	0.00	0.00		
0.08	56.34	0.08	0.05	0.52	22.54	0.12	0.00	7.51	115.18	12.52	10.02	15.02	0.68	0.15	0.00	0.00		
	0.00							10.00							0.00	0.00		
								26.67							0.00	0.00		
0.00	9.64	0.01	0.05	0.04	4.94	0.01	0.00	7.42	37.08	7.42	4.94	4.94	0.40	0.10	0.00	0.00	0.00	0.00
0.02	12.90	0.02	0.07	0.05	2.48	0.02	0.00	7.44	49.60	9.92	7.44	4.96	0.52	0.07	0.00	0.00		
0.00	5.93	0.00	0.01	0.02	2.47	0.01	0.00	4.94	22.25	7.42	2.47	2.47	0.02	0.02	0.00	0.00	0.00	0.00
								1173.70		60.50			1.74		0.00	0.00		
	0.00							60.00		0.00			0.00		0.00	0.00	0.00	0.00
	0.00	0.15	0.17	2.00	40.00	0.20	0.60	2.00		60.00		40.00	1.08	2.25	0.00	0.00		
0.00	0.00	0.00	0.03	0.00	11.84	0.00	0.00	7.10	87.62	0.00	2.37	7.10	0.05	0.05	47.36	0.00	0.00	0.00
	0.00							0.00		0.00			0.00		30.00	0.00	0.00	0.00
	0.00							10.00							18.00	0.00		
0.00	0.00	0.02	0.01	0.00	2.37	0.00	0.00	2.37	21.31	4.74	0.00	2.37	0.19	0.09				
0.00	0.00	0.00	0.00	0.05	0.00	0.00	0.00	23.68	30.78	7.10	2.37	2.37	0.12	0.02	16.58	0.00	0.00	0.00
0.00	0.00	0.00	0.02	0.09	0.00	0.00	0.00	14.28	49.98	4.76	2.38	4.76	0.02	0.07	26.18	0.00	0.00	0.00
0.00	23.31	0.00	0.05	0.09	10.36	0.01	0.00	7.77	49.21	5.18	2.59	5.18	0.05	0.08	28.49	0.00	0.00	0.00
	0.00							50.00		0.00			0.00		5.00	0.00	0.00	0.00
0.00	0.00	0.00	0.00	0.09	0.00	0.00	0.00	7.10	47.36	7.10	2.37	4.74	0.05	0.02	30.78	0.00	0.00	0.00
0.00	0.00	0.00	0.00	0.00	0.00	0.00	0.00	2.37	0.00	33.12	0.00	0.00	0.00	0.00	0.00	0.00	0.00	0.00
0.00	0.00	0.00	0.00	0.00	0.00	0.00	0.00	9.76	0.00	2.44	0.00	0.00	0.02	0.24	0.00	0.00	0.00	0.00
0.00	0.00	0.00	0.00	0.00	0.00	0.00	0.00	0.28	0.56	0.00	1.11	0.00	0.01	0.01	0.00	9.29	0.00	0.00
0.00	0.00	0.02	0.09	1.83	21.38	0.16	0.07	14.26	96.23	14.26	49.90	21.38	0.07	0.04	0.00	12.83	Sol	Insol
							0.00	8.94							0.00	13.50		
		0.03	0.03	1.41				10.99	59.00	10.99					0.00	14.11	0.00	0.00
0.00	0.00	0.02	0.05	1.38	21.24	0.12	0.32	14.16	74.34	14.16	42.48	17.70	0.11	0.04	0.00	10.97	0.00	0.00
	0.00		0.08	1.64		0.18	0.00	9.00	90.00	11.00	139.01	17.09			0.00	15.30		
		0.03	0.07	1.41				10.00	54.01	19.00					0.00	1.78	0.00	0.00
0.00	0.00	0.00	0.00	0.00	0.00	0.00	0.00	0.28	0.56	0.00	1.11	0.00	0.01	0.01	0.00	9.29	0.00	0.00
0.00	0.00	0.00	0.00	0.00	0.00	0.00	0.00	0.28	0.56	0.00	1.11	0.00	0.01	0.01	0.00	9.29	0.00	0.00
0.00	0.00	0.00	0.00	0.05	0.00	0.00	0.00	2.78	10.44	0.35	2.09	1.04	0.02	0.01	9.05	7.55	0.00	0.00
0.00	2.70	0.00	0.00	0.03	2.07	0.01	0.00	82.96	22.81	0.00	4.15	2.07	0.02	0.06	0.00	19.91	0.00	0.00
0.00	0.00	0.00	0.00	0.01	0.00	0.00	0.00	0.85	4.51	0.28	0.56	0.56	0.01	0.00	0.00	9.56	0.00	0.00
0.07	3.33	0.04	0.01	0.23	13.30	0.04	0.00	157.39	183.99	2.22	79.80	13.30	0.07	0.44	0.00	19.95		
0.00	3.35	0.02	0.01	0.04	0.00	0.00	0.00	92.15	23.04	0.00	12.57	2.09	0.02	0.13	0.00	19.90		
0.00	0.00	0.00	0.00	0.00	0.00	0.00	0.00	0.28	0.56	0.00	1.11	0.00	0.01	0.01	0.00	9.29	0.00	0.00
0.00	0.00	0.00	0.00	0.00	0.00	0.00	0.00	0.28	0.28	0.00	1.39	0.00	0.00	0.00	0.00	9.29	0.00	0.00
0.00	0.00	0.00	0.03	0.13	1.77	0.04	0.01	10.62	148.68	14.16	23.01	15.93	0.62	0.10	0.00	16.46	0.00	0.00
0.01	4.05	0.01	0.02	0.10	2.69	0.03	0.01	19.04	102.23	12.83	14.77	11.93	0.62	0.13	0.00	8.82		

Food Name	Amount	Measure	Weight (g)	Calories	Protein (g)	Total Carb (g)	Dietary Fiber (g)	Total Fat (g)	Sat Fat (g)	Mono Fat (g)	Poly Fat (g)	Chol (mg)	Vit A (mcg RAE)	Vit D (mcg)
CANDIES AND CONFECTIONS, GUM														
Candy Bar, 3 Musketeers, 2.13 oz bar	1	Each	60.39	251.20	1.93	46.38	1.09	7.79	3.93	2.59	0.27	6.64	9.06	
Candy Bar, 5th Avenue, 2oz bar	1	Each	56.70	273.29	4.98	35.54	1.76	13.60	3.77	6.01	1.92	3.40	7.94	
Candy Bar, almond chocolate, Golden Collection, 2.8oz pkg	1	Each	79.38	458.02	10.18	36.63	3.02	30.53	13.23	14.05	3.10	10.32		
Candy Bar, Almond Joy, 1.7oz	1	Each	48.19	230.85	1.99	28.68	2.41	12.98	8.48	2.54	0.57	1.93		
Candy Bar, Baby Ruth, 2.1 oz bar	1	Each	59.53	276.24	4.23	36.79	1.43	14.88	7.32	3.84	1.97	1.19		
Candy Bar, Butterfinger, 2.16oz bar	1	Each	61.24	291.48	3.55	44.39	1.04	11.63	6.27	2.99	1.51	0.00		
Candy Bar, Caramello, 1.6oz bar	1	Each	45.36	209.56	2.81	28.94	0.54	9.61	5.77	2.40	0.29	12.25		0.00
Candy Bar, carob, 3oz bar	1	Each	85.05	459.27	6.93	47.87	3.23	26.67	24.68	0.41	0.25	2.55		
Candy Bar, Chunky, 1.25oz bar	1	Each	35.44	175.42	3.19	20.23	1.70	10.35	8.23	0.11	1.56	3.90		
Candy Bar, Kit Kat, 1.625oz bar	1	Each	46.07	238.64	3.00	29.76	0.46	11.97	8.27	2.69	0.41	5.07	11.06	
Candy Bar, Krackel, 2.2oz bar	1	Each	62.37	319.33	4.13	39.89	1.37	16.58	9.93	3.90	0.36	6.86		
Candy Bar, Mars almond, 1.76oz bar	1	Each	50.00	233.50	4.05	31.35	1.00	11.50	3.63	5.35	1.99	8.50	7.50	
Candy Bar, milk chocolate, w/almonds, bites Hershey's Bites	17	Piece	39.00	214.50	3.81	19.89	1.40	13.93	6.78	5.61	0.94	7.41		
Candy Bar, Milky Way, 2.1oz bar	1	Each	59.53	251.83	2.68	42.69	1.01	9.59	4.64	3.58	0.36	8.33	10.72	
Candy Bar, Mounds, 1.9oz bar	1	Each	53.86	261.78	2.48	31.56	1.99	14.33	11.09	0.21	0.08	1.08	0.00	
Candy Bar, Mr. Goodbar, 1.75oz bar	1	Each	49.61	266.92	5.07	26.96	1.89	16.48	7.01	4.07	2.17	4.96	17.36	
Candy Bar, Nestle Crunch, 1.4 oz bar	1	Each	39.69	207.18	2.38	25.88	1.03	10.44	6.03	3.42	0.35	5.16		
Candy Bar, Skor, toffee bar, 1.4oz bar	1	Each	39.69	212.34	1.24	24.50	0.52	12.77	7.45	3.69	0.51	21.04		
Candy Bar, Snickers, 2oz bar	1	Each	56.70	264.79	5.17	36.64	1.42	10.86	4.17	4.67	1.53	7.94	22.11	
Candy Bar, Special Dark, sweet chocolate, 1.45oz bar	1	Each	41.11	218.28	2.28	24.42	2.67	13.32	7.89	2.11	0.18	2.06		
Candy Bar, Sweet Escapes, triple chocolate	1	Each	19.00	81.70	0.89	13.93	0.78	2.50	1.50	0.44	0.24	0.00	1.90	
Candy Bar, Symphony, milk chocolate, 1.5oz bar	1	Each	42.53	225.81	3.62	24.67	0.72	13.00	7.80	3.36	0.29	10.21		0.00
Candy Bar, Twix, caramel, 2oz bar	1	Each	56.70	282.93	2.61	37.18	0.62	13.83	5.05	7.60	0.48	2.84	14.74	
Candy, candy corn, prep f/recipe	10	Piece	10.80	40.39	0.00	10.09	0.00	0.00	0.00	0.00	0.00	0.00	0.00	
Candy, caramels	1	Piece	10.10	38.58	0.46	7.78	0.12	0.82	0.66	0.09	0.02	0.71	0.10	
Candy, chocolate cvrd, dietetic/low cal	1	Ounce-weight	28.35	163.01	3.57	12.05	1.02	11.17	6.21	3.10	1.23	5.95	15.59	
Candy, fruit snacks, w/vit A C & E, pouch Farley Candy Company	1	Each	26.00	88.66	1.14	21.03		0.00	0.00	0.00	0.00			
Candy, Goobers, chocolate cvrd peanuts, 1.375oz pkg	1	Each	38.98	199.97	5.34	18.98	2.38	13.06	4.76	5.75	1.99	3.51	0.00	
Candy, gumdrops, sml, 1/2"	1	Each	3.20	12.67	0.00	3.16	0.00	0.00	0.00	0.00	0.00	0.00	0.00	
Candy, halavah, plain	1	Ounce-weight	28.35	132.96	3.54	17.15	1.28	6.10	1.17	2.32	2.40	0.00		0.00
Candy, hard, all flvrs, sml	1	Piece	3.00	11.82	0.00	2.94	0.00	0.01	0.00	0.00	0.00	0.00	0.00	
Candy, jellybeans, sml	10	Piece	11.00	41.25	0.00	10.29	0.02	0.01	0.00	0.00	0.00	0.00	0.00	
Candy, milk chocolate peanut, 1.67oz pkg	1	Each	47.34	244.30	4.48	28.62	1.61	12.42	4.89	5.21	1.99	4.26	12.31	
Candy, milk chocolate, mini, 5oz pkg	1	Each	141.75	705.92	6.77	95.15	3.83	33.10	20.48	10.77	0.99	21.26		
Candy, mints, After Eight	5	Piece	41.00	146.78	0.90	31.49	0.86	5.62	3.35	1.81	0.21	0.00	0.41	
Candy, peanut brittle, prep f/recipe	1.5	Ounce-weight	42.53	205.82	3.22	30.05	1.06	8.07	1.76	3.43	1.94	5.10	16.58	
Candy, peanut butter cups, .6oz single pkg Reese's	1	Each	17.01	87.60	1.74	9.42	0.61	5.19	1.83	2.23	0.95	1.02	2.89	
Candy, peanut butter cups, 1.6oz double pkg Reese's	1	Each	45.36	233.60	4.64	25.11	1.63	13.85	4.87	5.94	2.54	2.72	7.71	
Candy, peanuts, milk chocolate cvrd, pces	10	Piece	40.00	207.60	5.24	19.76	1.88	13.40	5.84	5.17	1.73	3.60	13.60	
Candy, Pieces, 1.6oz pkg Reese's	1	Each	45.36	225.44	5.65	27.15	1.36	11.24	7.45	2.02	0.85	0.00	0.00	
Candy, plain chocolate, 1.69oz pkg	1	Each	47.91	235.72	2.07	34.12	1.20	10.12	6.27	1.69	0.18	6.71	12.94	
Candy, plain chocolate, pces	10	Piece	7.00	34.44	0.30	4.98	0.18	1.48	0.92	0.25	0.03	0.98	1.89	
Candy, Raisinets, chocolate cvrd raisins, 1.58oz pkg	1	Each	44.79	184.55	2.11	31.89	2.28	7.12	3.29	2.66	0.85	1.79		
Candy, raisins, milk chocolate cvrd	1.5	Ounce-weight	42.53	165.85	1.74	29.04	1.79	6.29	3.74	2.02	0.22	1.28	10.21	
Candy, Rolo, caramels in milk chocolate, 1.91oz roll	1	Each	54.15	256.66	2.75	36.79	0.49	11.33	7.81	2.04	0.21	6.50	18.41	
Candy, Skittles, original bite size candies, 2.3oz pkg	1	Each	65.21	264.08	0.12	59.10	0.00	2.85	0.57	1.93	0.08	0.00	0.00	

Vit E (mg)	Vit C	Vit B₁-Thia (mg)	Vit B₂-Ribo (mg)	Vit B₃-Nia (mg)	Fol (mcg)	Vit B₆ (mg)	Vita B₁₂ (mcg)	Sodi (mg)	Pota (mg)	Cal (mg)	Phos (mg)	Magn (mg)	Iron (mg)	Zinc (mg)	Caff (mg)	Alco (g)	Sol Fiber (g)	Insol Fiber (g)
0.56	0.24	0.02	0.08	0.14	0.00	0.01	0.11	117.15	80.31	50.72	54.95	17.51	0.44	0.33	4.83	0.00		
1.53	0.23	0.08	0.05	2.21	20.41	0.06	0.10	127.58	196.75	41.39	79.95	35.15	0.68	0.64	2.84	0.00		
0.48	0.00	0.05	0.42	0.84		0.04	0.34	50.80	373.88	152.41	214.33	88.11	1.47	1.35		0.00		
0.01	0.34	0.01	0.07	0.23		0.03	0.06	68.44	122.42	30.84	53.98	31.81	0.61	0.39		0.00		
1.11	0.06	0.06	0.05	1.65	18.46	0.04	0.02	127.40	211.94	26.79	82.16	43.46	0.42	0.71	2.38	0.00		
1.06	0.00	0.07	0.05	1.89	20.21	0.06	0.01	131.05	241.88	21.43	82.67	50.83	0.47	0.73	3.06	0.00		
0.10	0.77	0.02	0.18	0.52		0.02	0.29	55.34	154.68	96.62	68.04	19.05	0.49	0.43	1.81	0.00		
1.00	0.43	0.09	0.15	0.88	17.86	0.11	0.85	91.00	538.37	257.70	107.16	30.62	1.10	3.00	0.00	0.00		
0.53	0.11	0.03	0.14	0.67	7.80	0.04	0.13	18.78	189.24	50.68	73.71	25.87	0.44	0.65	10.28	0.00		
0.16	0.00	0.05	0.10	0.23	6.45	0.01	0.26	24.88	106.42	57.59	62.19	17.05	0.46	0.04	6.45	0.00		
0.05	0.50	0.03	0.12	0.16	3.74	0.02	0.36	122.25	202.70	98.54	76.72	8.11	0.66	0.31		0.00		
3.88	0.35	0.02	0.16	0.47	4.50	0.03	0.18	85.00	162.50	84.00	117.00	36.00	0.55	0.56	2.00	0.00		
0.15	0.70	0.03	0.15	0.24	6.24	0.03		28.86	183.69	85.80	88.53	23.01	0.58	0.52		0.00		
0.74	0.60	0.02	0.13	0.21	3.57	0.03	0.19	142.88	143.48	77.40	85.73	20.24	0.45	0.42	4.76	0.00		
0.10	0.38	0.00	0.00	0.00	0.00	0.00	0.00	78.10	172.91	11.31	0.00	0.00	1.13	0.00	9.16	0.00		
1.57	0.45	0.07	0.07	1.71	18.85	0.03	0.16	20.34	195.47	54.57	80.87	23.32	0.69	0.46	8.93	0.00		
0.44	0.12	0.13	0.22	1.57	31.36	0.16	0.15	52.79	136.53	67.08	80.17	23.02	0.20	0.57	9.53	0.00		
0.02	0.20	0.01	0.04	0.05	1.19	0.01	0.11	125.82	60.73	51.60	24.21	3.97	0.23	0.07		0.00		
0.85	0.00	0.03	0.07	2.04	15.31	0.05	0.09	129.28	183.14	59.54	107.73	40.82	0.68	1.42	4.54	0.00		
0.08	0.00	0.00	0.00	0.00	0.00	0.00	0.00	2.47	206.36	12.33	20.96	12.74	0.88	0.00	20.55	0.00		
0.17	0.00	0.01	0.02	0.09	1.71	0.00	0.03	30.02	67.45	99.94	25.27	12.35	0.43	0.22	2.28	0.00		
0.09	0.94	0.04	0.16	0.14		0.02	0.17	42.95	186.26	106.74	87.60	23.39	0.39	0.48	28.07	0.00		
1.10	0.23	0.07	0.11	0.43	10.77	0.01	0.16	109.43	107.16	51.03	61.80	18.14	0.46	0.57	1.70	0.00		
0.00	0.00	0.00	0.00	0.00	0.00	0.00	0.00	1.73	0.43	0.22	0.00	0.00	0.00	0.00	0.00	0.00	0.00	0.00
0.28	0.05	0.00	0.03	0.03	0.50	0.00	0.00	24.74	21.61	13.94	11.51	1.72	0.02	0.05	0.00	0.00		
0.83	0.40	0.06	0.13	0.64	7.37	0.04	0.24	30.90	171.80	85.90	94.12	28.35	0.41	0.77	2.55	0.00		
10.40	23.48							9.36								0.00	0.00	
0.99	0.00	0.05	0.08	2.03	3.12	0.08	0.11	15.98	195.69	49.51	115.38	46.39	0.52	0.85	8.58	0.00		
0.00	0.00	0.00	0.00	0.00	0.00	0.00	0.00	1.41	0.16	0.10	0.03	0.03	0.01	0.00	0.00	0.00		
0.81	0.03	0.12	0.03	0.81	18.43	0.10	0.01	55.28	53.01	9.36	172.08	61.80	1.28	1.23	0.00	0.00		
0.00	0.00	0.00	0.00	0.00	0.00	0.00	0.00	1.14	0.15	0.09	0.09	0.09	0.01	0.00	0.00	0.00	0.00	0.00
0.00	0.00	0.00	0.00	0.00	0.00	0.00	0.00	5.50	4.07	0.33	0.44	0.22	0.00	0.01	0.00	0.00		
1.21	0.24	0.05	0.07	1.94	17.99	0.04	0.08	22.73	164.29	47.82	110.31	35.98	0.54	1.14	5.21	0.00		
1.35	0.85	0.07	0.32	0.35	7.09	0.04	0.43	96.39	415.33	164.43	235.31	65.21	1.74	1.49		0.00		
0.16	0.00	0.02	0.02	0.12	0.41	0.01	0.00	4.92	68.88	9.43	23.37	18.45	0.63	0.24	8.20	0.00		
1.09	0.00	0.06	0.02	1.13	19.56	0.03	0.00	189.24	71.44	11.48	45.08	17.86	0.52	0.37	0.00	0.00		
0.03	0.05	0.03	0.02	0.76	8.51	0.02	0.10	53.41	58.34	13.27	27.39	10.55	0.21	0.22	3.06	0.00		
0.07	0.14	0.07	0.05	2.04	22.68	0.05	0.25	142.43	155.58	35.38	73.03	28.12	0.55	0.58	8.16	0.00		
1.38	0.00	0.05	0.07	1.70	3.20	0.08	0.18	16.40	200.80	41.60	84.80	38.40	0.52	0.96	8.80	0.00		
0.49	0.00	0.08	0.10	2.75	24.95	0.05	0.05	88.00	162.84	31.30	93.90	39.92	0.22	0.52	0.00	0.00		
0.53	0.24	0.03	0.08	0.10	2.87	0.01	0.16	29.23	97.26	50.31	54.62	16.29	0.53	0.53	5.27	0.00		
0.08	0.04	0.00	0.01	0.01	0.42	0.00	0.02	4.27	14.21	7.35	7.98	2.38	0.08	0.08	0.77	0.00		
0.47	0.09	0.04	0.10	0.18	2.24	0.05	0.09	16.13	230.24	48.38	64.50	20.16	0.53	0.35	11.20	0.00		
0.43	0.09	0.04	0.07	0.17	2.98	0.03	0.08	15.31	218.58	36.57	60.81	19.14	0.73	0.34	10.63	0.00		
0.48	0.49	0.01	0.06	0.02	0.00	0.00	0.15	101.80	101.80	78.52	38.45	0.00	0.23	0.00	1.62	0.00		
0.29	43.62	0.00	0.01	0.01	0.00	0.00	0.00	10.43	5.87	0.00	1.30	0.65	0.01	0.01	0.00	0.00	0.00	0.00

Food Name	Amount	Measure	Weight (g)	Calories	Protein (g)	Total Carb (g)	Dietary Fiber (g)	Total Fat (g)	Sat Fat (g)	Mono Fat (g)	Poly Fat (g)	Chol (mg)	Vit A (mcg RAE)	Vit D (mcg)
CANDIES AND CONFECTIONS, GUM *(continued)*														
Candy, Sno Caps, sweet chocolate, box	1	Each	65.20	300.00	2.00	48.00	3.00	13.00	8.00			0.00	0.00	
Candy, Starburst, fruit chews, 2.07oz pkg	1	Each	58.68	232.39	0.23	49.59	0.00	4.87	0.73	2.09	1.83	0.00	0.00	
Candy, strawberry twists, 5 oz pkg	4	Piece	38.00	133.00	0.97	30.30	0.00	0.88	0.00			0.00	0.00	
Candy, Turtles, chocolate caramel pecans, 6oz pkg, Demet's	1	Piece	17.00	82.45	1.09	9.86	0.44	4.73	1.84	1.88	0.79	3.74		
Candy, York peppermint patty, sml, .5oz	1	Each	14.18	54.43	0.31	11.48	0.28	1.02	0.62	0.06	0.01	0.14		0.00
Chewing Gum, stick	1	Piece	3.00	7.41	0.00	1.98	0.07	0.01	0.00	0.00	0.00	0.00	0.00	0.00
Chewing Gum, sugarless	1	Piece	2.00	5.36	0.00	1.90	0.05	0.01	0.00	0.00	0.00	0.00	0.00	
Fruit Leather, cherry	1	Ounce-weight	28.35	104.89	0.15	22.68	0.40	1.70	0.68	0.88	0.00	0.00		
Fudge, chocolate, prep f/recipe	1	Piece	17.00	69.87	0.41	13.00	0.29	1.77	1.01	0.46	0.04	2.38	7.48	0.07
Fudge, vanilla, prep f/recipe	1	Piece	16.00	61.44	0.17	13.16	0.00	0.87	0.45	0.19	0.01	2.40	7.36	0.06
Marshmallows	4	Each	28.80	91.58	0.52	23.41	0.03	0.06	0.01	0.02	0.01	0.00	0.00	
Marshmallows, miniature Jet-Puffed	0.5	Cup	30.00	100.00	1.00	25.00	0.00	0.00	0.00	0.00	0.00	0.00	0.00	
CEREALS, BREAKFAST TYPE														
Cereals, Cooked and Dry														
Cereal, hot, apple spice Kashi Company	0.5	Cup	140.00	270.00	7.00	56.00	6.00	3.00				0.00	0.00	
Cereal, hot, Cream Of Rice, ckd w/water w/o salt	0.5	Cup	122.00	63.44	1.10	13.91	0.12	0.12	0.04	0.04	0.04	0.00	0.00	0.00
Cereal, hot, Cream Of Wheat, ckd w/water w/o salt	0.5	Cup	125.30	62.65	1.83	13.44	0.50	0.24	0.04	0.03	0.13	0.00	0.00	0.00
Cereal, hot, Cream Of Wheat, mix 'n eat, prep w/water f/pkt	1	Each	142.00	102.24	2.70	21.44	0.43	0.28	0.05	0.04	0.16	0.00	376.30	0.00
Cereal, hot, Malt-O-Meal, choc, ckd w/water & salt	0.5	Cup	120.00	61.20	1.80	12.96	0.48	0.12	0.02	0.03	0.02	0.00	0.00	0.00
Cereal, hot, Malt-O-Meal, plain, ckd w/water w/o salt	0.5	Cup	120.00	61.20	1.80	12.84	0.48	0.12	0.05	0.03	0.02	0.00	0.00	0.00
Cereal, hot, oat bran, prep w/water w/o salt Quaker Oats	0.5	Cup	109.50	47.08	2.22	8.20	1.86	1.04	0.18	0.34	0.40		1.10	0.00
Cereal, hot, oatmeal, apple spice, inst Nutrition for Women	1	Each	47.00	169.20	4.97	34.78	3.24	1.96	0.33	0.66	0.59	0.00	336.99	3.93
Cereal, hot, oatmeal, bkd apple, inst, prep w/water Quaker Oats	1	Each	177.00	169.92	3.58	34.43	3.19	1.96	0.34	0.68	0.57	0.00	368.16	
Cereal, hot, oatmeal, fruit & cream, inst, prep w/water Quaker Oats	1	Each	154.00	110.88	2.23	20.88	1.69	2.09	0.44	0.67	0.36	0.00	263.34	0.00
Cereal, hot, oatmeal, plain, inst, fort, prep w/water	1	Each	177.00	97.35	4.11	16.97	2.83	1.61	0.26	0.51	0.59	0.00	284.97	0.00
Cereal, hot, oatmeal, plain, quick, dry Quaker Oats	0.5	Cup	40.00	148.40	5.48	27.27	3.76	2.75	0.44	0.79	0.92	Chol	0.00	0.00
Cereal, hot, oatmeal, plain, unfort, prep w/water & salt	0.5	Cup	117.00	72.54	3.04	12.64	1.99	1.17	0.21	0.38	0.44	0.00	0.00	0.00
Cereal, hot, Ralston, ckd w/water & salt	0.5	Cup	126.50	67.04	2.78	14.17	3.04	0.38	0.07	0.05	0.18	0.00	0.00	
Grits, corn, white, quick, unenrich, ckd w/water & salt	0.5	Cup	121.00	72.60	1.70	15.73	0.24	0.24	0.04	0.06	0.10	0.00	0.00	0.00
Grits, hominy, white, quick, dry Quaker Oats	0.25	Cup	37.00	128.39	3.16	29.29	1.78	0.50	0.10	0.07	0.25	0.00	0.00	
Cereals, Ready To Eat														
Cereal, 100% Bran C.W. Post	0.33	Cup	29.00	83.23	3.68	22.68	8.29	0.61	0.09			0.00		0.00
Cereal, All-Bran Kellogg's Company	0.5	Cup	30.00	78.00	3.94	22.27	8.79	1.47	0.19	0.20	0.63	0.00	157.50	1.28
Cereal, bran, malted flour	0.33	Cup	29.00	83.23	3.68	22.68	8.29	0.61	0.09	0.09	0.32	0.00	225.04	0.00
Cereal, Cap'N Crunch	0.75	Cup	27.00	108.27	1.17	22.90	0.68	1.57	0.41	0.29	0.20	0.00	1.89	0.00
Cereal, Cheerios General Mills, Inc.	1	Cup	30.00	110.70	3.55	22.20	3.57	1.77	0.36	0.64	0.22	0.00	150.30	1.00
Cereal, Chex, corn General Mills, Inc.	1	Cup	30.00	111.90	2.10	25.80	0.60	0.27	0.06	0.06	0.10	0.00	137.10	0.00
Cereal, Chex, multi-bran General Mills, Inc.	1	Cup	49.00	165.62	3.43	41.16	6.37	1.23	0.25	0.30	0.54	0.00	116.62	0.89
Cereal, Chex, rice General Mills, Inc.	1.25	Cup	31.00	116.87	1.86	26.66	0.31	0.31	0.12	0.07	0.07	0.00	155.31	0.00

Vit E (mg)	Vit C	Vit B₁-Thia (mg)	Vit B₂-Ribo (mg)	Vit B₃-Nia (mg)	Fol (mcg)	Vit B₆ (mg)	Vita B₁₂ (mcg)	Sodi (mg)	Pota (mg)	Cal (mg)	Phos (mg)	Magn (mg)	Iron (mg)	Zinc (mg)	Caff (mg)	Alco (g)	Sol Fiber (g)	Insol Fiber (g)
	0.00	0.03	0.03	0.18				0.00	21.10	0.00			1.08		22.62	0.00		
0.41	31.04	0.00	0.00	0.00	0.00	0.00	0.00	32.86	1.17	2.35	4.11	0.59	0.08	0.00	0.00	0.00	0.00	0.00
	0.00							109.06		0.00			0.19		0.00	0.00	0.00	0.00
	0.12	0.03	0.04	0.06	1.70	0.01	0.07	15.98	52.36	26.86	33.49	8.84	0.23	0.24	0.68	0.00		
0.00	0.00	0.00	0.01	0.12		0.00	0.07	3.97	15.73	1.56	0.00	8.93	0.13	0.11	1.42	0.00		
0.00	0.00	0.00	0.00	0.00	0.00	0.00	0.00	0.03	0.06	0.00	0.00	0.00	0.00	0.00	0.00	0.00		
0.00	0.00	0.00	0.00	0.00	0.00	0.00	0.00	0.14	0.00	0.40	0.00	0.00	0.00	0.00	0.00	0.00		
		0.00	0.00	0.00				55.57	45.64	6.52			0.08		0.00	0.00		
0.03	0.00	0.00	0.01	0.03	0.68	0.00	0.02	7.99	22.27	7.65	11.73	6.12	0.30	0.19	1.36	0.00		
0.02	0.00	0.00	0.01	0.01	0.16	0.00	0.01	8.16	7.36	5.44	4.48	0.48	0.00	0.02	0.00	0.00	0.00	0.00
0.00	0.00	0.00	0.00	0.02	0.29	0.00	0.00	23.04	1.44	0.86	2.30	0.58	0.06	0.01	0.00	0.00		
	0.00							30.00	0.00	0.00			0.00		0.00	0.00	0.00	0.00
	0.00	0.07	0.13	1.97	11.90	0.13		0.00	253.00	20.00	148.40		2.70		0.00	0.00		
0.02	0.00	0.00	0.00	0.49	3.66	0.04	0.00	1.22	24.40	3.66	20.74	3.66	0.24	0.20	0.00	0.00		
0.03	0.00	0.07	0.03	0.68	15.04	0.01	0.00	72.67	22.55	56.39	47.61	6.27	4.87	0.17	0.00	0.00		
0.01	0.00	0.43	0.28	4.97	100.82	0.57	0.00	241.40	38.34	19.88	19.88	7.10	8.09	0.24	0.00	0.00		
0.02	0.00	0.24	0.12	2.88	2.40	0.01	0.00	162.00	15.60	2.40	12.00	2.40	4.80	0.08	1.20	0.00		
0.01	0.00	0.24	0.12	2.88	2.40	0.01	0.00	1.20	15.60	2.40	12.00	2.40	4.80	0.08	1.20	0.00		
0.06	0.00	0.12	0.04	0.10	5.48	0.02	0.00	3.28	75.56	12.04	90.88	32.85	1.06	0.58	0.00	0.00		
5.31	0.38	0.33	0.38	4.49	156.98	0.78	1.34	315.84	137.24	397.62	133.48	36.19	7.08	0.86	0.00	0.00		
0.18	0.35	0.33	0.39	4.67	99.12	0.49	0.00	254.88	134.52	249.57	123.90	37.17	4.42	0.83	0.00	0.00		
0.12	0.15	0.24	0.28	3.34	70.84	0.35	0.02	144.76	78.54	90.86	83.16	23.10	3.17	0.49	0.00	0.00		
0.18	0.00	0.26	0.31	3.60	76.11	0.38	0.00	79.65	93.81	99.12	95.58	40.71	7.68	0.81	0.00	0.00		
0.28	0.00	0.22	0.05	0.33	12.80	0.04	0.00	1.20	143.20	18.80	183.20	108.00	1.86	1.28	0.00	0.00		
0.12	0.00	0.13	0.02	0.15	4.68	0.02	0.00	187.20	65.52	9.36	88.92	28.08	0.80	0.57	0.00	0.00	1.17	0.82
0.12	0.00	0.10	0.09	1.02	8.86	0.06	0.05	237.82	77.17	6.32	73.37	29.10	0.82	0.71	0.00	0.00		
0.02	0.00	0.02	0.01	0.24	1.21	0.03	0.00	269.83	26.62	0.00	14.52	4.84	0.24	0.08	0.00	0.00	0.20	0.04
	0.00	0.21	0.12	1.78	56.98	0.10	0.00	0.74	54.02	1.48	61.42	18.13	1.30	0.34	0.00	0.00		
	0.00	0.37	0.43	5.00	100.05	0.50	0.00	120.93	274.63	22.04	235.77	80.62	8.10	3.75	0.00	0.00		
0.38	6.00	0.68	0.81	4.44	393.00	3.60	5.64	72.60	306.00	116.70	345.00	108.60	5.28	3.72	0.00	0.00		
0.67	0.00	0.37	0.43	5.00	100.05	0.50	0.00	120.93	274.63	22.04	235.77	80.62	8.10	3.75	0.00	0.00		
0.25	0.00	0.43	0.48	5.71	420.12	0.57	0.00	202.23	54.00	4.05	45.09	15.12	5.16	4.28	0.00	0.00	0.22	0.45
0.11	6.00	0.54	0.50	5.76	200.10	0.66	1.43	213.30	208.80	121.50	132.30	39.30	10.32	4.62	0.00	0.00	2.28	1.29
0.05	6.00	0.38	0.43	5.01	200.10	0.50	1.50	287.70	24.90	99.90	21.60	8.40	9.00	3.75	0.00	0.00	0.00	0.60
0.15	5.39	0.33	0.38	4.46	356.23	0.45	1.32	321.93	189.63	89.18	178.36	53.41	14.46	3.33	0.00	0.00		
0.02	6.20	0.39	0.44	5.18	206.77	0.52	1.55	291.71	30.38	103.23	35.34	9.30	9.30	3.88	0.00	0.00	0.21	0.10

Food Name	Amount	Measure	Weight (g)	Calories	Protein (g)	Total Carb (g)	Dietary Fiber (g)	Total Fat (g)	Sat Fat (g)	Mono Fat (g)	Poly Fat (g)	Chol (mg)	Vit A (mcg RAE)	Vit D (mcg)
CEREALS, BREAKFAST TYPE *(continued)*														
Cereal, Chex, wheat General Mills, Inc.	1	Cup	30.00	103.50	3.00	24.30	3.30	0.60	0.12	0.08	0.24	0.00	90.00	0.00
Cereal, Cocoa Krispies Kellogg's Company	0.75	Cup	31.00	118.11	1.62	26.68	0.59	0.90	0.62	0.12	0.07	0.00	152.52	1.01
Cereal, Cookie Crisp Ralston Foods	1	Cup	30.00	116.70	1.20	26.40	0.45	0.90	0.18	0.44	0.21	0.00	143.10	1.00
Cereal, corn and oat, puffed, w/add sug	1.33	Cup	29.00	114.55	1.51	25.78	0.72	0.61	0.17	0.14	0.20	0.00	216.92	1.00
Cereal, corn flakes Kellogg's Company	1	Cup	28.00	101.08	1.85	24.39	0.70	0.17	0.05	0.03	0.09	0.00	127.68	1.06
Cereal, corn flakes, low sod	1	Cup	25.00	99.75	1.92	22.20	0.28	0.08	0.01	0.02	0.03	0.00	2.50	
Cereal, Cracklin' Oat Bran Kellogg's Company	0.75	Cup	55.00	224.95	4.57	39.27	6.44	8.03	2.31	4.57	1.16	0.00	252.45	1.12
Cereal, Crispix Kellogg's Company	1	Cup	29.00	109.33	1.97	24.94	0.14	0.23	0.06	0.06	0.12	0.00	142.97	1.00
Cereal, Crunchy Bran Quaker Oats	0.75	Cup	27.00	90.45	1.47	23.31	4.73	1.02	0.21	0.23	0.27	0.00	2.16	0.00
Cereal, Fiber One General Mills, Inc.	0.5	Cup	30.00	59.10	2.40	24.30	14.40	0.81	0.12	0.13	0.41	0.00	0.00	0.00
Cereal, Froot Loops Kellogg's Company	1	Cup	30.00	117.90	1.51	26.24	0.75	0.93	0.46	0.13	0.20	0.00	140.70	0.94
Cereal, Frosted Flakes, sugar Krusteaz	0.75	Cup	31.00	110.00	1.00	25.00	0.00	0.00	0.00	0.00	0.00	0.00		
Cereal, Frosted Mini Wheats, bite size Kellogg's Company	1	Cup	55.00	189.20	5.56	44.55	5.50	0.88	0.20	0.13	0.55	0.00	0.00	0.00
Cereal, Go Lean Kashi	0.75	Cup	40.00	113.60	10.44	23.20	7.84	0.76	0.16	0.16	0.44	0.00		
Cereal, Go Lean Crunch Kashi	1	Ounce-weight	28.35	106.88	4.97	19.26	4.31	1.64	0.13	0.91	0.60	0.00		
Cereal, Golden Grahams General Mills, Inc.	0.75	Cup	30.00	111.60	1.50	24.90	0.90	1.05	0.18	0.40	0.39	0.00	150.30	1.00
Cereal, granola, fruit, low fat Nature Valley	0.66	Cup	55.00	212.30	4.40	44.00	2.75	2.53	0.47	1.16	0.63	0.00	0.00	0.00
Cereal, granola, homemade, w/oats & wheat germ	0.5	Cup	61.00	298.90	9.07	32.30	5.25	14.86	2.77	4.66	6.53	0.00	0.61	0.00
Cereal, granola, tstd oats Nature Valley	0.5	Cup	56.50	254.81	5.96	37.22	3.62	9.96	1.31	6.67	1.92	0.00	0.00	
Cereal, Grape Nuts C.W. Post	0.5	Cup	58.00	208.22	6.26	47.15	5.05	1.10	0.23	0.20	0.67	0.00		1.00
Cereal, Heart to Heart Kashi	1	Ounce-weight	28.35	98.66	3.57	21.55	4.03	1.34	0.26	0.32	0.34	0.00	322.62	
Cereal, Honey Graham Oh!s Quaker Oats	0.75	Cup	27.00	110.97	1.07	22.62	0.57	2.00	0.54	0.36	0.19	0.00	177.12	0.00
Cereal, Just Right, crunchy nuggets Kellogg's Company	1	Cup	55.00	204.05	4.24	46.04	2.81	1.49	0.11	0.28	1.05	0.00	375.65	
Cereal, Kix General Mills, Inc.	1.33	Cup	30.00	113.10	1.80	25.80	0.90	0.60	0.15	0.16	0.20	0.00	152.40	1.06
Cereal, Life, plain Quaker Oats	0.75	Cup	32.00	120.00	3.17	24.99	2.11	1.40	0.26	0.48	0.45	0.00	0.64	0.00
Cereal, Lucky Charms General Mills, Inc.	1	Cup	30.00	114.00	2.10	24.90	1.50	1.14	0.24	0.25	0.29	0.00	150.30	1.00
Cereal, Nutri-Grain, wheat Nutri Grain	1	Ounce-weight	28.35	102.06	2.48	23.98	1.80	0.28	0.06	0.04	0.11	0.00	0.00	
Cereal, Oatmeal Crisp, w/almonds General Mills, Inc.	1	Cup	55.00	218.35	5.50	41.80	4.40	4.62	0.61	2.44	1.18	0.00	0.00	0.00
Cereal, Oatmeal Crisp, w/apples General Mills, Inc.	1	Cup	55.00	207.35	4.95	45.10	3.85	2.15	0.44	0.79	0.67	0.00	0.00	0.00
Cereal, Product 19 Kellogg's Company	1	Cup	30.00	99.90	2.31	24.90	0.99	0.42	0.09	0.12	0.21	0.00	214.20	0.98
Cereal, puffed rice Quaker Oats	1	Cup	14.00	53.62	0.98	12.29	0.20	0.13	0.04	0.03	0.05	0.00	0.00	0.00
Cereal, puffed rice, fort	1	Cup	14.00	56.28	0.88	12.57	0.24	0.07	0.02	0.01	0.02	0.00	0.00	0.47
Cereal, puffed wheat Kellogg's Company	1	Cup	15.00	49.80	1.37	12.27	1.71	0.24	0.05	0.12	0.08	0.00		
Cereal, puffed wheat, fort	1	Cup	12.00	43.68	1.76	9.55	0.53	0.14	0.02	0.02	0.07	0.00	0.00	0.40
Cereal, raisin bran	1	Cup	61.00	194.59	5.19	46.54	7.26	1.53	0.34	0.31	0.88	0.00	154.94	1.00
Cereal, raisin bran	1	Cup	56.00	210.00	4.00	45.00	6.00	1.50	0.00			0.00		
Cereal, Raisin Nut Bran General Mills, Inc.	1	Cup	55.00	209.00	5.16	41.45	5.06	4.40	0.77	2.36	0.88	0.00	0.00	0.00
Cereal, Raisin Squares, mini wheats Kellogg's Company	0.75	Cup	55.00	185.90	4.62	43.84	5.17	0.88	0.19	0.19	0.50	0.00	0.00	0.00
Cereal, Rice Krispies Kellogg's Company	1.25	Cup	33.00	118.80	2.29	28.03	0.13	0.36	0.13	0.09	0.13	0.00	153.12	1.02
Cereal, Shredded Wheat, bite size, frosted C.W. Post	1	Cup	52.00	183.04	4.06	43.58	4.99	0.99	0.16			0.00	0.00	0.00
Cereal, Shredded Wheat, spoon size C.W. Post	1	Cup	49.00	166.60	5.05	40.67	5.59	0.54	0.10			0.00	0.00	0.00
Cereal, Special K Kellogg's Company	1	Cup	31.00	117.49	6.98	22.01	0.74	0.48	0.11	0.12	0.25	0.00	230.33	1.25
Cereal, Tasteeos	1	Cup	24.00	94.32	3.07	18.98	2.54	0.67	0.23	0.17	0.18	0.00	317.76	0.00
Cereal, Total, wheat General Mills, Inc.	0.75	Cup	30.00	97.20	2.66	22.50	2.73	0.72	0.16	0.12	0.27	0.00	150.30	1.00
Cereal, Trix General Mills, Inc.	1	Cup	30.00	117.30	0.90	26.70	0.90	1.14	0.18	0.60	0.27	0.00	150.30	1.00

Vit E (mg)	Vit C	Vit B₁- Thia (mg)	Vit B₂- Ribo (mg)	Vit B₃- Nia (mg)	Fol (mcg)	Vit B₆ (mg)	Vita B₁₂ (mcg)	Sodi (mg)	Pota (mg)	Cal (mg)	Phos (mg)	Magn (mg)	Iron (mg)	Zinc (mg)	Caff (mg)	Alco (g)	Sol Fiber (g)	Insol Fiber (g)
0.22	3.60	0.23	0.26	3.00	240.00	0.30	0.90	267.30	112.50	60.00	90.00	24.00	8.70	2.40	0.00	0.00	0.56	2.74
0.08	15.00	0.46	0.70	4.96	197.47	1.02	2.15	196.85	61.07	39.68	31.62	11.78	6.88	1.49	1.55	0.00		
0.08	6.00	0.38	0.43	5.01	99.90	0.50	1.50	178.20	27.00	99.90	39.90	8.40	4.50	3.75	0.60	0.00		
0.06	0.00	0.37	0.43	5.00	100.05	0.50	1.50	215.47	34.80	4.93	26.97	10.73	2.70	1.50	0.00	0.00		
0.04	6.16	0.60	0.74	6.83	134.40	0.96	2.65	202.44	22.12	1.12	10.36	2.52	8.12	0.05	0.00	0.00		
0.04		0.00	0.04	0.10	8.25	0.02	0.00	2.50	18.25	10.75	12.25	3.25	0.56	0.07	0.00	0.00		
0.79	17.60	0.42	0.48	5.67	112.75	0.56	1.71	157.30	247.50	22.55	178.75	67.65	2.04	1.71	0.00	0.00		
0.04	5.80	0.55	0.61	6.99	279.85	0.70	2.09	209.96	37.70	6.09	26.39	7.25	8.12	1.45	0.00	0.00		
0.18	0.00	0.14	0.47	5.50	399.87	0.55	0.00	231.66	56.16	19.17	35.64	14.31	8.32	4.13	0.00	0.00	0.00	4.73
0.21	6.00	0.38	0.43	5.01	99.90	0.50	1.50	128.70	232.20	99.90	150.00	60.00	4.50	3.75	0.00	0.00		
0.09	14.10	0.68	0.58	7.26	105.60	1.10	2.12	150.30	36.00	4.20	33.60	9.90	6.12	5.70	0.00	0.00		
	15.00							170.00	35.00	0.00			4.50		0.00	0.00	0.00	0.00
0.00	0.00	0.41	0.46	5.39	107.80	0.54	1.62	4.40	189.75	17.60	161.70	64.90	15.40	1.76	0.00	0.00		
0.24	0.00	0.14	0.06	1.30	25.60	0.13	0.00	66.00	370.40	56.00	190.00	66.00	2.00	0.28	0.00	0.00		
0.51	0.00	0.02	0.00	0.09	0.57	0.00	0.00	109.15	160.46	24.66	60.39	23.53	1.00	0.26	0.00	0.00		
0.11	6.00	0.38	0.43	5.01	99.90	0.50	1.50	268.50	49.50	350.10	200.10	8.10	4.50	3.75	0.00	0.00	0.46	0.44
0.83	0.00	0.09	0.03	0.95	7.15	0.06	0.00	206.80	153.45	19.80	150.15	24.20	1.10	0.61	0.00	0.00		
3.59	0.73	0.45	0.18	1.29	50.63	0.19	0.00	13.42	327.57	47.58	278.77	106.75	2.59	2.51	0.00	0.00		
3.98	0.00	0.18	0.06	0.63	8.47	0.08	0.00	91.53	187.58	42.37	164.41	53.67	1.76	1.14			2.32	1.30
	0.00	0.38	0.42	5.00	99.76	0.50	1.50	353.80	178.06	19.72	138.62	58.00	16.20	1.20	0.00	0.00	2.78	2.27
11.60	25.80	0.15	0.06	0.53	343.60	1.74	5.16	0.85	85.05	15.31	24.95	85.05	1.85	1.30	0.00	0.00		
0.21	7.07	0.44	0.50	5.90	420.12	0.59	0.00	162.00	42.39	3.24	38.34	0.00	5.31	4.42	0.00	0.00		
1.47	0.00	0.39	0.44	5.01	102.30	0.50	1.49	337.70	121.00	14.30	106.15	34.10	16.23	0.88	0.00	0.00		
0.07	6.30	0.38	0.43	5.01	200.10	0.50	1.50	267.30	35.10	150.00	39.90	8.10	8.10	3.75	0.00	0.00	0.00	0.90
0.18	0.00	0.40	0.47	5.50	416.00	0.55	0.00	164.16	91.20	112.00	132.80	30.72	8.95	4.13	0.00	0.00	1.16	0.95
0.09	6.00	0.38	0.43	5.01	200.10	0.50	1.50	203.40	57.30	99.90	60.00	15.90	4.50	3.75	0.00	0.00	0.81	0.69
7.48	15.03	0.38	0.43	4.99	100.08	0.51	1.51	192.78	77.11	7.94	106.03	22.11	0.79	3.74	0.00	0.00		
1.90	6.05	0.37	0.42	5.01	100.10	0.50	1.49	236.50	184.25	19.80	150.15	59.95	4.51	3.74	0.00	0.00		
0.26	6.05	0.37	0.42	5.01	100.10	0.50	1.49	253.00	170.50	19.80	100.10	40.15	4.51	3.75	0.00	0.00		
13.50	61.20	1.50	1.71	20.01	399.90	2.07	6.00	207.00	50.10	4.80	39.90	15.90	18.09	15.30	0.00	0.00		
0.02	0.00	0.06	0.04	0.49	21.56	0.00	0.00	0.70	16.24	1.26	16.52	4.20	0.40	0.15	0.00	0.00	0.09	0.10
0.01	0.00	0.36	0.25	4.94	2.66	0.01	0.00	0.42	15.82	0.84	13.72	3.50	4.44	0.14	0.00	0.00	0.11	0.13
								0.45	71.10	6.00	63.15				0.00	0.00		
0.04	0.00	0.31	0.22	4.24	3.84	0.02	0.00	0.48	41.76	3.36	42.60	17.40	3.80	0.28	0.00	0.00		
0.41	0.43	0.39	0.44	5.19	103.70	0.52	1.55	361.73	372.10	29.28	258.64	82.96	4.64	1.55	0.00	0.00		
	6.00							320.00	300.00	40.00			18.00		0.00	0.00		
2.04	0.00	0.37	0.42	5.01	100.10	0.50	1.49	250.25	238.15	19.80	150.15	40.15	4.51	3.74	0.00	0.00		
0.36	0.00	0.39	0.44	5.17	103.95	0.52	1.60	3.30	264.55	21.45	155.65	43.45	15.40	1.54	0.00	0.00		
0.04	6.37	0.87	0.79	7.10	151.14	0.92	2.01	318.78	39.27	4.62	38.61	9.57	2.65	0.46	0.00	0.00		
	0.00	0.37	0.43	5.00	99.84	0.50	1.50	9.88	170.04	6.76	143.52	48.36	1.80	1.50	0.00	0.00		
	0.00	0.13	0.06	2.73	20.58	0.20	0.00	3.43	203.35	21.07	174.93	56.84	1.56	1.31	0.00	0.00		
4.74	20.99	0.53	0.59	7.13	399.90	1.98	6.05	223.51	60.76	9.30	67.89	19.22	8.37	0.90	0.00	0.00		
0.08	12.72	0.31	0.36	4.22	84.72	0.43	1.27	182.88	71.04	11.04	95.76	26.16	6.86	0.69	0.00	0.00	1.70	0.84
13.50	60.00	2.11	2.42	26.43	477.00	2.82	6.42	191.70	103.20	1104.00	88.80	39.30	22.35	17.46	0.00	0.00		
0.60	6.00	0.38	0.43	5.01	99.90	0.50	1.50	194.10	17.40	99.90	20.10	3.60	4.50	3.75	0.00	0.00	0.52	0.38

Food Name	Amount	Measure	Weight (g)	Calories	Protein (g)	Total Carb (g)	Dietary Fiber (g)	Total Fat (g)	Sat Fat (g)	Mono Fat (g)	Poly Fat (g)	Chol (mg)	Vit A (mcg RAE)	Vit D (mcg)
CEREALS, BREAKFAST TYPE *(continued)*														
Cereal, wheat, shredd, w/o sug & salt, spoon size	1	Cup	49.00	166.60	5.05	40.67	5.59	0.54	0.10	0.06	0.22	0.00	0.00	0.00
Cereal, Wheaties General Mills, Inc.	1	Cup	30.00	106.50	3.00	24.30	3.00	0.96	0.18	0.29	0.35	0.00	150.30	1.00
CHEESE AND CHEESE SUBSTITUTES														
Natural Cheeses														
Cheese, asiago, fresh, shredded Stella Foods	0.25	Cup	28.00	110.00	6.00	1.00	0.50	9.00	5.00			25.00		
Cheese, blue, 1" cube	1	Each	17.30	61.07	3.70	0.40	0.00	4.97	3.23	1.34	0.14	12.97	34.25	
Cheese, brick, 1" cube	1	Each	17.20	63.81	4.00	0.48	0.00	5.10	3.23	1.48	0.14	16.17	50.22	
Cheese, brie, 1" cube	1	Each	17.00	56.78	3.53	0.08	0.00	4.70	2.96	1.36	0.14	17.00	29.58	
Cheese, camembert, 1" cube	1	Each	17.00	51.00	3.37	0.08	0.00	4.12	2.59	1.19	0.12	12.24	40.97	0.05
Cheese, caraway	1	Ounce-weight	28.35	106.60	7.13	0.87	0.00	8.28	5.27	2.34	0.24	26.37	76.83	
Cheese, cheddar & monterey jack, shredded Sargento Food Inc.	0.25	Cup	28.00	110.00	7.00	1.00	0.00	9.00	5.00			30.00		
Cheese, cheddar, fancy, shredded Healthy Choice	0.25	Cup	28.00	50.00	8.00	1.00	1.00	1.50	1.00			5.00		
Cheese, cheddar, low sod, 1" cube	1	Each	17.30	68.85	4.22	0.33	0.00	5.65	3.59	1.59	0.17	17.30	45.67	
Cheese, cheddar, mild, shredded Sargento Fancy	0.25	Cup	28.00	110.00	7.00	1.00	0.00	9.00	5.00			30.00		
Cheese, cheddar, sharp Cracker Barrel	1	Ounce-weight	28.35	120.00	6.00	0.00	0.00	10.00	7.00			30.00		
Cheese, colby Kraft General Foods, Inc.	1	Ounce-weight	28.35	110.00	7.00	1.00	0.00	9.00	6.00			30.00		
Cheese, colby, low fat, 1" cube	1	Each	17.30	29.93	4.22	0.33	0.00	1.21	0.75	0.36	0.04	3.63	10.38	
Cheese, colby, slice, 1oz each	1	Each	28.35	111.70	6.74	0.73	0.00	9.10	5.73	2.63	0.27	26.93	74.84	
Cheese, edam	1	Ounce-weight	28.35	101.21	7.09	0.41	0.00	7.88	4.98	2.31	0.19	25.23	68.89	0.26
Cheese, feta, 1" cube	1	Each	17.00	44.88	2.41	0.70	0.00	3.62	2.54	0.79	0.10	15.13	21.25	
Cheese, fondue	2	Tablespoon	26.88	61.56	3.83	1.01	0.00	3.62	2.35	0.96	0.13	12.10	29.30	
Cheese, fontina, 1" cube	1	Each	15.00	58.35	3.84	0.24	0.00	4.67	2.88	1.30	0.25	17.40	39.15	
Cheese, four cheese, Mexican style, finely shredded Kraft General Foods, Inc.	0.33	Cup	32.00	120.00	7.00	1.00	0.00	10.00	7.00			30.00		
Cheese, goat, semi soft	1	Ounce-weight	28.35	103.19	6.11	0.72	0.00	8.46	5.85	1.93	0.20	22.40	115.38	
Cheese, gouda	1	Ounce-weight	28.35	100.93	7.07	0.63	0.00	7.78	4.99	2.19	0.19	32.32	46.78	0.07
Cheese, gruyere, 1" cube	1	Each	15.00	61.95	4.47	0.06	0.00	4.85	2.84	1.50	0.26	16.50	40.65	0.04
Cheese, Mexican, queso anejo, crumbled, cup	0.25	Cup	33.00	123.09	7.07	1.53	0.00	9.89	6.28	2.82	0.30	34.65	17.82	
Cheese, monterey jack, 1" cube	1	Each	17.20	64.16	4.21	0.11	0.00	5.21	3.28	1.51	0.15	15.31	34.06	
Cheese, monterey jack, hot pepper Land O'Lakes Incorporated	1	Ounce-weight	28.35	110.00	6.00	1.00	0.00	9.00	6.00			30.00		
Cheese, monterey, low fat, shredd	0.25	Cup	28.25	88.42	7.97	0.20	0.00	6.10	3.96	1.59	0.24	18.36	40.11	
Cheese, mozzarella, low moist, part skim Kraft General Foods, Inc.	1	Ounce-weight	28.35	80.00	8.00	1.00	0.00	5.00	3.50			15.00		
Cheese, mozzarella, part skm, shredded	0.25	Cup	28.25	71.75	6.86	0.78	0.00	4.50	2.85	1.27	0.13	18.08	35.88	0.04
Cheese, mozzarella, whole milk, slice, 1oz each	1	Each	34.00	102.00	7.54	0.74	0.00	7.60	4.47	2.23	0.26	26.86	60.86	
Cheese, muenster, 1" cube	1	Each	17.50	64.40	4.09	0.20	0.00	5.26	3.34	1.52	0.12	16.80	52.15	
Cheese, neufchatel	1	Ounce-weight	28.35	73.71	2.83	0.83	0.00	6.64	4.20	1.92	0.19	21.55	84.48	0.05
Cheese, parmesan, grated	1	Tablespoon	5.00	21.55	1.92	0.20	0.00	1.43	0.87	0.42	0.06	4.40	6.00	
Cheese, parmesan, hard, 1" cube	1	Each	10.30	40.38	3.69	0.33	0.00	2.66	1.69	0.78	0.06	7.00	11.12	0.08
Cheese, parmesan, shredded	1	Tablespoon	5.00	20.75	1.89	0.17	0.00	1.37	0.87	0.44	0.03	3.60	6.10	
Cheese, provolone, diced	0.25	Cup	33.00	115.83	8.44	0.70	0.00	8.79	5.63	2.44	0.25	22.77	77.88	
Cheese, ricotta, fat free Sargento Food Inc.	0.25	Cup	62.00	49.99	5.01	5.01	0.00	0.00	0.00	0.00	0.00	10.00	0.00	
Cheese, ricotta, part skim	0.25	Cup	62.00	85.56	7.06	3.19	0.00	4.90	3.05	1.43	0.16	19.22	66.34	
Cheese, ricotta, whole milk	0.25	Cup	62.00	107.88	6.99	1.88	0.00	8.04	5.15	2.25	0.25	31.62	74.40	
Cheese, romano, 100%, shredded Di Giorno	2	Tablespoon	5.00	20.00	2.00	0.00	0.00	1.50	1.00			5.00	0.00	
Cheese, roquefort, 3oz pkg	1	Ounce-weight	28.35	104.61	6.10	0.57	0.00	8.68	5.46	2.40	0.38	25.51	83.35	

Vit E (mg)	Vit C	Vit B₁-Thia (mg)	Vit B₂-Ribo (mg)	Vit B₃-Nia (mg)	Fol (mcg)	Vit B₆ (mg)	Vita B₁₂ (mcg)	Sodi (mg)	Pota (mg)	Cal (mg)	Phos (mg)	Magn (mg)	Iron (mg)	Zinc (mg)	Caff (mg)	Alco (g)	Sol Fiber (g)	Insol Fiber (g)
0.00	0.00	0.13	0.06	2.73	20.58	0.20	0.00	3.43	203.35	21.07	174.93	56.84	1.56	1.31	0.00	0.00		
0.19	6.00	0.75	0.85	9.99	200.10	1.00	3.00	217.50	111.00	0.00	99.90	32.10	8.10	7.50	0.00	0.00	1.02	1.98
	0.00							270.00		200.00		0.00			0.00	0.00		
0.05	0.00	0.01	0.06	0.17	6.23	0.03	0.21	241.33	44.29	91.34	66.95	3.98	0.05	0.46	0.00	0.00	0.00	0.00
0.05	0.00	0.00	0.06	0.02	3.44	0.01	0.22	96.32	23.39	115.93	77.57	4.13	0.07	0.45	0.00	0.00	0.00	0.00
0.04	0.00	0.01	0.09	0.06	11.05	0.04	0.28	106.93	25.84	31.28	31.96	3.40	0.08	0.40	0.00	0.00	0.00	0.00
0.04	0.00	0.00	0.08	0.11	10.54	0.04	0.22	143.14	31.79	65.96	58.99	3.40	0.06	0.40	0.00	0.00	0.00	0.00
0.14	0.00	0.01	0.13	0.05	5.10	0.02	0.08	195.61	26.37	190.80	138.91	6.24	0.18	0.83	0.00	0.00	0.00	0.00
	0.00							180.00		200.00		0.00			0.00	0.00	0.00	0.00
	0.00							220.00		100.00		0.00			0.00	0.00		
0.05	0.00	0.01	0.06	0.02	3.11	0.01	0.14	3.63	19.38	121.62	83.73	4.67	0.13	0.54	0.00	0.00	0.00	0.00
	0.00							180.00		200.00		0.00			0.00	0.00	0.00	0.00
	0.00		0.07					180.00	30.00	200.00	150.00		0.00	0.90	0.00	0.00	0.00	0.00
	0.00		0.10				0.24	180.00	15.00	200.00	150.00	0.00	0.00	0.90	0.00	0.00	0.00	0.00
0.01	0.00	0.00	0.04	0.01	1.90	0.01	0.09	105.88	11.42	71.79	83.73	2.77	0.07	0.32	0.00	0.00	0.00	0.00
0.08	0.00	0.00	0.11	0.03	5.10	0.02	0.24	171.23	36.00	194.20	129.56	7.37	0.22	0.87	0.00	0.00	0.00	0.00
0.07	0.00	0.01	0.11	0.02	4.54	0.02	0.43	273.58	53.30	207.24	151.96	8.50	0.12	1.07	0.00	0.00	0.00	0.00
0.03	0.00	0.03	0.14	0.17	5.44	0.07	0.29	189.72	10.54	83.81	57.29	3.23	0.11	0.49	0.00	0.00	0.00	0.00
0.06	0.00	0.01	0.05	0.05	2.15	0.02	0.22	35.48	28.22	127.95	82.25	6.18	0.11	0.53	0.00	0.08	0.00	0.00
0.04	0.00	0.00	0.03	0.02	0.90	0.01	0.25	120.00	9.60	82.50	51.90	2.10	0.04	0.52	0.00	0.00	0.00	0.00
	0.00		0.10					210.00	25.00	200.00	150.00		0.00	0.90	0.00	0.00	0.00	0.00
0.08	0.00	0.02	0.19	0.32	0.57	0.02	0.07	146.00	44.79	84.48	106.31	8.22	0.46	0.19	0.00	0.00	0.00	0.00
0.07	0.00	0.01	0.09	0.02	5.95	0.02	0.43	232.19	34.30	198.45	154.79	8.22	0.07	1.11	0.00	0.00	0.00	0.00
0.04	0.00	0.01	0.04	0.02	1.50	0.01	0.24	50.40	12.15	151.65	90.75	5.40	0.02	0.58	0.00	0.00	0.00	0.00
0.09	0.00	0.01	0.07	0.01	0.33	0.01	0.45	373.23	28.71	224.40	146.52	9.24	0.15	0.97	0.00	0.00	0.00	0.00
0.05	0.00	0.00	0.07	0.02	3.10	0.01	0.14	92.19	13.93	128.31	76.37	4.64	0.13	0.52	0.00	0.00	0.00	0.00
	0.00							140.00		200.00		0.00			0.00	0.00	0.00	0.00
0.06	0.00	0.01	0.10	0.03	5.08	0.02	0.24	159.33	22.88	199.16	125.43	7.63	0.21	0.85	0.00	0.00	0.00	0.00
	0.00		0.07				0.36	200.00	20.00	200.00	150.00	0.00	0.00	1.20	0.00	0.00	0.00	0.00
0.04	0.00	0.01	0.08	0.03	2.54	0.02	0.24	174.87	23.73	220.91	130.80	6.50	0.07	0.78	0.00	0.00	0.00	0.00
0.06	0.00	0.01	0.10	0.04	2.38	0.01	0.78	213.18	25.84	171.70	120.36	6.80	0.15	0.99	0.00	0.00	0.00	0.00
0.05	0.00	0.00	0.06	0.02	2.10	0.01	0.26	109.90	23.45	125.47	81.90	4.72	0.07	0.49	0.00	0.00	0.00	0.00
0.26	0.00	0.00	0.06	0.04	3.12	0.01	0.08	113.12	32.32	21.26	38.56	2.27	0.08	0.15	0.00	0.00	0.00	0.00
0.01	0.00	0.00	0.02	0.01	0.50	0.00	0.11	76.45	6.25	55.45	36.45	1.90	0.05	0.19	0.00	0.00	0.00	0.00
0.02	0.00	0.00	0.04	0.02	0.72	0.00	0.12	165.01	9.48	121.95	71.48	4.53	0.08	0.29	0.00	0.00	0.00	0.00
0.04	0.00	0.00	0.02	0.01	0.40	0.01	0.07	84.80	4.85	62.65	36.75	2.55	0.04	0.16	0.00	0.00	0.00	0.00
0.08	0.00	0.01	0.11	0.06	3.30	0.02	0.48	289.08	45.54	249.48	163.68	9.24	0.18	1.07	0.00	0.00	0.00	0.00
	0.00							65.00		100.00		0.00			0.00	0.00	0.00	0.00
0.05	0.00	0.01	0.11	0.05	8.06	0.01	0.18	77.50	77.50	168.64	113.46	9.30	0.27	0.83	0.00	0.00	0.00	0.00
0.06	0.00	0.00	0.12	0.06	7.44	0.02	0.21	52.08	65.10	128.34	97.96	6.82	0.23	0.72	0.00	0.00	0.00	0.00
	0.00	0.00	0.00	0.00				70.00	0.00	40.00	40.00	0.00	0.00		0.00	0.00	0.00	0.00
0.22	0.00	0.01	0.17	0.21	13.89	0.04	0.18	512.85	25.80	187.68	111.13	8.50	0.16	0.59	0.00	0.00	0.00	0.00

Food Name	Amount	Measure	Weight (g)	Calories	Protein (g)	Total Carb (g)	Dietary Fiber (g)	Total Fat (g)	Sat Fat (g)	Mono Fat (g)	Poly Fat (g)	Chol (mg)	Vit A (mcg RAE)	Vit D (mcg)
CHEESE AND CHEESE SUBSTITUTES *(continued)*														
Cheese, Swiss, 1" cube	1	Each	15.00	57.00	4.04	0.80	0.00	4.17	2.66	1.09	0.14	13.80	33.00	0.16
Cottage Cheese, 1% fat	0.5	Cup	113.00	81.36	14.00	3.07	0.00	1.15	0.73	0.33	0.04	4.52	12.43	
Cottage Cheese, 2% fat	0.5	Cup	113.00	101.70	15.53	4.10	0.00	2.18	1.38	0.62	0.07	9.04	23.73	
Cottage Cheese, 4% fat, lrg curd Knudsen	0.5	Cup	127.00	130.00	16.00	4.00	0.00	5.00	3.50			30.00		
Cottage Cheese, creamed, lrg curd, not packed	0.5	Cup	105.00	108.15	13.11	2.81	0.00	4.74	3.00	1.35	0.15	15.75	46.20	
Cottage Cheese, creamed, sml curd, not packed	0.5	Cup	112.50	115.88	14.05	3.02	0.00	5.07	3.21	1.45	0.16	16.88	49.50	
Cottage Cheese, creamed, w/fruit	0.5	Cup	113.00	109.61	12.08	5.21	0.23	4.35	2.61	1.17	0.14	14.69	42.94	
Cottage Cheese, fat free Breakstone's	0.5	Cup	124.00	80.00	13.00	6.00	0.00	0.00	0.00	0.00	0.00	5.00		
Cottage Cheese, nonfat, lrg curd, dry	0.5	Cup	113.00	96.05	19.52	2.09	0.00	0.47	0.31	0.12	0.02	7.91	10.17	
Cottage Cheese, nonfat, sml curd, dry	0.5	Cup	113.00	96.05	19.52	2.09	0.00	0.47	0.31	0.12	0.02	7.91	10.17	
Cream Cheese	2	Tablespoon	29.00	101.21	2.19	0.77	0.00	10.11	6.37	2.85	0.37	31.90	106.14	
Cream Cheese, fat free	2	Tablespoon	29.00	27.84	4.18	1.68	0.00	0.39	0.26	0.10	0.02	2.32	80.91	
Cream Cheese, light, soft Philadelphia	2	Tablespoon	32.00	70.00	3.00	2.00	0.00	5.00	3.50			15.00		
Cream Cheese, soft Philadelphia	2	Tablespoon	30.00	100.00	2.00	1.00	0.00	10.00	7.00			30.00		
Cream Cheese, w/chives, whipped Philadelphia	2	Tablespoon	21.00	70.00	1.00	1.00	0.00	6.00	4.00			20.00		
Cream Cheese, whipped Philadelphia	2	Tablespoon	21.00	70.00	1.00	1.00	0.00	7.00	4.50			25.00		
Process Cheese and Cheese Substitutes														
Cheese Food, American, cold pack	1	Ounce-weight	28.35	93.84	5.58	2.36	0.00	6.94	4.36	2.03	0.21	18.14	45.08	
Cheese Food, American, past, proc, 1.2oz slice Kraft General Foods, Inc.	1	Each	34.00	113.33	6.48	3.24	0.00	8.10	5.67			24.29		
Cheese Food, American, white, past, proc, rducd fat, slice Kraft Singles	1	Piece	21.00	50.00	4.00	2.00	0.00	3.00	2.00			10.00		
Cheese Food, monterey, past, proc, slice Kraft Singles	1	Piece	21.00	70.00	4.00	2.00	0.00	5.00	3.50			15.00		
Cheese Food, sharp, past, proc, slice Kraft Singles	1	Piece	21.00	70.00	4.00	1.00	0.00	6.00	3.50			20.00		
Cheese Product, past, proc, light Kraft General Foods, Inc.	2	Tablespoon	35.00	75.25	5.70	5.67	0.07	3.32	2.24			12.25		
Cheese Sauce, past, proc, squeezable Kraft General Foods, Inc.	2	Tablespoon	33.00	100.00	2.00	4.00	0.00	8.00	4.00			15.00		
Cheese Spread, American, w/disod phosphate, 5oz jar	1	Ounce-weight	28.35	82.21	4.65	2.48	0.00	6.02	3.78	1.77	0.18	15.59	50.75	
Cheese Substitute, mozzarella, 1" cube	1	Each	17.60	43.65	2.02	4.17	0.00	2.15	0.65	1.10	0.31	0.00	76.91	
Cheese, American, past, proc, w/disod phosphate, shredded	0.25	Cup	28.25	105.94	6.26	0.45	0.00	8.83	5.56	2.53	0.28	26.55	71.75	
Cheese, American, yellow, low fat, singles Healthy Choice	1	Piece	21.00	40.00	5.00	2.00	0.00	1.00	0.50			5.00		
Cheese, pimento, past, proc, shredded	0.25	Cup	28.25	105.94	6.25	0.49	0.03	8.81	5.55	2.52	0.28	26.55	70.06	
Cheese, Swiss, past, proc, w/disod phosphate, shredded	0.25	Cup	28.25	94.35	6.99	0.59	0.00	7.07	4.53	1.99	0.18	24.01	55.93	
DAIRY PRODUCTS AND SUBSTITUTES														
Creams and Substitutes														
Cream Substitute, hydrog veg oil & soy prot, liquid	1	Tablespoon	15.00	20.40	0.15	1.71	0.00	1.50	0.29	1.13	0.00	0.00	0.15	
Cream Substitute, pwd	1	Teaspoon	1.96	10.70	0.09	1.08	0.00	0.70	0.64	0.02	0.00	0.00	0.04	
Cream, half & half	2	Tablespoon	30.00	39.00	0.89	1.29	0.00	3.45	2.15	1.00	0.13	11.10	29.10	
Cream, whipping, heavy	2	Tablespoon	29.75	102.64	0.61	0.83	0.00	11.01	6.85	3.18	0.41	40.76	122.27	0.39
Cream, whipping, light	2	Tablespoon	29.88	87.25	0.65	0.88	0.00	9.24	5.78	2.72	0.26	33.17	83.37	
Creamer, non-dairy Carnation Coffee Mate	1	Tablespoon	17.00	20.00	0.00	2.00	0.00	1.00	0.00	0.50	0.00	0.00	0.00	
Creamer, non-dairy, Cafe Mocha flvr Carnation Coffee Mate	1	Tablespoon	17.00	40.00	0.00	5.00	0.00	2.00	0.00	1.00	0.00	0.00	0.00	

Vit E (mg)	Vit C	Vit B$_1$-Thia (mg)	Vit B$_2$-Ribo (mg)	Vit B$_3$-Nia (mg)	Fol (mcg)	Vit B$_6$ (mg)	Vita B$_{12}$ (mcg)	Sodi (mg)	Pota (mg)	Cal (mg)	Phos (mg)	Magn (mg)	Iron (mg)	Zinc (mg)	Caff (mg)	Alco (g)	Sol Fiber (g)	Insol Fiber (g)
0.06	0.00	0.01	0.04	0.02	0.90	0.01	0.50	28.80	11.55	118.65	85.05	5.70	0.03	0.66	0.00	0.00	0.00	0.00
0.01	0.00	0.02	0.19	0.14	13.56	0.08	0.71	458.78	97.18	68.93	151.42	5.65	0.16	0.43	0.00	0.00	0.00	0.00
0.02	0.00	0.03	0.21	0.16	14.69	0.09	0.80	458.78	108.48	77.97	170.63	6.78	0.18	0.47	0.00	0.00	0.00	0.00
	0.00	0.03	0.26				0.48	330.00	90.00	80.00	150.00		0.00		0.00	0.00	0.00	0.00
0.04	0.00	0.02	0.17	0.13	12.60	0.07	0.65	425.25	88.20	63.00	138.60	5.25	0.15	0.39	0.00	0.00	0.00	0.00
0.04	0.00	0.02	0.18	0.14	13.50	0.08	0.70	455.62	94.50	67.50	148.50	5.62	0.16	0.42	0.00	0.00	0.00	0.00
0.05	1.58	0.04	0.16	0.17	12.43	0.08	0.60	388.72	101.70	59.89	127.69	7.91	0.18	0.37	0.00	0.00		
	0.00		0.26				0.48	440.00	150.00	80.00	150.00		0.00		0.00	0.00	0.00	0.00
0.00	0.00	0.03	0.16	0.18	16.95	0.09	0.94	14.69	36.16	36.16	117.52	4.52	0.26	0.53	0.00	0.00	0.00	0.00
0.00	0.00	0.03	0.16	0.18	16.95	0.09	0.94	14.69	36.16	36.16	117.52	4.52	0.26	0.53	0.00	0.00	0.00	0.00
0.09	0.00	0.00	0.06	0.03	3.77	0.01	0.12	85.84	34.51	23.20	30.16	1.74	0.35	0.16	0.00	0.00	0.00	0.00
0.00	0.00	0.01	0.05	0.05	10.73	0.01	0.16	158.05	47.27	53.65	125.86	4.06	0.05	0.26	0.00	0.00	0.00	0.00
	0.00		0.03				0.00	150.00	55.00	40.00	40.00	0.00	0.00	0.00	0.00	0.00	0.00	0.00
	0.00		0.03				0.00	100.00	40.00	20.00	40.00	0.00	0.00	0.00	0.00	0.00	0.00	0.00
	0.00		0.03					130.00	30.00	20.00	20.00		0.00	0.00	0.00	0.00	0.00	0.00
	0.00		0.03				0.00	85.00	25.00	0.00	20.00	0.00	0.00	0.00	0.00	0.00	0.00	0.00
0.19	0.00	0.01	0.12	0.02	1.42	0.04	0.36	273.86	102.91	140.90	113.40	8.50	0.24	0.85	0.00	0.00	0.00	0.00
	0.00		0.17				0.19	453.33	80.95	161.90	161.90	0.00	0.00	0.97	0.00	0.00	0.00	0.00
	0.00		0.10				0.24	320.00	60.00	150.00	100.00	0.00	0.00	0.60	0.00	0.00	0.00	0.00
	0.00		0.10				0.24	290.00	55.00	100.00	100.00	0.00	0.00	0.60	0.00	0.00	0.00	0.00
	0.00		0.07				0.12	300.00	25.00	100.00	100.00	0.00	0.00	0.60	0.00	0.00	0.00	0.00
	0.14		0.12				0.12	596.75	103.95	146.30	330.05	8.00	0.06	0.83	0.00	0.00		
	0.00		0.07				0.00	470.00	30.00	60.00	200.00	0.00	0.00	0.30	0.00	0.00	0.00	0.00
0.09	0.00	0.01	0.12	0.04	1.98	0.04	0.11	460.69	68.61	159.33	248.06	8.22	0.09	0.74	0.00	0.00	0.00	0.00
0.02	0.02	0.01	0.08	0.06	1.94	0.01	0.14	120.56	80.08	107.36	102.61	7.22	0.07	0.34	0.00	0.00	0.00	0.00
0.08	0.00	0.01	0.10	0.02	2.26	0.02	0.20	420.64	47.74	155.94	144.92	7.63	0.05	0.80	0.00	0.00	0.00	0.00
	0.00	0.02	0.05	0.00				200.00		150.00			0.00		0.00	0.00	0.00	0.00
0.08	0.65	0.01	0.10	0.02	2.26	0.02	0.20	403.41	45.76	173.45	210.18	6.21	0.12	0.84	0.00	0.00		
0.10	0.00	0.00	0.08	0.01	1.69	0.01	0.35	387.02	61.02	218.09	215.26	8.19	0.17	1.02	0.00	0.00	0.00	0.00
0.12	0.00	0.00	0.00	0.00	0.00	0.00	0.00	11.85	28.65	1.35	9.60	0.00	0.00	0.00	0.00	0.00	0.00	0.00
0.01	0.00	0.00	0.00	0.00	0.00	0.00	0.00	3.55	15.92	0.43	8.27	0.08	0.02	0.01	0.00	0.00	0.00	0.00
0.10	0.27	0.01	0.04	0.02	0.90	0.01	0.10	12.30	39.00	31.50	28.50	3.00	0.02	0.15	0.00	0.00	0.00	0.00
0.32	0.18	0.01	0.03	0.01	1.19	0.01	0.05	11.31	22.31	19.34	18.45	2.08	0.01	0.07	0.00	0.00	0.00	0.00
0.26	0.18	0.01	0.04	0.01	1.20	0.01	0.06	10.16	28.98	20.62	18.23	2.09	0.01	0.07	0.00	0.00	0.00	0.00
	0.00							0.00	25.00	0.00		0.00			0.00	0.00	0.00	0.00
	0.00							5.00	30.00	0.00		0.00			0.00	0.00	0.00	0.00

Food Name	Amount	Measure	Weight (g)	Calories	Protein (g)	Total Carb (g)	Dietary Fiber (g)	Total Fat (g)	Sat Fat (g)	Mono Fat (g)	Poly Fat (g)	Chol (mg)	Vit A (mcg RAE)	Vit D (mcg)
DAIRY PRODUCTS AND SUBSTITUTES *(continued)*														
Creamer, non-dairy, cinnamon hazelnut flvr, fat free International Delight	1	Tablespoon	17.00	30.00	0.00	7.00	0.00	0.00	0.00	0.00	0.00	0.00	0.00	
Sour Cream, cultured	2	Tablespoon	28.75	61.52	0.91	1.23	0.00	6.03	3.75	1.74	0.22	12.65	50.89	
Sour Cream, imitation, cultured	2	Tablespoon	28.75	59.80	0.69	1.91	0.00	5.61	5.11	0.17	0.02	0.00	0.00	
Sour Cream, rducd fat, cultured	2	Tablespoon	30.00	40.50	0.88	1.28	0.00	3.60	2.24	1.04	0.13	11.70	30.60	
Milks and Non-Dairy Milks														
Buttermilk, dried	1	Tablespoon	7.50	29.03	2.57	3.68	0.00	0.43	0.27	0.13	0.02	5.18	3.68	
Buttermilk, low fat, cultured	1	Cup	245.00	98.00	8.11	11.74	0.00	2.16	1.34	0.62	0.08	9.80	17.15	
Eggnog	1	Cup	254.00	342.90	9.68	34.39	0.00	19.00	11.29	5.67	0.86	149.86	114.30	
Eggnog, prep f/dry mix w/milk	1	Cup	272.00	258.40	7.97	38.62	0.00	8.21	4.63	2.09	0.51	29.92	70.72	
Milk Substitute, fluid, w/hydrog veg oil	1	Cup	244.00	148.84	4.27	15.03	0.00	8.32	1.87	4.88	1.19	0.00	0.00	
Milk Substitute, fluid, w/lauric acid oil	1	Cup	244.00	148.84	4.27	15.03	0.00	8.32	7.41	0.43	0.02	0.00	0.00	
Milk, 1%, prot fort, w/add vit A & D	1	Cup	246.00	118.08	9.67	13.58	0.00	2.88	1.79	0.83	0.11	9.84	150.06	2.46
Milk, 1%, w/add vit A & D	1	Cup	244.00	102.48	8.22	12.18	0.00	2.37	1.54	0.68	0.09	12.20	141.52	3.17
Milk, 2%, prot fort, w/add vit A, ckd	1	Cup	244.00	135.46	9.64	13.40	0.00	4.83	3.01	1.40	0.18	18.79		2.44
Milk, 2%, prot fort, w/vit D	1	Cup	246.00	137.76	9.72	13.51	0.00	4.87	3.03	1.41	0.18	19.68	0.62	2.46
Milk, 2%, w/add nonfat milk solids, not fortified	1	Cup	245.00	137.20	9.68	13.45	0.00	4.85	3.02	0.16	0.02	19.60	41.65	
Milk, 2%, w/add vit A & D Darigold, Inc.	1	Cup	245.00	130.00	8.00	13.00	0.00	5.00	3.00			20.00		2.50
Milk, chocolate, cmrcl	1	Cup	250.00	207.50	7.92	25.85	2.00	8.48	5.26	2.48	0.31	30.00	65.00	2.50
Milk, chocolate, prep w/syrup	1	Cup	282.00	253.80	8.66	36.04	0.85	8.35	4.74	2.09	0.49	25.38	70.50	4.23
Milk, cond, swtnd, cnd	2	Tablespoon	38.25	122.78	3.03	20.81	0.00	3.33	2.10	0.93	0.13	13.00	28.30	
Milk, evaporated, w/add vit A, cnd	2	Tablespoon	31.50	42.21	2.15	3.16	0.00	2.38	1.45	0.74	0.08	9.13	35.28	
Milk, goat	1	Cup	244.00	168.36	8.69	10.86	0.00	10.10	6.51	2.71	0.36	26.84	139.08	0.73
Milk, Indian buffalo	1	Cup	244.00	236.68	9.15	12.64	0.00	16.81	11.22	4.36	0.36	46.36	129.32	
Milk, low fat, chocolate, cmrcl	1	Cup	250.00	157.50	8.10	26.10	1.25	2.50	1.54	0.75	0.09	7.50	145.00	2.50
Milk, nonfat/skim, prot fort, w/vit A	1	Cup	246.00	100.86	9.74	13.68	0.00	0.62	0.40	0.16	0.02	4.92	150.06	2.46
Milk, nonfat/skim, w/add vit A	1	Cup	245.00	83.30	8.26	12.15	0.00	0.20	0.13	0.05	0.01	4.90	149.45	2.54
Milk, nonfat/skim, w/add vit A, inst, dry pwd	1	Tablespoon	4.25	15.22	1.49	2.22	0.00	0.03	0.02	0.01	0.00	0.77	30.13	0.47
Milk, nonfat/skim, w/o add vit A, dry mix	1	Tablespoon	7.50	27.15	2.71	3.90	0.00	0.06	0.04	0.02	0.00	1.50	0.45	0.62
Milk, sheep	1	Cup	245.00	264.60	14.65	13.13	0.00	17.15	11.28	4.22	0.75	66.15	107.80	
Milk, whole, 3.25%	1	Cup	244.00	146.40	7.86	11.03	0.00	7.93	4.55	1.98	0.48	24.40	68.32	2.47
Milk, whole, dry pwd	1	Tablespoon	8.00	39.68	2.11	3.07	0.00	2.14	1.34	0.63	0.05	7.76	20.56	0.62
Rice Milk, original Imagine Foods	1	Cup	244.80	119.95	0.42	24.82	0.00	1.98	0.17	1.34	0.31	0.00	0.24	0.00
Soy Milk	1	Cup	245.00	127.40	10.98	12.08	3.19	4.70	0.57	0.94	1.88	0.00	75.95	0.98
Soy Milk, chocolate, enrich Imagine Foods	1	Cup	244.00	201.73	6.72	35.54	0.96	3.36	0.48			0.00		2.40
Soy Milk, original, light Vitasoy Incorporated	1	Cup	228.30	90.00	4.00	15.00		2.00	0.00	0.50	1.00	0.00		
Yogurt														
Yogurt, fruit, low fat, 10g prot/8oz ctn	1	Each	226.80	231.34	9.91	43.21	0.00	2.45	1.58	0.67	0.07	9.07	22.68	
Yogurt, plain, low fat, 12g prot/8oz ctn	1	Each	226.80	142.88	11.91	15.97	0.00	3.52	2.27	0.97	0.10	13.61	31.75	
Yogurt, plain, skim, 13g prot/8oz ctn	1	Each	226.80	127.01	13.00	17.42	0.00	0.41	0.26	0.11	0.01	4.54	4.54	
Yogurt, plain, whole milk, 8g prot/8oz ctn	1	Each	226.80	138.35	7.87	10.57	0.00	7.37	4.75	2.03	0.21	29.48	61.24	
Yogurt, soy, plain, 8oz ctn Silk	1	Each	170.10	90.00	3.75	16.50	0.75	1.88	0.00			0.00		
Yogurt, vanilla, low fat, 8oz ctn	1	Each	226.80	192.78	11.18	31.30	0.00	2.84	1.83	0.78	0.08	11.34	27.22	
Yogurt, vanilla, nonfat, 8oz ctn	1	Each	227.00	206.56	11.62	39.70	0.00	0.37	0.24	0.10	0.01	3.65	4.06	0.06
DESSERTS														
Brownies and Bars														
Bar, wafer, w/peanut butter, chocolate cvrd, Nutty Bars Little Debbies	1	Each	57.00	312.36	4.56	31.46		18.70	3.59					
Brownie, dry mix Gold Medal	1	Ounce-weight	28.35	124.17	1.70	21.55	0.94	3.69	1.25	1.33	0.31	9.64		

Vit E (mg)	Vit C	Vit B₁-Thia (mg)	Vit B₂-Ribo (mg)	Vit B₃-Nia (mg)	Fol (mcg)	Vit B₆ (mg)	Vita B₁₂ (mcg)	Sodi (mg)	Pota (mg)	Cal (mg)	Phos (mg)	Magn (mg)	Iron (mg)	Zinc (mg)	Caff (mg)	Alco (g)	Sol Fiber (g)	Insol Fiber (g)
	0.00							5.00		0.00			0.00		0.00	0.00	0.00	0.00
0.17	0.26	0.01	0.04	0.02	3.16	0.00	0.09	15.24	41.40	33.35	24.44	3.16	0.02	0.08	0.00	0.00	0.00	0.00
0.21	0.00	0.00	0.00	0.00	0.00	0.00	0.00	29.32	46.29	0.86	12.94	1.72	0.11	0.34	0.00	0.00	0.00	0.00
0.10	0.27	0.01	0.04	0.02	3.30	0.00	0.09	12.30	38.70	31.20	28.50	3.00	0.02	0.15	0.00	0.00	0.00	0.00
0.01	0.43	0.03	0.12	0.07	3.53	0.03	0.29	38.78	119.40	88.80	69.98	8.25	0.02	0.30	0.00	0.00	0.00	0.00
0.12	2.45	0.08	0.38	0.14	12.25	0.08	0.54	257.25	369.95	284.20	218.05	26.95	0.12	1.03	0.00	0.00	0.00	0.00
0.51	3.81	0.09	0.48	0.27	2.54	0.13	1.14	137.16	419.10	330.20	276.86	48.26	0.51	1.17	0.00	0.00	0.00	0.00
0.16	0.00	0.11	0.45	0.30	13.60	0.09	1.06	149.60	329.12	250.24	209.44	27.20	0.33	0.95	0.00	0.00	0.00	0.00
0.68	0.00	0.03	0.21	0.00	0.00	0.00	0.00	190.32	278.16	80.52	180.56	14.64	0.95	2.88	0.00	0.00	0.00	0.00
2.56	0.00	0.03	0.21	0.00	0.00	0.00	0.00	190.32	278.16	80.52	180.56	14.64	0.95	2.88	0.00	0.00	0.00	0.00
0.10	2.95	0.11	0.47	0.25	14.76	0.12	1.06	142.68	442.80	349.32	273.06	39.36	0.15	1.11	0.00	0.00	0.00	0.00
0.02	0.00	0.05	0.45	0.23	12.20	0.09	1.07	107.36	366.00	290.36	231.80	26.84	0.07	1.02	0.00	0.00	0.00	0.00
0.08	1.37	0.10	0.43	0.25	11.71	0.11	1.00	143.47	443.35	349.16	273.28	39.24	0.15	1.10	0.00	0.00	0.00	0.00
0.10	2.71	0.11	0.48	0.25	14.76	0.13	1.06	145.14	447.72	351.78	275.52	39.36	0.15	1.11	0.00	0.00	0.00	0.00
0.17	2.70	0.11	0.48	0.25	12.25	0.11	0.96	144.55	445.90	350.35	274.40	36.75	0.15	1.00	0.00	0.00	0.00	0.00
	1.20		0.45					125.00		250.00			0.00		0.00	0.00	0.00	0.00
0.15	2.25	0.09	0.40	0.31	12.50	0.10	0.82	150.00	417.50	280.00	252.50	32.50	0.60	1.02	5.00	0.00		
0.14	0.00	0.11	0.47	0.39	14.10	0.09	1.07	132.54	408.90	250.98	253.80	50.76	0.90	1.21	5.64	0.00		
0.06	0.99	0.03	0.16	0.08	4.21	0.02	0.17	48.58	141.91	108.63	96.77	9.94	0.07	0.36	0.00	0.00	0.00	0.00
0.06	0.60	0.01	0.10	0.06	2.52	0.02	0.05	33.39	95.44	82.21	63.94	7.56	0.06	0.24	0.00	0.00	0.00	0.00
0.17	3.17	0.12	0.34	0.68	2.44	0.11	0.17	122.00	497.76	326.96	270.84	34.16	0.12	0.73	0.00	0.00	0.00	0.00
	5.61	0.13	0.33	0.22	14.64	0.06	0.88	126.88	434.32	412.36	285.48	75.64	0.29	0.54	0.00	0.00	0.00	0.00
0.05	2.25	0.10	0.42	0.32	12.50	0.10	0.85	152.50	425.00	287.50	257.50	32.50	0.60	1.02	5.00	0.00		
0.10	2.71	0.11	0.48	0.25	14.76	0.12	1.06	145.14	447.72	351.78	275.52	39.36	0.15	1.11	0.00	0.00	0.00	0.00
0.02	0.00	0.11	0.45	0.23	12.25	0.09	1.30	102.90	382.20	306.25	247.45	26.95	0.07	1.03	0.00	0.00	0.00	0.00
0.00	0.24	0.02	0.07	0.04	2.13	0.01	0.17	23.33	72.46	52.32	41.86	4.97	0.01	0.19	0.00	0.00	0.00	0.00
0.00	0.51	0.03	0.12	0.07	3.75	0.03	0.30	40.13	134.55	94.28	72.60	8.25	0.02	0.31	0.00	0.00	0.00	0.00
0.25	10.29	0.16	0.87	1.02	17.15	0.15	1.74	107.80	335.65	472.85	387.10	44.10	0.25	1.32	0.00	0.00	0.00	0.00
0.15	0.00	0.11	0.45	0.26	12.20	0.09	1.07	97.60	348.92	275.72	222.04	24.40	0.07	0.98	0.00	0.00	0.00	0.00
0.04	0.69	0.02	0.10	0.05	2.96	0.02	0.26	29.68	106.40	72.96	62.08	6.80	0.04	0.27	0.00	0.00	0.00	0.00
1.76	1.22	0.08	0.01	1.91	90.58	0.04	0.00	85.68	68.54	19.58	34.27	9.79	0.20	0.24	0.00	0.00	0.00	0.00
3.31	0.00	0.15	0.12	0.71	39.20	0.24	2.99	134.75	303.80	93.10	134.75	61.25	2.70	1.08	0.00	0.00	0.47	2.72
4.83	0.00	0.14	0.07	0.77	57.64	0.12	2.88	153.70	336.22	288.19	240.16	57.64	1.73	0.58		0.00		
		0.09	0.07					95.00	125.00	80.00						0.00	0.00	
0.05	1.59	0.08	0.40	0.22	20.41	0.09	1.07	131.54	442.26	344.74	269.89	34.02	0.16	1.68	0.00	0.00	0.00	0.00
0.07	1.81	0.10	0.49	0.26	24.95	0.11	1.27	158.76	530.71	415.04	326.59	38.56	0.18	2.02	0.00	0.00	0.00	0.00
0.00	2.04	0.11	0.53	0.28	27.22	0.12	1.38	174.64	578.34	451.33	356.08	43.09	0.20	2.20	0.00	0.00	0.00	0.00
0.14	1.13	0.07	0.32	0.17	15.88	0.07	0.84	104.33	351.54	274.43	215.46	27.22	0.11	1.34	0.00	0.00	0.00	0.00
	0.00							22.50		525.00				0.68	0.00	0.00		
0.05	1.81	0.10	0.46	0.24	24.95	0.10	1.20	149.69	496.69	387.83	306.18	36.29	0.16	1.88	0.00	0.00	0.00	0.00
0.01	1.76	0.10	0.48	0.25	24.75	0.11	1.24	155.43	517.56	404.13	317.96	38.75	0.20	1.97	0.00	0.00	0.00	0.00
	1.14							127.11									0.00	
	0.00	0.04	0.05	0.37				83.63	100.08	6.80			0.85				0.00	

Food Name	Amount	Measure	Weight (g)	Calories	Protein (g)	Total Carb (g)	Dietary Fiber (g)	Total Fat (g)	Sat Fat (g)	Mono Fat (g)	Poly Fat (g)	Chol (mg)	Vit A (mcg RAE)	Vit D (mcg)
DESSERTS *(continued)*														
Brownie, fudge, chewy, dry mix, svg Martha White	1	Ounce-weight	28.35	115.67	1.34	23.53		1.78	0.45					
Brownie, nut, w/o icing & nut topping Keebler Company Incorporated	1	Each	35.00	151.20	1.40	22.05	0.70	6.30	1.61			8.05		
Brownie, prep f/recipe, 2" square	1	Each	24.00	111.84	1.49	12.05	0.53	6.98	1.76	2.60	2.26	17.52	42.24	
Brownie, special dietary, prep f/dry mix, 2" square	1	Each	22.00	84.48	0.84	15.69	0.81	2.44	1.12	1.01	0.18	0.00	0.00	
Cakes														
Cake, angel food, cmrcl prep, 9" whl or 1/12 pce	1	Piece	28.35	73.14	1.67	16.39	0.43	0.23	0.03	0.02	0.10	0.00	0.00	
Cake, angel food, prep f/dry mix, tube, 10" whl or 1/12 pce	1	Piece	50.00	128.50	3.05	29.35	0.10	0.15	0.02	0.01	0.06	0.00	0.00	
Cake, Boston cream pie, cmrcl prep, 9" whl or 1/6 pce	1	Piece	92.00	231.84	2.21	39.47	1.29	7.82	2.25	4.18	0.93	34.04	22.08	
Cake, carrot, layer, w/cream cheese frosting, whl or 1/24pce Mrs. Smith's	1	Piece	76.00	300.00	3.00	35.00	1.00	16.00	4.00			20.00		
Cake, chocolate mousse, enchantment, 9" whl or 1/14 pce Mrs. Smith's	1	Piece	130.00	510.00	5.00	68.00	2.00	25.00	12.00			35.00		
Cake, chocolate, prep f/rec, w/o frosting 9" whl or 1/12 pce	1	Piece	95.00	340.10	5.03	50.73	1.52	14.34	5.16	5.74	2.62	55.10	38.00	
Cake, chocolate, w/chocolate icing, cmrcl prep 1/8th of 18oz	1	Piece	64.00	234.88	2.62	34.94	1.79	10.50	3.05	5.61	1.18	26.88	16.64	
Cake, coffee, cheese, 1/6 of 16oz	1	Piece	76.00	257.64	5.32	33.67	0.76	11.55	4.10	5.42	1.25	64.60	65.36	
Cake, coffee, cinnamon, w/crumb topping prep f/mix 8" or 1/8	1	Piece	56.00	178.08	3.08	29.57	0.67	5.38	1.04	2.16	1.77	27.44	19.60	
Cake, coffee, cinnamon, w/crumb topping, enrich, indv cake	1	Each	57.00	238.26	3.88	26.62	1.14	13.28	3.30	7.40	1.78	18.24	18.81	
Cake, coffee, fruit, 1/8	1	Piece	50.00	155.50	2.60	25.75	1.25	5.10	1.25	2.78	0.74	3.50	3.50	
Cake, Ding Dongs, w/cream filling, Hostess Ralston Foods	1	Each	80.00	368.00	3.12	45.36	1.84	19.36	11.04	3.99	1.20	13.60		
Cake, gingerbread, prep f/rec, 1/9 of 8" square	1	Piece	74.00	263.44	2.89	36.41	0.61	12.14	3.05	5.27	3.12	23.68	10.36	
Cake, krimpet, Kreme Krimpies, sponge cake w/filling TastyKake, Inc.	2	Each	57.00	230.00	2.00	37.00	0.00	8.00	1.50			40.00		
Cake, pineapple upside down, prep f/rec, 1/9th of 8" square	1	Piece	115.00	366.85	4.02	58.07	0.92	13.91	3.35	5.97	3.77	25.30	71.30	
Cake, pound, w/butter, cmrcl prep, 1/10 pce	1	Piece	30.00	116.40	1.65	14.64	0.15	5.97	3.47	1.77	0.32	66.30	44.70	
Cake, sponge, cmrcl prep, 1/12 of 16oz	1	Piece	38.00	109.82	2.05	23.22	0.19	1.03	0.30	0.36	0.17	38.76	16.72	
Cake, white, dry mix, 18.5 oz pkg	1	Ounce-weight	28.35	120.77	1.28	22.11	0.26	3.09	0.46	1.30	1.16	0.00		
Cake, white, w/o frosting, prep f/recipe, 9" or 1/12 pce	1	Piece	74.00	264.18	4.00	42.33	0.59	9.18	2.42	3.93	2.33	1.48	11.10	
Cake, yellow, w/chocolate icing, cmrcl prep, 1/8 of 18oz	1	Piece	64.00	242.56	2.43	35.46	1.15	11.14	2.98	6.14	1.35	35.20	21.12	
Cake, yellow, w/vanilla icing, cmrcl prep, 1/8 of 18oz	1	Piece	64.00	238.72	2.24	37.63	0.19	9.28	1.52	3.91	3.30	35.20	12.16	
Cheesecake, amaretto The Cheesecake Lady	1	Each	113.40	420.00	7.00	30.00	1.00	31.00	16.00			100.00		
Cheesecake, cmrcl prep, 1/6 of 17oz	1	Piece	80.00	256.80	4.40	20.40	0.32	18.00	7.94	6.91	1.28	44.00	113.60	
Cheesecake, no bake, prep f/dry mix, 1/12 of 9"	1	Piece	99.00	271.26	5.45	35.15	1.88	12.57	6.62	4.47	0.80	28.71	95.04	
Muffin, coffee coffee, fzn Krusteaz	1	Each	57.00	229.14	3.53	28.50	1.14	11.17	2.04	3.35	5.78	41.04		
Cookies														
Cookie, anisette sponge, w/o lemon juice & rind 4" × 1 1/8" × 7/8	2	Each	26.00	94.90	2.76	15.52	0.26	2.37	0.88	1.07	0.41	94.90	43.42	
Cookie, biscotti, almond Perugina	1	Each	26.77	120.00	1.00	17.00	1.00	5.00	2.00			25.00	0.00	

Vit E (mg)	Vit C	Vit B₁-Thia (mg)	Vit B₂-Ribo (mg)	Vit B₃-Nia (mg)	Fol (mcg)	Vit B₆ (mg)	Vita B₁₂ (mcg)	Sodi (mg)	Pota (mg)	Cal (mg)	Phos (mg)	Magn (mg)	Iron (mg)	Zinc (mg)	Caff (mg)	Alco (g)	Sol Fiber (g)	Insol Fiber (g)
								140.05					1.10			0.00		
	0.00	0.09	0.07	0.60	7.35			101.50		9.41			0.35			0.00		
0.70	0.07	0.04	0.05	0.23	6.96	0.02	0.04	82.32	42.24	13.68	31.68	12.72	0.44	0.23		0.00		
0.00	0.00	0.02	0.03	0.22	9.46	0.00	0.01	20.68	69.08	2.64	11.44	1.32	0.30	0.03	0.44	0.00		
0.03	0.00	0.03	0.14	0.25	9.92	0.01	0.02	212.34	26.37	39.69	9.07	3.40	0.15	0.02	0.00	0.00	0.13	0.30
0.00	0.00	0.05	0.10	0.09	9.50	0.00	0.02	254.50	67.50	42.00	116.00	4.00	0.12	0.06	0.00	0.00	0.03	0.07
0.14	0.18	0.38	0.25	0.18	12.88	0.02	0.15	132.48	35.88	21.16	45.08	5.52	0.35	0.15	0.00	0.00		
								380.00							0.00	0.00		
								250.00								0.00		
1.51	0.19	0.13	0.20	1.08	25.65	0.04	0.15	299.25	133.00	57.00	100.70	30.40	1.53	0.66		0.00	0.35	1.17
0.01	0.06	0.02	0.09	0.37	10.88	0.03	0.09	213.76	128.00	27.52	78.08	21.76	1.41	0.44	7.42	0.00		
1.19	0.08	0.08	0.09	0.52	29.64	0.04	0.26	257.64	219.64	44.84	76.76	11.40	0.49	0.45	0.00	0.00	0.16	0.60
0.11	0.11	0.09	0.10	0.85	26.88	0.03	0.08	235.76	62.72	76.16	120.40	10.08	0.80	0.25	0.00	0.00	0.14	0.53
1.94	0.17	0.12	0.13	0.96	34.77	0.02	0.10	200.07	70.11	30.78	61.56	12.54	1.09	0.46	0.00	0.00	0.24	0.90
0.42	0.40	0.02	0.10	1.29	23.50	0.02	0.01	192.50	45.00	22.50	59.00	8.50	1.22	0.32	0.00	0.00	0.25	1.00
								240.80		3.20			1.84			0.00		
1.78	0.07	0.14	0.12	1.29	24.42	0.14	0.04	241.98	324.86	52.54	39.96	51.80	2.13	0.29	0.00	0.00		
	0.00							160.00		20.00			0.72		0.00	0.00	0.00	0.00
1.54	1.38	0.18	0.18	1.37	29.90	0.04	0.09	366.85	128.80	138.00	94.30	14.95	1.70	0.36	0.00	0.00		
0.20	0.00	0.04	0.07	0.39	12.30	0.01	0.08	119.40	35.70	10.50	41.10	3.30	0.41	0.14	0.00	0.00	0.04	0.11
0.09	0.00	0.09	0.10	0.73	17.86	0.02	0.09	92.72	37.62	26.60	52.06	4.18	1.03	0.19	0.00	0.00	0.05	0.14
0.25	0.09	0.07	0.06	0.30	25.80	0.01	0.05	188.24	33.17	54.43	95.54	3.12	0.40	0.13	0.00	0.00	0.06	0.20
0.09	0.15	0.14	0.18	1.13	28.12	0.02	0.06	241.98	70.30	96.20	68.82	8.88	1.12	0.24	0.00	0.00	0.12	0.47
1.45	0.00	0.08	0.10	0.80	14.08	0.02	0.11	215.68	113.92	23.68	103.04	19.20	1.33	0.40		0.00	0.24	0.91
1.22	0.00	0.06	0.04	0.32	17.28	0.02	0.10	220.16	33.92	39.68	91.52	3.84	0.68	0.16	0.00	0.00	0.04	0.15
	0.00							260.00		80.00			1.80			0.00		
1.26	0.32	0.02	0.15	0.16	14.40	0.04	0.14	165.60	72.00	40.80	74.40	8.80	0.50	0.41	0.00	0.00		
1.09	0.50	0.12	0.26	0.49	29.70	0.05	0.31	376.20	208.89	170.28	231.66	18.81	0.47	0.46	0.00	0.00		
	0.00							249.66	56.43	18.92	80.94		0.87		0.00	0.00		
0.33	0.00	0.08	0.11	0.55	20.02	0.03	0.20	38.22	29.38	12.22	44.98	3.12	0.93	0.29	0.00	0.00		
	0.00							45.00		0.00			0.36			0.00	0.00	

Food Name	Amount	Measure	Weight (g)	Calories	Protein (g)	Total Carb (g)	Dietary Fiber (g)	Total Fat (g)	Sat Fat (g)	Mono Fat (g)	Poly Fat (g)	Chol (mg)	Vit A (mcg RAE)	Vit D (mcg)
DESSERTS *(continued)*														
Cookie, biscuit, shortbread, intl collection Pepperidge Farm	2	Each	27.00	140.00	25.00	5.00	2.00	7.00	5.00			17.00	0.00	
Cookie, bordeaux, distinctive Pepperidge Farm	4	Each	28.00	130.00	1.00	20.00	1.00	5.00	2.50	1.50	0.00	10.00	0.00	
Cookie, butter, enrich, cmrcl prep	5	Each	25.00	116.75	1.52	17.23	0.20	4.70	2.76	1.38	0.25	29.25	41.25	
Cookie, chocolate chip Archway Cookies	3	Each	27.00	130.00	1.00	17.00	0.00	7.00	2.00			10.00	0.00	
Cookie, chocolate chip, dry mix Arrowhead Mills, Inc.	1	Ounce-weight	28.35	113.40	1.42	22.68	0.00	2.12	0.72			0.00	0.00	
Cookie, chocolate chip, enrich, higher fat cmrcl lrg 3.5"-4"	1	Each	40.00	195.60	2.20	25.63	1.16	9.89	3.07	5.31	0.55	0.00	0.00	
Cookie, chocolate chip, fudge, big, homestyle Grandma's	1	Each	39.00	170.00	1.00	26.00	1.00	7.00	2.50			5.00	0.00	
Cookie, chocolate chip, lower fat, cmrcl prep	3	Each	30.00	135.90	1.74	21.99	1.08	4.62	1.14	1.83	1.39	0.00		
Cookie, chocolate chip, prep w/butter f/recipe 2 1/4"	2	Each	32.00	156.16	1.82	18.62	0.80	9.08	4.50	2.64	1.46	22.40	44.48	
Cookie, chocolate chip, refrig dough, svg, spooned f/roll	1	Each	29.00	128.47	1.28	17.81	0.43	5.92	1.95	3.02	0.63	6.96	5.22	
Cookie, chocolate chip, soft, cmrcl prep	2	Each	30.00	137.40	1.05	17.73	0.96	7.29	2.22	3.91	1.05	0.00		
Cookie, chocolate chip, special dietary, cmrcl prep, 1 5/8"	4	Each	28.00	126.00	1.09	20.55	0.45	4.70	1.17	1.89	1.41	0.00	0.28	
Cookie, chocolate sandwich, creme filled	3	Each	30.00	139.80	1.60	21.50	0.87	5.72	1.10	3.19	0.68	0.00		
Cookie, chocolate sandwich, creme filled, special dietary	3	Each	30.00	138.30	1.35	20.31	1.23	6.63	1.15	2.77	2.38	0.00	0.30	
Cookie, coconut macaroon, prep f/recipe, 2"	1	Each	24.00	96.96	0.86	17.33	0.43	3.05	2.70	0.13	0.03	0.00	0.00	
Cookie, fig bar	2	Each	32.00	111.36	1.18	22.69	1.47	2.34	0.36	0.96	0.89	0.00	2.88	
Cookie, fortune	3	Each	24.00	90.72	1.01	20.16	0.38	0.65	0.16	0.32	0.11	0.48	0.24	
Cookie, gingersnap	4	Each	28.00	116.48	1.57	21.53	0.62	2.74	0.69	1.50	0.38	0.00	0.03	
Cookie, graham, Goldfish Pepperidge Farm	19	Each	30.00	150.00	2.00	20.00	2.00	7.00	2.50			15.00	0.00	
Cookie, lemon nut crunch, old fash Pepperidge Farm	3	Each	31.00	170.00	2.00	18.00	2.00	9.00	2.00	4.50	1.50	5.00	0.00	
Cookie, marshmallow pie, chocolate coated .75" × 3"	1	Each	39.00	164.19	1.56	26.40	0.78	6.59	1.84	3.64	0.76	0.00	0.39	
Cookie, molasses, lrg, 3 1/2" to 4"	1	Each	32.00	137.60	1.79	23.62	0.32	4.10	1.03	2.28	0.55	0.00	0.00	
Cookie, oatmeal raisin, big, homestyle Grandma's	1	Each	39.00	160.00	1.00	26.00	1.00	6.00	1.50			5.00	0.00	
Cookie, oatmeal raisin, special dietary, cmrcl prep, 1 5/8"	4	Each	28.00	125.72	1.34	19.57	0.81	5.04	0.76	2.12	1.90	0.00	0.28	
Cookie, oatmeal, cmrcl prep, big, 3 1/2" to 4"	1	Each	25.00	112.50	1.55	17.18	0.70	4.53	1.13	2.51	0.64	0.00	1.25	
Cookie, oatmeal, prep f/recipe, 2 5/8"	2	Each	30.00	134.10	2.04	19.92	0.86	5.37	1.07	2.30	1.68	10.80	48.00	
Cookie, oatmeal, refrig dough, each	2	Each	32.00	135.68	1.73	18.91	0.80	6.05	1.53	3.37	0.83	7.68	1.28	
Cookie, Oreo chocolate sandwich Nabisco	3	Each	33.00	160.00	2.00	23.00	1.00	7.00	1.50			0.00		
Cookie, peanut butter bar TastyKake, Inc.	1	Each	43.00	240.00	2.00	18.00	1.00	11.00	3.00			5.00	0.00	
Cookie, peanut butter sandwich	2	Each	28.00	133.84	2.46	18.37	0.53	5.91	1.40	3.14	1.06	0.00	0.28	
Cookie, peanut butter sandwich, special dietary	3	Each	30.00	160.50	3.00	15.24	0.49	10.20	1.48	4.62	3.61	0.00	0.00	
Cookie, peanut butter, big Grandma's	1	Each	39.00	190.00	2.00	22.00	1.00	9.00	2.00			5.00	0.00	
Cookie, peanut butter, cmrcl prep	2	Each	30.00	143.10	2.88	17.67	0.54	7.08	1.35	3.71	1.66	0.30	0.90	
Cookie, peanut butter, prep f/recipe, 3"	1	Each	20.00	95.00	1.80	11.78	0.40	4.76	0.89	2.17	1.45	6.20	27.40	
Cookie, peanut butter, refrig dough, each	2	Each	32.00	146.56	2.62	16.67	0.35	8.00	1.86	4.20	1.54	8.64	4.48	
Cookie, raisin, soft type	2	Each	30.00	120.30	1.23	20.40	0.36	4.08	1.04	2.29	0.53	0.60	2.40	
Cookie, shortbread, old fash Pepperidge Farm	2	Each	26.00	140.00	2.00	16.00	1.00	7.00	2.50	3.50	0.50	5.00	0.00	

Vit E (mg)	Vit C	Vit B₁-Thia (mg)	Vit B₂-Ribo (mg)	Vit B₃-Nia (mg)	Fol (mcg)	Vit B₆ (mg)	Vita B₁₂ (mcg)	Sodi (mg)	Pota (mg)	Cal (mg)	Phos (mg)	Magn (mg)	Iron (mg)	Zinc (mg)	Caff (mg)	Alco (g)	Sol Fiber (g)	Insol Fiber (g)
	0.00	0.00	0.00	0.00				0.50		0.00			0.00		0.00	0.00		
	0.00	0.08	0.68	0.80				95.00		0.00			0.36		0.00	0.00		
0.14	0.00	0.09	0.08	0.80	19.00	0.01	0.09	87.75	27.75	7.25	25.50	3.00	0.56	0.10	0.00	0.00	0.07	0.13
	0.00							70.00		0.00			0.72			0.00	0.00	0.00
	0.00	0.04	0.06	0.57				155.92	42.52	0.00			1.02			0.00	0.00	0.00
0.64	0.00	0.09	0.09	0.96	25.20	0.01	0.00	118.80	59.20	14.00	46.40	19.20	1.43	0.29	4.40	0.00		
	0.00							160.00		0.00			1.08			0.00		
0.54	0.00	0.09	0.08	0.83	21.00	0.08	0.00	113.10	36.90	5.70	25.20	8.40	0.92	0.21	2.10	0.00		
0.28	0.06	0.06	0.06	0.44	10.56	0.02	0.02	109.12	70.72	12.16	32.00	17.60	0.80	0.30		0.00		
0.68	0.00	0.06	0.06	0.57	16.53	0.01	0.02	60.61	52.20	7.25	20.01	6.96	0.66	0.14	2.61	0.00		
0.87	0.00	0.03	0.06	0.49	11.70	0.05	0.00	97.80	27.90	4.50	15.00	10.50	0.72	0.14	2.10	0.00		
0.30	0.00	0.10	0.06	0.79	15.12	0.01	0.00	3.08	55.72	12.88	30.52	5.88	0.98	0.13	2.24	0.00		
0.52	0.00	0.05	0.04	0.80	15.90	0.00	0.01	144.90	56.10	6.30	27.60	14.40	3.16	0.29	3.90	0.00		
0.55	0.00	0.16	0.09	1.19	21.60	0.01	0.01	72.90	88.50	29.40	60.00	7.80	1.42	0.17	0.90	0.00		
0.04	0.00	0.00	0.03	0.03	0.96	0.02	0.01	59.28	37.44	1.68	10.32	5.04	0.18	0.17	0.00	0.00		
0.21	0.10	0.05	0.07	0.60	11.20	0.02	0.03	112.00	66.24	20.48	19.84	8.64	0.93	0.13	0.00	0.00		
0.01	0.00	0.04	0.03	0.44	15.84	0.00	0.00	65.76	9.84	2.88	8.40	1.68	0.34	0.04	0.00	0.00		
0.27	0.00	0.06	0.08	0.91	24.36	0.03	0.00	183.12	96.88	21.56	23.24	13.72	1.79	0.16	0.00	0.00		
	0.00	0.09	0.07	0.80				150.00					0.72		0.00	0.00		
	0.00	0.06	0.03	0.40				60.00		0.00			0.36		0.00	0.00		
0.05	0.04	0.04	0.08	0.31	8.97	0.02	0.07	65.52	70.98	17.94	37.83	14.04	0.99	0.25	1.95	0.00		
0.04	0.00	0.11	0.08	0.97	28.48	0.03	0.00	146.88	110.72	23.68	30.40	16.64	2.06	0.14	0.00	0.00		
	0.00							250.00		100.00			1.08		0.00	0.00		
0.43	0.08	0.13	0.06	0.91	12.88	0.01	0.00	2.52	49.00	15.12	34.16	4.76	1.14	0.14	0.00	0.00		
0.06	0.12	0.07	0.06	0.56	14.75	0.02	0.00	95.75	35.50	9.25	34.50	8.25	0.64	0.20	0.00	0.00		
0.81	0.06	0.08	0.05	0.39	9.90	0.02	0.03	179.40	54.60	31.50	50.10	12.90	0.81	0.28	0.00	0.00		
0.82	0.00	0.07	0.04	0.60	11.20	0.01	0.01	94.08	47.04	9.92	33.28	8.96	0.68	0.20	0.00	0.00		
								220.00	60.00				0.72			0.00		
	0.00							110.00		0.00			0.72		0.00	0.00		
0.52	0.03	0.09	0.07	1.05	17.08	0.04	0.07	103.04	53.76	14.84	52.64	13.72	0.73	0.30	0.00	0.00		
1.72	0.00	0.10	0.04	1.58	16.20	0.02	0.00	123.60	88.20	12.90	46.20	15.30	0.77	0.31	0.00	0.00		
	0.00							200.00		0.00			0.72		0.00	0.00		
0.66	0.00	0.05	0.05	1.28	21.60	0.03	0.01	124.50	50.10	10.50	25.80	13.50	0.75	0.16	0.00	0.00		
0.76	0.02	0.05	0.04	0.70	11.00	0.02	0.02	103.60	46.20	7.80	23.20	7.80	0.45	0.17	0.00	0.00		
1.30	0.00	0.06	0.06	1.32	18.24	0.04	0.01	127.04	98.56	32.32	77.12	11.84	0.54	0.21	0.00	0.00		
0.67	0.12	0.06	0.06	0.59	9.60	0.02	0.01	101.40	42.00	13.80	24.90	6.30	0.69	0.10	0.00	0.00		
	0.00	0.06	0.03	0.80				105.00		0.00			0.36		0.00	0.00		

DESSERTS (continued)

Food Name	Amount	Measure	Weight (g)	Calories	Protein (g)	Total Carb (g)	Dietary Fiber (g)	Total Fat (g)	Sat Fat (g)	Mono Fat (g)	Poly Fat (g)	Chol (mg)	Vit A (mcg RAE)	Vit D (mcg)
Cookie, shortbread, pecan, cmrcl prep, 2"	2	Each	28.00	151.76	1.37	16.32	0.50	9.10	2.30	5.22	1.16	9.24	0.28	
Cookie, shortbread, plain, cmrcl prep, 1 5/8" square	4	Each	32.00	160.64	1.95	20.64	0.58	7.71	1.95	4.29	1.03	6.40	5.76	
Cookie, sugar wafer, creme filled, lrg, 3 1/2" × 1" × 1/2"	3	Each	27.00	137.97	1.11	18.93	0.16	6.56	0.98	2.79	2.47	0.00	0.00	
Cookie, sugar wafer, creme filled, special dietary	7	Each	28.00	140.56	0.87	18.48	0.49	7.20	1.07	3.06	2.72	0.00	0.00	
Cookie, sugar, bkd f/refrig dough, rolled	2	Each	30.00	145.20	1.41	19.68	0.24	6.93	1.77	3.90	0.87	9.60	3.60	
Cookie, sugar, cmrcl prep	2	Each	30.00	143.40	1.53	20.37	0.24	6.33	1.63	3.55	0.80	15.30	7.80	
Cookie, Thin Mints Little Brownie Bakers	4	Each	28.35	140.00	1.00	18.00	1.00	8.00	2.00			0.00	0.00	
Cookie, vanilla sandwich, creme filled, oval 3 1/8" × 1 1/4"	2	Each	30.00	144.90	1.35	21.63	0.45	6.00	0.89	2.53	2.27	0.00	0.00	
Cookie, vanilla wafer, golden, art flvr Keebler Company Incorporated	8	Each	31.00	147.25	1.61	21.61		6.05	1.11	3.53	0.52			
Cookie, vanilla wafer, higher fat	4	Each	24.00	113.52	1.03	17.06	0.48	4.66	1.18	2.66	0.58	0.00		0.03
Cookie, vanilla wafer, lower fat, lrg	5	Each	30.00	132.30	1.50	22.08	0.57	4.56	1.15	1.96	1.17	15.30	2.40	
Crackers, animal, 2oz box	1	Each	56.70	252.88	3.91	42.01	0.62	7.82	1.97	4.35	1.06	0.00	0.00	

Doughnuts

Food Name	Amount	Measure	Weight (g)	Calories	Protein (g)	Total Carb (g)	Dietary Fiber (g)	Total Fat (g)	Sat Fat (g)	Mono Fat (g)	Poly Fat (g)	Chol (mg)	Vit A (mcg RAE)	Vit D (mcg)
Doughnut, buttermilk, glazed Entenmann's	1	Each	64.00	270.00	3.00	35.00	0.00	13.00	3.00			15.00	0.00	
Doughnut, cake, chocolate, glazed/sugared, med, 3"	1	Each	42.00	175.14	1.89	24.11	0.92	8.36	2.16	4.74	1.04	23.94	5.04	
Doughnut, cake, glazed/sugared, med, 3"	1	Each	45.00	191.70	2.34	22.86	0.67	10.30	2.67	5.71	1.31	14.40	1.35	
Doughnut, cake, w/chocolate icing, sml, 2"	1	Each	28.00	132.72	1.40	13.44	0.56	8.68	2.27	4.90	1.06	17.08	1.96	
Doughnut, cream puff, choc, custard filled, prep f/rec 3.5 × 2	1	Each	112.00	293.44	7.17	27.10	0.67	17.58	4.61	7.26	4.42	142.24	222.88	
Doughnut, cream puff, custard filled, miniature, prep f/rec	1	Each	23.00	59.34	1.54	5.27	0.09	3.57	0.85	1.50	0.96	30.82	32.66	
Doughnut, creme filled, 3 1/2" oval	1	Each	85.00	306.85	5.44	25.50	0.68	20.83	4.62	10.27	2.62	20.40	9.35	
Doughnut, French crullers, glazed, 3"	1	Each	41.00	168.92	1.27	24.39	0.49	7.50	1.91	4.28	0.94	4.51	0.82	
Doughnut, glazed, enrich, extra lrg, 5"	1	Each	122.00	491.66	7.81	54.05	1.46	27.82	7.09	15.70	3.54	7.32	4.88	
Doughnut, jelly filled, 3 1/2" oval	1	Each	85.00	289.00	5.02	33.15	0.77	15.90	4.12	8.69	2.02	22.10	14.45	
Doughnut, powdered sugar, mini TastyKake, Inc.	1	Each	11.83	48.32	0.67	6.66	0.17	2.00	0.42				4.17	0.00

Frozen Desserts

Food Name	Amount	Measure	Weight (g)	Calories	Protein (g)	Total Carb (g)	Dietary Fiber (g)	Total Fat (g)	Sat Fat (g)	Mono Fat (g)	Poly Fat (g)	Chol (mg)	Vit A (mcg RAE)	Vit D (mcg)
Frozen Dessert Bar, ice novelty, fruit, rducd cal, w/asp	1	Each	51.00	12.24	0.26	3.16	0.00	0.05	0.00			0.00	0.02	
Frozen Dessert Bar, orange, all nat, fat free Good Humor-Breyers	1	Each	52.00	50.00	0.00	13.00	0.00	0.00	0.00	0.00	0.00	0.00	0.00	
Frozen Dessert Bar, skim milk, dietary	1	Each	81.00	88.49	2.23	18.71	0.00	1.00	0.23	0.13	0.39	1.25	38.13	
Frozen Dessert Bar, tropical, no sug add, fat free Good Humor-Breyers	1	Each	45.00	25.00	0.00	5.00	0.00	0.00	0.00	0.00	0.00	0.00	0.00	
Frozen Dessert Pop, double stick	1	Each	128.00	92.16	0.00	24.19	0.00	0.00	0.00	0.00	0.00	0.00	0.00	
Frozen Dessert Sandwich, van choc chip Tofutti Brands, Inc.	1	Each	77.00	230.00	3.00	30.00	0.00	11.00	3.00			0.00	0.00	
Frozen Dessert Sandwich, vanilla Tofutti Brands, Inc.	1	Each	77.00	215.00	3.00	28.00	0.00	10.00	3.00			0.00	0.00	
Frozen Dessert, carob Imagine Foods	0.5	Cup	92.00	150.00	1.00	24.00	2.00	6.00	0.50			0.00		
Frozen Dessert, ice novelty, Italian, restaurant prep	0.5	Cup	116.00	61.48	0.04	15.67	0.00	0.03	0.00	0.00	0.00	0.00	9.28	
Frozen Dessert, ice novelty, lime	0.5	Cup	99.00	126.72	0.40	32.27	0.00	0.00	0.00	0.00	0.00	0.00	0.00	
Frozen Yogurt Bar, carob coated	1	Each	41.00	100.18	2.02	12.87	0.35	4.66	3.75	0.55	0.09	0.91	18.07	
Frozen Yogurt Bar, chocolate coated	1	Each	41.00	109.04	1.32	11.84	0.10	6.73	5.34	0.81	0.16	0.64	17.34	
Frozen Yogurt, chocolate, low fat	0.5	Cup	96.50	109.65	5.05	20.84	1.50	1.88	1.18	0.56	0.06	4.81	11.89	
Frozen Yogurt, chocolate, soft serve, cup	0.5	Cup	72.00	115.20	2.88	17.93	1.58	4.32	2.61	1.26	0.16	3.60	31.68	

Vit E (mg)	Vit C	Vit B₁-Thia (mg)	Vit B₂-Ribo (mg)	Vit B₃-Nia (mg)	Fol (mcg)	Vit B6 (mg)	Vita B12 (mcg)	Sodi (mg)	Pota (mg)	Cal (mg)	Phos (mg)	Magn (mg)	Iron (mg)	Zinc (mg)	Caff (mg)	Alco (g)	Sol Fiber (g)	Insol Fiber (g)
1.06	0.00	0.08	0.07	0.69	17.64	0.01	0.00	78.68	20.44	8.40	23.80	5.04	0.68	0.16	0.00	0.00		
0.11	0.00	0.11	0.11	1.07	22.40	0.03	0.03	145.60	32.00	11.20	34.56	5.44	0.88	0.17	0.00	0.00	0.21	0.37
0.53	0.00	0.03	0.05	0.66	14.04	0.00	0.00	39.69	15.93	4.86	15.12	2.97	0.53	0.10	0.00	0.00		
1.14	0.00	0.05	0.03	0.43	11.76	0.00	0.00	2.52	17.08	14.84	9.52	1.68	0.40	0.06	0.00	0.00		
0.06	0.00	0.05	0.04	0.72	21.00	0.01	0.02	140.40	48.90	27.00	56.10	2.40	0.55	0.08	0.00	0.00	0.09	0.15
0.08	0.03	0.07	0.06	0.81	15.90	0.02	0.06	107.10	18.90	6.30	24.00	3.60	0.64	0.13	0.00	0.00	0.09	0.15
	0.00							80.00		200.00					0.00	0.00		
0.48	0.00	0.08	0.07	0.81	15.00	0.01	0.00	104.70	27.30	8.10	22.50	4.20	0.66	0.12	0.00	0.00		
	0.00	0.05	0.03	0.47	13.02			119.66		11.16			0.74		0.00	0.00		
0.34	0.00	0.09	0.05	0.71	10.32	0.01	0.01	73.44	25.68	6.00	15.36	2.88	0.53	0.08	0.00	0.00		
0.07	0.00	0.08	0.10	0.93	18.00	0.02	0.04	93.60	29.10	14.40	31.20	4.20	0.71	0.11	0.00	0.00		
0.08	0.00	0.21	0.19	1.97	58.40	0.02	0.04	222.83	56.70	24.38	64.64	10.21	1.57	0.36	0.00	0.00		
	0.00							290.00		60.00			1.08		0.00	0.00	0.00	0.00
0.09	0.04	0.02	0.03	0.20	18.90	0.01	0.04	142.80	44.52	89.46	68.04	14.28	0.95	0.24	0.42	0.00	0.21	0.71
0.45	0.04	0.10	0.09	0.68	20.70	0.01	0.11	180.90	45.90	27.00	52.65	7.65	0.48	0.20	0.00	0.00	0.24	0.44
0.10	0.06	0.04	0.03	0.36	13.16	0.01	0.07	120.12	54.88	9.80	56.56	11.20	0.69	0.17	0.56	0.00	0.17	0.39
2.25	0.34	0.13	0.30	0.89	48.16	0.07	0.38	377.44	131.04	70.56	119.84	16.80	1.32	0.68	2.24	0.00	0.16	0.51
0.33	0.07	0.03	0.06	0.19	8.51	0.01	0.08	78.43	26.45	15.18	25.07	2.76	0.27	0.14	0.00	0.00	0.03	0.06
0.25	0.00	0.29	0.13	1.91	59.50	0.06	0.12	262.65	68.00	21.25	64.60	17.00	1.56	0.68	0.00	0.00	0.20	0.48
0.07	0.00	0.07	0.09	0.87	17.22	0.01	0.02	141.45	31.98	10.66	50.43	4.92	0.99	0.11	0.00	0.00	0.17	0.32
0.43	0.12	0.44	0.26	3.48	59.78	0.07	0.11	417.24	131.76	52.46	113.46	26.84	2.49	0.94	0.00	0.00	0.48	0.98
0.37	0.00	0.27	0.12	1.82	57.80	0.09	0.19	249.05	67.15	21.25	72.25	17.00	1.50	0.64	0.00	0.00	0.18	0.59
	0.00							58.32		3.33			0.06		0.00	0.00		
0.00	0.00	0.00	0.00	0.08	0.00	0.00	0.00	2.55	13.26	1.02	0.00	1.02	0.07	0.02	0.00	0.00	0.00	0.00
	4.80							5.00		0.00			0.00		0.00	0.00	0.00	0.00
0.07	0.63	0.03	0.11	0.06	3.38	0.03	0.24	43.90	107.23	81.05	65.36	9.25	0.04	0.26	0.00	0.00		
	2.40							0.00		0.00			0.00		0.00	0.00	0.00	0.00
0.00	0.00	0.00	0.00	0.00	0.00	0.00	0.00	15.36	5.12	0.00	0.00	1.28	0.00	0.03	0.00	0.00		
	0.00							155.00	4.00	0.00			0.00		0.00	0.00	0.00	
	0.00							141.00	4.00	0.00			0.00		0.00	0.00	0.00	
	1.20							100.00		20.00			0.72		0.00	0.00		
0.00	0.59	0.00	0.01	0.83	5.80	0.00	0.00	4.64	6.96	1.16	0.00	0.00	0.11	0.04	0.00	0.00	0.00	0.00
0.00	0.99	0.00	0.00	0.01	0.00	0.00	0.00	21.78	2.97	1.98	0.99	0.99	0.16	0.02	0.00	0.00	0.00	0.00
0.22	0.30	0.02	0.09	0.19	4.48	0.04	0.18	37.51	125.26	73.32	52.61	7.76	0.21	0.46		0.00		
0.03	0.25	0.01	0.07	0.10	2.02	0.03	0.09	27.78	74.41	45.89	43.30	5.82	0.14	0.15	3.28	0.00		
0.06	0.64	0.05	0.19	0.22	10.44	0.05	0.44	56.49	310.70	149.82	150.05	37.66	0.85	1.02	2.89	0.00		
0.10	0.22	0.03	0.15	0.22	7.92	0.05	0.21	70.56	187.92	105.84	100.08	19.44	0.90	0.35	2.16	0.00		

Food Name	Amount	Measure	Weight (g)	Calories	Protein (g)	Total Carb (g)	Dietary Fiber (g)	Total Fat (g)	Sat Fat (g)	Mono Fat (g)	Poly Fat (g)	Chol (mg)	Vit A (mcg RAE)	Vit D (mcg)
DESSERTS (continued)														
Frozen Yogurt, coffee, nonfat, soft serve, mix Haagen Dazs	0.5	Cup	95.00	110.00	5.00	22.00	0.00	0.00	0.00	0.00	0.00	3.00	0.00	
Frozen Yogurt, vanilla, soft serve	0.5	Cup	72.00	117.36	2.88	17.42	0.00	4.03	2.46	1.14	0.15	1.44	42.48	
Ice Cream Bar, chocolate & dark chocolate Haagen Dazs	1	Each	83.00	284.80	4.07	22.78	1.63	19.53	12.21			69.17		
Ice Cream Bar, cookie sandwich	1	Each	59.00	143.63	2.62	21.75	0.55	5.61	3.24	1.65	0.36	19.78	50.14	0.06
Ice Cream Bar, vanilla, chocolate coated	1	Each	91.00	280.00	3.00	24.00	0.00	19.00	14.00			20.00		
Ice Cream Bar, vanilla, dark chocolate coated, Eskimo Pie	1	Each	50.00	165.50	2.05	12.25		12.05	7.25			14.00		
Ice Cream Bar, vanilla, uncoated Haagen Dazs	1	Each	78.00	190.00	3.00	15.00	0.00	13.00	8.00			85.00		
Ice Cream Sandwich	1	Each	59.00	143.63	2.62	21.75	0.55	5.61	3.24	1.65	0.36	19.78	50.14	0.06
Ice Cream, butter pecan Ben & Jerry's	0.5	Cup	100.00	290.00	4.00	20.00	1.00	21.00	10.00			70.00		
Ice Cream, chocolate Haagen Dazs	0.5	Cup	106.00	270.00	5.00	22.00	1.00	18.00	9.90			115.00		
Ice Cream, chocolate, 3.5 fl oz indv pkg	1	Each	58.00	125.28	2.20	16.36	0.70	6.38	3.94	1.86	0.24	19.72	68.44	
Ice Cream, chocolate, light, no sugar add	3	Ounce-weight	85.05	129.28	3.01	21.60	0.77	4.88	3.07	0.79	0.45	13.61	63.79	
Ice Cream, French vanilla, soft serve	0.5	Cup	86.00	190.92	3.53	19.09	0.60	11.18	6.43	3.00	0.39	78.26	139.32	
Ice Cream, strawberry, 3.5 fl oz indv pkg	1	Each	58.00	111.36	1.86	16.01	0.53	4.87	3.01	1.39	0.18	16.82	55.68	
Ice Cream, vanilla	0.5	Cup	66.00	132.66	2.31	15.58	0.47	7.26	4.48	1.96	0.30	29.04	77.88	0.57
Ice Cream, vanilla, light, 50% less fat	0.5	Cup	66.00	108.90	3.15	17.03	0.20	3.19	1.93	0.85	0.15	17.82	41.58	0.43
Ice Cream, vanilla, light, 50% less fat, soft serve	0.5	Cup	88.00	110.88	4.32	19.18	0.00	2.29	1.44	0.67	0.09	10.56	25.52	
Ice Cream, vanilla, light, no add sug, w/asp	0.5	Cup	65.00	100.75	2.58	13.93	0.46	4.84	2.63	1.21	0.48	17.55	55.90	
Ice Cream, vanilla, rich	0.5	Cup	74.00	184.26	2.59	16.50	0.00	11.99	7.64	3.30	0.50	68.08	134.68	0.81
Milk Shake, chocolate, fast food, 10 fl oz each	1	Each	208.00	264.16	7.07	42.64	3.95	7.70	4.81	2.24	0.29	27.04	54.08	1.80
Milk Shake, chocolate, thick, 10.6 fl oz	1	Each	300.00	357.00	9.15	63.45	0.90	8.10	5.04	2.34	0.30	33.00	54.00	3.00
Milk Shake, vanilla, thick, 11 fl oz	1	Each	313.00	350.56	12.08	55.56	0.00	9.48	5.90	2.74	0.35	37.56	78.25	
Sherbet, orange	0.5	Cup	74.00	106.56	0.81	22.50	2.44	1.48	0.86	0.39	0.06	0.00	7.40	
Sorbet, chocolate Haagen Dazs	0.5	Cup	105.00	120.00	2.00	28.00	2.00	0.00	0.00	0.00	0.00	0.00	0.00	
Sorbet, mango Haagen Dazs	0.5	Cup	113.00	120.00	0.00	31.00	1.00	0.00	0.00	0.00	0.00	0.00		
Sorbet, raspberry Haagen Dazs	0.5	Cup	105.00	120.00	0.00	30.00	2.00	0.00	0.00	0.00	0.00	0.00	0.00	
Fruit Desserts														
Cobbler, apple, fzn, whl or 1/18 pce Mrs. Smith's	1	Piece	126.00	280.00	2.00	42.00	2.00	12.00	2.50			0.00		
Cobbler, peach crumb, fzn Pet Ritz	1	Piece	123.00	230.00	2.00	38.00	1.00	7.00	3.00	3.00	1.00	5.00	0.00	
Strudel, apple	1	Piece	71.00	194.54	2.34	29.18	1.56	7.95	1.45	2.32	3.77	4.26	4.26	
Gelatin Desserts														
Gelatin Substitute, cherry gel, low prot, prep f/dry mix Kingsmill Foods Company, Ltd.	0.5	Cup	120.00	86.40	0.02	22.24		0.02						
Gelatin, lemon, prep f/dry mix Jell-O	0.5	Cup	140.00	80.00	2.00	19.00	0.00	0.00	0.00	0.00	0.00	0.00	0.00	
Gelatin, orange, snack cup Juicy Gels	1	Each	99.22	99.99	0.00	25.00	0.00	0.00	0.00	0.00	0.00	0.00	0.00	
Gelatin, orange, sug free, low cal, snack cup Jell-O	1	Each	92.00	10.00	1.00	0.00	0.00	0.00	0.00	0.00	0.00	0.00	0.00	
Gelatin, rducd cal, w/asp add minerals & vit C dry mix svg	1	Each	2.50	8.63	1.38	0.83	0.00	0.00	0.00	0.00	0.00	0.00	0.00	
Pastries and Sweet Rolls														
Croissant, cheese, sml	1	Each	42.00	173.88	3.86	19.74	1.09	8.78	4.46	2.73	1.00	23.94	85.68	
Danish, almond, 15oz ring or 1/8 pce	1	Piece	53.16	228.59	3.77	24.29	1.06	13.40	3.09	7.27	2.28	24.45	4.78	
Danish, apple cinnamon, enrich, lrg, 7"	1	Each	142.00	526.82	7.67	67.88	2.70	26.27	6.90	14.24	3.36	161.88	21.30	
Danish, apple cinnamon, enrich, med, 4 1/4"	1	Each	71.00	263.41	3.83	33.94	1.35	13.13	3.45	7.12	1.68	80.94	10.65	
Fritter, apple	1	Each	24.00	87.01	1.44	8.05	0.35	5.55	1.23	2.39	1.60	20.25	12.53	

Vit E (mg)	Vit C	Vit B₁- Thia (mg)	Vit B₂- Ribo (mg)	Vit B₃- Nia (mg)	Fol (mcg)	Vit B₆ (mg)	Vita B₁₂ (mcg)	Sodi (mg)	Pota (mg)	Cal (mg)	Phos (mg)	Magn (mg)	Iron (mg)	Zinc (mg)	Caff (mg)	Alco (g)	Sol Fiber (g)	Insol Fiber (g)
	0.00							75.00		150.00			0.00			0.00	0.00	0.00
0.08	0.58	0.03	0.16	0.20	4.32	0.06	0.21	62.64	151.92	102.96	92.88	10.08	0.22	0.30	0.00	0.00	0.00	0.00
	0.00		0.08					48.82	177.80	81.37	83.00		2.20			0.00		
0.07	0.27	0.03	0.12	0.18	4.83	0.03	0.18	36.37	122.38	60.02	63.68	12.67	0.28	0.43		0.00		
	1.20							75.00		100.00			0.36			0.00	0.00	0.00
								34.00	59.50							0.00		
	0.00							65.00		100.00			0.00			0.00	0.00	0.00
0.07	0.27	0.03	0.12	0.18	4.83	0.03	0.18	36.37	122.38	60.02	63.68	12.67	0.28	0.43		0.00		
	0.00							80.00		150.00			0.72			0.00		
	0.00	0.18	0.85	0.85				75.00	238.50	150.00	106.00		1.08			0.00		
0.17	0.41	0.02	0.11	0.13	9.28	0.03	0.17	44.08	144.42	63.22	62.06	16.82	0.54	0.34	1.74	0.00		
0.26	0.60	0.04	0.15	0.09	4.25	0.04	0.32	63.79	166.70	102.91	90.15	12.76	0.41	0.34	0.00	0.00		
0.52	0.69	0.04	0.16	0.08	7.74	0.04	0.43	52.46	152.22	112.66	99.76	10.32	0.18	0.45	0.00	0.00		
0.03	4.47	0.03	0.15	0.10	6.96	0.03	0.18	34.80	109.04	69.60	58.00	8.12	0.12	0.20	0.00	0.00		
0.20	0.40	0.02	0.16	0.08	3.30	0.03	0.26	52.80	131.34	84.48	69.30	9.24	0.06	0.46	0.00	0.00		
0.08	0.79	0.04	0.17	0.09	3.96	0.03	0.31	48.84	137.28	106.26	67.98	9.24	0.12	0.48	0.00	0.00		
0.05	0.80	0.04	0.18	0.10	4.40	0.04	0.45	61.60	194.48	138.16	106.48	12.32	0.05	0.47	0.00	0.00	0.00	0.00
0.19	0.59	0.02	0.08	0.05	2.60	0.02	0.34	62.40	127.40	88.40	48.75	5.85	0.12	0.20	0.00	0.00		
0.37	0.00	0.03	0.12	0.06	5.92	0.03	0.29	45.14	116.18	86.58	77.70	8.14	0.25	0.35	0.00	0.00	0.00	0.00
0.23	0.83	0.12	0.51	0.33	10.40	0.10	0.71	201.76	416.00	235.04	212.16	35.36	0.64	0.85	2.08	0.00		
0.15	0.00	0.14	0.67	0.37	15.00	0.08	0.96	333.00	672.00	396.00	378.00	48.00	0.93	1.44	6.00	0.00		
0.16	0.00	0.09	0.61	0.46	21.91	0.13	1.63	297.35	572.79	456.98	359.95	37.56	0.31	1.22	0.00	0.00	0.00	0.00
0.02	4.29	0.02	0.07	0.06	5.18	0.02	0.09	34.04	71.04	39.96	29.60	5.92	0.10	0.36	0.00	0.00		
	0.00							70.00		0.00			1.08			0.00		
	12.00							0.00		0.00			0.00			0.00	0.00	
	2.40							0.00	55.70	0.00			0.00			0.00	0.00	
	0.00							260.00		0.00			0.36			0.00	0.00	
	6.00							170.00		0.00			0.00			0.00	0.00	
1.01	1.21	0.03	0.02	0.23	19.88	0.03	0.16	190.99	105.79	10.65	23.43	6.39	0.30	0.13	0.00	0.00		
								4.96	166.88		13.28					0.00	0.00	
	0.00							120.00	0.00	0.00	40.00		0.00			0.00	0.00	0.00	0.00
	0.00							40.00		0.00			0.00			0.00	0.00	0.00	0.00
	0.00							45.00	0.00	0.00	0.00		0.00			0.00	0.00	0.00	0.00
0.00	12.25	0.00	0.00	0.00	0.35	0.00	0.00	68.78	49.63	0.05	0.00	0.03	0.00	0.00	0.00	0.00	0.00	0.00
0.60	0.08	0.22	0.14	0.91	31.08	0.03	0.13	233.10	55.44	22.26	54.60	10.08	0.90	0.39	0.00	0.00	0.37	0.72
0.44	0.90	0.12	0.13	1.22	44.12	0.06	0.11	192.97	50.50	49.97	58.48	17.01	0.96	0.46	0.00	0.00		
0.48	5.54	0.37	0.31	2.83	66.74	0.06	0.13	502.68	117.86	65.32	126.38	21.30	2.51	0.77	0.00	0.00		
0.24	2.77	0.19	0.16	1.41	33.37	0.03	0.06	251.34	58.93	32.66	63.19	10.65	1.26	0.38	0.00	0.00		
0.69	0.35	0.04	0.06	0.32	2.95	0.02	0.06	9.70	33.80	12.64	22.37	3.03	0.35	0.12	0.00	0.00		

Food Name	Amount	Measure	Weight (g)	Calories	Protein (g)	Total Carb (g)	Dietary Fiber (g)	Total Fat (g)	Sat Fat (g)	Mono Fat (g)	Poly Fat (g)	Chol (mg)	Vit A (mcg RAE)	Vit D (mcg)
DESSERTS *(continued)*														
Fruit Burrito, apple, sml	1	Each	74.00	230.88	2.50	34.98		9.52	4.57	3.42	1.06	3.70	20.72	
Pastry, apple cinnamon, frosted, low fat Pop Tarts	1	Each	52.00	191.36	2.18	39.99	0.57	2.86	0.57	1.46	0.83	0.00		
Pastry, blueberry Pop Tarts	1	Each	52.00	212.16	2.39	35.56	0.57	6.92	1.05	3.37	2.50	0.00		
Pastry, brown sugar cinnamon Pop Tarts	1	Each	50.00	219.00	2.70	32.20	0.75	9.20	1.04	3.57	4.57	0.00		
Pastry, brown sugar cinnamon, frosted Pop Tarts	1	Each	50.00	211.00	2.50	34.16	0.65	7.40	1.12	3.91	2.36	0.00		
Pastry, brown sugar cinnamon, frosted, low fat Pop Tarts	1	Each	50.00	188.00	2.35	39.15	0.60	2.75	0.60	1.45	0.65	0.00		
Pastry, cherry Pop Tarts	1	Each	52.00	204.36	2.39	37.02	0.57	5.41	0.87	2.98	1.56	0.00		
Pastry, cherry, low fat Pop Tarts	1	Each	52.00	191.88	2.34	39.78	0.62	2.86	0.62	1.56	0.68	0.00		
Pastry, chocolate fudge, frosted Pop Tarts	1	Each	52.00	201.24	2.65	37.34	0.57	4.84	0.99	2.70	1.14	0.00		
Pastry, s'mores	1	Each	52.00	203.84	3.22	36.19	0.73	5.46	1.46	3.07	0.94	0.00		
Pastry, strawberry, frosted Pop Tarts	1	Each	52.00	202.80	2.29	37.65	0.52	4.99	1.35	2.91	0.73	0.00		
Pastry, strawberry, low fat Pop Tarts	1	Each	52.00	191.88	2.34	39.78	0.62	2.86	0.62	1.56	0.68	0.00		
Sweet Roll, cinnamon raisin, cmrcl, 2 3/4" square	1	Each	60.00	223.20	3.72	30.54	1.44	9.84	1.85	2.88	4.48	39.60	37.20	
Sweet Roll, cinnamon, w/icing, refrig dough Pillsbury	1	Each	44.00	150.04	2.38	23.89		5.02	1.25	2.71	0.31			
Turnover, apple, fzn, rtb Pepperidge Farm	1	Each	89.00	283.91	3.74	31.24	1.60	16.02	4.03	8.55	0.79			
Pastry, Pie, Dessert Crusts, and Cones														
Cone, ice cream, sugar, rolled type	1	Each	10.00	40.20	0.79	8.41	0.17	0.38	0.06	0.15	0.15	0.00	0.00	
Cone, ice cream, wafer/cake type	1	Each	4.00	16.68	0.32	3.16	0.12	0.28	0.05	0.07	0.13	0.00	0.00	
Crust, cookie, chocolate, prep f/rec, chilled, 9" or 1/8 pce	1	Piece	28.00	141.68	1.43	15.23	0.42	8.71	1.88	4.12	2.16	0.28	59.08	
Crust, pastry, cream puff shell, prep f/recipe, 3 1/2"	1	Each	66.00	238.92	5.94	15.05	0.53	17.09	3.70	7.34	4.87	129.36	183.48	0.00
Crust, pastry, eclair shell, prep f/recipe, 5" × 2" × 1 3/4"	1	Each	48.00	173.76	4.32	10.94	0.38	12.43	2.69	5.34	3.54	94.08	133.44	0.00
Crust, pie, bkd f/fzn, 9" whl or 1/8 pce	1	Piece	16.00	82.24	0.70	7.94	0.16	5.25	1.69	2.51	0.65	0.00	0.00	
Crust, pie, prep f/recipe, bkd, 9" whl or 1/8 pce	1	Piece	23.00	121.21	1.47	10.93	0.39	7.96	1.98	3.49	2.10	0.00	0.00	
Crust, pie, chocolate, 1/8 of 9", Ready Crust Keebler Company Incorporated	1	Piece	18.00	87.12	1.08	12.24	0.54	3.96	0.86			0.18		
Crust, pie, Nilla, rtu, svg Nabisco	1	Each	28.00	143.64	0.98	17.67	0.25	7.59	1.44	5.24	0.38	2.80		
Crust, pie, rtb, enrich, fzn, 9" whl or 1/8 pce	1	Piece	18.00	82.26	0.70	7.94	0.16	5.26	0.78	2.24	1.98	0.00		
Crust, pie, single, prep f/rec, unbkd, 9" whl or 1/8 pce	1	Piece	24.25	113.73	1.38	10.26	0.82	7.47	1.86	3.27	1.97	0.00	0.00	
Pies														
Pie, apple, fzn Amy's Kitchen Inc	0.5	Each	114.00	240.00	2.00	37.00	2.00	8.00	4.50			25.00		
Pie, apple, prep f/recipe, 9" whl or 1/8 pce	1	Piece	155.00	410.75	3.72	57.50	2.17	19.37	4.73	8.36	5.17	0.00	17.05	
Pie, banana cream, fzn Pet Ritz	1	Piece	99.00	270.00	3.00	37.00	1.00	13.00	8.00			5.00	0.00	
Pie, banana cream, no bake, prep f/mix, 9" whl or 1/8 pce	1	Piece	92.00	230.92	3.13	29.07	0.55	11.87	6.35	4.19	0.70	26.68	87.40	
Pie, banana cream, prep f/recipe, 9" whl or 1/8 pce	1	Piece	144.00	387.36	6.34	47.38	1.01	19.58	5.41	8.24	4.74	73.44	87.84	
Pie, blackberry, prep f/recipe, 9" whl or 1/8 pce	1	Piece	150.00	402.27	3.80	56.15	4.71	18.81	3.70	8.26	5.85	0.00	24.33	0.00
Pie, blueberry, cmrcl prep, 8" whl or 1/6 pce	1	Piece	117.00	271.44	2.11	40.83	1.17	11.70	1.96	4.97	4.12	0.00	51.48	
Pie, blueberry, prep f/recipe, 9" whl or 1/8 pce	1	Piece	147.00	360.15	3.97	49.25	2.06	17.49	4.28	7.53	4.53	0.00	2.94	
Pie, cherry, cmrcl prep, 8" whl or 1/6 pce	1	Piece	117.00	304.20	2.34	46.57	0.94	12.87	3.00	6.83	2.40	0.00	60.84	

Vit E (mg)	Vit C	Vit B₁-Thia (mg)	Vit B₂-Ribo (mg)	Vit B₃-Nia (mg)	Fol (mcg)	Vit B₆ (mg)	Vita B₁₂ (mcg)	Sodi (mg)	Pota (mg)	Cal (mg)	Phos (mg)	Magn (mg)	Iron (mg)	Zinc (mg)	Caff (mg)	Alco (g)	Sol Fiber (g)	Insol Fiber (g)
	0.74	0.17	0.18	1.86	24.42	0.07	0.51	211.64	104.34	15.54	14.80	7.40	1.07	0.40	0.00	0.00		
0.00	0.00	0.16	0.16	1.98	52.00	0.21	0.00	205.92	28.08	5.72	21.32	4.68	1.82	0.16	0.00	0.00		
0.00	0.00	0.15	0.17	1.98	41.60	0.20	0.00	206.96	49.40	12.48	45.76	8.32	1.82	0.66	0.00	0.00		
0.00	0.00	0.15	0.17	2.00	40.00	0.20	0.00	214.00	67.50	15.50	31.50	8.00	1.80	0.61	0.00	0.00		
0.00	0.00	0.15	0.17	2.00	40.00	0.20	0.00	184.50	55.50	14.50	46.50	7.50	1.80	1.21	0.00	0.00		
0.00	0.00	0.15	0.15	2.00	50.00	0.20	0.00	209.50	30.50	7.00	22.50	5.00	1.80	0.15	0.00	0.00		
0.00	0.00	0.15	0.17	1.98	41.60	0.20	0.00	219.96	59.28	14.56	44.20	8.32	1.82	0.64	0.00	0.00		
0.00	0.00	0.16	0.16	1.98	52.00	0.21	0.00	221.52	29.64	5.72	22.36	4.68	1.82	0.16	0.00	0.00		
0.00	0.00	0.16	0.16	1.98	52.00	0.21	0.00	202.80	82.16	19.76	43.68	15.08	1.82	0.26		0.00		
0.00	0.00	0.16	0.16	1.98	52.00	0.21	0.00	198.64	65.00	15.08	39.00	10.92	1.82	0.21		0.00		
0.00	0.00	0.16	0.16	1.98	52.00	0.21	0.00	169.00	44.20	11.44	26.52	5.20	1.82	0.16	0.00	0.00		
0.00	0.00	0.16	0.16	1.98	52.00	0.21	0.00	221.52	29.64	5.72	22.88	4.68	1.82	0.16	0.00	0.00		
1.19	1.20	0.19	0.16	1.43	43.20	0.06	0.08	229.80	66.60	43.20	45.60	10.20	0.96	0.35	0.00	0.00	0.72	0.72
								334.40							0.00	0.00		
	0.00							176.22					1.22		0.00	0.00		
0.01	0.00	0.05	0.04	0.51	14.00	0.01	0.00	32.00	14.50	4.40	10.30	3.10	0.44	0.08	0.00	0.00		
0.03	0.00	0.01	0.01	0.18	6.92	0.00	0.00	5.72	4.48	1.00	3.88	1.04	0.14	0.03	0.00	0.00		
0.79	0.00	0.04	0.06	0.60	14.84	0.00	0.01	188.16	47.04	8.40	29.40	11.20	0.84	0.23	1.40	0.00		
1.85	0.00	0.14	0.24	1.03	34.98	0.05	0.26	367.62	64.02	23.76	78.54	7.92	1.33	0.48	0.00	0.00	0.17	0.35
1.35	0.00	0.10	0.17	0.75	25.44	0.04	0.19	267.36	46.56	17.28	57.12	5.76	0.97	0.35	0.00	0.00	0.13	0.26
0.42	0.00	0.04	0.06	0.39	8.80	0.01	0.00	103.52	17.60	3.36	9.44	2.88	0.36	0.05	0.00	0.00	0.05	0.11
0.07	0.00	0.09	0.06	0.76	15.41	0.01	0.00	124.66	15.41	2.30	15.41	3.22	0.66	0.10	0.00	0.00	0.13	0.26
	0.00							86.22		7.38			0.40			0.00		
		0.05	0.05	0.70	8.40	0.01	0.03	62.72	19.32	11.48	23.24	2.24	0.50	0.08	0.00	0.00		
0.42	0.00	0.06	0.07	0.43	12.60	0.01	0.01	103.68	17.64	3.24	9.54	2.88	0.36	0.05	0.00	0.00	0.06	0.11
0.07	0.00	0.08	0.06	0.71	17.22	0.01	0.00	116.89	14.31	2.18	14.55	2.91	0.62	0.09	0.00	0.00	0.29	0.54
	4.80							135.00		20.00			0.72		0.00	0.00		
2.94	2.63	0.23	0.17	1.91	37.20	0.05	0.00	327.05	122.45	10.85	43.40	10.85	1.74	0.29	0.00	0.00		
	0.00							250.00		20.00			0.72		0.00	0.00		
1.47	0.46	0.09	0.13	0.65	19.32	0.03	0.19	266.80	103.96	67.16	153.64	11.04	0.42	0.30	0.00	0.00		
0.58	2.30	0.20	0.30	1.52	38.88	0.19	0.36	345.60	237.60	108.00	132.48	23.04	1.50	0.69	0.00	0.00		
2.92	13.40	0.22	0.17	1.93	20.74	0.05	0.00	26.52	166.22	28.22	50.52	21.82	1.89	0.43	0.00	0.00		
1.22	3.16	0.01	0.04	0.35	31.59	0.04	0.01	380.25	58.50	9.36	26.91	5.85	0.35	0.19	0.00	0.00		
3.09	1.03	0.22	0.19	1.76	33.81	0.05	0.00	271.95	73.50	10.29	44.10	11.76	1.81	0.29	0.00	0.00		
0.89	1.05	0.03	0.03	0.23	31.59	0.05	0.01	287.82	94.77	14.04	33.93	9.36	0.56	0.21	0.00	0.00		

Food Name	Amount	Measure	Weight (g)	Calories	Protein (g)	Total Carb (g)	Dietary Fiber (g)	Total Fat (g)	Sat Fat (g)	Mono Fat (g)	Poly Fat (g)	Chol (mg)	Vit A (mcg RAE)	Vit D (mcg)
DESSERTS *(continued)*														
Pie, cherry, old fash, rtb, 10" whl or 1/10 pce Mrs. Smith's	1	Piece	133.00	370.00	3.00	55.00	1.00	16.00	3.50			0.00		
Pie, chocolate cream, gourmet, 10" whl or 1/12 pce Mrs. Smith's	1	Piece	116.00	320.00	3.00	39.00	1.00	18.00	10.00			15.00		
Pie, chocolate mousse, no bake, prep f/mix, 9"whl or 1/8 pce	1	Piece	95.00	247.00	3.32	28.12		14.63	7.79	4.83	0.77	33.25	117.80	
Pie, coconut cream, cmrcl prep, 7" whl or 1/6 pce	1	Piece	64.00	190.72	1.34	23.81	0.83	10.62	4.46	4.65	0.99	0.00	17.28	
Pie, coconut cream, gourmet, 10" whl or 1/12 pce Mrs. Smith's	1	Piece	116.00	340.00	2.00	38.00		20.00	13.00			15.00	0.00	
Pie, egg custard, cmrcl prep, 8" whl or 1/6 pce	1	Piece	105.00	220.50	5.77	21.84	1.68	12.18	2.47	5.04	3.91	34.65	59.85	
Pie, fruit, fried, 5" × 3 3/4"	1	Each	128.00	404.48	3.84	54.53	3.33	20.61	3.14	9.53	6.88	0.00	6.40	
Pie, lemon meringue, prep f/recipe, 9" whl or 1/8 pce	1	Piece	127.00	361.95	4.83	49.66	1.52	16.38	4.04	7.09	4.23	67.31	54.61	
Pie, mincemeat, prep f/recipe, 9" whl or 1/8 pce	1	Piece	165.00	476.85	4.29	79.20	4.29	17.82	4.43	7.68	4.69	0.00	1.65	
Pie, peach, 8" whl or 1/6 pce	1	Piece	117.00	260.91	2.22	38.49	0.94	11.70	1.76	4.96	4.39	0.00	11.70	
Pie, peach, old fash, 10" whl or 1/10 pce Mrs. Smith's	1	Piece	133.00	330.00	3.00	46.00	2.00	15.00	3.00			0.00		
Pie, pecan, 10" whl or 1/8 pce Mrs. Smith's	1	Piece	128.00	550.00	7.00	75.00	2.00	26.00	6.00			85.00		
Pie, pecan, cmrcl prep, 8" whl or 1/6 pce	1	Piece	113.00	452.00	4.52	64.64	3.95	20.90	4.01	12.14	3.60	36.16	57.63	
Pie, pineapple TastyKake, Inc.	1	Each	113.00	290.00	3.00	45.00	1.00	12.00	1.00			20.00	0.00	
Pie, pumpkin, 10" whl or 1/10 pce Mrs. Smith's	1	Piece	125.00	310.00	5.00	47.00	2.00	12.00	3.00			45.00		
Pie, pumpkin, cmrcl prep, 8" whl or 1/6 pce	1	Piece	109.00	228.90	4.25	29.76	2.94	10.36	1.95	4.39	3.43	21.80	488.32	
Pie, strawberry TastyKake, Inc.	1	Each	106.00	310.00	2.00	50.00	1.00	12.00	3.00			0.00	0.00	
Puddings, Custards, and Pie Fillings														
Custard, chocolate, dry mix, 2oz pkg	1	Tablespoon	9.00	32.67	0.22	8.24	0.46	0.30	0.17	0.10	0.01	0.00		
Custard, chocolate, prep f/dry mix w/whole milk	0.5	Cup	136.00	130.56	4.35	18.14	0.68	4.54	2.72	1.27	0.16	16.32	36.72	1.22
Custard, egg, prep f/dry mix w/2% milk	0.5	Cup	133.00	147.63	5.43	23.17	0.00	3.64	1.80	1.13	0.26	63.84	81.13	
Custard, flan, dry mix, 3oz pkg	1	Tablespoon	9.00	31.32	0.00	8.24	0.00	0.00	0.00	0.00	0.00	0.00	0.00	
Custard, vanilla, prep f/dry mix w/2% milk	0.5	Cup	133.00	102.41	4.07	16.41	0.00	2.35	1.41	0.64	0.09	9.31	67.83	1.22
Custard, vanilla, prep f/dry mix w/whole milk	0.5	Cup	133.00	118.37	4.03	16.24	0.00	4.08	2.46	1.12	0.15	17.29	35.91	1.22
Filling, poppy seed, Solo Sokol & Company	2	Tablespoon	36.00	119.52	1.73	20.92		3.21	0.37	0.47	2.01			
Pie Filling, apple, 21oz can	0.5	Cup	127.50	128.77	0.12	33.41	1.27	0.12	0.02	0.00	0.03	0.00	0.00	
Pie Filling, cherry, 21 oz can	0.5	Cup	132.00	151.80	0.50	36.96	0.80	0.09	0.02	0.04	0.04	0.00	13.20	
Pie Filling, pumpkin, cnd, cup	0.5	Cup	135.00	140.40	1.47	35.63	11.21	0.17	0.09	0.02	0.01	0.00	560.25	
Pudding, banana, inst, dry mix, svg, makes 1/2 cup prep	1	Each	25.00	91.75	0.00	23.18	0.00	0.15	0.02	0.04	0.09	0.00	0.00	
Pudding, chocolate, rte, 4oz snack can	1	Each	113.40	157.63	3.06	26.08	1.13	4.54	0.81	1.93	1.62	3.40	11.34	
Pudding, chocolate, sug free, rducd cal, dry mix Jell-O	1	Ounce-weight	28.35	85.05	2.84	19.85	2.84	0.00	0.00	0.00	0.00	0.00	0.00	
Pudding, coconut cream, inst, prep f/dry mix w/2% milk	0.5	Cup	147.00	157.29	4.26	28.22	0.15	3.38	2.01	0.91	0.28	8.82	66.15	
Pudding, corn, prep f/recipe	0.5	Cup	125.00	136.25	5.49	15.95	1.88	6.65	3.17	2.15	0.86	125.00	67.50	
Pudding, flan, prep f/dry mix w/2% milk Jello-O	0.5	Cup	144.00	140.00	4.00	26.00	0.00	2.50	1.50			10.00		
Pudding, lemon, rte, 5oz can	1	Each	141.75	177.19	0.14	35.44	0.14	4.25	0.64	1.84	1.62	0.00	0.00	

Vit E (mg)	Vit C	Vit B₁-Thia (mg)	Vit B₂-Ribo (mg)	Vit B₃-Nia (mg)	Fol (mcg)	Vit B₆ (mg)	Vita B₁₂ (mcg)	Sodi (mg)	Pota (mg)	Cal (mg)	Phos (mg)	Magn (mg)	Iron (mg)	Zinc (mg)	Caff (mg)	Alco (g)	Sol Fiber (g)	Insol Fiber (g)
	0.00	0.05	0.06	0.16				260.00	159.00	0.00			0.72		0.00	0.00		
	0.00							180.00		0.00			1.08			0.00		
1.42	0.47	0.05	0.14	0.57	24.70	0.03	0.20	437.00	270.75	73.15	219.45	30.40	1.03	0.57	0.95	0.00		
0.10	0.00	0.03	0.05	0.13	4.48	0.04	0.08	163.20	41.60	18.56	54.40	12.80	0.51	0.30	0.00	0.00		
	0.00							260.00		0.00			0.00		0.00	0.00		
0.99	0.63	0.04	0.22	0.31	21.00	0.05	0.45	252.00	111.30	84.00	117.60	11.55	0.61	0.55	0.00	0.00		
2.20	1.66	0.18	0.14	1.82	23.04	0.04	0.10	478.72	83.20	28.16	55.04	12.80	1.56	0.29	0.00	0.00		
2.29	4.19	0.15	0.20	1.20	31.75	0.03	0.15	307.34	82.55	15.24	53.34	7.62	1.27	0.36	0.00	0.00		
0.25	9.73	0.25	0.17	1.96	37.95	0.11	0.00	419.10	334.95	36.30	69.30	23.10	2.46	0.36	0.00	0.00		
1.10	1.05	0.07	0.04	0.23	33.93	0.03	0.00	315.90	146.25	9.36	25.74	7.02	0.58	0.11	0.00	0.00		
	0.00							290.00	159.00	0.00			0.00		0.00	0.00		
	0.00							510.00	90.00	0.00			0.72		0.00	0.00		
0.36	1.24	0.10	0.14	0.28	38.42	0.02	0.11	479.12	83.62	19.21	87.01	20.34	1.18	0.64	0.00	0.00		
	1.20							310.00		20.00			1.08		0.00	0.00		
	0.00	0.05	0.20	0.49				390.00	193.00	80.00			1.44		0.00	0.00		
1.12	1.09	0.06	0.17	0.20	26.16	0.06	0.28	307.38	167.86	65.40	77.39	16.35	0.86	0.49	0.00	0.00		
	9.00							300.00		20.00			1.08		0.00	0.00		
0.01	0.00	0.00	0.01	0.03	0.54	0.00	0.00	6.30	38.70	14.94	11.61	7.29	0.23	0.14	1.17	0.00		
0.13	1.09	0.05	0.21	0.14	6.80	0.06	0.44	69.36	243.44	168.64	131.92	27.20	0.41	0.68	1.36	0.00		
0.27	1.06	0.07	0.28	0.17	11.97	0.09	0.60	118.37	297.92	192.85	183.54	25.27	0.47	0.69	0.00	0.00	0.00	0.00
0.00	0.00	0.00	0.00	0.00	0.00	0.00	0.00	38.88	13.77	2.16	0.09	0.00	0.01	0.00	0.00	0.00	0.00	0.00
0.09	1.20	0.05	0.20	0.11	6.65	0.05	0.44	61.18	188.86	160.93	126.35	17.29	0.07	0.48	0.00	0.00	0.00	
0.12	1.20	0.05	0.20	0.10	6.65	0.05	0.44	61.18	186.20	158.27	123.69	15.96	0.07	0.47	0.00	0.00	0.00	0.00
								26.64		115.92					0.00	0.00		
0.00	0.12	0.02	0.02	0.05	0.00	0.02	0.00	56.09	57.38	5.11	8.93	2.55	0.38	0.05	0.00	0.00	0.48	0.79
0.28	4.75	0.04	0.02	0.18	5.29	0.05	0.00	23.77	138.60	14.53	19.79	9.24	0.32	0.07	0.00	0.00		
1.08	4.73	0.02	0.16	0.51	47.25	0.22	0.00	280.80	186.30	49.95	60.75	21.60	1.44	0.37	0.00	0.00		
0.01	0.00	0.00	0.00	0.00	0.00	0.00	0.00	374.75	3.75	1.50	201.00	0.50	0.03	0.01	0.00	0.00	0.00	0.00
0.33	2.04	0.03	0.18	0.39	3.40	0.03	0.00	146.29	204.12	102.06	90.72	23.81	0.58	0.48	5.67	0.00		
	0.00							311.85	396.90	0.00			3.06			0.00		
0.06	1.18	0.05	0.20	0.13	5.88	0.06	0.44	361.62	194.04	149.94	295.47	20.58	0.22	0.49	0.00	0.00		
0.26	3.50	0.52	0.16	1.23	31.25	0.15	0.11	68.75	201.25	50.00	71.25	18.75	0.70	0.62	0.00	0.00	0.12	1.75
	0.00							65.00	200.00	150.00	100.00		0.00		0.00	0.00	0.00	0.00
0.18	0.14	0.00	0.01	0.00	0.00	0.00	0.00	198.45	1.42	2.84	7.09	1.42	0.10	0.04	0.00	0.00		

Food Name	Amount	Measure	Weight (g)	Calories	Protein (g)	Total Carb (g)	Dietary Fiber (g)	Total Fat (g)	Sat Fat (g)	Mono Fat (g)	Poly Fat (g)	Chol (mg)	Vit A (mcg RAE)	Vit D (mcg)
DESSERTS *(continued)*														
Pudding, pistachio, inst, prep w/2% milk Jell-O	0.5	Cup	147.00	160.00	4.00	29.00	0.00	3.00	1.50			10.00		
Pudding, rice, rte, 5oz can	1	Each	141.75	231.05	2.84	31.19	0.14	10.63	1.66	4.55	3.95	1.42	35.44	
Pudding, tapioca, fat free, rte	0.5	Cup	125.00	111.25	2.25	25.50	0.00	0.05	0.00	0.00	0.00	1.25	40.00	
Pudding, tapioca, rte, 5oz can	1	Each	141.75	168.68	2.84	27.50	0.14	5.24	0.85	2.24	1.93	1.42	0.07	
Pudding, vanilla, fat free, rte	0.5	Cup	125.00	116.25	2.75	28.35	0.00	0.08	0.03	0.03	0.01	1.25	50.00	
Pudding, vanilla, rte, 4oz snack can	1	Each	113.40	146.29	2.61	24.83	0.00	4.08	0.65	1.75	1.52	7.94	6.80	
DESSERT TOPPINGS														
Frosting, chocolate fudge, rte Creamy Supreme	2	Tablespoon	34.00	140.00	0.00	21.00	0.00	6.00	1.50			0.00	0.00	
Frosting, chocolate, creamy, dry mix, pkg	1	Ounce-weight	28.35	110.28	0.36	26.08	0.68	1.47	0.34	0.65	0.42	0.00	0.00	
Frosting, cream cheese, rte Creamy Supreme	2	Tablespoon	35.00	150.00	0.00	24.00	0.00	6.00	1.50			0.00	0.00	
Frosting, cream cheese, rte, 16oz can	1	Ounce-weight	28.35	117.65	0.03	19.09	0.00	4.90	1.29	1.06	1.75	0.00	0.00	
Frosting, glaze, prep f/recipe	1	Ounce-weight	28.35	101.78	0.17	20.83	0.00	2.24	0.49	0.96	0.66	0.57	24.66	
Frosting, vanilla, creamy, rte, 16oz pkg	1	Ounce-weight	28.35	119.07	0.00	19.14	0.03	4.71	0.84	1.38	2.25	0.00	0.00	
Frosting, white, fluffy, prep f/dry mix w/water	1	Ounce-weight	28.35	69.17	0.42	17.75	0.00	0.00	0.00	0.00	0.00	0.00	0.00	
Syrup, chocolate, tbsp Hershey's	2	Tablespoon	39.00	100.00	1.00	24.00		0.00	0.00	0.00	0.00	0.00	0.00	
Topping, caramel	2	Tablespoon	41.00	103.32	0.61	27.02	0.37	0.04	0.03	0.01	0.00	0.41	11.07	
Topping, hot fudge	2	Tablespoon	41.00	140.00	1.00	24.00	1.00	4.50	2.00			0.00	0.00	
Topping, marshmallow creme Jet-Puffed	2	Tablespoon	12.00	40.00	0.00	10.00	0.00	0.00	0.00	0.00	0.00	0.00	0.00	
Topping, strawberry	2	Tablespoon	42.50	107.95	0.09	28.18	0.30	0.04	0.00	0.01	0.02	0.00	0.43	
Topping, whipped, fat free, Cool Whip	2	Tablespoon	9.00	15.00	0.00	3.00	0.00	0.00	0.00	0.00	0.00	0.00	0.00	
Topping, whipped, pressurized	2	Tablespoon	8.75	23.10	0.09	1.41	0.00	1.95	1.65	0.17	0.02	0.00	0.35	
Topping, whipped, semi-solid, fzn	2	Tablespoon	9.38	29.81	0.12	2.16	0.00	2.37	2.04	0.15	0.05	0.00	0.66	
EGGS, SUBSTITUTES, AND EGG DISHES														
Egg Substitute, fzn, cup	0.25	Cup	60.00	96.00	6.77	1.92	0.00	6.67	1.16	1.46	3.74	1.20	6.60	
Egg Substitute, liquid, cup	0.25	Cup	62.75	52.71	7.53	0.40	0.00	2.08	0.41	0.56	1.01	0.63	11.29	
Egg Substitute, scrambled, prep f/fzn	0.25	Cup	35.00	57.67	3.60	1.41	0.00	4.13	0.74	1.15	2.05	0.75	33.74	0.40
Egg Whites, pwd Ener-G Foods	1	Tablespoon	15.00	56.40	12.36	0.67	0.00	0.01				0.00	0.00	0.00
Egg Whites, raw, lrg, each	1	Each	33.40	17.37	3.64	0.24	0.00	0.06	0.00	0.00	0.00	0.00	0.00	0.00
Egg Yolks, raw, lrg, each	1	Each	16.60	53.45	2.63	0.60	0.00	4.41	1.59	1.95	0.70	204.84	63.25	0.45
Eggs, deviled	1	Each	31.00	62.67	3.60	0.39	0.00	5.08	1.23	1.75	1.48	121.94	49.89	0.38
Eggs, hard bld, lrg, each	1	Each	50.00	77.50	6.29	0.56	0.00	5.30	1.63	2.04	0.71	212.00	84.50	
Eggs, poached, lrg, each	1	Each	50.00	73.50	6.26	0.38	0.00	4.95	1.54	1.90	0.68	211.00	69.50	0.43
Eggs, scrambled, fast food	1	Each	47.00	99.64	6.50	0.98	0.00	7.60	2.89	2.77	0.92	200.22	104.81	0.80
Eggs, scrambled, prep f/one lrg egg butter & milk	1	Each	61.00	101.26	6.76	1.34	0.00	7.45	2.24	2.91	1.31	214.72	87.23	0.53
Eggs, whole, lrg, fried	1	Each	46.00	92.46	6.27	0.40	0.00	7.04	1.98	2.92	1.22	210.22	91.08	0.43
Eggs, whole, raw, lrg, each	1	Each	50.00	73.50	6.29	0.38	0.00	4.97	1.55	1.90	0.68	211.50	70.00	0.43
Omelette, plain, prep w/one lrg egg margarine & salt	1	Each	61.00	93.33	6.48	0.42	0.00	7.33	2.05	3.04	1.28	217.16	94.55	0.76
ETHNIC FOODS														
Italian Foods														
Mexican Foods														
Oriental Foods														
Dish, edamame soybeans Ace Sushi Inc.	0.5	Cup	75.00	90.00	9.00	3.00		5.00	1.00			0.00	0.00	
Dish, fish curry, Thai, prep f/recipe, svg	1	Each	187.58	256.01	16.67	10.81	1.62	17.06	11.20			32.36		0.00
Dish, inari, svg Ace Sushi Inc.	3	Piece	144.00	264.00	8.40	48.00	1.20	6.00	1.20			0.00	0.00	
Dish, pad Thai, w/chicken & shrimp, prep f/recipe, svg	1	Each	317.08	590.14	30.88	41.75	4.87	35.84	6.09			161.99		1.18

Vit E (mg)	Vit C	Vit B₁-Thia (mg)	Vit B₂-Ribo (mg)	Vit B₃-Nia (mg)	Fol (mcg)	Vit B₆ (mg)	Vita B₁₂ (mcg)	Sodi (mg)	Pota (mg)	Cal (mg)	Phos (mg)	Magn (mg)	Iron (mg)	Zinc (mg)	Caff (mg)	Alco (g)	Sol Fiber (g)	Insol Fiber (g)
	0.00							410.00	200.00	150.00	300.00		0.00		0.00	0.00	0.00	0.00
1.96	0.71	0.03	0.10	0.23	4.25	0.04	0.30	120.49	85.05	73.71	96.39	11.34	0.43	0.69	0.00	0.00		
0.00	0.00	0.02	0.12	0.06	2.50	0.02	0.19	265.00	66.25	62.50	50.00	6.25	0.44	0.58	0.00	0.00	0.00	0.00
0.43	0.57	0.03	0.14	0.44	4.25	0.03	0.30	225.38	136.08	119.07	111.98	11.34	0.33	0.38	0.00	0.00	0.04	0.10
0.00	0.00	0.03	0.16	0.11	3.75	0.02	0.24	266.25	90.00	75.00	61.25	8.75	0.45	0.70	0.00	0.00	0.00	0.00
0.00	0.00	0.02	0.16	0.29	0.00	0.01	0.11	153.09	128.14	99.79	77.11	9.07	0.15	0.28	0.00	0.00	0.00	0.00
	0.00							75.00		0.00			0.72		0.00	0.00	0.00	
0.28	0.00	0.00	0.01	0.04	0.85	0.02	0.00	21.55	51.03	3.12	17.58	10.77	0.34	0.23	1.70	0.00		
	0.00							70.00		0.00			0.00		0.00	0.00	0.00	0.00
1.20	0.00	0.00	0.00	0.00	0.00	0.00	0.00	54.15	9.92	0.85	0.85	0.56	0.05	0.01	0.00	0.00	0.00	0.00
0.22	0.06	0.00	0.01	0.01	0.28	0.00	0.02	26.65	8.51	6.24	5.10	0.85	0.02	0.02	0.00	0.00	0.00	0.00
0.59	0.00	0.00	0.08	0.06	2.27	0.00	0.00	52.16	9.64	0.85	5.11	0.29	0.05	0.02	0.00	0.00		
0.00	0.00	0.00	0.01	0.18	0.57	0.00	0.00	44.23	21.83	1.13	1.41	0.57	0.02	0.01	0.00	0.00	0.00	0.00
	0.00							25.00		0.00			0.36		7.00	0.00		
0.00	0.12	0.00	0.04	0.02	0.82	0.01	0.04	143.09	34.44	21.73	19.27	2.87	0.08	0.08	0.00	0.00		
	0.00							100.00	85.00	40.00	60.00		0.36					
0.00	0.00							10.00	0.00	0.00			0.00		0.00	0.00	0.00	0.00
0.04	5.82	0.00	0.01	0.07	2.55	0.01	0.00	8.93	21.68	2.55	2.13	1.70	0.12	0.03	0.00	0.00		
	0.00							5.00	0.00	0.00	0.00		0.00		0.00	0.00	0.00	0.00
0.07	0.00	0.00	0.00	0.00	0.00	0.00	0.00	5.42	1.66	0.44	1.57	0.09	0.00	0.00	0.00	0.00	0.00	0.00
0.09	0.00	0.00	0.00	0.00	0.00	0.00	0.00	2.34	1.69	0.56	0.75	0.19	0.01	0.00	0.00	0.00	0.00	0.00
0.95	0.30	0.07	0.23	0.08	9.60	0.08	0.20	119.40	127.80	43.80	43.20	9.00	1.19	0.59	0.00	0.00	0.00	0.00
0.17	0.00	0.07	0.19	0.07	9.41	0.00	0.19	111.07	207.07	33.26	75.93	5.65	1.32	0.82	0.00	0.00	0.00	0.00
0.75	0.20	0.03	0.12	0.05	4.04	0.04	0.12	73.24	78.21	33.43	30.83	5.46	0.58	0.32	0.00	0.00	0.00	0.00
0.00	0.00	0.01	0.35	0.11	14.40	0.00	0.08		167.40	13.35	13.35	10.80	0.04	0.02	0.00	0.00	0.00	0.00
0.00	0.00	0.00	0.15	0.04	1.34	0.00	0.03	55.44	54.44	2.34	5.01	3.67	0.03	0.01	0.00	0.00	0.00	0.00
0.43	0.00	0.03	0.09	0.00	24.24	0.06	0.32	7.97	18.09	21.41	64.74	0.83	0.45	0.38	0.00	0.00	0.00	0.00
0.61	0.00	0.02	0.15	0.02	12.69	0.05	0.32	50.01	36.66	14.67	49.57	2.87	0.35	0.30	0.00	0.00	0.00	0.00
0.52	0.00	0.03	0.26	0.03	22.00	0.06	0.56	62.00	63.00	25.00	86.00	5.00	0.60	0.52	0.00	0.00	0.00	0.00
0.48	0.00	0.03	0.24	0.04	23.50	0.07	0.64	147.00	66.50	26.50	95.00	6.00	0.92	0.55	0.00	0.00	0.00	0.00
0.45	1.55	0.04	0.24	0.10	26.32	0.09	0.48	105.28	69.09	26.79	113.74	6.58	1.22	0.78	0.00	0.00	0.00	0.00
0.52	0.12	0.03	0.27	0.05	18.30	0.07	0.47	170.80	84.18	43.31	103.70	7.32	0.73	0.61	0.00	0.00	0.00	0.00
0.56	0.00	0.03	0.24	0.04	23.46	0.07	0.64	93.84	67.62	27.14	95.68	5.98	0.91	0.55	0.00	0.00	0.00	0.00
0.48	0.00	0.03	0.24	0.04	23.50	0.07	0.64	70.00	67.00	26.50	95.50	6.00	0.92	0.56	0.00	0.00	0.00	0.00
0.58	0.00	0.04	0.25	0.04	23.79	0.07	0.66	98.21	69.54	28.67	98.82	6.10	0.94	0.57	0.00	0.00	0.00	0.00
	2.40							0.00		40.00			1.44		0.00	0.00		
1.75	24.08	0.14	0.13	1.88	24.58	0.43	12.09	206.04	501.21	49.20	259.64	80.31	4.26	1.31	0.00	0.00		
	2.88							396.00		96.00			1.30		0.00	0.00		
2.93	10.89	0.33	0.26	4.82	119.08	0.41	0.79	2281.84	569.15	618.37	382.30	163.12	5.37	2.89	0.00	0.00		

Food Name	Amount	Measure	Weight (g)	Calories	Protein (g)	Total Carb (g)	Dietary Fiber (g)	Total Fat (g)	Sat Fat (g)	Mono Fat (g)	Poly Fat (g)	Chol (mg)	Vit A (mcg RAE)	Vit D (mcg)
ETHNIC FOODS (*continued*)														
Dish, spring roll, vegetable, Thai, prep f/recipe	1	Piece	63.22	158.50	4.24	19.89	0.95	6.92	0.92			2.85		0.21
Dish, sushi combo, Fujiyama Aurora Hissho Sushi	1	Each	226.00	349.00	12.00	56.00	3.00	4.00	1.00			8.00		
Dish, sushi combo, Kobe Meridian Hissho Sushi	1	Each	198.00	355.00	15.00	53.00	2.00	4.00	1.00			32.00		
Dish, sushi, California roll & inari Ace Sushi Inc.	3	Piece	117.00	200.00	6.00	36.00	1.00	4.00	1.00			3.00	0.00	
Dish, sushi, futomaki & inari Ace Sushi Inc.	3	Piece	120.00	210.00	2.00	38.00	2.00	4.00	1.00			10.00		
Dish, sushi, golden vgtrn combo Ace Sushi Inc.	4	Piece	128.00	250.00	7.00	44.00	2.00	5.00	1.00			0.00		
Dish, sweet noodles, Thai, prep f/recipe, svg	1	Each	141.75	339.25	14.47	36.92	1.69	15.46	2.44			121.49		1.27
Dish, tofu w/sour curry, Thai, prep f/recipe, svg	1	Each	297.67	421.86	25.07	15.79	4.96	31.72	4.28			0.00		0.00
Dumpling, shumai, pork, rth Ace Sushi Inc.	9	Piece	135.00	220.00	11.00	21.00	2.00	10.00	4.00			30.00	0.00	
Miso	1	Cup	275.00	547.25	32.15	72.79	14.85	16.53	3.13	3.42	8.81	0.00	11.00	
Sushi, California roll Ace Sushi Inc.	3	Piece	90.00	125.00	3.00	24.00	1.00	2.00	0.50			3.00		
Sushi, cucumber & imit crab Hissho Sushi	3	Ounce-weight	85.05	128.58	3.50	23.01	0.50	0.50	0.00			1.50		
Sushi, cucumber roll Ace Sushi Inc.	6	Piece	85.00	120.00	3.00	25.00	2.00	1.00	0.00			0.00		
Sushi, dynamite roll	3	Ounce-weight	85.05	141.75	5.58	20.62	0.86	2.15	0.43			6.87		
Sushi, eel roll Ace Sushi Inc.	3	Piece	85.00	130.00	4.00	24.00	2.00	2.50	0.50			20.00		
Sushi, salmon roll, spicy Hissho Sushi	3	Ounce-weight	85.05	143.03	6.01	18.47	0.43	3.01	0.43			14.61		
Sushi, shrimp roll, spicy Hissho Sushi	3	Ounce-weight	85.05	128.01	6.01	18.47	0.43	1.29	0.00			33.08		
Sushi, tuna roll Lwin Family Co.	3	Ounce-weight	85.05	148.59	8.00	21.01	0.50	1.50	0.50			9.51		
Sushi, yellowtail roll, spicy Hissho Sushi	3	Ounce-weight	85.05	135.74	6.44	18.47	0.43	2.15	0.43			13.75		
FAST FOODS/RESTAURANTS														
Generic Fast Food														
Brownie, 2" square	1	Each	60.00	243.00	2.74	38.97		10.11	3.14	3.82	2.64	9.60	3.00	
Cheeseburger, double, lrg, w/condiments & veg	1	Each	258.00	704.34	37.98	39.65		43.65	17.67	17.35	4.70	141.90	61.92	
Cheeseburger, double, plain	1	Each	155.00	457.25	27.67	22.06		28.47	13.00	11.01	1.91	110.05	99.20	
Cheeseburger, double, reg, w/condiments & veg	1	Each	166.00	416.66	21.25	35.19		21.08	8.72	7.81	2.66	59.76	71.38	
Cheeseburger, lrg, plain	1	Each	185.00	608.65	30.14	47.42		32.99	14.84	12.74	2.44	96.20	185.00	0.56
Cheeseburger, reg, plain	1	Each	102.00	319.26	14.77	31.75		15.15	6.47	5.77	1.54	49.98	45.90	0.31
Chicken, wing, pieces, hot	6	Each	134.00	450.00	24.00	23.00	1.00	29.00	6.00			145.00		
Cole Slaw, fast food	0.75	Cup	99.00	146.52	1.46	12.75		10.97	1.61	2.42	6.39	4.95	35.64	
Cornbread, hush puppies, svg	5	Piece	78.00	256.62	4.88	34.90	2.67	11.59	2.68	7.81	0.38	134.94	8.58	
Danish, cheese	1	Each	91.00	353.08	5.83	28.69		24.62	5.12	15.60	2.42	20.02	44.59	
Danish, cinnamon	1	Each	88.00	349.36	4.80	46.85	0.29	16.72	3.48	10.59	1.65	27.28	5.28	
Danish, fruit	1	Each	94.00	334.64	4.76	45.06		15.93	3.32	10.10	1.57	18.80	25.38	
Dish, corn, cob, w/butter	1	Each	146.00	154.76	4.47	31.94		3.43	1.64	1.00	0.61	5.84	33.58	
Dish, crab cake	1	Each	60.00	159.60	11.25	5.11	0.24	10.35	2.24	4.31	3.08	82.20	93.00	
Dish, mashed potatoes	0.5	Cup	121.00	100.43	2.79	19.51		1.46	0.58	0.42	0.35	2.42	13.31	
Fish, fillet, brd/batter fried	3	Ounce-weight	85.05	197.32	12.47	14.43	0.43	10.45	2.40	2.19	5.33	28.92	9.36	
French Toast, sticks	5	Piece	141.00	513.24	8.28	57.85	2.68	29.05	4.70	12.65	9.95	74.73	0.36	
Frozen Dessert, ice milk cone, vanilla, soft serve	1	Each	103.00	163.77	3.89	24.11	0.11	6.12	3.53	1.82	0.36	27.81	59.74	0.21
Hamburger, double, reg, plain	1	Each	176.00	543.84	29.92	42.93		27.90	10.38	12.11	2.34	98.56	0.00	0.70
Hamburger, double, reg, w/condiment	1	Each	215.00	576.20	31.82	38.74		32.47	12.00	14.13	2.76	103.20	2.15	
Hamburger, lrg, w/condiment	1	Each	171.50	425.32	23.03	36.72	2.06	20.94	7.90	9.28	1.59	70.32	5.15	

Vit E (mg)	Vit C	Vit B₁-Thia (mg)	Vit B₂-Ribo (mg)	Vit B₃-Nia (mg)	Fol (mcg)	Vit B₆ (mg)	Vita B₁₂ (mcg)	Sodi (mg)	Pota (mg)	Cal (mg)	Phos (mg)	Magn (mg)	Iron (mg)	Zinc (mg)	Caff (mg)	Alco (g)	Sol Fiber (g)	Insol Fiber (g)
1.30	0.95	0.18	0.14	1.89	31.74	0.03	0.01	262.83	74.59	58.25	42.36	11.89	1.79	0.39	0.00	0.00		
	5.40							1114.00		30.00			1.62		0.00	0.00		
	4.20							1046.00		20.00			1.44		0.00	0.00		
	1.20							320.00		50.00			0.72		0.00	0.00		
	1.80							280.00		50.00			0.72		0.00	0.00		
	1.20							490.00		60.00			1.44		0.00	0.00		
1.63	4.63	0.07	0.09	1.02	15.24	0.14	0.56	376.51	176.40	277.32	169.71	40.07	2.92	1.29	0.00	0.00		
4.26	19.10	0.31	0.21	1.34	61.98	0.25	0.00	409.84	625.11	1046.06	323.62	107.11	4.53	2.57	0.00	0.00		
	0.00							460.00		20.00			1.80		0.00	0.00		
0.03	0.00	0.27	0.64	2.49	52.25	0.55	0.22	10252.00	577.50	156.75	437.25	132.00	6.85	7.04	0.00	0.00	7.12	7.73
	0.00							240.00		0.00			0.00		0.00	0.00		
	1.80							459.27		5.00			0.45		0.00	0.00		
	0.00							90.00		0.00			0.36		0.00	0.00		
	1.55							418.81		8.60			0.54		0.00	0.00		
	2.40							85.00		0.00			0.00		0.00	0.00		
	2.06							376.28		8.60			0.46		0.00	0.00		
	1.80							393.89		17.18			0.85		0.00	0.00		
	1.20							388.23		5.00			0.63		0.00	0.00		
	1.80							372.42		12.89			0.46		0.00	0.00		
	3.18	0.08	0.12	0.58	17.40	0.03	0.15	153.00	83.40	25.20	87.60	16.20	1.29	0.56	1.20	0.00		
	1.03	0.36	0.49	7.25	74.82	0.41	3.41	1148.10	595.98	239.94	394.74	51.60	5.91	6.68	0.00	0.00		
1.19	0.00	0.25	0.37	6.01	68.20	0.25	2.31	635.50	308.45	232.50	373.55	32.55	3.41	4.96	0.00	0.00		
	1.66	0.35	0.28	8.05	61.42	0.18	1.93	1050.78	335.32	170.98	242.36	29.88	3.42	3.49	0.00	0.00		
	0.00	0.48	0.57	11.17	74.00	0.28	2.53	1589.15	643.80	90.65	421.80	38.85	5.46	5.55	0.00	0.00		
0.41	0.00	0.40	0.40	3.70	54.06	0.09	0.97	499.80	164.22	140.76	195.84	21.42	2.44	2.37	0.00	0.00		
	3.60							1120.00		80.00			1.80		0.00	0.00		
3.96	8.32	0.04	0.03	0.08	38.61	0.11	0.18	267.30	177.21	33.66	35.64	8.91	0.72	0.20	0.00	0.00		
	0.00	0.00	0.03	2.03	57.72	0.10	0.17	964.86	187.98	68.64	190.32	16.38	1.43	0.43	0.00	0.00		
	2.64	0.26	0.21	2.55	54.60	0.05	0.23	319.41	116.48	70.07	80.08	15.47	1.85	0.63	0.00	0.00		
0.79	2.55	0.26	0.19	2.20	54.56	0.05	0.22	326.48	95.92	36.96	73.92	14.08	1.80	0.48	0.00	0.00		
0.85	1.60	0.29	0.21	1.80	31.02	0.06	0.23	332.76	109.98	21.62	68.62	14.10	1.40	0.48	0.00	0.00		
	6.86	0.25	0.10	2.18	43.80	0.32	0.00	29.20	359.16	4.38	108.04	40.88	0.88	0.91	0.00	0.00		
	0.18	0.06	0.08	1.17	24.60	0.15	4.40	491.40	162.00	202.20	226.80	25.20	1.12	2.12	0.00	0.00		
	0.48	0.11	0.06	1.45	9.68	0.28	0.06	274.67	355.74	25.41	66.55	21.78	0.57	0.39	0.00	0.00		
	0.00	0.09	0.09	1.79	14.46	0.09	0.94	452.47	272.16	15.31	145.44	20.41	1.79	0.37	0.00	0.00		
2.33	0.00	0.23	0.26	2.96	197.40	0.26	0.08	499.14	126.90	77.55	122.67	26.79	2.96	0.94	0.00	0.00		
0.38	1.14	0.05	0.25	0.32	12.36	0.06	0.21	91.67	168.92	153.47	139.05	15.45	0.16	0.57	0.00	0.00		
1.32	0.00	0.33	0.37	8.25	77.44	0.32	2.92	554.40	362.56	86.24	234.08	36.96	4.56	5.72	0.00	0.00		
1.61	1.08	0.34	0.41	6.73	83.85	0.37	3.33	741.75	526.75	92.45	283.80	45.15	5.55	5.81	0.00	0.00		
0.03	2.57	0.34	0.28	6.54	61.74	0.25	2.57	728.88	394.45	133.77	212.66	34.30	4.13	4.75	0.00	0.00		

Food Name	Amount	Measure	Weight (g)	Calories	Protein (g)	Total Carb (g)	Dietary Fiber (g)	Total Fat (g)	Sat Fat (g)	Mono Fat (g)	Poly Fat (g)	Chol (mg)	Vit A (mcg RAE)	Vit D (mcg)
Hamburger, reg, plain	1	Each	90.00	274.50	12.32	30.51		11.82	4.14	5.46	0.92	35.10	0.00	0.27
Hot Dog, plain, w/bun	1	Each	98.00	242.06	10.39	18.03		14.54	5.11	6.85	1.71	44.10	0.00	
Hot Dog, w/chili & bun	1	Each	114.00	296.40	13.51	31.29		13.44	4.85	6.59	1.19	51.30	3.42	
Milk Shake, strawberry, fast food	1	Cup	283.00	319.79	9.62	53.49	1.13	7.92	4.91	2.21	0.31	31.13	73.58	0.57
Nachos, w/cheese	7	Piece	113.00	345.78	9.10	36.33		18.95	7.78	7.99	2.23	18.08	149.16	
Nachos, w/cheese & jalapeno peppers	7	Piece	204.00	607.92	16.81	60.08		34.15	14.02	14.40	4.02	83.64	573.24	
Nachos, w/cheese beans beef & peppers	7	Piece	225.00	501.75	17.46	49.25		27.09	11.02	9.69	5.02	18.00	384.75	
Onion Rings, breaded, fried, svg	8	Piece	78.11	259.33	3.48	29.47		14.60	6.54	6.26	0.62	13.28	0.78	
Oysters, brd/battered, fried	3	Ounce-weight	85.05	225.38	7.67	24.40	0.32	10.97	2.80	4.23	2.84	66.34	66.34	
Pancakes, w/butter & syrup	1	Each	116.00	259.84	4.13	45.45	0.60	6.99	2.92	2.64	0.98	29.00	40.60	
Potatoes, hash browns	0.5	Cup	72.00	151.20	1.94	16.15		9.22	4.32	3.86	0.47	9.36	1.44	
Sandwich, breakfast, egg bacon, w/biscuit	1	Each	150.00	457.50	17.00	28.59	0.75	31.10	7.95	13.44	7.47	352.50	106.50	
Sandwich, breakfast, egg cheese bacon, w/biscuit	1	Each	144.00	476.64	16.26	33.42	0.35	31.39	11.40	14.23	3.49	260.64	190.08	
Sandwich, breakfast, egg ham, w/biscuit	1	Each	192.00	441.60	20.43	30.32	0.77	27.03	5.91	10.96	7.70	299.52	236.16	
Sandwich, breakfast, egg sausage, w/biscuit	1	Each	180.00	581.40	19.15	41.15	0.90	38.70	14.98	16.40	4.45	302.40	160.20	
Sandwich, breakfast, egg steak, w/biscuit	1	Each	148.00	409.96	17.94	21.27		28.43	8.60	11.71	5.85	272.32	205.72	
Sandwich, breakfast, egg, w/biscuit	1	Each	136.00	372.64	11.60	31.91	0.82	22.07	4.73	9.07	6.40	244.80	179.52	
Sandwich, croissant, w/egg & cheese	1	Each	127.00	368.30	12.79	24.31		24.70	14.07	7.54	1.37	215.90	276.86	
Sandwich, croissant, w/egg cheese & bacon	1	Each	129.00	412.80	16.23	23.65		28.35	15.43	9.18	1.76	215.43	141.90	
Sandwich, croissant, w/egg cheese & ham	1	Each	152.00	474.24	18.92	24.20		33.58	17.48	11.39	2.36	212.80	130.72	
Sandwich, english muffin, w/cheese & sausage	1	Each	115.00	393.30	15.34	29.16	1.49	24.26	9.85	10.08	2.69	58.65	101.20	
Sandwich, english muffin, w/egg cheese & Canadian bacon	1	Each	146.00	308.06	17.78	28.50	1.61	13.42	4.97	4.98	1.66	249.66	188.34	1.17
Shrimp, brd, fried, fast food, each	4	Each	93.70	259.55	10.79	22.85		14.22	3.07	9.93	0.36	114.31	20.61	

A&W Restaurants

Food Name	Amount	Measure	Weight (g)	Calories	Protein (g)	Total Carb (g)	Dietary Fiber (g)	Total Fat (g)	Sat Fat (g)	Mono Fat (g)	Poly Fat (g)	Chol (mg)	Vit A (mcg RAE)	Vit D (mcg)
Cheeseburger, deluxe, w/bacon	1	Each	277.50	600.00	32.00	44.00	4.00	33.00	12.00			110.00		

Arby's

Food Name	Amount	Measure	Weight (g)	Calories	Protein (g)	Total Carb (g)	Dietary Fiber (g)	Total Fat (g)	Sat Fat (g)	Mono Fat (g)	Poly Fat (g)	Chol (mg)	Vit A (mcg RAE)	Vit D (mcg)
Cheese, mozzarella sticks, svg	1	Each	137.00	470.00	18.00	34.00	2.00	29.00	14.00			60.00		
Sandwich, beef melt, w/cheddar	1	Each	150.00	320.00	16.00	36.00	2.00	14.00	6.00			45.00		
Sandwich, ham swiss, hot	1	Each	170.00	340.00	23.00	35.00	1.00	13.00	4.50			90.00		
Sandwich, roast beef, giant	1	Each	228.00	440.00	32.00	42.00	3.00	20.00	11.00			45.00		
Sandwich, roast beef, jr	1	Each	129.00	290.00	16.00	34.00	2.00	12.00	5.00			40.00		
Sandwich, turkey, rstd, deluxe, light	1	Each	194.00	260.00	23.00	33.00	3.00	5.00	0.50	2.20	2.30	40.00		

Burger King

Food Name	Amount	Measure	Weight (g)	Calories	Protein (g)	Total Carb (g)	Dietary Fiber (g)	Total Fat (g)	Sat Fat (g)	Mono Fat (g)	Poly Fat (g)	Chol (mg)	Vit A (mcg RAE)	Vit D (mcg)
Cheeseburger, Whopper, double	1	Each	378.00	1020.00	53.00	55.00	4.00	65.00	25.00			170.00		
Chicken, Tenders, 6 pce svg	6	Piece	92.00	250.00	16.00	15.00	1.00	14.00	4.00			35.00	0.00	
Dish, Jalapeno Poppers, 4 pce svg	4	Piece	77.00	230.00	7.00	22.00	2.00	13.00	5.00			20.00		
Hamburger, Whopper Jr	1	Each	167.00	410.00	18.00	32.00	2.00	23.00	7.00			50.00		
Milk Shake, vanilla, med	1	Each	397.00	440.00	12.00	79.00	2.00	8.00	5.00			25.00		
Sandwich, chicken tenders	1	Each	148.00	450.00	14.00	37.00	2.00	27.00	5.00			30.00		
Sandwich, chicken, club	1	Each	256.00	740.00	30.00	55.00	4.00	44.00	10.00			85.00		

Carl's Junior

Food Name	Amount	Measure	Weight (g)	Calories	Protein (g)	Total Carb (g)	Dietary Fiber (g)	Total Fat (g)	Sat Fat (g)	Mono Fat (g)	Poly Fat (g)	Chol (mg)	Vit A (mcg RAE)	Vit D (mcg)
Bacon, ckd, 2 strip svg	2	Each	9.00	50.00	3.00	0.00	0.00	4.00	1.50			10.00	0.00	
Cheeseburger, double, Western Bacon	1	Each	308.00	900.00	51.00	64.00	2.00	49.00	21.00			155.00		

Chick-Fil-A

Food Name	Amount	Measure	Weight (g)	Calories	Protein (g)	Total Carb (g)	Dietary Fiber (g)	Total Fat (g)	Sat Fat (g)	Mono Fat (g)	Poly Fat (g)	Chol (mg)	Vit A (mcg RAE)	Vit D (mcg)
Chicken, strips, Chick-N-Strips, 4 pce svg	4	Piece	108.00	250.00	25.00	12.00	0.00	11.00	2.50			70.00	0.00	

Dairy Queen

Food Name	Amount	Measure	Weight (g)	Calories	Protein (g)	Total Carb (g)	Dietary Fiber (g)	Total Fat (g)	Sat Fat (g)	Mono Fat (g)	Poly Fat (g)	Chol (mg)	Vit A (mcg RAE)	Vit D (mcg)
Frozen Dessert Bar, Starkiss, non dairy	1	Each	85.00	80.00	0.00	21.00	0.00	0.00	0.00	0.00	0.00	0.00	0.00	
Frozen Dessert, banana split, Royal Treats	1	Each	369.00	510.00	8.00	96.00	3.00	12.00	8.00			30.00		

Vit E (mg)	Vit C	Vit B₁-Thia (mg)	Vit B₂-Ribo (mg)	Vit B₃-Nia (mg)	Fol (mcg)	Vit B₆ (mg)	Vita B₁₂ (mcg)	Sodi (mg)	Pota (mg)	Cal (mg)	Phos (mg)	Magn (mg)	Iron (mg)	Zinc (mg)	Caff (mg)	Alco (g)	Sol Fiber (g)	Insol Fiber (g)
0.49	0.00	0.33	0.27	3.72	53.10	0.06	0.89	387.00	144.90	63.00	102.60	18.90	2.40	2.00	0.00	0.00		
0.27	0.10	0.24	0.27	3.65	48.02	0.05	0.51	670.32	143.08	23.52	97.02	12.74	2.31	1.98	0.00	0.00		
	2.74	0.22	0.40	3.74	72.96	0.05	0.30	479.94	166.44	19.38	191.52	10.26	3.28	0.78	0.00	0.00		
0.37	2.26	0.13	0.55	0.50	8.49	0.12	0.88	234.89	515.06	319.79	283.00	36.79	0.31	1.02	0.00	0.00		
	1.24	0.19	0.37	1.54	10.17	0.20	0.82	815.86	171.76	272.33	275.72	55.37	1.28	1.79	0.00	0.00		
	1.02	0.12	0.49	2.84	18.36	0.37	1.02	1736.04	293.76	620.16	393.72	108.12	2.45	2.90	0.00	0.00		
	4.27	0.20	0.61	2.95	33.75	0.36	0.90	1588.50	398.25	339.75	342.00	85.50	2.45	3.22	0.00	0.00		
0.31	0.55	0.08	0.09	0.87	51.55	0.06	0.11	404.61	121.85	68.74	81.23	14.84	0.80	0.33	0.00	0.00		
	2.55	0.19	0.21	2.70	18.71	0.02	0.62	414.19	111.42	17.01	119.92	14.46	2.73	9.57	0.00	0.00		
0.70	1.74	0.20	0.27	1.70	25.52	0.06	0.12	552.16	125.28	63.80	237.80	24.36	1.31	0.51	0.00	0.00		
0.12	5.47	0.08	0.01	1.07	7.92	0.17	0.01	290.16	267.12	7.20	69.12	15.84	0.48	0.22	0.00	0.00		
1.96	2.70	0.14	0.22	2.40	60.00	0.14	1.03	999.00	250.50	189.00	238.50	24.00	3.74	1.64	0.00	0.00		
1.44	1.58	0.30	0.43	2.30	53.28	0.10	1.05	1260.00	230.40	164.16	459.36	20.16	2.55	1.54	0.00	0.00		
2.28	0.00	0.67	0.60	2.00	65.28	0.27	1.19	1382.40	318.72	220.80	316.80	30.72	4.55	2.23	0.00	0.00		
2.84	0.00	0.50	0.45	3.60	64.80	0.20	1.37	1141.20	320.40	154.80	489.60	25.20	3.96	2.16	0.00	0.00		
	0.15	0.36	0.52	3.06	56.24	0.18	1.41	888.00	306.36	137.64	224.96	25.16	5.30	2.80	0.00	0.00		
3.26	0.14	0.30	0.49	2.15	57.12	0.11	0.63	890.80	238.00	81.60	387.60	19.04	2.90	0.99	0.00	0.00		
	0.13	0.19	0.38	1.51	46.99	0.10	0.77	551.18	173.99	243.84	347.98	21.59	2.20	1.75	0.00	0.00		
	2.19	0.35	0.34	2.19	45.15	0.12	0.86	888.81	201.24	150.93	276.06	23.22	2.19	1.90	0.00	0.00		
	11.40	0.52	0.30	3.19	45.60	0.23	1.00	1080.72	272.08	144.40	335.92	25.84	2.13	2.17	0.00	0.00		
1.26	1.26	0.70	0.25	4.14	66.70	0.15	0.68	1036.15	215.05	167.90	186.30	24.15	2.25	1.68	0.00	0.00		
0.60	1.90	0.53	0.48	3.55	73.00	0.16	0.72	776.72	211.70	160.60	287.62	24.82	2.60	1.66	0.00	0.00		
	0.00	0.12	0.52	0.00	57.16	0.03	0.09	826.43	104.95	47.79	196.78	22.49	1.69	0.69	0.00	0.00		
	6.00							1390.00		200.00			5.40		0.00	0.00		
	1.20							1330.00		400.00			0.72		0.00	0.00		
	0.00							850.00		80.00			2.70		0.00	0.00		
	1.20	0.83	0.37	7.80	26.00	0.31		1450.00	382.00	150.00	405.00	31.00	2.70	0.90	0.00	0.00		
	0.00	0.41	0.75	16.80				1330.00	599.00	60.00			5.40	6.00	0.00	0.00		
		0.26	0.37	9.57	10.14	0.14		700.00	291.30	60.00	86.96	11.60	2.70	2.17	0.00	0.00		
	1.20	0.08	0.41	15.32	19.90	0.52		1030.00	351.00	80.00	249.00	29.80	1.80	1.50	0.00	0.00		
	9.00							1460.00		300.00			7.20		0.00	0.00		
	0.00							630.00		0.00			0.72		0.00	0.00		
	0.00							790.00		150.00			0.72		0.00	0.00		
	4.80							520.00		80.00			3.60		0.00	0.00		
	6.00							340.00		400.00			0.00		0.00	0.00		
	3.60							680.00		60.00			1.80		0.00	0.00		
	6.00							1530.00		80.00			3.60		0.00	0.00		
	0.00							140.00		0.00			0.00		0.00	0.00	0.00	0.00
	1.20							1770.00		300.00			6.30		0.00	0.00		
	0.00							570.00		40.00			1.08		0.00	0.00	0.00	0.00
	0.00							10.00		0.00			0.00			0.00	0.00	0.00
	15.00							180.00		250.00			1.80			0.00		

Food Name	Amount	Measure	Weight (g)	Calories	Protein (g)	Total Carb (g)	Dietary Fiber (g)	Total Fat (g)	Sat Fat (g)	Mono Fat (g)	Poly Fat (g)	Chol (mg)	Vit A (mcg RAE)	Vit D (mcg)
FAST FOODS/RESTAURANTS *(continued)*														
Frozen Dessert, chocolate chip cookie dough, med	1	Each	439.00	950.00	17.00	143.00	2.00	36.00	19.00			75.00		
Frozen Dessert, Lemon Freez'r	0.5	Cup	92.00	80.00	0.00	20.00	0.00	0.00	0.00	0.00	0.00	0.00	0.00	
Frozen Dessert, Misty Slush, med	1	Each	595.00	290.00	0.00	74.00	0.00	0.00	0.00	0.00	0.00	0.00	0.00	
Frozen Dessert, parfait, Peanut Buster, Royal Treats	1	Each	305.00	730.00	16.00	99.00	2.00	31.00	17.00			35.00		
Hot Dog	1	Each	99.00	240.00	9.00	19.00	1.00	14.00	5.00			25.00		
Ice Cream Bar, Buster Bar	1	Each	149.00	450.00	10.00	41.00	2.00	28.00	12.00			15.00		
Ice Cream Bar, Dilly, chocolate	1	Each	85.00	210.00	3.00	21.00	0.00	13.00	7.00			10.00		
Ice Cream Cone, chocolate, med	1	Each	198.00	340.00	8.00	53.00	0.00	11.00	7.00			30.00		
Ice Cream Cone, chocolate, sml	1	Each	142.00	240.00	6.00	37.00	0.00	8.00	5.00			20.00		
Ice Cream Cone, dipped, med	1	Each	220.00	490.00	8.00	59.00	1.00	24.00	13.00			30.00		
Ice Cream Cone, dipped, sml	1	Each	156.00	340.00	6.00	42.00	1.00	17.00	9.00			20.00		
Ice Cream Sandwich	1	Each	85.00	200.00	4.00	31.00	1.00	6.00	3.00			10.00		
Milk Shake, chocolate malt, med	1	Each	567.00	880.00	19.00	153.00	0.00	22.00	14.00			70.00		
Potatoes, french fries, sml, svg	1	Each	113.00	350.00	4.00	42.00	3.00	18.00	3.50			0.00	0.00	
Dennys														
Quesadilla, chicken	1	Each	454.00	827.00	50.00	43.00	2.00	55.00	23.00			181.00		
Sandwich, club	1	Each	312.00	718.00	32.00	62.00	3.00	38.00	7.00			75.00		
Sauce, barbecue, svg	1	Each	46.00	47.00	0.00	11.00	0.00	1.00	0.00			0.00		
Dominos Pizza														
Chicken, buffalo wings, hot	1	Each	24.90	44.92	5.46	0.50	0.19	2.39	0.65			25.58		
Dunkin' Donuts														
Bagel, poppy seed	1	Each	125.00	340.00	12.00	68.00	3.00	2.50	0.00			0.00	0.00	
Bagel, whole wheat	1	Each	125.00	320.00	12.00	63.00	5.00	1.50	0.00			0.00	0.00	
Doughnut, cake, chocolate	1	Each	59.00	210.00	3.00	19.00	1.00	14.00	3.00			0.00	0.00	
Doughnut, cake, cinnamon	1	Each	66.00	300.00	3.00	29.00	1.00	19.00	4.00			0.00	0.00	
Doughnut, cake, old fash	1	Each	60.00	280.00	3.00	24.00	1.00	19.00	4.00			0.00	0.00	
Doughnut, raised, glazed	1	Each	46.00	160.00	3.00	23.00	1.00	7.00	2.00			0.00	0.00	
Muffin, bran, low fat	1	Each	95.00	260.00	4.00	59.00	4.00	1.50	0.00			0.00	0.00	
Muffin, corn, low fat	1	Each	95.00	250.00	4.00	55.00	1.00	2.00	0.00			0.00	0.00	
El Pollo Loco														
Salad, garden, reg	1	Each	113.00	104.63	4.98	6.98	1.00	6.98	2.99			14.95		
Hardees														
Biscuit, Made from Scratch	1	Each	83.00	390.00	6.00	44.00		21.00	6.00			0.00		
Cheeseburger	1	Each	124.00	313.00	16.00	26.00	1.00	14.00	7.00			40.00		
Hamburger, Six Dollar	1	Each	353.00	911.00	41.00	50.00	2.00	61.00	27.00			137.00		
Milk Shake, chocolate	12.3	Fluid ounce	349.00	370.00	13.00	67.00	0.00	5.00	3.00			30.00		
Potatoes, french fries, Crispy Curls, reg svg	1	Each	96.00	340.00	5.00	41.00	0.00	18.00	4.00			0.00		
Potatoes, french fries, reg svg	1	Each	113.00	340.00	4.00	45.00	0.00	16.00	2.00			0.00		
Sandwich, roast beef, big	1	Each	165.00	411.46	24.02	27.15	2.09	22.97	9.40			67.88		
In-N-Out Burgers														
Cheeseburger, Double Double, w/spread	1	Each	328.00	670.00	37.00	40.00	3.00	41.00	18.00			120.00		
Cheeseburger, protein style, wrapped w/lettuce, no bun	1	Each	300.00	330.00	18.00	11.00	2.00	25.00	9.00			60.00		
Jack in the Box														
Cheeseburger, w/bacon, ultimate	1	Each	302.00	1020.00	58.00	37.00	1.00	71.00	26.00			210.00		
Dish, fish & chips	1	Each	281.00	780.00	19.00	86.00	6.00	39.00	9.00			45.00		
Sandwich, sausage, w/croissant	1	Each	181.00	660.00	20.00	37.00	0.00	48.00	15.00			240.00		
Taco, monster	1	Each	138.00	270.00	12.00	19.00	4.00	17.00	6.00			30.00		

Vit E (mg)	Vit C	Vit B₁- Thia (mg)	Vit B₂- Ribo (mg)	Vit B₃- Nia (mg)	Fol (mcg)	Vit B₆ (mg)	Vita B₁₂ (mcg)	Sodi (mg)	Pota (mg)	Cal (mg)	Phos (mg)	Magn (mg)	Iron (mg)	Zinc (mg)	Caff (mg)	Alco (g)	Sol Fiber (g)	Insol Fiber (g)
	1.20							660.00	450.00				2.70			0.00		
	0.00							10.00	0.00				0.00		0.00	0.00	0.00	0.00
	0.00							30.00	0.00				0.00		0.00	0.00	0.00	0.00
	1.20							400.00	300.00				1.80			0.00		
	3.60							730.00	60.00				1.80		0.00	0.00		
	0.00							280.00	150.00				1.08			0.00		
	0.00							75.00	100.00				0.36			0.00	0.00	0.00
	1.20							160.00	250.00				1.80			0.00	0.00	0.00
	0.00							115.00	150.00				1.08			0.00	0.00	0.00
	2.40							190.00	250.00				1.80			0.00		
	1.20							130.00	200.00				1.08			0.00		
	0.00							140.00	80.00				1.08			0.00		
	2.40							500.00	600.00				2.70			0.00	0.00	0.00
	3.60							880.00	20.00				1.08		0.00	0.00		
	54.00							1982.00	640.00				1.80		0.00	0.00		
	13.20							1666.00	120.00				4.32		0.00	0.00		
	2.40							595.00	10.00				0.18		0.00	0.00	0.00	0.00
	1.13							354.40	5.44				0.30		0.00	0.00		
	3.60							680.00	80.00				4.50		0.00	0.00		
	6.00							630.00	40.00				3.60		0.00	0.00		
	3.60							270.00	0.00				1.44			0.00		
	1.20							350.00	0.00				1.08		0.00	0.00		
	1.20							350.00	0.00				1.08		0.00	0.00		
	1.20							200.00	0.00				0.36		0.00	0.00		
	0.00							440.00	60.00				2.70		0.00	0.00		
	0.00							460.00	0.00				1.08		0.00	0.00		
	6.58							98.65	109.61				0.36		0.00	0.00		
								1000.00							0.00	0.00		
								895.00							0.00	0.00		
								1584.00							0.00	0.00		
								270.00								0.00	0.00	0.00
								950.00							0.00	0.00	0.00	0.00
								390.00							0.00	0.00	0.00	0.00
								1127.85							0.00	0.00		
	15.00							1430.00	350.00				5.40		0.00	0.00		
	18.00							720.00	200.00				1.08		0.00	0.00		
	0.60							1740.00	630.00	300.00			7.20		0.00	0.00		
	15.00							1740.00	1060.00	20.00			2.70		0.00	0.00		
	0.00							860.00	160.00	100.00			1.80		0.00	0.00	0.00	0.00
	2.40							630.00	365.00	200.00	217.00	49.30	1.44	1.80	0.00	0.00		

Food Name	Amount	Measure	Weight (g)	Calories	Protein (g)	Total Carb (g)	Dietary Fiber (g)	Total Fat (g)	Sat Fat (g)	Mono Fat (g)	Poly Fat (g)	Chol (mg)	Vit A (mcg RAE)	Vit D (mcg)
FAST FOODS/RESTAURANTS *(continued)*														
Kentucky Fried Chicken														
Beans, green, svg	4	Ounce-weight	113.40	50.18	5.02	5.02	2.01	1.51	0.50			5.02		
Chicken, breast, extra crispy	1	Each	162.00	460.00	34.00	19.00	0.00	28.00	8.00			135.00	0.00	
Chicken, breast, hot & spicy	1	Each	179.00	460.00	33.00	20.00	0.00	27.00	8.00			130.00	0.00	
Chicken, breast, original rec	1	Each	161.00	380.00	40.00	11.00	0.00	19.00	6.00			145.00	0.00	
Chicken, drumstick, extra crispy	1	Each	60.00	160.00	12.00	5.00	0.00	10.00	2.50			70.00	0.00	
Chicken, drumstick, original rec	1	Each	59.00	140.00	14.00	4.00	0.00	8.00	2.00			75.00	0.00	
Chicken, thigh, extra crispy	1	Each	114.00	370.00	21.00	12.00	0.00	26.00	7.00			120.00	0.00	
Chicken, thigh, original rec	1	Each	126.00	360.00	22.00	12.00	0.00	25.00	7.00			165.00	0.00	
Chicken, wing, extra crispy	1	Each	52.00	190.00	10.00	10.00	0.00	12.00	4.00			55.00	0.00	
Chicken, wing, original rec	1	Each	47.00	150.00	11.00	5.00	0.00	9.00	2.50			60.00	0.00	
Long John Silvers														
Cheese, cheesesticks, brd, fried	3	Each	45.00	140.00	4.00	12.00	1.00	8.00	2.00			10.00		
Chicken, strips, plank, battered	1	Piece	52.50	140.00	8.00	9.00	0.00	8.00	2.50			20.00	0.00	
Fish, batter dipped, reg	1	Piece	92.00	230.00	11.00	16.00	0.00	13.00	4.00			30.00	0.00	
McDonalds														
Cheeseburger, Big Mac	1	Each	219.00	571.59	26.15	47.15	3.07	30.88	10.95	11.30	8.50	78.84		
Chicken, nuggets, McNuggets, 4 pce svg	4	Piece	72.00	190.00	10.00	13.00	1.00	11.00	2.50			35.00	0.00	
Cookie, chocolate chip, pkg	1	Each	56.00	280.00	3.00	37.00	1.00	14.00	8.00			40.00		
Cookie, McDonaldland, pkg	1	Each	57.00	230.00	3.00	38.00	1.00	8.00	2.00			0.00	0.00	
Danish, apple	1	Each	105.00	340.00	5.00	47.00	2.00	15.00	3.00			20.00		
Frozen Dessert, McFlurry, Nestle Crunch, svg	1	Each	348.00	630.00	16.00	89.00	1.00	24.00	16.00			75.00		
Hamburger	1	Each	105.00	269.85	13.03	32.34	1.68	9.76	3.64	4.06	1.27	27.30		
Milk Shake, strawberry, sml	1	Each	294.00	360.00	11.00	60.00	0.00	9.00	6.00			40.00		
Milk Shake, vanilla, sml	1	Each	293.40	360.00	11.00	59.00	0.00	9.00	6.00			40.00		
Potatoes, french fries, lrg svg	1	Each	171.00	617.31	6.67	73.29	6.50	32.95	7.40	17.34	6.65		0.00	
Sandwich, ham egg cheese, w/bagel	1	Each	218.00	550.00	26.00	58.00	2.00	23.00	8.00			255.00		
Pizza Hut														
Pizza, cheese, 6"	1	Piece	63.00	160.00	7.00	18.00	1.00	7.00	3.00			15.00		
Pizza, cheese, med, 12"	1	Piece	79.00	200.00	10.00	21.00	1.00	8.00	4.50			25.00		
Pizza, Pepperoni Lover's, med, 12"	1	Piece	92.00	260.00	13.00	21.00	2.00	14.00	7.00			40.00		
Pizza, Pepperoni Lover's, pan, med, 12"	1	Piece	118.00	340.00	15.00	29.00	2.00	19.00	7.00			40.00		
Pizza, pepperoni, 6"	1	Piece	61.00	170.00	7.00	18.00	1.00	8.00	3.00			15.00		
Pizza, supreme, 6"	1	Piece	77.00	190.00	8.00	19.00	1.00	9.00	3.50			20.00		
Pizza, supreme, med, 12"	1	Piece	106.00	240.00	11.00	22.00	2.00	11.00	5.00			25.00		
Pizza, supreme, pan, med, 12"	1	Piece	127.00	320.00	13.00	30.00	2.00	16.00	6.00			25.00		
Pizza, supreme, super, med, 12"	1	Piece	119.00	260.00	13.00	23.00	2.00	13.00	6.00			35.00		
Pizza, supreme, super, pan, med, 12"	1	Piece	139.00	340.00	14.00	30.00	2.00	18.00	6.00			35.00		
Taco Bell														
Burrito, bean	1	Each	198.00	370.00	14.00	55.00	8.00	10.00	3.50			10.00		
Burrito, beef, grilled, Stuft	1	Each	325.00	730.00	28.00	79.00	10.00	33.00	11.00			55.00		
Burrito, beef, supreme	1	Each	248.00	440.00	18.00	51.00	7.00	18.00	8.00			40.00		
Burrito, chicken, fiesta	1	Each	184.00	370.00	18.00	48.00	3.00	12.00	3.50			30.00		
Burrito, chicken, supreme	1	Each	248.00	410.00	21.00	50.00	5.00	14.00	6.00			45.00		
Burrito, seven layer	1	Each	283.00	530.00	18.00	67.00	10.00	22.00	8.00			25.00		
Chalupa, beef, supreme	1	Each	153.00	390.00	14.00	31.00	3.00	24.00	10.00			40.00		
Gordita, chicken, Baja	1	Each	153.00	320.00	17.00	29.00	2.00	15.00	3.50			40.00		
Quesadilla, cheese	1	Each	142.00	490.00	19.00	39.00	3.00	28.00	13.00			55.00		
Salad, taco, w/salsa, w/o shell	1	Each	462.00	420.00	24.00	33.00	11.00	21.00	11.00			65.00		
Taco	1	Each	78.00	170.00	8.00	13.00	3.00	10.00	4.00			25.00		
Taco Johns														
Burrito, bean	1	Each	170.10	340.00	14.80	45.20		11.10	3.00			15.00		
Burrito, beef	1	Each	170.10	415.00	22.40	39.40		18.90	6.41			43.10		

Vit E (mg)	Vit C	Vit B₁-Thia (mg)	Vit B₂-Ribo (mg)	Vit B₃-Nia (mg)	Fol (mcg)	Vit B6 (mg)	Vita B12 (mcg)	Sodi (mg)	Pota (mg)	Cal (mg)	Phos (mg)	Magn (mg)	Iron (mg)	Zinc (mg)	Caff (mg)	Alco (g)	Sol Fiber (g)	Insol Fiber (g)
	1.20							461.63		0.00			0.72		0.00	0.00		
	0.00							1230.00		0.00			1.44		0.00	0.00	0.00	0.00
	0.00							1450.00		0.00			1.14		0.00	0.00	0.00	0.00
	0.00							1150.00		0.00			1.80		0.00	0.00	0.00	0.00
	0.00							420.00		0.00			0.72		0.00	0.00	0.00	0.00
	0.00							440.00		0.00			0.72		0.00	0.00	0.00	0.00
	0.00							710.00		0.00			1.14		0.00	0.00	0.00	0.00
	0.00							1060.00		0.00			1.14		0.00	0.00	0.00	0.00
	0.00							390.00		0.00			0.38		0.00	0.00	0.00	0.00
	0.00							370.00		0.00			0.38		0.00	0.00	0.00	0.00
	0.00							320.00		100.00			0.72		0.00	0.00		
	2.40							400.00		0.00			0.36		0.00	0.00	0.00	0.00
	4.80							700.00		20.00			1.80		0.00	0.00	0.00	0.00
0.13	0.66	0.40	0.44	7.95	59.13	0.37	2.78	1062.15	398.58	278.13	297.84	54.75	3.07	4.73	0.00	0.00		
0.94	0.00			4.94			0.20	360.00	201.60	9.10	191.10	16.38	0.71	0.66	0.00	0.00		
0.92	0.00	0.14	0.16	1.48				170.00	142.20	20.00	83.44	23.80	1.44	0.40	3.00	0.00		
1.00	0.00			2.04				250.00	62.70	20.00	71.25	11.34	1.80	0.39	0.00	0.00		
	15.00	0.30	0.17	2.00				340.00	113.40	60.00	0.00		1.44		0.00	0.00		
	2.40							230.00		500.00			0.36			0.00		
0.10	0.31	0.31	0.07	4.56	29.40	0.10	1.18	501.90	203.70	130.20	112.35	25.20	1.78	2.03	0.00	0.00		
	6.00							180.00	542.00	350.00	328.60		0.72		0.00	0.00	0.00	0.00
	1.20							250.00	533.70	350.00	326.70		0.36		0.00	0.00	0.00	0.00
1.33	3.59	0.30	0.18	4.56	13.68	0.98		292.41	1031.13	29.07	227.43	63.27	1.50	0.94	0.00	0.00		
	0.00							1490.00		200.00			4.50		0.00	0.00		
	0.00							310.00		100.00			1.44		0.00	0.00		
	1.20							490.00		200.00			1.08		0.00	0.00		
	2.40							690.00		200.00			1.44		0.00	0.00		
	2.40							700.00		200.00			2.70		0.00	0.00		
	1.20							340.00		80.00			1.44		0.00	0.00		
	3.60							420.00		80.00			1.80		0.00	0.00		
	9.00							640.00		150.00			1.80		0.00	0.00		
	6.00							650.00		150.00			2.70		0.00	0.00		
	12.00							760.00		150.00			1.80		0.00	0.00		
	9.00							760.00		150.00			2.70		0.00	0.00		
	4.80							1200.00		200.00			2.70		0.00	0.00		
	6.00							2080.00		350.00			4.50		0.00	0.00		
	9.00							1330.00		200.00			2.70		0.00	0.00		
	3.60							1090.00		200.00			2.70		0.00	0.00		
	9.00							1270.00		200.00			2.70		0.00	0.00		
	4.80							1360.00		300.00			3.60		0.00	0.00		
	4.80							600.00		150.00			1.80		0.00	0.00		
	3.60							690.00		100.00			1.80		0.00	0.00		
	0.00							1150.00		500.00			1.44		0.00	0.00		
	21.00							1400.00		250.00			3.60		0.00	0.00		
	2.40							350.00		60.00			1.08		0.00	0.00		
	0.69							654.00		260.00			6.29		0.00	0.00		
	0.86							703.00		250.00			5.98		0.00	0.00		

Food Name	Amount	Measure	Weight (g)	Calories	Protein (g)	Total Carb (g)	Dietary Fiber (g)	Total Fat (g)	Sat Fat (g)	Mono Fat (g)	Poly Fat (g)	Chol (mg)	Vit A (mcg RAE)	Vit D (mcg)
FAST FOODS/RESTAURANTS *(continued)*														
Taco Time														
Burrito, veggie	1	Each	321.40	491.00	21.00	70.00	10.00	16.00	6.00			24.00		
Wendy's														
Cheeseburger, deluxe, jr	1	Each	179.00	350.00	17.00	37.00	2.00	15.00	6.00			45.00		
Cheeseburger, jr	1	Each	129.00	310.00	17.00	34.00	2.00	12.00	6.00			45.00		
Cheeseburger, w/bacon, jr	1	Each	165.00	380.00	20.00	34.00	2.00	19.00	7.00			55.00		
Frozen Dessert, Frosty, dairy, jr	1	Each	113.00	170.00	4.00	28.00	0.00	4.00	2.50			20.00		
Hamburger, Big Bacon Classic	1	Each	282.00	570.00	34.00	46.00	3.00	29.00	12.00			100.00		
Hamburger, jr	1	Each	117.00	270.00	14.00	34.00	2.00	9.00	3.00			30.00		
Hamburger, single, w/everything	1	Each	218.00	410.00	24.00	37.00	2.00	19.00	7.00			70.00		
FATS, OILS, MARGARINES, SHORTENINGS, AND SUBSTITUTES														
Fat Substitutes														
Butter Substitute, Butterlike, dried Mrs. Bateman's	0.5	Teaspoon	5.00	20.60	0.02	4.10	0.00	0.50	0.30			1.27		0.00
Butter Substitute, plain, soy, vegetarian Veggie	1	Tablespoon	14.00	40.00	1.00	2.00		3.00	0.00			0.00		
Fats and Oils, Animal														
Butter, salted, pat, 1" square × 1/3" high	1	Each	5.00	35.85	0.04	0.00	0.00	4.06	2.57	1.05	0.15	10.75	34.20	0.07
Butter, salted, whipped, pat, 1" square × 1/3" high	1	Each	3.80	27.25	0.03	0.00	0.00	3.08	1.92	0.89	0.11	8.32	25.99	
Butter, unsalted, pat, 1" square × 1/3" high	1	Each	5.00	35.85	0.04	0.00	0.00	4.06	2.57	1.05	0.15	10.75	34.20	
Fat, lard	1	Tablespoon	12.80	115.46	0.00	0.00	0.00	12.80	5.02	5.77	1.43	12.16	0.00	
Oil, fish, herring	1	Tablespoon	13.60	122.67	0.00	0.00	0.00	13.60	2.90	7.69	2.12	104.18	0.00	20.40
Fats and Oils, Vegetable														
Oil, canola, pure Crisco	1	Tablespoon	14.00	120.00	0.00	0.00	0.00	14.00	1.00	8.00	4.00	0.00	0.00	
Oil, cocoa butter	1	Tablespoon	13.60	120.22	0.00	0.00	0.00	13.60	8.12	4.47	0.41	0.00	0.00	
Oil, coconut	1	Tablespoon	13.60	117.23	0.00	0.00	0.00	13.60	11.76	0.79	0.24	0.00	0.00	
Oil, cooking spray, 0.33 second spray, svg Crisco	1	Each	0.25	2.25	0.00	0.00	0.00	0.25	0.00			0.00	0.00	
Oil, corn & canola	1	Tablespoon	14.00	123.76	0.00	0.00	0.00	14.00	1.30	5.85	6.24	0.00	0.00	
Oil, grapeseed	1	Tablespoon	13.60	120.22	0.00	0.00	0.00	13.60	1.31	2.19	9.51	0.00	0.00	0.00
Oil, oat	1	Tablespoon	13.60	120.22	0.00	0.00	0.00	13.60	2.67	4.77	5.56	0.00	0.00	0.00
Oil, olive, extra virgin Natural Oils International	1	Tablespoon	14.00	126.00	0.00	0.00	0.00	14.00	1.96	10.78	1.26	0.00		
Oil, palm kernel	1	Tablespoon	13.60	117.23	0.00	0.00	0.00	13.60	11.08	1.55	0.22	0.00	0.00	
Oil, peanut, salad or cooking	1	Tablespoon	13.50	119.34	0.00	0.00	0.00	13.50	2.28	6.24	4.32	0.00	0.00	
Oil, rice bran	1	Tablespoon	13.60	120.22	0.00	0.00	0.00	13.60	2.68	5.34	4.76	0.00	0.00	0.00
Oil, safflower Saffola	1	Tablespoon	14.00	120.00	0.00	0.00	0.00	14.00	1.00	11.00	2.00	0.00	0.00	
Oil, sesame Eden Foods, Inc.	1	Tablespoon	14.00	130.00	0.00	0.00	0.00	14.00	2.00	6.00	6.00	0.00	0.00	0.00
Oil, soybean lecithin	1	Tablespoon	13.60	103.77	0.00	0.00	0.00	13.60	2.04	1.49	6.16	0.00	0.00	
Oil, soybean, partially hydrog, winterized Archer Daniels Midland Company	1	Tablespoon	13.75	121.83	0.00	0.00	0.00	13.75	2.20	4.26	6.12	0.00	0.00	
Oil, soybean, salad or cooking	1	Tablespoon	13.60	120.22	0.00	0.00	0.00	13.60	1.96	3.17	7.87	0.00	0.00	
Oil, sunflower, greater than 60% linoleic	1	Tablespoon	13.60	120.22	0.00	0.00	0.00	13.60	1.40	2.65	8.94	0.00	0.00	
Oil, sunflower, less than 60% linoleic	1	Tablespoon	13.60	120.22	0.00	0.00	0.00	13.60	1.37	6.17	5.45	0.00	0.00	
Oil, sunflower, mid oleic, transfree, NuSun	1	Tablespoon	13.60	122.40	0.00	0.00	0.00	13.60	1.50	7.07	4.76	0.00	0.00	0.00
Oil, veg, pure Crisco	1	Tablespoon	14.00	120.00	0.00	0.00	0.00	14.00	1.50	6.00	6.00	0.00	0.00	
Margarines and Spreads														
Margarine & Butter, blend, w/60% corn oil & 40% butter	1	Tablespoon	14.20	101.96	0.12	0.09	0.00	11.46	4.04	4.65	2.26	12.50	116.30	
Margarine, 80% fat	1	Tablespoon	14.10	99.41	0.03	0.27	0.00	11.11	2.08	5.25	3.26	0.00	115.48	

Vit E (mg)	Vit C	Vit B$_1$-Thia (mg)	Vit B$_2$-Ribo (mg)	Vit B$_3$-Nia (mg)	Fol (mcg)	Vit B$_6$ (mg)	Vita B$_{12}$ (mcg)	Sodi (mg)	Pota (mg)	Cal (mg)	Phos (mg)	Magn (mg)	Iron (mg)	Zinc (mg)	Caff (mg)	Alco (g)	Sol Fiber (g)	Insol Fiber (g)
								643.00							0.00	0.00		
	9.00							890.00	320.00	150.00			3.60		0.00	0.00		
	3.60							820.00	230.00	150.00			3.60		0.00	0.00		
	9.00							890.00	320.00	150.00			3.60		0.00	0.00		
	0.00							100.00	290.00	150.00			0.72			0.00	0.00	0.00
	15.00							1460.00	580.00	200.00			5.40		0.00	0.00		
	3.60							600.00	220.00	100.00			3.60		0.00	0.00		
	9.00							890.00	440.00	100.00			5.40		0.00	0.00		
0.00	0.02	0.00	0.00	0.00	0.02	0.00	0.00	15.85	1.02	0.85	0.57	0.22	0.02	0.00	0.00	0.00	0.00	0.00
								120.00	5.00	60.00	90.00				0.00	0.00		
0.12	0.00	0.00	0.00	0.00	0.15	0.00	0.01	28.80	1.20	1.20	1.20	0.10	0.00	0.00	0.00	0.00	0.00	0.00
0.09	0.00	0.00	0.00	0.00	0.11	0.00	0.00	31.43	0.99	0.91	0.87	0.08	0.01	0.00	0.00	0.00	0.00	0.00
0.12	0.00	0.00	0.00	0.00	0.15	0.00	0.01	0.55	1.20	1.20	1.20	0.10	0.00	0.00	0.00	0.00	0.00	0.00
0.08	0.00	0.00	0.00	0.00	0.00	0.00	0.00	0.00	0.00	0.00	0.00	0.00	0.00	0.01	0.00	0.00	0.00	0.00
1.25	0.00	0.00	0.00	0.00	0.00	0.00	0.00	0.00	0.00	0.00	0.00	0.00	0.00	0.00	0.00	0.00	0.00	0.00
4.03	0.00							0.00		0.00			0.00		0.00	0.00	0.00	0.00
0.24	0.00	0.00	0.00	0.00	0.00	0.00	0.00	0.00	0.00	0.00	0.00	0.00	0.00	0.00	0.00	0.00	0.00	0.00
0.01	0.00	0.00	0.00	0.00	0.00	0.00	0.00	0.00	0.00	0.00	0.00	0.00	0.01	0.00	0.00	0.00	0.00	0.00
	0.00							0.00		0.00			0.00		0.00	0.00	0.00	0.00
2.83	0.00	0.00	0.00	0.00	0.00	0.00	0.00	0.00	0.00	0.00	0.00	0.00	0.00	0.00	0.00	0.00	0.00	0.00
3.92	0.00	0.00	0.00	0.00	0.00	0.00	0.00	0.00	0.00	0.00	0.00	0.00	0.00	0.00	0.00	0.00	0.00	0.00
1.96	0.00	0.00	0.00	0.00	0.00	0.00	0.00	0.00	0.00	0.00	0.00	0.00	0.00	0.00	0.00	0.00	0.00	0.00
1.74															0.00	0.00	0.00	0.00
0.52	0.00	0.00	0.00	0.00	0.00	0.00	0.00	0.00	0.00	0.00	0.00	0.00	0.00	0.00	0.00	0.00	0.00	0.00
2.12	0.00	0.00	0.00	0.00	0.00	0.00	0.00	0.00	0.00	0.00	0.00	0.00	0.00	0.00	0.00	0.00	0.00	0.00
4.39	0.00	0.00	0.00	0.00	0.00	0.00	0.00	0.00	0.00	0.00	0.00	0.00	0.01	0.00	0.00	0.00	0.00	0.00
	0.00							0.00		0.00			0.00		0.00	0.00	0.00	0.00
0.57	0.00	0.00	0.00	0.00	0.00	0.00	0.00	0.00	0.00	0.00	0.00	0.00	0.00	0.00	0.00	0.00	0.00	0.00
1.25	0.00	0.00	0.00	0.00	0.00	0.00	0.00	0.00	0.00	0.00	0.00	0.00	0.00	0.00	0.00	0.00	0.00	0.00
	0.00	0.00	0.00	0.00				0.00	0.00	0.00			0.00		0.00	0.00	0.00	0.00
1.25	0.00	0.00	0.00	0.00	0.00	0.00	0.00	0.00	0.00	0.00	0.00	0.00	0.00	0.00	0.00	0.00	0.00	0.00
5.59	0.00	0.00	0.00	0.00	0.00	0.00	0.00	0.00	0.00	0.00	0.00	0.00	0.00	0.00	0.00	0.00	0.00	0.00
5.59	0.00	0.00	0.00	0.00	0.00	0.00	0.00	0.00	0.00	0.00	0.00	0.00	0.00	0.00	0.00	0.00	0.00	0.00
0.00	0.00							0.00	0.00	0.00			0.00		0.00	0.00	0.00	0.00
3.02	0.00							0.00		0.00			0.00		0.00	0.00	0.00	0.00
0.56	0.01	0.00	0.00	0.00	0.28	0.00	0.01	127.37	5.11	3.98	3.27	0.28	0.01	0.00	0.00	0.00	0.00	0.00
0.88	0.00	0.00	0.00	0.00	0.14	0.00	0.01	92.21	2.54	0.42	0.71	0.14	0.02	0.02	0.00	0.00	0.00	0.00

Food Name	Amount	Measure	Weight (g)	Calories	Protein (g)	Total Carb (g)	Dietary Fiber (g)	Total Fat (g)	Sat Fat (g)	Mono Fat (g)	Poly Fat (g)	Chol (mg)	Vit A (mcg RAE)	Vit D (mcg)
FATS, OILS, MARGARINES, SHORTENINGS, AND SUBSTITUTES *(continued)*														
Margarine, 80% fat, unsalted	1	Tablespoon	14.20	102.10	0.13	0.13	0.00	11.43	2.20	5.54	3.17	0.00	116.30	
Margarine, hard, corn cottonseed & hydrog soybean oil, stick	1	Tablespoon	14.10	101.38	0.13	0.13	0.00	11.35	2.12	5.19	3.54	0.00	115.48	
Margarine, hard, corn hydrog soybean & cttnsd oil, stick	1	Tablespoon	14.10	101.38	0.13	0.13	0.00	11.35	2.79	4.51	3.54	0.00	115.48	
Margarine, hard, hydrog & reg soybean & palm oil, stick	1	Tablespoon	14.10	101.38	0.13	0.13	0.00	11.35	2.47	4.40	3.98	0.00	115.48	
Margarine, hard, hydrog & reg soybean oil, stick	1	Tablespoon	14.10	101.38	0.13	0.13	0.00	11.35	1.85	5.30	3.69	0.00	115.48	
Margarine, hard, hydrog corn oil, stick	1	Tablespoon	14.10	101.38	0.13	0.13	0.00	11.35	1.86	6.46	2.54	0.00	115.48	
Margarine, hard, hydrog soybean & cottonseed oil, stick	1	Tablespoon	14.10	101.38	0.13	0.13	0.00	11.35	2.13	6.67	2.06	0.00	115.48	
Margarine, hard, hydrog soybean & palm oil, stick	1	Tablespoon	14.10	101.38	0.13	0.13	0.00	11.35	2.13	4.51	4.20	0.00	115.48	
Margarine, hard, safflower hydrog&reg soy & cttnsd oil stick	1	Tablespoon	14.10	101.38	0.13	0.13	0.00	11.35	2.03	4.27	4.55	0.00	115.48	
Margarine, hard, soy hydrog corn & cttnsd oil unsalted stick	1	Tablespoon	14.10	100.67	0.07	0.07	0.00	11.32	2.12	5.17	3.53	0.00	115.48	
Margarine, hard, soybean hydrog soybean & cttnsd oil, stick	1	Tablespoon	14.10	101.38	0.13	0.13	0.00	11.35	2.20	5.09	3.57	0.00	115.48	
Margarine, hard, sunflower hydrog soybean & cttnsd oil stick	1	Tablespoon	14.10	101.38	0.13	0.13	0.00	11.35	1.68	4.02	5.16	0.00	115.48	
Margarine, hard, unspecified oil, unsalted, stick	1	Tablespoon	14.10	100.67	0.07	0.07	0.00	11.32	2.12	5.17	3.53	0.00	115.48	0.00
Margarine, liquid, cttnsd hydrog & reg soy oil	1	Tablespoon	14.20	102.38	0.27	0.00	0.00	11.45	1.87	3.99	5.08	0.00	116.30	
Margarine, unspecified oil, stick	1	Tablespoon	14.10	101.38	0.13	0.13	0.00	11.35	2.23	5.05	3.58	0.00	115.48	
Spread, 40% fat, rducd cal, stick	1	Tablespoon	14.00	49.84	0.08	0.00	0.00	5.60	0.85	2.64	1.86	0.00	114.66	
Spread, 48% fat, tub	1	Tablespoon	14.00	59.36	0.03	0.12	0.00	6.65	1.23	2.30	2.83	0.14		
Spread, rducd cal	1	Tablespoon	14.20	49.02	0.07	0.06	0.00	5.51	1.09	2.23	1.96	0.00	147.18	0.00
Spread, rducd cal, cottonseed & soybean oil, 40% fat	1	Tablespoon	14.40	49.68	0.06	0.06	0.00	5.58	1.20	2.04	2.10	0.00	117.93	
Spread, rducd cal, hydrog soy & cttnsd oil, 60% fat	1	Tablespoon	14.40	77.76	0.09	0.00	0.00	8.76	1.74	5.61	1.02	0.00	117.93	
Spread, rducd cal, hydrog soybean oil, 40%fat	1	Tablespoon	14.40	49.68	0.06	0.06	0.00	5.58	0.93	2.40	1.98	0.00	117.93	1.53
Spread, rducd cal, unspecified oil, 40%fat	1	Tablespoon	14.40	49.68	0.06	0.06	0.00	5.58	1.11	2.25	1.98	0.00	117.93	
Spread, vegetable oil butter	1	Tablespoon	14.20	77.38	0.09	0.00	0.00	8.72	1.98	4.44	1.91	0.93	103.65	0.00
Spread, vegetable oil, tub	1	Tablespoon	14.00	50.68	0.14	0.14	0.00	5.60	1.01	2.58	1.76	0.00	114.66	
Shortenings														
Shortening, bread, hydrog soy & ctnsd oil	1	Tablespoon	12.80	113.15	0.00	0.00	0.00	12.80	2.82	4.22	5.20	0.00	0.00	
Shortening, frying, heavy duty, hydrog palm oil	1	Tablespoon	12.80	113.15	0.00	0.00	0.00	12.80	6.08	5.20	0.96	0.00	0.00	
FISH, SEAFOOD, AND SHELLFISH														
Abalone, raw, mixed species	4	Ounce-weight	113.40	119.07	19.39	6.82	0.00	0.86	0.17	0.12	0.12	96.39	2.27	
Clams, brd, fried	3	Ounce-weight	85.05	333.40	9.48	28.70		19.53	4.88	8.46	5.01	64.64	27.22	
Clams, brd, fried, mixed species, sml	3	Ounce-weight	85.05	171.80	12.11	8.79	0.14	9.48	2.28	3.87	2.44	51.88	77.40	
Clams, cnd, mixed species, drained	3	Ounce-weight	85.05	125.87	21.73	4.36	0.00	1.66	0.16	0.15	0.47	56.98	153.94	
Clams, minced, cnd S & W	3	Ounce-weight	85.05	30.93	6.19	1.55	0.00	0.00	0.00	0.00	0.00	15.46	0.00	
Clams, raw, mixed species, cup	4	Ounce-weight	113.40	83.92	14.48	2.91	0.00	1.10	0.11	0.09	0.32	38.56	102.06	0.11
Crab, Alaska king, imit f/surimi	3	Ounce-weight	85.05	86.75	10.22	8.69	0.00	1.11	0.22	0.17	0.57	17.01	17.01	
Crab, Alaska king, leg, raw	4	Ounce-weight	113.40	95.26	20.74	0.00	0.00	0.68	0.10	0.09	0.15	47.63	7.94	
Crab, bkd/brld	3	Ounce-weight	85.05	117.46	16.22	0.05	0.00	5.42	0.96	2.17	1.66	80.07	37.97	0.09
Crab, blue, raw	4	Ounce-weight	113.40	98.66	20.48	0.05	0.00	1.22	0.25	0.22	0.44	88.45	2.27	

Vit E (mg)	Vit C	Vit B₁-Thia (mg)	Vit B₂-Ribo (mg)	Vit B₃-Nia (mg)	Fol (mcg)	Vit B₆ (mg)	Vita B₁₂ (mcg)	Sodi (mg)	Pota (mg)	Cal (mg)	Phos (mg)	Magn (mg)	Iron (mg)	Zinc (mg)	Caff (mg)	Alco (g)	Sol Fiber (g)	Insol Fiber (g)
0.71	0.01	0.00	0.00	0.00	0.14	0.00	0.01	0.28	3.55	2.41	1.85	0.28	0.00	0.00	0.00	0.00	0.00	0.00
1.55	0.03	0.00	0.01	0.00	0.14	0.00	0.01	132.96	5.92	4.23	3.24	0.42	0.00	0.00	0.00	0.00	0.00	0.00
0.44	0.03	0.00	0.01	0.00	0.14	0.00	0.01	132.96	5.92	4.23	3.24	0.42	0.00	0.00	0.00	0.00	0.00	0.00
0.44	0.03	0.00	0.01	0.00	0.14	0.00	0.01	132.96	5.92	4.23	3.24	0.42	0.00	0.00	0.00	0.00	0.00	0.00
0.44	0.03	0.00	0.01	0.00	0.14	0.00	0.01	132.96	5.92	4.23	3.24	0.42	0.00		0.00	0.00	0.00	0.00
1.64	0.03	0.00	0.01	0.00	0.14	0.00	0.01	132.96	5.92	4.23	3.24	0.42	0.00		0.00	0.00	0.00	0.00
1.10	0.03	0.00	0.01	0.00	0.14	0.00	0.01	132.96	5.92	4.23	3.24	0.42	0.00	0.00	0.00	0.00	0.00	0.00
0.44	0.03	0.00	0.01	0.00	0.14	0.00	0.01	132.96	5.92	4.23	3.24	0.42	0.00	0.00	0.00	0.00	0.00	0.00
2.31	0.03	0.00	0.01	0.00	0.14	0.00	0.01	132.96	5.92	4.23	3.24	0.42	0.00	0.00	0.00	0.00	0.00	0.00
1.64	0.01	0.00	0.00	0.00	0.14	0.00	0.01	0.28	3.53	2.40	1.83	0.28	0.00	0.00	0.00	0.00	0.00	0.00
1.75	0.03	0.00	0.01	0.00	0.14	0.00	0.01	132.96	5.92	4.23	3.24	0.42	0.00	0.00	0.00	0.00	0.00	0.00
1.55	0.03	0.00	0.01	0.00	0.14	0.00	0.01	132.96	5.92	4.23	3.24	0.42	0.00	0.00	0.00	0.00	0.00	0.00
1.80	0.01	0.00	0.00	0.00	0.14	0.00	0.01	0.28	3.53	2.40	1.83	0.28	0.00	0.00	0.00	0.00	0.00	0.00
0.65	0.06	0.00	0.01	0.01	0.43	0.00	0.03	110.90	13.35	9.37	7.24	0.85	0.00	0.00	0.00	0.00	0.00	0.00
1.27	0.03	0.00	0.01	0.00	0.14	0.00	0.01	132.96	5.92	4.23	3.24	0.42	0.01	0.00	0.00	0.00	0.00	0.00
0.70	0.01	0.00	0.00	0.00	0.14	0.00	0.01	139.16	4.20	2.94	2.24	0.28	0.00	0.00	0.00	0.00	0.00	0.00
0.55	0.00	0.00	0.00	0.00	0.28	0.00		90.44	5.04	0.56	0.56	0.14	0.03	0.01	0.00	0.00	0.00	0.00
0.33	0.01	0.00	0.00	0.00	0.10	0.00	0.01	136.26	3.59	2.53	1.95	0.22	0.00	0.00	0.00	0.00	0.00	0.00
0.39	0.00	0.00	0.00	0.00	0.15	0.00	0.00	138.24	3.60	2.58	2.01	0.30	0.00	0.00	0.00	0.00	0.00	0.00
0.72	0.00	0.00	0.00	0.00	0.15	0.00	0.00	143.13	4.32	3.03	2.31	0.30	0.00	0.00	0.00	0.00	0.00	0.00
0.12	0.00	0.00	0.00	0.00	0.15	0.00	0.00	138.24	3.60	2.58	2.01	0.30	0.00	0.00	0.00	0.00	0.00	0.00
0.57	0.00	0.00	0.00	0.00	0.15	0.00	0.00	138.24	3.60	2.58	2.01	0.30	0.00	0.00	0.00	0.00	0.00	0.00
1.25	0.02	0.00	0.00	0.00	0.13	0.00	0.01	140.42	4.22	2.98	2.32	0.26	0.00	0.00	0.00	0.00	0.00	0.00
0.63	0.01	0.00	0.00	0.00	0.14	0.00	0.01	110.04	5.04	3.36	2.80	0.28	0.01	0.00	0.00	0.00	0.00	0.00
1.02	0.00	0.00	0.00	0.00	0.00	0.00	0.00	0.00	0.00	0.00	0.00	0.00	0.00	0.00	0.00	0.00	0.00	0.00
2.43	0.00	0.00	0.00	0.00	0.00	0.00	0.00	0.00	0.00	0.00	0.00	0.00	0.00	0.00	0.00	0.00	0.00	0.00
4.54	2.27	0.22	0.11	1.70	5.67	0.17	0.83	341.33	283.50	35.15	215.46	54.43	3.62	0.93	0.00	0.00	0.00	0.00
	0.00	0.15	0.20	2.12	31.47	0.03	0.82	616.61	196.47	15.31	176.05	22.96	2.25	1.21	0.00	0.00		
2.13	8.51	0.09	0.21	1.76	30.62	0.05	34.25	309.58	277.26	53.58	159.89	11.91	11.83	1.24	0.00	0.00	0.06	0.08
0.53	18.80	0.13	0.36	2.85	24.66	0.09	84.11	95.26	534.11	78.25	287.47	15.31	23.78	2.32	0.00	0.00	0.00	0.00
	0.00							556.69	0.00	0.00				1.11	0.00	0.00	0.00	0.00
0.35	14.74	0.09	0.24	2.00	18.14	0.07	56.06	63.50	356.08	52.16	191.65	10.21	15.85	1.55	0.00	0.00	0.00	0.00
0.09	0.00	0.03	0.02	0.15	1.70	0.03	1.36	715.27	76.55	11.06	239.84	36.57	0.33	0.28	0.00	0.00	0.00	0.00
1.02	7.94	0.05	0.05	1.25	49.90	0.17	10.21	948.02	231.34	52.16	248.35	55.57	0.67	6.75	0.00	0.00	0.00	0.00
1.40	2.65	0.08	0.04	2.64	40.73	0.14	5.85	270.34	261.52	84.77	166.09	26.57	0.73	3.38	0.00	0.00	0.00	0.00
1.13	3.40	0.09	0.05	3.06	49.90	0.17	10.21	332.26	373.09	100.93	259.69	38.56	0.84	4.01	0.00	0.00	0.00	0.00

Food Name	Amount	Measure	Weight (g)	Calories	Protein (g)	Total Carb (g)	Dietary Fiber (g)	Total Fat (g)	Sat Fat (g)	Mono Fat (g)	Poly Fat (g)	Chol (mg)	Vit A (mcg RAE)	Vit D (mcg)
Crab, dungeoness, raw	4	Ounce-weight	113.40	97.52	19.74	0.84	0.00	1.10	0.15	0.19	0.36	66.91	30.62	
Crab, soft shell, brd/floured, fried	1	Each	65.00	217.18	13.30	11.17	0.38	12.99	2.65	5.42	3.95	80.11	14.82	0.13
Eel, fillet, mixed species, raw	4	Ounce-weight	113.40	208.66	20.91	0.00	0.00	13.22	2.67	8.15	1.07	142.88	1182.76	
Eel, fillet, sashimi, mixed species	4	Ounce-weight	113.40	208.66	20.91	0.00	0.00	13.22	2.67	8.15	1.07	142.88	1182.76	
Escargot, stmd/poached	2	Each	10.00	27.40	4.77	1.55	0.00	0.08	0.01	0.01	0.00	13.00	4.68	
Fish Cake, brd, fried, heated f/fzn														
Universal Labs	1	Each	85.00	231.29	7.88	14.73		15.33	6.00	3.43	3.43	22.27		
Fish Cake, fried	1	Each	69.00	149.03	13.27	5.82	0.19	7.75	1.62	3.24	2.37	54.35	18.79	
Fish Paste, Japanese	1	Tablespoon	16.00	18.56	2.15	2.01	0.02	0.11	0.02	0.01	0.05	7.83	1.09	
Fish Sticks, brd, Healthy Treasures Mrs. Paul's	4	Piece	85.00	170.00	10.00	20.00	2.00	3.00	1.50			20.00	0.00	
Fish Sticks, oven breaded, fzn Van de Kamp's	6	Piece	114.00	290.00	13.00	23.00	0.00	17.00				35.00		
Fish, bass, freshwater, fillet, bkd/brld, mixed species	3	Ounce-weight	85.05	124.17	20.57	0.00	0.00	4.02	0.85	1.56	1.16	73.99	29.77	
Fish, bass, sea, fillet, bkd/brld, mixed species	3	Ounce-weight	85.05	105.46	20.10	0.00	0.00	2.18	0.56	0.46	0.81	45.08	54.43	
Fish, bass, striped, fillet, bkd/brld	3	Ounce-weight	85.05	105.46	19.33	0.00	0.00	2.54	0.55	0.72	0.85	87.60	26.37	
Fish, bluefish, fillet, bkd/brld	3	Ounce-weight	85.05	135.23	21.85	0.00	0.00	4.63	1.00	1.95	1.15	64.64	117.37	
Fish, carp, fillet, bkd/brld	3	Ounce-weight	85.05	137.78	19.44	0.00	0.00	6.10	1.18	2.54	1.56	71.44	8.51	
Fish, catfish, channel, fillet, bkd/brld, farmed	3	Ounce-weight	85.05	129.28	15.92	0.00	0.00	6.82	1.52	3.53	1.18	54.43	12.76	
Fish, catfish, channel, fillet, bkd/brld, wild	3	Ounce-weight	85.05	89.30	15.71	0.00	0.00	2.42	0.63	0.93	0.54	61.24	12.76	
Fish, cod, Atlantic, dried & salted, 5.5" x 1.5" x .5" pce	1	Piece	80.00	232.00	50.26	0.00	0.00	1.90	0.37	0.27	0.64	121.60	33.60	
Fish, cod, Atlantic, fillet, bkd/brld	3	Ounce-weight	85.05	89.30	19.42	0.00	0.00	0.73	0.14	0.11	0.25	46.78	11.91	
Fish, cod, Pacific, fillet, bkd/brld	3	Ounce-weight	85.05	89.30	19.52	0.00	0.00	0.69	0.09	0.09	0.27	39.97	8.51	
Fish, grouper, fillet, mixed species, bkd/brld	3	Ounce-weight	85.05	100.36	21.13	0.00	0.00	1.11	0.25	0.23	0.34	39.97	42.53	
Fish, haddock, fillet, bkd/brld	3	Ounce-weight	85.05	95.26	20.62	0.00	0.00	0.79	0.14	0.13	0.26	62.94	16.16	
Fish, haddock, smkd, 1" cube	3	Ounce-weight	85.05	98.66	21.46	0.00	0.00	0.80	0.15	0.15	0.25	65.49	18.71	
Fish, halibut, Atlantic/Pacific, fillet, bkd/brld	3	Ounce-weight	85.05	119.07	22.70	0.00	0.00	2.50	0.35	0.82	0.80	34.87	45.93	
Fish, halibut, Greenland, fillet, bkd/brld	3	Ounce-weight	85.05	203.27	15.67	0.00	0.00	15.09	2.64	9.14	1.49	50.18	15.31	12.76
Fish, herring, Atlantic, fillet, bkd/brld	3	Ounce-weight	85.05	172.65	19.59	0.00	0.00	9.86	2.22	4.07	2.33	65.49	30.62	
Fish, herring, Atlantic, pickled, pce, 1 3/4" x 7/8" x 1/2"	1	Piece	15.00	39.30	2.13	1.45	0.00	2.70	0.36	1.79	0.25	1.95	38.70	2.55
Fish, herring, Atlantic, smkd, kippered fillet 5" x 1.75" x .25"	1	Piece	40.00	86.80	9.83	0.00	0.00	4.95	1.12	2.04	1.17	32.80	16.00	1.20
Fish, mackerel, Atlantic, fillet, bkd/brld	3	Ounce-weight	85.05	222.83	20.28	0.00	0.00	15.15	3.55	5.96	3.66	63.79	45.93	
Fish, mackerel, king, fillet, bkd/brld	3	Ounce-weight	85.05	113.97	22.11	0.00	0.00	2.18	0.40	0.83	0.50	57.83	214.33	
Fish, monkfish, bkd/brld	3	Ounce-weight	85.05	82.50	15.79	0.00	0.00	1.66	0.46	0.32	0.82	27.22	11.91	
Fish, orange roughy, fillet, bkd/brld	3	Ounce-weight	85.05	75.69	16.03	0.00	0.00	0.77	0.02	0.52	0.01	22.11	20.41	
Fish, perch, fillet, bkd/brld, mixed species	3	Ounce-weight	85.05	99.51	21.14	0.00	0.00	1.00	0.20	0.17	0.40	97.81	8.51	
Fish, perch, ocean, Atlantic, fillet, bkd/brld	3	Ounce-weight	85.05	102.91	20.31	0.00	0.00	1.78	0.27	0.68	0.47	45.93	11.91	
Fish, pike, northen, fillet, bkd/brld	3	Ounce-weight	85.05	96.11	21.00	0.00	0.00	0.75	0.13	0.17	0.22	42.53	20.41	
Fish, pike, walleye, fillet, bkd/brld	3	Ounce-weight	85.05	101.21	20.87	0.00	0.00	1.33	0.27	0.32	0.49	93.56	20.41	
Fish, pollock, Atlantic, fillet, bkd/brld	3	Ounce-weight	85.05	100.36	21.19	0.00	0.00	1.07	0.14	0.12	0.53	77.40	10.21	
Fish, pollock, walleye, fillet, bkd/brld	3	Ounce-weight	85.05	96.11	20.00	0.00	0.00	0.95	0.20	0.15	0.45	81.65	21.26	
Fish, portions, heated f/fzn, 4" x 2" x 1/2"	1	Piece	57.00	155.04	8.92	13.54	0.80	6.97	1.79	2.89	1.80	63.84	17.67	0.10
Fish, pumpkinseed sunfish, fillet, bkd/brld	3	Ounce-weight	85.05	96.96	21.15	0.00	0.00	0.77	0.15	0.13	0.27	73.14	14.46	
Fish, salmon, Atlantic, fillet, bkd/brld, farmed	3	Ounce-weight	85.05	175.20	18.80	0.00	0.00	10.50	2.13	3.77	3.76	53.58	12.76	

Vit E (mg)	Vit C	Vit B₁-Thia (mg)	Vit B₂-Ribo (mg)	Vit B₃-Nia (mg)	Fol (mcg)	Vit B₆ (mg)	Vita B₁₂ (mcg)	Sodi (mg)	Pota (mg)	Cal (mg)	Phos (mg)	Magn (mg)	Iron (mg)	Zinc (mg)	Caff (mg)	Alco (g)	Sol Fiber (g)	Insol Fiber (g)
1.02	3.97	0.05	0.19	3.56	49.90	0.17	10.21	334.53	401.44	52.16	206.39	51.03	0.42	4.84	0.00	0.00	0.00	0.00
2.07	1.43	0.15	0.13	2.55	27.10	0.11	3.36	216.59	208.97	79.51	142.67	23.50	1.36	2.46	0.00	0.00	0.19	0.19
4.54	2.04	0.17	0.05	3.97	17.01	0.08	3.40	57.83	308.45	22.68	244.94	22.68	0.57	1.84	0.00	0.00	0.00	0.00
4.54	2.04	0.17	0.05	3.97	17.01	0.08	3.40	57.83	308.45	22.68	244.94	22.68	0.57	1.84	0.00	0.00	0.00	0.00
0.03	0.60	0.00	0.02	0.16	0.95	0.06	1.09	35.02	48.58	10.83	19.74	14.62	0.91	0.33	0.00	0.00	0.00	0.00
0.51	0.00	0.03	0.06	1.37	10.54	0.04	0.86		298.11	9.42	143.06	15.42	0.34	0.34	0.00	0.00		
1.29	0.27	0.09	0.09	1.72	6.10	0.10	1.33	127.32	256.65	29.51	206.97	32.49	0.74	0.45	0.00	0.00	0.09	0.09
0.03	0.00	0.00	0.02	0.36	0.31	0.03	0.33	9.77	39.35	6.72	24.67	7.49	0.06	0.05	0.00	0.00		
	1.20							350.00		40.00			1.08			0.00	0.00	
									110.00		100.00				0.00	0.00	0.00	0.00
0.63	1.79	0.07	0.08	1.29	14.46	0.12	1.96	76.55	387.83	87.60	217.73	32.32	1.62	0.71	0.00	0.00	0.00	0.00
0.54	0.00	0.11	0.13	1.62	5.10	0.39	0.26	73.99	278.96	11.06	210.92	45.08	0.31	0.44	0.00	0.00	0.00	0.00
0.52	0.00	0.10	0.03	2.18	8.51	0.29	3.75	74.84	278.96	16.16	216.03	43.38	0.92	0.43	0.00	0.00	0.00	0.00
0.54	0.00	0.06	0.08	6.16	1.70	0.39	5.29	65.49	405.69	7.65	247.50	35.72	0.53	0.88	0.00	0.00	0.00	0.00
0.91	1.36	0.12	0.06	1.79	14.46	0.19	1.25	53.58	363.16	44.23	451.62	32.32	1.35	1.62	0.00	0.00	0.00	0.00
1.12	0.68	0.36	0.06	2.14	5.95	0.14	2.38	68.04	273.01	7.65	208.37	22.11	0.70	0.89	0.00	0.00	0.00	0.00
	0.68	0.19	0.06	2.03	8.51	0.09	2.47	42.53	356.36	9.36	258.55	23.81	0.30	0.52	0.00	0.00	0.00	0.00
2.27	2.80	0.21	0.19	6.00	20.00	0.69	8.00	5621.60	1166.40	128.00	760.00	106.40	2.00	1.27	0.00	0.00	0.00	0.00
0.69	0.85	0.07	0.07	2.14	6.80	0.24	0.89	66.34	207.52	11.91	117.37	35.72	0.42	0.49	0.00	0.00	0.00	0.00
0.29	2.55	0.02	0.04	2.11	6.80	0.39	0.88	77.40	439.71	7.65	189.66	26.37	0.28	0.43	0.00	0.00	0.00	0.00
0.53	0.00	0.07	0.01	0.32	8.51	0.30	0.59	45.08	403.99	17.86	121.62	31.47	0.97	0.43	0.00	0.00	0.00	0.00
0.42	0.00	0.03	0.04	3.94	11.06	0.29	1.18	73.99	339.35	35.72	204.97	42.53	1.15	0.41	0.00	0.00	0.00	0.00
0.45	0.00	0.05	0.05	4.30	12.76	0.35	1.35	648.93	352.96	41.67	213.48	45.93	1.20	0.45	0.00	0.00	0.00	0.00
0.93	0.00	0.06	0.08	6.06	11.91	0.34	1.17	58.68	489.89	51.03	242.39	91.00	0.91	0.45	0.00	0.00	0.00	0.00
1.05	0.00	0.06	0.09	1.64	0.85	0.41	0.82	87.60	292.57	3.40	178.61	28.07	0.72	0.43	0.00	0.00	0.00	0.00
1.17	0.60	0.10	0.25	3.51	10.21	0.30	11.18	97.81	356.36	62.94	257.70	34.87	1.20	1.08	0.00	0.00	0.00	0.00
0.26	0.00	0.01	0.02	0.50	0.30	0.03	0.64	130.50	10.35	11.55	13.35	1.20	0.18	0.08	0.00	0.00	0.00	0.00
0.62	0.40	0.05	0.13	1.76	5.60	0.17	7.48	367.20	178.80	33.60	130.00	18.40	0.60	0.54	0.00	0.00	0.00	0.00
1.57	0.34	0.14	0.35	5.83	1.70	0.39	16.16	70.59	341.05	12.76	236.44	82.50	1.34	0.80	0.00	0.00	0.00	0.00
1.47	1.36	0.10	0.49	8.90	7.65	0.43	15.31	172.65	474.58	34.02	270.46	34.87	1.94	0.61	0.00	0.00	0.00	0.00
0.24	0.85	0.02	0.06	2.18	6.80	0.24	0.88	19.56	436.31	8.51	217.73	22.96	0.35	0.45	0.00	0.00	0.00	0.00
0.54	0.00	0.10	0.16	3.11	6.80	0.29	1.96	68.89	327.44	32.32	217.73	32.32	0.20	0.82	0.00	0.00	0.00	0.00
1.28	1.45	0.07	0.10	1.62	5.10	0.12	1.87	67.19	292.57	86.75	218.58	32.32	0.99	1.22	0.00	0.00	0.00	0.00
1.39	0.68	0.11	0.11	2.07	8.51	0.23	0.98	81.65	297.68	116.52	235.59	33.17	1.00	0.52	0.00	0.00	0.00	0.00
0.20	3.23	0.06	0.07	2.38	14.46	0.11	1.96	41.67	281.52	62.09	239.84	34.02	0.60	0.73	0.00	0.00	0.00	0.00
0.24	0.00	0.27	0.17	2.38	14.46	0.12	1.96	55.28	424.40	119.92	228.78	32.32	1.42	0.67	0.00	0.00	0.00	0.00
0.24	0.00	0.05	0.19	3.39	2.55	0.28	3.13	93.56	387.83	65.49	240.69	73.14	0.50	0.51	0.00	0.00	0.00	0.00
0.67	0.00	0.06	0.06	1.40	3.40	0.06	3.57	98.66	329.14	5.10	409.94	62.09	0.24	0.51	0.00	0.00	0.00	0.00
0.30	0.00	0.07	0.10	1.21	24.51	0.03	1.03	331.74	148.77	11.40	103.17	14.25	0.42	0.38	0.00	0.00		
0.22	0.85	0.08	0.07	1.24	14.46	0.12	1.96	87.60	381.87	87.60	196.47	32.32	1.31	1.69	0.00	0.00	0.00	0.00
0.75	3.15	0.29	0.11	6.84	28.92	0.55	2.38	51.88	326.59	12.76	214.33	25.52	0.29	0.37	0.00	0.00	0.00	0.00

Food Name	Amount	Measure	Weight (g)	Calories	Protein (g)	Total Carb (g)	Dietary Fiber (g)	Total Fat (g)	Sat Fat (g)	Mono Fat (g)	Poly Fat (g)	Chol (mg)	Vit A (mcg RAE)	Vit D (mcg)
Fish, salmon, Atlantic, fillet, bkd/brld, wild	3	Ounce-weight	85.05	154.79	21.64	0.00	0.00	6.91	1.07	2.29	2.77	60.39	11.06	5.95
Fish, salmon, chinook, fillet, bkd/brld	3	Ounce-weight	85.05	196.47	21.87	0.00	0.00	11.38	2.73	4.88	2.26	72.29	126.72	
Fish, salmon, chinook, smkd	3	Ounce-weight	85.05	99.51	15.55	0.00	0.00	3.67	0.79	1.72	0.85	19.56	22.11	
Fish, salmon, chum, w/bone, cnd, drained, unsalted	3	Ounce-weight	85.05	119.92	18.23	0.00	0.00	4.68	1.26	1.63	1.29	33.17	15.31	
Fish, salmon, coho, fillet, bkd/brld, farmed	3	Ounce-weight	85.05	151.39	20.67	0.00	0.00	7.00	1.65	3.08	1.67	53.58	50.18	
Fish, salmon, coho, fillet, bkd/brld, wild	3	Ounce-weight	85.05	118.22	19.94	0.00	0.00	3.66	0.90	1.34	1.08	46.78	32.32	
Fish, salmon, coho, fillet, stmd/poached, wild	3	Ounce-weight	85.05	156.49	23.27	0.00	0.00	6.38	1.36	2.30	2.15	48.48	27.22	
Fish, salmon, pink, fillet, bkd/brld	3	Ounce-weight	85.05	126.72	21.74	0.00	0.00	3.76	0.61	1.02	1.47	56.98	34.87	
Fish, salmon, pink, w/bone, cnd, not drained	3	Ounce-weight	85.05	118.22	16.82	0.00	0.00	5.15	1.31	1.54	1.74	46.78	14.46	13.27
Fish, sardines, Atlantic, w/bones, w/oil, drained	3	Ounce-weight	85.05	176.90	20.94	0.00	0.00	9.74	1.30	3.29	4.38	120.77	27.22	5.78
Fish, sardines, Pacific, w/bone & tomato sauce, drained	3	Ounce-weight	85.05	158.19	17.74	0.63	0.09	8.90	2.28	4.10	1.80	51.88	28.92	10.21
Fish, sea trout, fillet, bkd/brld, mixed species	3	Ounce-weight	85.05	113.12	18.25	0.00	0.00	3.94	1.10	0.96	0.79	90.15	29.77	
Fish, shad, American, fillet, bkd/brld	3	Ounce-weight	85.05	214.33	18.46	0.00	0.00	15.01	3.83	6.97	4.00	81.65	30.62	
Fish, shark, batter dipped, fried, mixed species	3	Ounce-weight	85.05	193.91	15.84	5.43	0.00	11.75	2.73	5.05	3.15	50.18	45.93	
Fish, shark, raw, mixed species	4	Ounce-weight	113.40	147.42	23.79	0.00	0.00	5.11	1.05	2.05	1.36	57.83	79.38	
Fish, snapper, fillet, bkd/brld, mixed species	3	Ounce-weight	85.05	108.86	22.37	0.00	0.00	1.46	0.31	0.27	0.50	39.97	29.77	
Fish, sole, fillet, natural, fzn Van de Kamp's	3	Ounce-weight	85.05	82.79	17.31	0.00	0.00	1.13	0.00	0.00	0.38	37.63	0.00	
Fish, swordfish, fillet, bkd/brld	3	Ounce-weight	85.05	131.83	21.59	0.00	0.00	4.37	1.20	1.68	1.01	42.53	34.87	
Fish, trout, fillet, bkd/brld, mixed species	3	Ounce-weight	85.05	161.60	22.65	0.00	0.00	7.20	1.25	3.55	1.63	62.94	16.16	
Fish, trout, rainbow, fillet, bkd/brld, farmed	3	Ounce-weight	85.05	143.73	20.64	0.00	0.00	6.12	1.79	1.78	1.98	57.83	73.14	
Fish, trout, rainbow, fillet, bkd/brld, wild	3	Ounce-weight	85.05	127.58	19.49	0.00	0.00	4.95	1.38	1.48	1.56	58.68	12.76	
Fish, tuna, bluefin, fillet, bkd/brld	3	Ounce-weight	85.05	156.49	25.44	0.00	0.00	5.34	1.37	1.75	1.57	41.67	643.83	
Fish, tuna, light, w/oil, drained, can	0.5	Cup	73.00	144.54	21.27	0.00	0.00	5.99	1.12	2.15	2.10	13.14	16.79	4.31
Fish, tuna, light, w/oil, drained, unsalted, cnd	3	Ounce-weight	85.05	168.40	24.78	0.00	0.00	6.98	1.30	2.51	2.45	15.31	19.56	
Fish, tuna, light, w/water, chunk, cnd S & W	3	Ounce-weight	85.05	105.00	22.50	0.00	0.00	0.08	0.00			52.50	0.00	
Fish, tuna, light, w/water, drained, can	0.5	Cup	77.00	89.32	19.65	0.00	0.00	0.63	0.18	0.13	0.26	23.10	13.09	
Fish, tuna, white, w/oil, drained, cnd	3	Ounce-weight	85.05	158.19	22.56	0.00	0.00	6.87	1.09	2.77	2.53	26.37	4.25	
Fish, tuna, white, w/water, drained, cnd	3	Ounce-weight	85.05	108.86	20.09	0.00	0.00	2.53	0.67	0.67	0.94	35.72	5.10	
Fish, tuna, yellowfin, fillet, bkd/brld	3	Ounce-weight	85.05	118.22	25.49	0.00	0.00	1.04	0.26	0.17	0.31	49.33	17.01	
Fish, turbot, European, fillet, bkd/brld	3	Ounce-weight	85.05	103.76	17.50	0.00	0.00	3.21				52.73	10.21	
Fish, whitefish, fillet, bkd/brld, mixed species	3	Ounce-weight	85.05	146.29	20.81	0.00	0.00	6.39	0.99	2.18	2.34	65.49	33.17	
Fish, whiting, fillet, bkd/brld, mixed species	3	Ounce-weight	85.05	98.66	19.97	0.00	0.00	1.44	0.34	0.38	0.50	71.44	28.92	
Fish, yellowtail, fillet, bkd/brld, mixed species	3	Ounce-weight	85.05	159.04	25.23	0.00	0.00	5.72				60.39	26.37	
Juice, clam, cnd, mixed species	1	Cup	240.00	4.80	0.96	0.24	0.00	0.05	0.00	0.00	0.01	7.20	21.60	
Lobster, northern, raw	4	Ounce-weight	113.40	102.06	21.32	0.57	0.00	1.02	0.20	0.29	0.17	107.73	23.81	
Lobster, spiny, raw, mixed species	4	Ounce-weight	113.40	127.01	23.36	2.76	0.00	1.71	0.27	0.31	0.67	79.38	5.67	
Mussels, blue, raw, cup	4	Ounce-weight	113.40	97.52	13.49	4.18	0.00	2.54	0.48	0.57	0.69	31.75	54.43	
Oysters, eastern, bkd/brld, farmed, med	3	Ounce-weight	85.05	67.19	5.95	6.19	0.00	1.80	0.58	0.20	0.61	32.32	16.16	
Oysters, eastern, bkd/brld, wild, med	3	Ounce-weight	85.05	61.24	7.02	4.08	0.00	1.62	0.47	0.20	0.69	41.67	0.00	
Oysters, eastern, raw, farmed, med	4	Ounce-weight	113.40	66.91	5.92	6.27	0.00	1.76	0.50	0.17	0.67	28.35	9.07	

Vit E (mg)	Vit C	Vit B₁-Thia (mg)	Vit B₂-Ribo (mg)	Vit B₃-Nia (mg)	Fol (mcg)	Vit B₆ (mg)	Vita B₁₂ (mcg)	Sodi (mg)	Pota (mg)	Cal (mg)	Phos (mg)	Magn (mg)	Iron (mg)	Zinc (mg)	Caff (mg)	Alco (g)	Sol Fiber (g)	Insol Fiber (g)
1.07	0.00	0.23	0.41	8.57	24.66	0.80	2.59	47.63	534.11	12.76	217.73	31.47	0.88	0.70	0.00	0.00	0.00	0.00
1.45	3.49	0.04	0.13	8.54	29.77	0.39	2.44	51.03	429.50	23.81	315.54	103.76	0.77	0.48	0.00	0.00	0.00	0.00
1.15	0.00	0.02	0.09	4.01	1.70	0.24	2.77	666.79	148.84	9.36	139.48	15.31	0.72	0.26	0.00	0.00	0.00	0.00
1.36	0.00	0.02	0.14	5.95	17.01	0.32	3.74	63.79	255.15	211.77	301.08	25.52	0.60	0.85	0.00	0.00	0.00	0.00
0.48	1.28	0.09	0.10	6.29	11.91	0.48	2.70	44.23	391.23	10.21	282.37	28.92	0.33	0.40	0.00	0.00	0.00	0.00
0.69	1.19	0.06	0.12	6.76	11.06	0.48	4.25	49.33	369.12	38.27	273.86	28.07	0.52	0.48	0.00	0.00	0.00	0.00
0.69	0.85	0.10	0.14	6.62	7.65	0.47	3.81	45.08	386.98	39.12	253.45	29.77	0.60	0.44	0.00	0.00	0.00	0.00
1.07	0.00	0.17	0.06	7.25	4.25	0.20	2.94	73.14	352.11	14.46	250.90	28.07	0.84	0.60	0.00	0.00	0.00	0.00
0.54	0.00	0.02	0.16	5.56	12.76	0.26	3.74	471.18	277.26	181.16	279.81	28.92	0.71	0.78	0.00	0.00	0.00	0.00
1.74	0.00	0.07	0.19	4.46	10.21	0.14	7.60	429.50	337.65	324.89	416.75	33.17	2.48	1.11	0.00	0.00	0.00	0.00
1.22	0.85	0.04	0.20	3.57	20.41	0.10	7.65	352.11	290.02	204.12	311.28	28.92	1.96	1.19	0.00	0.00		
0.21	0.00	0.06	0.18	2.49	5.10	0.39	2.94	62.94	371.67	18.71	273.01	34.02	0.30	0.49	0.00	0.00	0.00	0.00
1.07	0.00	0.16	0.26	9.16	14.46	0.39	0.12	55.28	418.45	51.03	296.82	32.32	1.05	0.40	0.00	0.00	0.00	0.00
0.89	0.00	0.06	0.08	2.37	12.76	0.26	1.03	103.76	131.83	42.53	165.00	36.57	0.94	0.41	0.00	0.00	0.00	0.00
1.13	0.00	0.05	0.07	3.33	3.40	0.45	1.69	89.59	181.44	38.56	238.14	55.57	0.95	0.49	0.00	0.00	0.00	0.00
0.54	1.36	0.05	0.00	0.29	5.10	0.39	2.98	48.48	443.96	34.02	170.95	31.47	0.20	0.37	0.00	0.00	0.00	0.00
		0.05	0.02	1.51				94.08	376.33	15.05	150.53		0.27		0.00	0.00	0.00	0.00
0.54	0.94	0.04	0.10	10.03	1.70	0.32	1.72	97.81	313.83	5.10	286.62	28.92	0.88	1.25	0.00	0.00	0.00	0.00
0.22	0.43	0.36	0.36	4.91	12.76	0.20	6.37	56.98	393.78	46.78	267.06	23.81	1.63	0.72	0.00	0.00	0.00	0.00
0.03	2.81	0.20	0.07	7.48	20.41	0.34	4.23	35.72	375.07	73.14	226.23	27.22	0.28	0.42	0.00	0.00	0.00	0.00
0.43	1.70	0.13	0.08	4.91	16.16	0.29	5.36	47.63	381.02	73.14	228.78	26.37	0.32	0.43	0.00	0.00	0.00	0.00
1.07	0.00	0.24	0.26	8.96	1.70	0.45	9.25	42.53	274.71	8.51	277.26	54.43	1.11	0.65	0.00	0.00	0.00	0.00
0.64	0.00	0.03	0.09	9.06	3.65	0.08	1.61	258.42	151.11	9.49	227.03	22.63	1.01	0.66	0.00	0.00	0.00	0.00
1.02	0.00	0.03	0.10	10.55	4.25	0.09	1.87	42.53	176.05	11.06	264.51	26.37	1.18	0.77	0.00	0.00	0.00	0.00
	0.00							345.00	0.00	0.00			0.00		0.00	0.00	0.00	0.00
0.25	0.00	0.03	0.05	10.22	3.08	0.27	2.30	260.26	182.49	8.47	125.51	20.79	1.18	0.59	0.00	0.00	0.00	0.00
1.96	0.00	0.01	0.07	9.95	4.25	0.37	1.87	336.80	283.22	3.40	227.08	28.92	0.55	0.40	0.00	0.00	0.00	0.00
0.72	0.00	0.01	0.04	4.93	1.70	0.18	1.00	320.64	201.57	11.91	184.56	28.07	0.82	0.41	0.00	0.00	0.00	0.00
0.54	0.85	0.43	0.05	10.15	1.70	0.88	0.51	39.97	483.93	17.86	208.37	54.43	0.80	0.57	0.00	0.00	0.00	0.00
0.21	1.45	0.06	0.08	2.28	7.65	0.21	2.16	163.30	259.40	19.56	140.33	55.28	0.39	0.24	0.00	0.00	0.00	0.00
0.21	0.00	0.15	0.13	3.27	14.46	0.29	0.82	55.28	345.30	28.07	294.27	35.72	0.40	1.08	0.00	0.00	0.00	0.00
0.26	0.00	0.06	0.05	1.42	12.76	0.15	2.21	112.27	369.12	52.73	242.39	22.96	0.36	0.45	0.00	0.00	0.00	0.00
0.21	2.47	0.15	0.04	7.41	3.40	0.16	1.06	42.53	457.57	24.66	170.95	32.32	0.54	0.57	0.00	0.00	0.00	0.00
0.74	2.40	0.02	0.05	0.43	4.80	0.02	12.00	516.00	357.60	31.20	273.60	26.40	0.72	0.24	0.00	0.00	0.00	0.00
1.67	0.00	0.01	0.05	1.65	10.21	0.07	1.05	335.66	311.85	54.43	163.30	30.62	0.34	3.42	0.00	0.00	0.00	0.00
1.67	2.27	0.01	0.05	4.81	1.13	0.17	3.97	200.72	204.12	55.57	269.89	45.36	1.38	6.43	0.00	0.00	0.00	0.00
0.62	9.07	0.18	0.24	1.81	47.63	0.06	13.61	324.32	362.88	29.48	223.40	38.56	4.48	1.81	0.00	0.00	0.00	0.00
0.68	5.10	0.11	0.05	1.52	20.41	0.06	20.67	138.63	129.28	47.63	97.81	28.07	6.61	38.40	0.00	0.00	0.00	0.00
0.72	3.49	0.07	0.07	1.42	15.31	0.08	23.64	207.52	142.88	38.27	115.67	39.12	3.68	62.60	0.00	0.00	0.00	0.00
0.77	5.33	0.12	0.07	1.44	20.41	0.07	18.37	201.85	140.62	49.90	105.46	37.42	6.55	43.00	0.00	0.00	0.00	0.00

Food Name	Amount	Measure	Weight (g)	Calories	Protein (g)	Total Carb (g)	Dietary Fiber (g)	Total Fat (g)	Sat Fat (g)	Mono Fat (g)	Poly Fat (g)	Chol (mg)	Vit A (mcg RAE)	Vit D (mcg)
FISH, SEAFOOD, AND SHELLFISH *(continued)*														
Pompano, Florida, fillet, bkd/brld	3	Ounce-weight	85.05	179.46	20.15	0.00	0.00	10.33	3.83	2.82	1.24	54.43	30.62	
Roe, black/red, granular	1	Tablespoon	16.00	40.32	3.94	0.64	0.00	2.86	0.65	0.74	1.18	94.08	89.76	0.93
Sashimi, mackerel, Pacific & jack, fillet	4	Ounce-weight	113.40	179.17	22.76	0.00	0.00	8.95	2.55	2.98	2.20	53.30	14.74	
Sashimi, salmon, chinook, fillet	4	Ounce-weight	113.40	202.99	22.60	0.00	0.00	11.83	3.52	4.99	3.17	56.70	154.22	
Sashimi, snapper, fillet, mixed species	4	Ounce-weight	113.40	113.40	23.26	0.00	0.00	1.52	0.32	0.28	0.52	41.96	34.02	
Sashimi, tuna, skipjack, fillet	4	Ounce-weight	113.40	116.80	24.95	0.00	0.00	1.15	0.37	0.22	0.36	53.30	18.14	
Sashimi, tuna, yellowfin, fillet, w/o bone, 1" cube	4	Ounce-weight	113.40	122.47	26.51	0.00	0.00	1.08	0.27	0.17	0.32	51.03	20.41	
Sashimi, yellowtail, fillet, mixed species	4	Ounce-weight	113.40	165.56	26.24	0.00	0.00	5.94	1.45	2.26	1.61	62.37	32.89	
Scallops, raw, mixed species, lrg	4	Ounce-weight	113.40	99.79	19.03	2.68	0.00	0.86	0.09	0.04	0.30	37.42	17.01	
Shrimp, ckd, lrg, mixed species, each	3	Ounce-weight	85.05	84.20	17.78	0.00	0.00	0.92	0.25	0.17	0.37	165.85	57.83	
Shrimp, imit f/surimi, mixed species	3	Ounce-weight	85.05	85.90	10.54	7.77	0.00	1.25	0.25	0.19	0.64	30.62	17.01	
Shrimp, raw, lrg, mixed species	4	Ounce-weight	113.40	120.20	23.03	1.03	0.00	1.96	0.37	0.29	0.76	172.37	61.24	4.31
Surimi	3	Ounce-weight	85.05	84.20	12.91	5.83	0.00	0.77	0.16	0.13	0.38	25.52	17.01	
FOOD ADDITIVES														
Gums, Fibers, Starches, Pectins, Emulsifiers														
Pectin, unswtnd, dry, 1.75oz pkg	1	Each	49.61	161.24	0.00	44.65	4.47	0.00	0.00	0.00	0.00	0.00	0.00	
Starch, corn	1	Tablespoon	8.00	30.48	0.02	7.30	0.07	0.00	0.00	0.00	0.00	0.00	0.00	
Ingredient Sweeteners														
Nutraceuticals														
Nutritional Additives														
Bee Pollen	1	Teaspoon	5.00	15.70	1.21	2.18	0.39	0.25	0.17	0.02	0.03	0.00	0.00	
Multi Vitamin & Mineral, active formula, tablet Bayer Corporation	1	Each	1.75	0.00	0.00	0.00	0.00	0.00	0.00	0.00	0.00			10.00
Multi Vitamin & Mineral, Daily One Caps, w/iron, capsule Twin Laboratories	1	Each	1.75	0.00	0.00	0.03	0.00	0.00	0.00	0.00	0.00		500.00	10.00
Multi Vitamin & Mineral, Daily One Caps, w/o iron, capsule Twin Laboratories	1	Each	1.75	0.00	0.00	0.03	0.00	0.00	0.00	0.00	0.00		500.00	10.00
Multi Vitamin & Mineral, Daily One Complete, w/iron, capsule Optimum Nutrition	1	Each	1.17	0.10	0.00	0.03	0.00	0.00	0.00	0.00	0.00	0.00		10.00
Multi Vitamin & Mineral, maximum formula, tablet Bayer Corporation	1	Each	1.75	0.00	0.00	0.00	0.00	0.00	0.00	0.00	0.00	3.00		10.00
Multi Vitamin & Mineral, men's formula, tablet Bayer Corporation	1	Each	1.75	0.00	0.00	0.00	0.00	0.00	0.00	0.00	0.00			10.00
Multi Vitamin & Mineral, One A Day, women's formula, tablet Bayer Corporation	1	Each	1.75	0.00	0.00	0.00	0.00	0.00	0.00	0.00	0.00			10.00
Multi Vitamin, essential formula, tablet Bayer Corporation	1	Each	1.75	0.00	0.00	0.00	0.00	0.00	0.00	0.00	0.00			10.00
Protein, soy, conc, produced by acid wash	1	Ounce-weight	28.35	93.84	16.48	8.76	1.56	0.13	0.02	0.02	0.06	0.00	0.00	
Protein, soy, isolate	1	Ounce-weight	28.35	95.82	22.88	2.09	1.59	0.96	0.12	0.18	0.46	0.00	0.00	
Protein, soy, isolate, Supro Protein Technologies International	1	Ounce-weight	28.35	110.00	24.88	0.00	0.00	1.13	0.25	0.19	0.49	0.00	0.00	
Yeast, nutritional, flakes Now Foods	2	Tablespoon	16.00	50.00	8.00	5.00	4.00	0.65	0.00			0.00	0.00	
FRUIT, VEGETABLE, AND BLENDED JUICES														
Juice, apple, unswtnd, w/vit C, cnd/btld	1	Cup	248.00	116.56	0.15	28.97	0.25	0.27	0.05	0.01	0.08	0.00	0.12	0.00
Juice, apple, unswtnd, w/vit C, prep f/fzn conc w/water	1	Cup	239.00	112.33	0.33	27.58	0.24	0.24	0.04	0.00	0.07	0.00	0.00	0.00
Juice, apricot nectar, w/add vit C, cnd	1	Cup	251.00	140.56	0.93	36.12	1.51	0.23	0.02	0.10	0.04	0.00	165.66	
Juice, carrot	1	Cup	236.00	49.56	1.49	11.49		0.35	0.07	0.02	0.17	0.00	257.59	
Juice, cranberry cocktail, btld	1	Cup	252.80	144.10	0.00	36.40	0.25	0.25	0.02	0.04	0.11	0.00	0.51	
Juice, cranberry cocktail, prep f/fzn conc w/water	1	Cup	249.60	137.28	0.00	34.94	0.25	0.00	0.00	0.00	0.00	0.00	2.50	0.00

Vit E (mg)	Vit C	Vit B$_1$-Thia (mg)	Vit B$_2$-Ribo (mg)	Vit B$_3$-Nia (mg)	Fol (mcg)	Vit B$_6$ (mg)	Vita B$_{12}$ (mcg)	Sodi (mg)	Pota (mg)	Cal (mg)	Phos (mg)	Magn (mg)	Iron (mg)	Zinc (mg)	Caff (mg)	Alco (g)	Sol Fiber (g)	Insol Fiber (g)
0.19	0.00	0.58	0.13	3.23	14.46	0.20	1.02	64.64	540.92	36.57	290.02	26.37	0.57	0.59	0.00	0.00	0.00	0.00
1.12	0.00	0.03	0.10	0.02	8.00	0.05	3.20	240.00	28.96	44.00	56.96	48.00	1.90	0.15	0.00	0.00	0.00	0.00
1.13	2.27	0.13	0.48	9.43	2.27	0.37	4.99	97.52	460.40	26.08	141.75	31.75	1.32	0.76	0.00	0.00	0.00	0.00
1.38	4.54	0.06	0.13	9.55	34.02	0.45	1.47	53.30	446.80	29.48	327.73	107.73	0.28	0.50	0.00	0.00	0.00	0.00
0.57	1.81	0.05	0.00	0.32	5.67	0.45	3.40	72.58	472.88	36.29	224.53	36.29	0.20	0.41	0.00	0.00	0.00	0.00
1.13	1.13	0.04	0.11	17.46	10.21	0.96	2.15	41.96	461.54	32.89	251.75	38.56	1.42	0.93	0.00	0.00	0.00	0.00
0.57	1.13	0.49	0.05	11.11	2.27	1.02	0.59	41.96	503.50	18.14	216.59	56.70	0.83	0.59	0.00	0.00	0.00	0.00
0.20	3.18	0.16	0.05	7.71	4.54	0.18	1.47	44.23	476.28	26.08	178.04	34.02	0.56	0.59	0.00	0.00	0.00	0.00
0.00	3.40	0.01	0.07	1.30	18.14	0.17	1.74	182.57	365.15	27.22	248.35	63.50	0.33	1.08	0.00	0.00	0.00	0.00
1.17	1.87	0.03	0.03	2.20	3.40	0.11	1.27	190.51	154.79	33.17	116.52	28.92	2.63	1.33	0.00	0.00	0.00	0.00
0.09	0.00	0.02	0.03	0.14	1.70	0.03	1.36	599.60	75.69	16.16	239.84	36.57	0.51	0.28	0.00	0.00	0.00	0.00
1.25	2.27	0.03	0.04	2.89	3.40	0.12	1.32	167.83	209.79	58.97	232.47	41.96	2.73	1.26	0.00	0.00	0.00	0.00
0.54	0.00	0.02	0.02	0.19	1.70	0.03	1.36	121.62	95.26	7.65	239.84	36.57	0.22	0.28	0.00	0.00	0.00	0.00
0.00	0.00	0.00	0.00	0.00	0.50	0.00	0.00	99.22	3.47	3.47	0.99	0.50	1.49	0.00	0.00	0.00		
0.00	0.00	0.00	0.00	0.00	0.00	0.00	0.00	0.72	0.24	0.16	1.04	0.24	0.04	0.00	0.00	0.00		
0.27	2.50	0.02	0.04	0.23	0.00	0.02	0.00	0.25	11.10	4.05	4.55	2.60	0.32	0.28	0.00	0.00		
27.27	120.00	4.50	5.10	40.00	400.00	6.00	18.00		200.00	110.00	48.00	40.00	9.00	15.00	0.00	0.00	0.00	0.00
67.11	150.00	25.00	25.00	100.00	400.00	25.00	100.00		5.00	25.00		7.20	10.00	15.00	0.00	0.00	0.00	0.00
67.11	150.00	25.00	25.00	100.00	400.00	25.00	100.00		5.00	25.00		7.20		15.00	0.00	0.00	0.00	0.00
67.11	150.00	25.00	25.00	100.00	400.00	25.00	100.00		5.00	25.00		7.20	10.00	15.00	0.00	0.00	0.00	0.00
13.64	60.00	1.50	1.70	20.00	400.00	2.00	6.00		80.00	162.00	109.00	100.00	18.00	15.00	0.00	0.00	0.00	0.00
20.45	90.00	2.25	2.55	20.00	400.00	3.00	9.00		37.50			100.00		15.00	0.00	0.00	0.00	0.00
13.64	60.00	1.50	1.70	20.00	400.00	2.00	6.00			450.00			27.00	15.00	0.00	0.00	0.00	0.00
13.64	60.00	1.50	1.70	20.00	400.00	2.00	6.00								0.00	0.00	0.00	0.00
0.00	0.00	0.09	0.04	0.20	96.39	0.04	0.00	255.15	127.57	102.91	237.86	39.69	3.05	1.25	0.00	0.00	0.14	1.42
0.00	0.00	0.05	0.03	0.41	49.90	0.03	0.00	284.92	22.96	50.46	220.00	11.06	4.11	1.14	0.00	0.00		
	0.00	0.06	0.03	0.09	56.70		0.00	336.80	28.35	56.70	244.38	11.34	4.54	1.13	0.00	0.00	0.00	0.00
	0.00	9.60	9.52	56.00	240.00	9.60	7.80	5.00	320.00				0.72		0.00	0.00		
0.02	103.17	0.05	0.04	0.25	0.00	0.07	0.00	7.44	295.12	17.36	17.36	7.44	0.92	0.07	0.00	0.00	0.25	0.00
0.02	59.75	0.01	0.04	0.09	0.00	0.08	0.00	16.73	301.14	14.34	16.73	11.95	0.62	0.10	0.00	0.00	0.24	0.00
0.23	136.54	0.02	0.04	0.65	2.51	0.06	0.00	7.53	286.14	17.57	22.59	12.55	0.95	0.23	0.00	0.00	0.75	0.75
	8.92						0.00	122.72	516.84	63.72	73.16				0.00	0.00		
0.00	89.49	0.02	0.02	0.09	0.00	0.05	0.00	5.06	45.50	7.58	5.06	5.06	0.38	0.18	0.00	0.00		
0.02	24.71	0.02	0.02	0.03	0.00	0.03	0.00	7.49	34.94	12.48	2.50	4.99	0.22	0.10	0.00	0.00		

Food Name	Amount	Measure	Weight (g)	Calories	Protein (g)	Total Carb (g)	Dietary Fiber (g)	Total Fat (g)	Sat Fat (g)	Mono Fat (g)	Poly Fat (g)	Chol (mg)	Vit A (mcg RAE)	Vit D (mcg)
FRUIT, VEGETABLE, AND BLENDED JUICES *(continued)*														
Juice, grape, swtnd, w/add vit C, prep f/fzn conc w/water	1	Cup	250.00	127.50	0.48	31.88	0.25	0.22	0.07	0.01	0.06	0.00	1.00	
Juice, grapefruit cocktail, ruby red, rtd Season's Best	1	Cup	247.20	130.00	1.00	33.00	0.00	0.00	0.00	0.00	0.00	0.00	0.00	
Juice, grapefruit, pink, fresh, cup	1	Cup	247.00	96.33	1.24	22.72	0.25	0.25	0.03	0.03	0.06	0.00	54.34	0.00
Juice, grapefruit, swtnd, cnd, cup	1	Cup	250.00	115.00	1.45	27.83	0.25	0.22	0.03	0.03	0.05	0.00	0.88	
Juice, grapefruit, unswtnd, cnd, cup	1	Cup	247.00	93.86	1.28	22.13	0.25	0.25	0.03	0.03	0.06	0.00	0.86	
Juice, grapefruit, unswtnd, prep f/fzn conc w/water	1	Cup	247.00	101.27	1.36	24.03	0.25	0.32	0.05	0.04	0.08	0.00	1.11	
Juice, grapefruit, white, fresh, yield per fruit	1	Each	196.00	76.44	0.98	18.03	0.20	0.20	0.03	0.03	0.05	0.00	3.92	
Juice, lemon, cnd/btld, cup	1	Cup	244.00	51.24	0.98	15.81	0.98	0.71	0.09	0.03	0.21	0.00	2.44	
Juice, lemon, fresh	1	Cup	244.00	61.00	0.93	21.06	0.98	0.00	0.00	0.00	0.00	0.00	2.44	
Juice, lime, fresh, yield per wedge	1	Each	5.00	1.25	0.02	0.42	0.02	0.00	0.00	0.00	0.00	0.00	0.10	
Juice, lime, unswtnd, cnd/btld, cup	1	Cup	246.00	51.66	0.62	16.46	0.98	0.57	0.06	0.05	0.16	0.00	2.46	
Juice, orange grapefruit, unswtnd, cnd, cup	1	Cup	247.00	106.21	1.48	25.39	0.25	0.25	0.03	0.04	0.05	0.00	14.82	
Juice, orange, fresh, yield per fruit	1	Each	86.00	38.70	0.60	8.94	0.17	0.17	0.02	0.03	0.03	0.00	8.60	
Juice, orange, unswtnd, cnd, cup	1	Cup	249.00	104.58	1.47	24.53	0.50	0.35	0.04	0.06	0.08	0.00	22.41	
Juice, orange, unswtnd, prep f/fzn conc w/water	1	Cup	249.00	112.05	1.69	26.84	0.50	0.15	0.02	0.02	0.03	0.00	12.45	
Juice, papaya nectar, cnd, cup	1	Cup	250.00	142.50	0.43	36.28	1.50	0.38	0.12	0.10	0.09	0.00	45.00	
Juice, passion fruit, purple, fresh	1	Cup	247.00	125.97	0.96	33.59	0.49	0.12	0.01	0.01	0.07	0.00	88.92	
Juice, peach nectar, w/add vit C, cnd	1	Cup	249.00	134.46	0.67	34.66	1.49	0.05	0.00	0.02	0.03	0.00	32.37	0.00
Juice, pear nectar, w/add vit C, cnd	1	Cup	250.00	150.00	0.28	39.40	1.50	0.02	0.00	0.01	0.01	0.00	0.12	0.00
Juice, pineapple, unswtnd, w/add vit C, cnd	1	Cup	250.00	140.00	0.80	34.45	0.50	0.20	0.01	0.02	0.07	0.00	0.62	0.00
Juice, tangerine, swtnd, cnd, cup	1	Cup	249.00	124.50	1.25	29.88	0.50	0.50	0.03	0.04	0.06	0.00	32.37	
Juice, tomato, cnd	1	Cup	243.00	41.31	1.85	10.30	0.97	0.12	0.02	0.02	0.06	0.00	55.89	
Juice, tomato, unsalted, cnd	1	Cup	243.00	41.31	1.85	10.30	0.97	0.12	0.02	0.02	0.06	0.00	55.89	
Juice, vegetable cocktail, cnd	1	Cup	242.00	45.98	1.52	11.01	1.94	0.22	0.03	0.03	0.09	0.00	188.76	
FRUITS														
Apples, fresh, med, 2 3/4"	1	Each	138.00	71.76	0.36	19.06	3.31	0.23	0.04	0.01	0.07	0.00	4.14	
Apples, fresh, peeled, med, 2 3/4"	1	Each	128.00	61.44	0.35	16.33	1.66	0.17	0.03	0.01	0.05	0.00	2.56	
Apples, slices, swtnd, drained, cnd, unheated	0.5	Cup	102.00	68.34	0.18	17.03	1.73	0.50	0.08	0.02	0.15	0.00	3.06	
Apples, sulfured, dehyd, unckd, cup	0.5	Cup	30.00	103.80	0.40	28.06	3.72	0.17	0.03	0.01	0.05	0.00	1.20	0.00
Apples, unswtnd, unheated, fzn	0.5	Cup	86.50	41.52	0.24	10.65	1.64	0.28	0.04	0.01	0.08	0.00	1.73	0.00
Applesauce, swtnd, cnd	0.5	Cup	127.50	96.90	0.23	25.38	1.53	0.23	0.04	0.01	0.07	0.00	1.27	0.00
Applesauce, unswtnd, w/o add Vit C, cnd	0.5	Cup	122.00	52.46	0.21	13.78	1.46	0.06	0.01	0.00	0.02	0.00	1.22	
Apricots, dried, California Sunsweet Growers Inc.	5	Each	40.00	100.00	1.00	24.00	4.00	0.00	0.00	0.00	0.00	0.00	90.00	
Apricots, fresh, whole, each	1	Each	35.00	16.80	0.49	3.89	0.70	0.14	0.01	0.06	0.03	0.00	33.60	
Apricots, halves, w/skin, w/juice, cnd	0.5	Cup	122.00	58.56	0.77	15.06	1.95	0.05	0.00	0.02	0.01	0.00	103.70	
Apricots, halves, w/skin, w/light syrup	0.5	Cup	126.50	79.69	0.67	20.86	2.02	0.06	0.00	0.03	0.01	0.00	83.49	
Apricots, swtnd, fzn	0.5	Cup	121.00	118.58	0.85	30.37	2.66	0.12	0.01	0.05	0.03	0.00	101.64	
Apricots, w/o skin, w/water, cnd	0.5	Cup	113.50	24.97	0.79	6.22	1.25	0.03	0.00	0.01	0.01	0.00	103.29	0.00
Apricots, whole, w/o skin & pit, w/heavy syrup, cnd	0.5	Cup	129.00	107.07	0.65	27.67	2.06	0.12	0.01	0.05	0.02	0.00	79.98	0.00
Avocado, avg, fresh, each	1	Each	201.00	321.60	4.02	17.15	13.47	29.47	4.27	19.70	3.65	0.00	14.07	
Avocado, Florida, fresh, each	1	Each	304.00	364.80	6.78	23.77	16.66	30.58	5.96	16.76	5.10	0.00	21.28	
Banana, chips	1	Ounce-weight	28.35	147.14	0.65	16.56	2.18	9.53	8.21	0.56	0.18	0.00	1.13	
Banana, fresh, extra lrg, 9" or longer, each	1	Each	152.00	135.28	1.66	34.72	3.95	0.50	0.17	0.05	0.11	0.00	4.56	
Banana, fresh, mashed, cup	0.5	Cup	112.50	100.12	1.23	25.70	2.92	0.37	0.13	0.03	0.08	0.00	3.37	
Banana, fresh, slices, cup	0.5	Cup	75.00	66.75	0.82	17.13	1.95	0.25	0.09	0.02	0.05	0.00	2.25	

Vit E (mg)	Vit C	Vit B₁-Thia (mg)	Vit B₂-Ribo (mg)	Vit B₃-Nia (mg)	Fol (mcg)	Vit B₆ (mg)	Vita B₁₂ (mcg)	Sodi (mg)	Pota (mg)	Cal (mg)	Phos (mg)	Magn (mg)	Iron (mg)	Zinc (mg)	Caff (mg)	Alco (g)	Sol Fiber (g)	Insol Fiber (g)
0.00	59.75	0.04	0.06	0.31	2.50	0.11	0.00	5.00	52.50	10.00	10.00	10.00	0.25	0.10	0.00	0.00	0.08	0.18
0.00	60.00	0.00		0.00	0.00	0.00		30.00	0.00	0.00			0.00		0.00	0.00	0.00	0.00
0.10	93.86	0.10	0.05	0.49	24.70	0.11	0.00	2.47	400.14	22.23	37.05	29.64	0.49	0.12	0.00	0.00		
0.10	67.25	0.10	0.06	0.80	25.00	0.05	0.00	5.00	405.00	20.00	27.50	25.00	0.90	0.15	0.00	0.00	0.08	0.18
0.10	72.12	0.10	0.05	0.57	24.70	0.05	0.00	2.47	377.91	17.29	27.17	24.70	0.49	0.22	0.00	0.00	0.07	0.17
0.10	83.24	0.10	0.05	0.54	9.88	0.11	0.00	2.47	335.92	19.76	34.58	27.17	0.35	0.12	0.00	0.00	0.07	0.17
0.43	74.48	0.08	0.04	0.39	19.60	0.09	0.00	1.96	317.52	17.64	29.40	23.52	0.39	0.10	0.00	0.00	0.06	0.14
0.37	60.51	0.10	0.02	0.48	24.40	0.10	0.00	51.24	248.88	26.84	21.96	19.52	0.32	0.15	0.00	0.00	0.46	0.51
0.37	112.24	0.07	0.02	0.24	31.72	0.12	0.00	2.44	302.56	17.08	14.64	14.64	0.07	0.12	0.00	0.00	0.46	0.51
0.01	1.50	0.00	0.00	0.01	0.50	0.00	0.00	0.10	5.85	0.70	0.70	0.40	0.00	0.00	0.00	0.00		
0.30	15.74	0.08	0.01	0.40	19.68	0.07	0.00	39.36	184.50	29.52	24.60	17.22	0.57	0.15	0.00	0.00		
0.35	71.88	0.14	0.07	0.83	34.58	0.06	0.00	7.41	390.26	19.76	34.58	24.70	1.14	0.17	0.00	0.00	0.05	0.20
0.03	43.00	0.08	0.03	0.34	25.80	0.03	0.00	0.86	172.00	9.46	14.62	9.46	0.17	0.04	0.00	0.00	0.05	0.12
0.50	85.66	0.15	0.07	0.78	44.82	0.22	0.00	4.98	435.75	19.92	34.86	27.39	1.10	0.17	0.00	0.00	0.10	0.40
0.50	96.86	0.20	0.04	0.50	109.56	0.11	0.00	2.49	473.10	22.41	39.84	24.90	0.25	0.12	0.00	0.00	0.16	0.34
0.60	7.50	0.02	0.01	0.38	5.00	0.02	0.00	12.50	77.50	25.00	0.00	7.50	0.85	0.38	0.00	0.00	0.70	0.80
0.02	73.61	0.00	0.32	3.61	17.29	0.12	0.00	14.82	686.66	9.88	32.11	41.99	0.59	0.12	0.00	0.00	0.25	0.25
0.20	66.73	0.01	0.03	0.72	2.49	0.02	0.00	17.43	99.60	12.45	14.94	9.96	0.47	0.20	0.00	0.00	1.00	0.50
0.25	67.50	0.00	0.03	0.32	2.50	0.04	0.00	10.00	32.50	12.50	7.50	7.50	0.65	0.18	0.00	0.00	0.30	1.20
0.05	60.00	0.14	0.05	0.64	57.50	0.24	0.00	2.50	335.00	42.50	20.00	32.50	0.65	0.28	0.00	0.00	0.15	0.35
0.37	54.78	0.15	0.05	0.25	12.45	0.08	0.00	2.49	443.22	44.82	34.86	19.92	0.50	0.07	0.00	0.00	0.15	0.35
0.78	44.47	0.11	0.08	1.64	48.60	0.27	0.00	653.67	556.47	24.30	43.74	26.73	1.04	0.36	0.00	0.00	0.24	0.73
0.78	44.47	0.11	0.08	1.64	48.60	0.27	0.00	24.30	556.47	24.30	43.74	26.73	1.04	0.36	0.00	0.00		
0.77	67.03	0.10	0.07	1.76	50.82	0.34	0.00	653.40	467.06	26.62	41.14	26.62	1.02	0.48	0.00	0.00		
0.25	6.35	0.02	0.04	0.13	4.14	0.06	0.00	1.38	147.66	8.28	15.18	6.90	0.17	0.06	0.00	0.00	0.33	2.98
0.06	5.12	0.02	0.04	0.12	0.00	0.05	0.00	0.00	115.20	6.40	14.08	5.12	0.09	0.06	0.00	0.00	0.22	1.45
0.21	0.41	0.01	0.01	0.07	0.00	0.04	0.00	3.06	69.36	4.08	5.10	2.04	0.23	0.03	0.00	0.00	0.51	1.22
0.22	0.66	0.02	0.04	0.20	0.30	0.08	0.00	37.20	192.00	5.70	16.50	6.60	0.60	0.09	0.00	0.00		
0.93	0.09	0.01	0.01	0.04	0.87	0.03	0.00	2.60	66.61	3.46	6.92	2.60	0.15	0.04	0.00	0.00		
0.06	2.17	0.02	0.04	0.24	1.27	0.04	0.00	35.70	77.77	5.10	8.92	3.82	0.45	0.05	0.00	0.00	0.38	1.15
0.25	1.46	0.02	0.03	0.23	1.22	0.03	0.00	2.44	91.50	3.66	8.54	3.66	0.15	0.03	0.00	0.00		
	1.20						0.00	0.00	520.00	20.00			1.08		0.00	0.00		
0.31	3.50	0.01	0.01	0.21	3.15	0.02	0.00	0.35	90.65	4.55	8.05	3.50	0.14	0.07	0.00	0.00		
0.73	5.98	0.03	0.03	0.42	2.44	0.07	0.00	4.88	201.30	14.64	24.40	12.20	0.37	0.13	0.00	0.00	0.84	1.12
0.76	3.42	0.02	0.03	0.39	2.53	0.07	0.00	5.06	174.57	13.91	16.44	10.12	0.50	0.14	0.00	0.00	0.77	1.26
1.08	10.89	0.03	0.05	0.97	2.42	0.07	0.00	4.84	277.09	12.10	22.99	10.89	1.09	0.12	0.00	0.00	0.93	1.73
1.01	2.04	0.02	0.02	0.49	2.27	0.06	0.00	12.49	174.79	9.08	18.16	10.22	0.62	0.12	0.00	0.00	0.85	0.40
1.15	3.61	0.03	0.03	0.53	2.58	0.07	0.00	14.19	172.86	11.61	16.77	10.32	0.55	0.13	0.00	0.00		
4.16	20.10	0.13	0.26	3.49	162.81	0.52	0.00	14.07	974.85	24.12	104.52	58.29	1.11	1.29	0.00	0.00		
8.09	52.90	0.06	0.16	2.04	106.40	0.24	0.00	6.08	1067.04	30.40	121.60	72.96	0.52	1.22	0.00	0.00		
0.07	1.79	0.03	0.01	0.20	3.97	0.08	0.00	1.70	151.96	5.10	15.88	21.55	0.36	0.22	0.00	0.00	0.60	1.59
0.15	13.22	0.05	0.11	1.01	30.40	0.56	0.00	1.52	544.16	7.60	33.44	41.04	0.40	0.23	0.00	0.00		
0.11	9.79	0.03	0.08	0.75	22.50	0.41	0.00	1.12	402.75	5.62	24.75	30.37	0.29	0.17	0.00	0.00		
0.07	6.52	0.02	0.05	0.50	15.00	0.27	0.00	0.75	268.50	3.75	16.50	20.25	0.19	0.11	0.00	0.00		

Food Name	Amount	Measure	Weight (g)	Calories	Protein (g)	Total Carb (g)	Dietary Fiber (g)	Total Fat (g)	Sat Fat (g)	Mono Fat (g)	Poly Fat (g)	Chol (mg)	Vit A (mcg RAE)	Vit D (mcg)
FRUITS *(continued)*														
Banana, fresh, sml, 6" to 6 7/8" long, each	1	Each	101.00	89.89	1.10	23.07	2.63	0.33	0.11	0.03	0.07	0.00	3.03	
Banana, pwd	1	Tablespoon	6.20	21.45	0.24	5.47	0.61	0.11	0.04	0.01	0.02	0.00	0.74	
Blackberries, unswtnd, fzn, cup	0.5	Cup	75.50	48.32	0.89	11.83	3.78	0.32	0.01	0.03	0.18	0.00	4.53	
Blueberries, fresh, cup	0.5	Cup	72.50	41.32	0.54	10.50	1.74	0.24	0.02	0.04	0.10	0.00	2.17	
Blueberries, unswtnd, fzn, pkg	0.5	Cup	77.50	39.52	0.33	9.43	2.09	0.50	0.04	0.07	0.22	0.00	1.55	
Blueberries, w/heavy syrup, cnd, not drained, cup	0.5	Cup	128.00	112.64	0.83	28.23	2.05	0.42	0.04	0.06	0.18	0.00	2.56	
Boysenberries, fresh, cup	0.5	Cup	72.00	30.96	1.00	6.92	3.67	0.35	0.01	0.04	0.20	0.00	7.92	
Boysenberries, unswtnd, fzn, pkg	0.5	Cup	66.00	33.00	0.73	8.05	3.50	0.17	0.00	0.01	0.10	0.00	1.98	
Breadfruit, fresh, each	0.25	Each	96.00	98.88	1.03	26.04	4.70	0.22	0.05	0.03	0.06	0.00	0.00	
Carambola, fresh, sml, 3" long, each	1	Each	70.00	21.70	0.73	4.71	1.95	0.23	0.01	0.02	0.13	0.00	2.10	
Carissa, fresh, w/o skin & seeds, each	1	Each	20.00	12.40	0.10	2.73		0.26				0.00	0.40	
Chayote, ckd, drained, 1" pces, cup	0.5	Cup	80.00	19.20	0.50	4.08	2.24	0.39	0.07	0.03	0.16	0.00	1.60	
Cherimoya, fresh, each	0.25	Each	136.75	101.20	2.26	24.20	3.15	0.85				0.00	0.00	
Cherries, maraschino, cnd, drained	1	Each	4.00	6.60	0.01	1.68	0.13	0.01	0.00	0.00	0.00	0.00	0.08	
Cherries, red, sour, fresh, cup	0.5	Cup	77.50	38.75	0.77	9.44	1.24	0.23	0.06	0.06	0.07	0.00	49.60	0.00
Cherries, red, sour, unswtnd, fzn	0.5	Cup	77.50	35.65	0.71	8.54	1.24	0.34	0.08	0.09	0.10	0.00	34.10	
Cherries, red, sour, w/light syrup, cnd, not drained	0.5	Cup	126.00	94.50	0.94	24.32	1.01	0.13	0.03	0.04	0.04	0.00	45.36	0.00
Cherries, red, sour/tart, w/water, cnd, not drained	0.5	Cup	122.00	43.92	0.94	10.91	1.34	0.12	0.03	0.03	0.03	0.00	46.36	
Cherries, sweet, fresh, cup	0.5	Cup	72.50	45.67	0.77	11.61	1.52	0.14	0.03	0.04	0.04	0.00	2.17	
Cherries, sweet, swtnd, fzn, pkg	1	Ounce-weight	28.35	25.23	0.33	6.34	0.60	0.04	0.01	0.01	0.01	0.00	2.55	
Cherries, sweet, w/light syrup, cnd, not drained	0.5	Cup	126.00	84.42	0.76	21.79	1.89	0.19	0.04	0.05	0.05	0.00	10.08	0.00
Cherries, swtnd, w/juice, cnd, not drained	0.5	Cup	125.00	67.50	1.13	17.26	1.87	0.03	0.01	0.01	0.01	0.00	7.50	0.00
Cranberries, fresh, whole, cup	0.5	Cup	47.50	21.85	0.18	5.80	2.18	0.06	0.00	0.01	0.02	0.00	1.42	
Cranberry Sauce, swtnd, cnd, slice, 1/2" thick	0.25	Cup	69.25	104.57	0.14	26.94	0.69	0.10	0.01	0.01	0.05	0.00	1.38	
Currants, black, European, fresh, cup	0.5	Cup	56.00	35.28	0.78	8.61	4.14	0.22	0.01	0.03	0.10	0.00	6.72	
Dates, Deglet Noor, whole, each	5	Each	41.50	117.03	1.02	31.14	3.32	0.17	0.01	0.01	0.01	0.00	0.21	
Figs, fresh, sml, 1 1/2" each	1	Each	40.00	29.60	0.30	7.67	1.16	0.12	0.02	0.03	0.06	0.00	2.80	
Figs, stwd f/dried, cup	0.5	Cup	129.50	138.57	1.84	35.71	5.44	0.52	0.08	0.09	0.19	0.00	0.26	0.00
Figs, w/light syrup, cnd, not drained, each or cup	0.5	Cup	126.00	86.94	0.49	22.62	2.27	0.13	0.03	0.03	0.06	0.00	2.52	0.00
Fruit Cocktail, w/extra heavy syrup, cnd, not drained, cup	0.5	Cup	130.00	114.40	0.51	29.76	1.43	0.09	0.01	0.02	0.04	0.00	13.00	0.00
Fruit Cocktail, w/extra light syrup, cnd, not drained, cup	0.5	Cup	123.00	55.35	0.49	14.30	1.35	0.09	0.01	0.02	0.04	0.00	14.76	0.00
Gooseberries, fresh, cup	0.5	Cup	75.00	33.00	0.66	7.63	3.22	0.43	0.03	0.04	0.24	0.00	11.25	
Grapefruit, pink, fresh, sections, cup	0.5	Cup	115.00	36.80	0.72	9.29	1.27	0.12	0.02	0.02	0.02	0.00	52.90	
Grapefruit, w/juice, cnd, not drained, sections, cup	0.5	Cup	124.50	46.06	0.87	11.46	0.50	0.11	0.02	0.02	0.02	0.00	0.00	0.00
Grapefruit, w/light syrup, cnd, not drained, sections, cup	0.5	Cup	127.00	76.20	0.71	19.61	0.51	0.12	0.02	0.02	0.03	0.00	0.00	
Grapes, concord, fresh, cup	0.5	Cup	46.00	30.82	0.29	7.89	0.41	0.16	0.05	0.01	0.05	0.00	2.30	
Grapes, red European type varieties, fresh, each	10	Each	50.00	34.50	0.36	9.05	0.45	0.08	0.03	0.00	0.03	0.00	1.50	
Grapes, Thompson seedless, fresh, cup	0.5	Cup	80.00	55.20	0.58	14.48	0.72	0.13	0.05	0.01	0.04	0.00	2.40	
Grapes, Thompson seedless, w/heavy syrup, cnd S & W	0.5	Cup	123.00	100.00	0.00	23.00	0.00	0.00	0.00	0.00	0.00	0.00	0.00	
Guava, fresh, cup	0.5	Cup	82.50	56.10	2.10	11.82	4.46	0.78	0.22	0.07	0.33	0.00	25.58	
Huckleberries, fresh, cup	0.5	Cup	72.50	41.32	0.54	10.51	1.74	0.24	0.02	0.04	0.10	0.00	2.17	
Kiwi, fresh, w/o skin, med	1	Each	76.00	46.36	0.87	11.14	2.28	0.40	0.02	0.04	0.22	0.00	3.04	
Kumquats, fresh, each	1	Each	19.00	13.49	0.36	3.02	1.23	0.16	0.02	0.03	0.03	0.00	2.85	
Leechees, fresh, cup	0.5	Cup	80.00	52.80	0.66	13.22	1.04	0.35	0.08	0.10	0.10	0.00	0.00	
Lemon, peeled, fresh, 2 1/8"	1	Each	58.00	16.82	0.64	5.41	1.62	0.17	0.02	0.01	0.05	0.00	0.58	

Vit E (mg)	Vit C	Vit B₁-Thia (mg)	Vit B₂-Ribo (mg)	Vit B₃-Nia (mg)	Fol (mcg)	Vit B₆ (mg)	Vita B₁₂ (mcg)	Sodi (mg)	Pota (mg)	Cal (mg)	Phos (mg)	Magn (mg)	Iron (mg)	Zinc (mg)	Caff (mg)	Alco (g)	Sol Fiber (g)	Insol Fiber (g)
0.10	8.79	0.03	0.07	0.67	20.20	0.37	0.00	1.01	361.58	5.05	22.22	27.27	0.26	0.15	0.00	0.00		
0.02	0.43	0.01	0.01	0.17	0.87	0.03	0.00	0.19	92.44	1.36	4.59	6.70	0.07	0.04	0.00	0.00		
0.88	2.34	0.02	0.03	0.91	25.67	0.05	0.00	0.76	105.70	21.90	22.65	16.61	0.60	0.19	0.00	0.00	0.87	2.91
0.42	7.04	0.02	0.03	0.30	4.35	0.04	0.00	0.72	55.82	4.35	8.70	4.35	0.20	0.12	0.00	0.00	0.20	1.54
0.37	1.94	0.02	0.03	0.40	5.42	0.04	0.00	0.77	41.85	6.20	8.52	3.87	0.14	0.06	0.00	0.00	0.62	1.47
0.48	1.41	0.05	0.06	0.15	2.56	0.05	0.00	3.84	51.20	6.40	12.80	5.12	0.42	0.09	0.00	0.00		
0.84	15.12	0.02	0.02	0.46	18.00	0.02	0.00	0.72	116.64	20.88	15.84	14.40	0.45	0.38	0.00	0.00		
0.58	2.05	0.03	0.02	0.50	41.58	0.04	0.00	0.66	91.74	17.82	17.82	10.56	0.56	0.15	0.00	0.00		
0.10	27.84	0.10	0.03	0.86	13.44	0.10	0.00	1.92	470.40	16.32	28.80	24.00	0.52	0.12	0.00	0.00		
0.10	24.08	0.01	0.01	0.26	8.40	0.01	0.00	1.40	93.10	2.10	8.40	7.00	0.06	0.08	0.00	0.00	0.14	1.81
	7.60	0.01	0.01	0.04			0.00	0.60	52.00	2.20	1.40	3.20	0.26		0.00	0.00		
0.09	6.40	0.02	0.03	0.34	14.40	0.09	0.00	0.80	138.40	10.40	23.20	9.60	0.18	0.24	0.00	0.00		
	15.73	0.13	0.17	0.78	24.62	0.29	0.00	5.47	367.86	10.94	35.56	21.88	0.41	0.24	0.00	0.00		
0.00	0.00	0.00	0.00	0.00	0.00	0.00	0.00	0.16	0.84	2.16	0.12	0.16	0.02	0.01	0.00	0.00		
0.06	7.75	0.02	0.03	0.31	6.20	0.03	0.00	2.32	134.07	12.40	11.62	6.97	0.25	0.08	0.00	0.00	0.58	0.66
0.04	1.32	0.03	0.03	0.11	3.87	0.05	0.00	0.77	96.10	10.07	12.40	6.97	0.41	0.08	0.00	0.00	0.58	0.66
0.07	2.52	0.02	0.04	0.22	10.08	0.05	0.00	8.82	119.70	12.60	12.60	7.56	1.66	0.09	0.00	0.00		
0.28	2.56	0.02	0.05	0.22	9.76	0.05	0.00	8.54	119.56	13.42	12.20	7.32	1.67	0.09	0.00	0.00	0.63	0.71
0.05	5.07	0.02	0.03	0.11	2.90	0.04	0.00	0.00	160.95	9.42	15.22	7.97	0.26	0.05	0.00	0.00		
0.02	0.28	0.01	0.01	0.05	1.13	0.01	0.00	0.28	56.42	3.40	4.54	2.84	0.10	0.01	0.00	0.00	0.45	0.15
0.29	4.66	0.03	0.05	0.50	5.04	0.04	0.00	3.78	186.48	11.34	22.68	11.34	0.45	0.13	0.00	0.00		
0.29	3.12	0.03	0.03	0.51	5.00	0.04	0.00	3.75	163.75	17.50	27.50	15.00	0.72	0.12	0.00	0.00	0.88	0.99
0.57	6.32	0.00	0.01	0.05	0.48	0.02	0.00	0.95	40.38	3.80	6.18	2.85	0.12	0.04	0.00	0.00		
0.57	1.38	0.01	0.01	0.07	0.69	0.01	0.00	20.08	18.00	2.77	4.15	2.08	0.15	0.03	0.00	0.00	0.28	0.42
0.56	101.36	0.03	0.03	0.17	1.95	0.04	0.00	1.12	180.32	30.80	33.04	13.44	0.87	0.15	0.00	0.00	0.67	3.47
0.02	0.17	0.02	0.03	0.53	7.89	0.07	0.00	0.83	272.24	16.19	25.73	17.85	0.43	0.12	0.00	0.00		
0.04	0.80	0.02	0.02	0.16	2.40	0.05	0.00	0.40	92.80	14.00	5.60	6.80	0.15	0.06	0.00	0.00		
0.19	5.70	0.02	0.14	0.83	1.30	0.18	0.00	5.18	380.73	90.65	37.56	37.56	1.14	0.31	0.00	0.00		
0.13	1.26	0.03	0.04	0.55	2.52	0.09	0.00	1.26	128.52	34.02	12.60	12.60	0.37	0.13	0.00	0.00	0.45	1.82
0.38	2.47	0.03	0.03	0.48	3.90	0.06	0.00	7.80	111.80	7.80	14.30	6.50	0.36	0.10	0.00	0.00		
0.36	3.69	0.04	0.01	0.62	3.69	0.06	0.00	4.92	127.92	9.84	14.76	7.38	0.37	0.10	0.00	0.00		
0.28	20.77	0.03	0.02	0.22	4.50	0.06	0.00	0.75	148.50	18.75	20.25	7.50	0.23	0.09	0.00	0.00	1.09	2.13
0.15	39.56	0.04	0.02	0.29	11.50	0.05	0.00	0.00	159.85	13.80	9.20	9.20	0.11	0.08	0.00	0.00	0.94	0.33
0.11	42.20	0.04	0.02	0.31	11.20	0.02	0.00	8.72	210.40	18.68	14.94	13.70	0.26	0.10	0.00	0.00	0.20	0.30
0.12	27.05	0.05	0.02	0.31	11.43	0.02	0.00	2.54	163.83	17.78	12.70	12.70	0.51	0.10	0.00	0.00	0.20	0.30
0.09	1.84	0.04	0.03	0.14	1.84	0.05	0.00	0.92	87.86	6.44	4.60	2.30	0.13	0.02	0.00	0.00		
0.10	5.40	0.04	0.04	0.09	1.00	0.04	0.00	1.00	95.50	5.00	10.00	3.50	0.18	0.04	0.00	0.00		
0.15	8.64	0.06	0.06	0.15	1.60	0.07	0.00	1.60	152.80	8.00	16.00	5.60	0.29	0.06	0.00	0.00		
	0.00						0.00	20.00	120.00	0.00			1.44		0.00	0.00	0.00	0.00
0.60	188.35	0.05	0.04	0.90	40.43	0.09	0.00	1.65	344.03	14.85	33.00	18.15	0.21	0.19	0.00	0.00	2.23	2.23
0.41	7.03	0.03	0.03	0.31	4.35	0.04	0.00	0.72	55.82	4.35	8.70	4.35	0.20	0.11	0.00	0.00	0.20	1.54
1.11	70.45	0.02	0.02	0.26	19.00	0.05	0.00	2.28	237.12	25.84	25.84	12.92	0.24	0.11	0.00	0.00		
0.03	8.34	0.01	0.02	0.08	3.23	0.01	0.00	1.90	35.34	11.78	3.61	3.80	0.16	0.03	0.00	0.00	0.07	1.16
0.06	57.20	0.01	0.05	0.48	11.20	0.08	0.00	0.80	136.80	4.00	24.80	8.00	0.25	0.06	0.00	0.00		
0.09	30.74	0.02	0.01	0.06	6.38	0.05	0.00	1.16	80.04	15.08	9.28	4.64	0.35	0.03	0.00	0.00	0.52	1.10

Food Name	Amount	Measure	Weight (g)	Calories	Protein (g)	Total Carb (g)	Dietary Fiber (g)	Total Fat (g)	Sat Fat (g)	Mono Fat (g)	Poly Fat (g)	Chol (mg)	Vit A (mcg RAE)	Vit D (mcg)
FRUITS *(continued)*														
Limes, med, fresh FDA	1	Each	67.00	20.00	0.00	7.00	2.00	0.00	0.00	0.00	0.00	0.00	0.00	
Litchis, dried, each	1	Each	2.50	6.93	0.10	1.77	0.12	0.03	0.01	0.01	0.01	0.00	0.00	
Loganberries, w/heavy syrup, cnd, cup	0.5	Cup	128.00	112.64	1.27	28.55	3.33	0.16	0.01	0.02	0.09	0.00	2.56	
Mandarin Oranges, fresh, sections, cup	1	Cup	195.00	103.35	1.58	26.01	3.51	0.60	0.08	0.12	0.13	0.00	66.30	
Mango, dried Sunsweet Growers Inc.	0.33	Cup	40.00	140.00	0.00	34.00	1.00	0.00	0.00	0.00	0.00	0.00	25.00	
Mango, fresh, whole, each	0.5	Each	103.50	67.27	0.52	17.59	1.86	0.28	0.07	0.10	0.05	0.00	39.33	
Melon, balls, fzn, cup	0.5	Cup	86.50	28.55	0.73	6.87	0.61	0.22	0.06	0.01	0.09	0.00	76.99	
Melon, casaba, fresh, cubes, cup	0.5	Cup	85.00	23.80	0.94	5.59	0.77	0.09	0.02	0.00	0.03	0.00	0.00	
Melon, honeydew, fresh, balls, cup	0.5	Cup	88.50	31.86	0.48	8.05	0.71	0.13	0.03	0.00	0.05	0.00	2.65	
Mixed Fruit, peach pear & pine, w/heavy syrup, cnd undrained	0.5	Cup	127.50	91.80	0.47	23.92	1.27	0.13	0.02	0.03	0.05	0.00	12.75	0.00
Mixed Fruit, prunes apricots & pears, dried, pkg	1	Ounce-weight	28.35	68.89	0.70	18.16	2.21	0.14	0.01	0.07	0.03	0.00	34.59	
Nectarines, fresh, 2 1/2" each	1	Each	136.00	59.84	1.44	14.35	2.31	0.44	0.03	0.12	0.15	0.00	23.12	
Oranges, Calif, navels, fresh, 2 7/8" each	1	Each	140.00	68.60	1.27	17.56	3.08	0.21	0.02	0.04	0.04	0.00	16.80	
Oranges, Calif, valencias, fresh, 2 5/8" each	1	Each	121.00	59.29	1.26	14.39	3.03	0.36	0.04	0.07	0.07	0.00	14.52	
Papaya, fresh, cubes, cup	0.5	Cup	70.00	27.30	0.42	6.86	1.26	0.10	0.03	0.02	0.02	0.00	38.50	
Passion Fruit, purple, fresh, each	1	Each	18.00	17.46	0.40	4.21	1.87	0.13	0.01	0.02	0.07	0.00	11.52	
Peaches, fresh, lrg, w/o skin, 2 3/4" each	1	Each	157.00	61.23	1.43	14.98	2.34	0.39	0.03	0.11	0.14	0.00	25.12	
Peaches, halves, dried, sulfured, unckd	0.5	Cup	80.00	191.20	2.88	49.06	6.56	0.60	0.06	0.22	0.30	0.00	86.40	
Peaches, halves, w/heavy syrup, cnd, not drained, each	1	Each	98.00	72.52	0.44	19.54	1.27	0.10	0.01	0.03	0.05	0.00	16.66	
Peaches, halves, w/juice, cnd, not drained	0.5	Cup	124.00	54.56	0.78	14.35	1.61	0.04	0.01	0.02	0.02	0.00	23.56	
Peaches, halves, w/light syrup, cnd, not drained	0.5	Cup	125.50	67.77	0.56	18.26	1.63	0.04	0.00	0.02	0.02	0.00	22.59	
Peaches, slices, swtnd, fzn, each	5	Each	77.50	72.85	0.49	18.58	1.39	0.10	0.01	0.04	0.05	0.00	10.85	
Pears, fresh, d'anjou, lrg, each	1	Each	209.00	121.22	0.79	32.31	6.48	0.25	0.01	0.05	0.06	0.00	2.09	
Pears, halves, w/juice, cnd, not drained	0.5	Cup	124.00	62.00	0.43	16.05	1.98	0.09	0.01	0.02	0.02	0.00	0.37	
Pears, halves, w/light syrup, cnd, not drained	0.5	Cup	125.50	71.54	0.24	19.04	2.01	0.04	0.00	0.01	0.01	0.00	0.00	
Pears, sulfured, halves, ckd f/dried	0.5	Cup	90.00	235.80	1.68	62.73	6.75	0.57	0.03	0.12	0.13	0.00	0.13	
Persimmon, native, fresh	1	Each	25.00	31.75	0.20	8.38	0.38	0.10				0.00		
Pineapple, chunks, swtnd, fzn, cup	0.5	Cup	122.50	105.35	0.49	27.20	1.35	0.12	0.01	0.02	0.04	0.00	2.45	
Pineapple, chunks, w/juice, cnd, not drained, cup	0.5	Cup	124.50	74.70	0.52	19.55	1.00	0.10	0.01	0.01	0.04	0.00	2.49	
Pineapple, chunks, w/light syrup, cnd, not drained, cup	0.5	Cup	126.00	65.52	0.45	16.95	1.01	0.15	0.01	0.01	0.05	0.00	2.52	
Pineapple, fresh, dices, cup	0.5	Cup	77.50	37.20	0.42	9.79	1.08	0.09	0.01	0.01	0.03	0.00	2.32	
Pitanga, fresh, each	1	Each	7.00	2.31	0.06	0.52		0.03				0.00	5.25	
Plantain, fresh, med, each	1	Each	179.00	218.38	2.33	57.08	4.12	0.66	0.26	0.06	0.12	0.00	100.24	
Plums, fresh, 2 1/8", each	1	Each	66.00	30.36	0.46	7.54	0.92	0.18	0.01	0.09	0.03	0.00	11.22	
Plums, purple, w/juice, cnd, not drained, cup	0.5	Cup	126.00	73.08	0.64	19.09	1.13	0.03	0.00	0.02	0.01	0.00	63.00	
Plums, purple, w/light syrup, cnd, not drained, cup	0.5	Cup	126.00	79.38	0.47	20.51	1.13	0.13	0.01	0.09	0.03	0.00	15.12	
Pomegranate, fresh, 3 3/8"	1	Each	154.00	104.72	1.46	26.44	0.92	0.46	0.06	0.07	0.10	0.00	7.70	
Prickly Pears, fresh, each	1	Each	103.00	42.23	0.75	9.86	3.71	0.53	0.07	0.08	0.22	0.00	2.06	
Prunes, dried, each	5	Each	42.00	100.80	0.91	26.83	2.98	0.16	0.04	0.02	0.02	0.00	16.38	
Prunes, stwd f/dried w/o add sug	0.5	Cup	124.00	132.68	1.19	34.82	3.84	0.19	0.02	0.13	0.04	0.00	21.08	
Quince, fresh, each	1	Each	92.00	52.44	0.37	14.08	1.75	0.09	0.01	0.03	0.05	0.00	1.84	
Raisins, golden, seedless, packed cup All American Foods	0.25	Cup	41.25	124.58	1.40	32.80	1.65	0.19	0.06	0.01	0.05	0.00	0.00	
Raisins, seedless, packed cup	0.25	Cup	41.25	123.34	1.27	32.66	1.53	0.19	0.02	0.02	0.01	0.00	0.00	
Raspberries, fzn, swtnd, 10oz pkg or cup	0.5	Cup	125.00	128.75	0.87	32.70	5.50	0.20	0.01	0.02	0.11	0.00	3.75	
Raspberries, red, fresh, cup	0.5	Cup	61.50	31.98	0.74	7.34	4.00	0.40	0.01	0.04	0.23	0.00	1.23	

Vit E (mg)	Vit C	Vit B_1-Thia (mg)	Vit B_2-Ribo (mg)	Vit B_3-Nia (mg)	Fol (mcg)	Vit B_6 (mg)	Vita B_{12} (mcg)	Sodi (mg)	Pota (mg)	Cal (mg)	Phos (mg)	Magn (mg)	Iron (mg)	Zinc (mg)	Caff (mg)	Alco (g)	Sol Fiber (g)	Insol Fiber (g)
	21.00						0.00	0.00	75.00	0.00			0.00		0.00	0.00		
0.01	4.58	0.00	0.01	0.08	0.30	0.00	0.00	0.08	27.75	0.83	4.53	1.05	0.04	0.01	0.00	0.00		
0.91	7.94	0.04	0.04	0.29	43.52	0.05	0.00	3.84	115.20	23.04	12.80	14.08	0.55	0.25	0.00	0.00	0.38	2.94
0.39	52.07	0.11	0.07	0.73	31.20	0.15	0.00	3.90	323.70	72.15	39.00	23.40	0.29	0.14	0.00	0.00	2.11	1.40
	1.20						0.00	20.00	10.00	80.00			0.36		0.00	0.00		
1.16	28.67	0.06	0.06	0.61	14.49	0.14	0.00	2.07	161.46	10.35	11.38	9.31	0.13	0.04	0.00	0.00	1.08	0.78
0.12	5.36	0.14	0.02	0.56	22.49	0.09	0.00	26.82	242.20	8.65	10.38	12.11	0.25	0.15	0.00	0.00	0.15	0.45
0.04	18.53	0.01	0.02	0.19	6.80	0.14	0.00	7.65	154.70	9.35	4.25	9.35	0.29	0.06	0.00	0.00		
0.02	15.93	0.03	0.01	0.37	16.81	0.08	0.00	15.93	201.78	5.31	9.73	8.85	0.15	0.08	0.00	0.00		
0.51	87.97	0.02	0.05	0.76	3.82	0.05	0.00	5.10	107.10	1.27	12.75	6.37	0.46	0.09	0.00	0.00		
0.18	1.08	0.01	0.04	0.55	1.13	0.05	0.00	5.10	225.67	10.77	21.83	11.06	0.77	0.14	0.00	0.00		
1.05	7.34	0.05	0.04	1.53	6.80	0.03	0.00	0.00	273.36	8.16	35.36	12.24	0.38	0.23	0.00	0.00	0.76	1.55
0.21	82.74	0.10	0.07	0.59	47.60	0.11	0.00	1.40	232.40	60.20	32.20	15.40	0.18	0.11	0.00	0.00	0.56	2.52
0.36	58.69	0.11	0.05	0.33	47.19	0.08	0.00	0.00	216.59	48.40	20.57	12.10	0.11	0.07	0.00	0.00	1.75	1.27
0.51	43.26	0.02	0.02	0.24	26.60	0.02	0.00	2.10	179.90	16.80	3.50	7.00	0.07	0.05	0.00	0.00		
0.00	5.40	0.00	0.02	0.27	2.52	0.02	0.00	5.04	62.64	2.16	12.24	5.22	0.29	0.02	0.00	0.00	0.94	0.94
1.15	10.36	0.04	0.05	1.27	6.28	0.04	0.00	0.00	298.30	9.42	31.40	14.13	0.39	0.27	0.00	0.00		
0.16	3.84	0.00	0.16	3.50	0.00	0.06	0.00	5.60	796.80	22.40	95.20	33.60	3.24	0.46	0.00	0.00	2.62	3.94
0.48	2.74	0.01	0.02	0.60	2.94	0.02	0.00	5.88	90.16	2.94	10.78	4.90	0.27	0.09	0.00	0.00	0.66	0.61
0.61	4.46	0.01	0.02	0.72	3.72	0.03	0.00	4.96	158.72	7.44	21.08	8.68	0.34	0.13	0.00	0.00	0.45	1.16
0.62	3.01	0.01	0.03	0.74	3.77	0.03	0.00	6.28	121.74	3.77	13.81	6.28	0.45	0.12	0.00	0.00	0.85	0.78
0.48	73.00	0.01	0.03	0.50	2.32	0.02	0.00	4.65	100.75	2.32	8.52	3.87	0.29	0.04	0.00	0.00	0.73	0.67
0.25	8.78	0.03	0.05	0.33	14.63	0.06	0.00	2.09	248.71	18.81	22.99	14.63	0.36	0.21	0.00	0.00	1.35	5.13
0.10	1.98	0.02	0.02	0.25	1.24	0.02	0.00	4.96	119.04	11.16	14.88	8.68	0.36	0.12	0.00	0.00	0.56	1.43
0.10	0.88	0.01	0.02	0.20	1.26	0.02	0.00	6.28	82.83	6.28	8.79	5.02	0.35	0.10	0.00	0.00	0.20	1.81
0.05	6.30	0.01	0.13	1.23	0.00	0.06	0.00	5.40	479.70	30.60	53.10	29.70	1.89	0.35	0.00	0.00	1.35	5.40
0.25	16.50				2.00		0.00	0.25	77.50	6.75	6.50		0.62		0.00	0.00	0.10	0.28
0.03	9.80	0.12	0.04	0.37	13.48	0.09	0.00	2.45	122.50	11.02	4.90	12.25	0.49	0.13	0.00	0.00	0.37	0.98
0.01	11.83	0.12	0.03	0.36	6.23	0.09	0.00	1.25	151.89	17.43	7.47	17.43	0.35	0.12	0.00	0.00	0.25	0.75
0.01	9.45	0.12	0.03	0.37	6.30	0.09	0.00	1.26	132.30	17.64	8.82	20.16	0.49	0.15	0.00	0.00	0.25	0.76
0.02	28.05	0.06	0.02	0.38	11.62	0.08	0.00	0.77	89.12	10.07	6.20	9.30	0.22	0.08	0.00	0.00		
	1.84	0.00	0.00	0.02			0.00	0.21	7.21	0.63	0.77	0.84	0.01		0.00	0.00		
0.25	32.94	0.09	0.10	1.23	39.38	0.54	0.00	7.16	893.21	5.37	60.86	66.23	1.07	0.25	0.00	0.00	1.38	2.74
0.17	6.27	0.02	0.02	0.28	3.30	0.02	0.00	0.00	103.62	3.96	10.56	4.62	0.11	0.07	0.00	0.00	0.30	0.62
0.22	3.53	0.03	0.07	0.59	3.78	0.04	0.00	1.26	194.04	12.60	18.90	10.08	0.43	0.13	0.00	0.00		
0.22	0.50	0.02	0.04	0.38	3.78	0.04	0.00	25.20	117.18	11.34	16.38	6.30	1.08	0.10	0.00	0.00		
0.92	9.39	0.05	0.05	0.46	9.24	0.16	0.00	4.62	398.86	4.62	12.32	4.62	0.46	0.18	0.00	0.00	0.18	0.74
0.01	14.42	0.01	0.06	0.47	6.18	0.06	0.00	5.15	226.60	57.68	24.72	87.55	0.31	0.12	0.00	0.00	0.11	3.59
0.18	0.25	0.02	0.07	0.79	1.68	0.08	0.00	0.84	307.44	18.06	28.98	17.22	0.39	0.19	0.00	0.00	1.25	1.73
0.24	3.60	0.03	0.12	0.89	0.00	0.27	0.00	1.24	398.04	23.56	37.20	22.32	0.50	0.24	0.00	0.00		
0.51	13.80	0.02	0.03	0.18	2.76	0.04	0.00	3.68	181.24	10.12	15.64	7.36	0.64	0.04	0.00	0.00	0.41	1.33
0.05	1.32	0.00	0.08	0.47	1.24	0.13	0.00	4.95	307.73	21.86	47.44	14.44	0.74	0.13	0.00	0.00	0.50	1.16
0.05	0.95	0.04	0.05	0.32	2.06	0.07	0.00	4.54	308.96	20.62	41.66	13.20	0.77	0.09	0.00	0.00	0.22	1.31
0.90	20.62	0.03	0.05	0.29	32.50	0.04	0.00	1.25	142.50	18.75	21.25	16.25	0.81	0.22	0.00	0.00	1.74	3.76
0.54	16.11	0.02	0.02	0.37	12.92	0.04	0.00	0.62	92.87	15.38	17.84	13.53	0.43	0.26	0.00	0.00		

Food Name	Amount	Measure	Weight (g)	Calories	Protein (g)	Total Carb (g)	Dietary Fiber (g)	Total Fat (g)	Sat Fat (g)	Mono Fat (g)	Poly Fat (g)	Chol (mg)	Vit A (mcg RAE)	Vit D (mcg)
FRUITS (continued)														
Raspberries, red, w/heavy syrup, cnd, not drained	0.5	Cup	128.00	116.48	1.06	29.90	4.22	0.16	0.01	0.02	0.09	0.00	2.56	
Rhubarb, ckd f/fzn w/sugar	0.5	Cup	120.00	139.20	0.47	37.44	2.40	0.07	0.02	0.01	0.03	0.00	4.80	
Rhubarb, fresh, diced, cup	0.5	Cup	61.00	12.81	0.55	2.77	1.10	0.12	0.03	0.02	0.06	0.00	3.05	
Strawberries, fresh, halves, cup	0.5	Cup	76.00	24.32	0.51	5.84	1.52	0.23	0.01	0.03	0.12	0.00	0.76	
Strawberries, fzn, unswtnd, cup	0.5	Cup	74.50	26.08	0.32	6.80	1.56	0.08	0.01	0.01	0.04	0.00	1.49	
Strawberries, w/ heavy syrup, cnd, not drained, cup	0.5	Cup	127.00	116.84	0.71	29.88	2.16	0.33	0.02	0.05	0.16	0.00	1.27	0.00
Tamar Hindi, fresh, 3" × 1", each	1	Each	2.00	4.78	0.06	1.25	0.10	0.01	0.01	0.00	0.00	0.00	0.04	
Tangerines, fresh, med, 2 3/8", each	1	Each	84.00	44.52	0.68	11.21	1.51	0.26	0.03	0.05	0.05	0.00	28.56	
Watermelon, fresh, balls, cup	0.5	Cup	77.00	23.10	0.47	5.81	0.31	0.12	0.01	0.03	0.04	0.00	21.56	
GRAINS, FLOURS, AND FRACTIONS														
Barley, pearled, ckd	0.5	Cup	78.50	96.56	1.78	22.15	2.98	0.35	0.07	0.05	0.17	0.00	0.28	
Bran, corn, crude	1	Tablespoon	4.75	10.64	0.40	4.07	3.75	0.04	0.01	0.01	0.02	0.00	0.19	
Bran, oat, ckd	1	Tablespoon	13.69	5.48	0.44	1.57	0.36	0.12	0.02	0.04	0.05	0.00	0.00	
Bran, wheat, crude	1	Tablespoon	3.63	7.84	0.56	2.34	1.55	0.15	0.02	0.02	0.08	0.00	0.02	
Buckwheat	0.25	Cup	42.50	145.77	5.63	30.38	4.25	1.44	0.31	0.44	0.44	0.00	0.00	
Buckwheat, groats, rstd, dry	0.25	Cup	41.00	141.86	4.81	30.73	4.22	1.11	0.25	0.34	0.34	0.00	0.00	
Corn, yellow, dry	0.25	Cup	41.50	151.47	3.91	30.82	3.03	1.96	0.28	0.53	0.90	0.00	4.56	
Cornmeal, white, bolted, w/wheat flour, enrich, self rising	0.25	Cup	42.50	147.90	3.57	31.21	2.68	1.22	0.17	0.33	0.55	0.00	0.00	
Cornmeal, white, degermed, enrich, self rising	0.25	Cup	34.50	122.47	2.90	25.81	2.45	0.60	0.08	0.15	0.25	0.00	0.00	
Cornmeal, white, degermed, unenrich	0.25	Cup	34.50	126.27	2.92	26.79	2.55	0.57	0.08	0.14	0.24	0.00	0.00	
Cornmeal, yellow, bolted, w/wheat flour, enrich, self rising	0.25	Cup	42.50	147.90	3.57	31.21	2.68	1.22	0.17	0.33	0.55	0.00	5.95	
Cornmeal, yellow, degermed, enrich, self rising	0.25	Cup	34.50	122.47	2.90	25.81	2.45	0.60	0.08	0.15	0.25	0.00	7.13	
Cornmeal, yellow, whole grain	0.25	Cup	30.50	110.41	2.48	23.45	2.23	1.10	0.15	0.28	0.50	0.00	3.35	
Flour, acorn, full fat	1	Ounce-weight	28.35	142.03	2.12	15.50	0.62	8.56	1.12	5.42	1.64	0.00	0.85	
Flour, all purpose, white, bleached, enrich	0.25	Cup	31.25	113.75	3.23	23.84	0.84	0.30	0.05	0.03	0.12	0.00	0.00	
Flour, all purpose, white, self rising, enrich	0.25	Cup	31.25	110.62	3.09	23.20	0.84	0.30	0.05	0.03	0.12	0.00	0.00	
Flour, amaranth, whole grain Arrowhead Mills, Inc.	0.25	Cup	22.70	90.80	3.03	15.13	1.51	1.89	0.00			0.00	0.00	
Flour, arrowroot	0.25	Cup	32.00	114.24	0.10	28.21	1.09	0.03	0.01	0.00	0.01	0.00	0.00	
Flour, barley, cup	0.25	Cup	37.00	127.65	3.89	27.58	3.74	0.59	0.12	0.07	0.28	0.00	0.00	
Flour, barley, malt	0.25	Cup	40.50	146.21	4.16	31.71	2.88	0.74	0.16	0.11	0.39	Chol	0.41	
Flour, bread, white, enrich	0.25	Cup	34.25	123.64	4.10	24.84	0.82	0.57	0.08	0.05	0.25	0.00	0.03	
Flour, buckwheat, whole groat	0.25	Cup	30.00	100.50	3.79	21.18	3.00	0.93	0.20	0.28	0.28	0.00	0.00	
Flour, cake, white, enrich, unsifted	0.25	Cup	34.25	123.98	2.81	26.73	0.58	0.30	0.05	0.02	0.13	0.00	0.00	
Flour, corn, masa, enrich	0.25	Cup	28.50	104.02	2.66	21.74	2.74	1.07	0.15	0.28	0.49	0.00	0.05	
Flour, corn, white, whole grain	0.25	Cup	29.25	105.59	2.03	22.48	2.81	1.13	0.16	0.30	0.52	0.00	0.05	
Flour, corn, yellow, degermed, unenrich, cup	0.25	Cup	31.50	118.12	1.76	26.07	0.60	0.44	0.05	0.08	0.22	0.00	3.46	
Flour, corn, yellow, whole grain	0.25	Cup	29.25	105.59	2.03	22.48	3.92	1.13	0.16	0.30	0.52	0.00	3.22	
Flour, garbanzo, tstd Arrowhead Mills, Inc.	0.25	Cup	23.00	82.80	4.60	13.80	2.76	0.92	0.00			0.00	0.00	
Flour, millet, whole grain Arrowhead Mills, Inc.	0.25	Cup	26.50	98.43	3.03	19.69	2.27	1.14	0.00			0.00	0.00	
Flour, oat, whole grain Arrowhead Mills, Inc.	0.25	Cup	22.70	90.80	3.03	15.89	2.27	2.27	0.38			0.00	0.00	
Flour, peanut, defatted	0.25	Cup	15.00	49.05	7.83	5.20	2.37	0.08	0.01	0.04	0.02	0.00	0.00	
Flour, peanut, low fat	0.25	Cup	15.00	64.20	5.07	4.69	2.37	3.28	0.46	1.63	1.04	0.00	0.00	
Flour, potato	0.25	Cup	40.00	142.80	2.76	33.23	2.36	0.13	0.04	0.00	0.07	0.00	0.00	

Vit E (mg)	Vit C	Vit B1-Thia (mg)	Vit B2-Ribo (mg)	Vit B3-Nia (mg)	Fol (mcg)	Vit B6 (mg)	Vita B12 (mcg)	Sodi (mg)	Pota (mg)	Cal (mg)	Phos (mg)	Magn (mg)	Iron (mg)	Zinc (mg)	Caff (mg)	Alco (g)	Sol Fiber (g)	Insol Fiber (g)
0.76	11.14	0.03	0.04	0.57	14.08	0.05	0.00	3.84	120.32	14.08	11.52	15.36	0.54	0.20	0.00	0.00	0.42	3.80
0.33	3.96	0.02	0.03	0.24	6.00	0.02	0.00	1.20	115.20	174.00	9.60	14.40	0.25	0.10	0.00	0.00	0.74	1.66
0.23	4.88	0.01	0.02	0.18	4.27	0.01	0.00	2.44	175.68	52.46	8.54	7.32	0.14	0.06	0.00	0.00	0.34	0.76
0.22	44.69	0.02	0.02	0.29	18.24	0.04	0.00	0.76	116.28	12.16	18.24	9.88	0.32	0.11	0.00	0.00	0.34	1.18
0.22	30.69	0.02	0.03	0.35	12.67	0.02	0.00	1.49	110.26	11.92	9.69	8.20	0.56	0.10	0.00	0.00	0.48	1.08
0.24	40.26	0.03	0.05	0.07	35.56	0.06	0.00	5.08	109.22	16.51	15.24	10.16	0.63	0.12	0.00	0.00		
0.00	0.07	0.01	0.00	0.04	0.28	0.00	0.00	0.56	12.56	1.48	2.26	1.84	0.06	0.00	0.00	0.00		
0.17	22.43	0.05	0.03	0.32	13.44	0.07	0.00	1.68	139.44	31.08	16.80	10.08	0.13	0.06	0.00	0.00	0.91	0.60
0.04	6.24	0.02	0.02	0.14	2.31	0.04	0.00	0.77	86.24	5.39	8.47	7.70	0.18	0.08	0.00	0.00	0.08	0.23
0.00	0.00	0.07	0.05	1.62	12.56	0.09	0.00	2.36	73.01	8.64	42.39	17.27	1.05	0.65	0.00	0.00	0.84	2.15
0.02	0.00	0.00	0.01	0.13	0.19	0.01	0.00	0.33	2.09	1.99	3.42	3.04	0.13	0.07	0.00	0.00	0.04	3.71
0.01	0.00	0.02	0.01	0.02	0.82	0.00	0.00	0.14	12.59	1.37	16.29	5.48	0.12	0.07	0.00	0.00	0.18	0.17
0.05	0.00	0.02	0.02	0.49	2.87	0.05	0.00	0.07	42.91	2.65	36.77	22.18	0.38	0.26	0.00	0.00	0.11	1.44
0.43	0.00	0.05	0.18	2.98	12.75	0.08	0.00	0.42	195.50	7.65	147.47	98.17	0.93	1.02	0.00	0.00		
0.42	0.00	0.09	0.11	2.10	17.22	0.15	0.00	4.51	131.20	6.97	130.79	90.61	1.01	0.99	0.00	0.00		
0.21	0.00	0.17	0.08	1.51	7.88	0.26	0.00	14.52	119.10	2.90	87.15	52.70	1.12	0.91	0.00	0.00		
0.11	0.00	0.30	0.18	2.21	112.20	0.17	0.00	560.57	87.97	127.07	276.67	22.95	2.11	0.59	0.00	0.00		
0.06	0.00	0.23	0.14	1.58	80.38	0.14	0.00	465.06	58.65	120.75	214.93	16.90	1.63	0.34	0.00	0.00	0.64	1.82
0.11	0.00	0.05	0.02	0.34	16.56	0.09	0.00	1.03	55.89	1.72	28.98	13.80	0.38	0.25	0.00	0.00	0.64	1.92
0.11	0.00	0.30	0.18	2.21	112.20	0.17	0.00	560.57	87.97	127.07	276.67	22.95	2.11	0.59	0.00	0.00		
0.06	0.00	0.23	0.14	1.58	80.38	0.14	0.00	465.06	58.65	120.75	214.93	16.90	1.63	0.34	0.00	0.00	0.74	1.71
0.13	0.00	0.12	0.06	1.11	7.62	0.09	0.00	10.67	87.53	1.83	73.50	38.73	1.06	0.56	0.00	0.00	1.28	0.95
	0.00	0.04	0.04	0.68	32.32	0.19	0.00	0.00	201.85	12.19	29.20	31.18	0.34	0.19	0.00	0.00		
0.02	0.00	0.25	0.16	1.84	57.19	0.01	0.00	0.62	33.44	4.69	33.75	6.87	1.45	0.22	0.00	0.00	0.32	0.52
0.02	0.00	0.21	0.12	1.82	61.25	0.02	0.00	396.87	38.75	105.62	185.94	5.94	1.46	0.20	0.00	0.00	0.28	0.56
	0.00		0.05	0.30				0.00	83.23	30.27	45.40		2.04		0.00	0.00		
0.00	0.00	0.00	0.00	0.00	2.24	0.00	0.00	0.64	3.52	12.80	1.60	0.96	0.11	0.02	0.00	0.00		
0.21	0.00	0.14	0.04	2.32	2.96	0.15	0.00	1.48	114.33	11.84	109.52	35.52	0.99	0.74	0.00	0.00		
0.23	0.24	0.12	0.12	2.28	15.39	0.27	0.00	4.46	90.72	14.99	122.72	39.29	1.90	0.84	0.00	0.00		
0.14	0.00	0.27	0.17	2.59	62.68	0.01	0.00	0.68	34.25	5.14	33.22	8.56	1.51	0.30	0.00	0.00		
0.10	0.00	0.13	0.06	1.85	16.20	0.17	0.00	3.30	173.10	12.30	101.10	75.30	1.22	0.94	0.00	0.00		
0.01	0.00	0.31	0.15	2.33	63.70	0.01	0.00	0.68	35.96	4.79	29.11	5.48	2.51	0.22	0.00	0.00	0.21	0.38
0.05	0.00	0.41	0.22	2.80	66.40	0.10	0.00	1.42	84.93	40.18	63.55	31.35	2.05	0.50	0.00	0.00	0.83	1.91
0.13	0.00	0.07	0.02	0.56	7.31	0.11	0.00	1.46	92.14	2.05	79.56	27.20	0.69	0.51	0.00	0.00	0.70	2.11
0.05	0.00	0.02	0.02	0.84	15.12	0.03	0.00	0.31	28.35	0.63	18.90	5.67	0.28	0.12	0.00	0.00		
0.13	0.00	0.07	0.02	0.56	7.31	0.11	0.00	1.46	92.14	2.05	79.56	27.20	0.69	0.51	0.00	0.00	0.99	2.93
	0.00	0.08	0.03	0.37			0.00	0.00	184.00	36.80	78.66		1.66		0.00	0.00		
	0.00	0.17	0.11	0.61				0.00	113.57	0.00			2.04		0.00	0.00		
	0.00	0.11						0.00	79.45	15.13			1.09		0.00	0.00		
0.01	0.00	0.10	0.07	4.05	37.20	0.08	0.00	27.00	193.50	21.00	114.00	55.50	0.32	0.76	0.00	0.00	0.07	2.30
0.30	0.00	0.07	0.02	1.72	19.95	0.04	0.00	0.15	203.70	19.50	76.20	7.20	0.71	0.90	0.00	0.00	0.07	2.30
0.11	1.52	0.09	0.03	1.40	10.00	0.31	0.00	22.00	400.40	26.00	67.20	26.00	0.55	0.21	0.00	0.00		

Food Name	Amount	Measure	Weight (g)	Calories	Protein (g)	Total Carb (g)	Dietary Fiber (g)	Total Fat (g)	Sat Fat (g)	Mono Fat (g)	Poly Fat (g)	Chol (mg)	Vit A (mcg RAE)	Vit D (mcg)
Flour, rice, brown	0.25	Cup	39.50	143.39	2.86	30.20	1.82	1.09	0.22	0.40	0.40	0.00	0.00	
Flour, rice, white	0.25	Cup	39.50	144.57	2.36	31.65	0.95	0.57	0.16	0.17	0.14	0.00	0.00	
Flour, rye wheat, Bohemian style, enrich Pillsbury	0.25	Cup	30.00	100.00	3.00	22.00	2.00	0.00	0.00	0.00	0.00	0.00	0.00	
Flour, rye, dark	0.25	Cup	32.00	103.68	4.49	21.99	7.23	0.86	0.10	0.11	0.38	0.00	0.32	
Flour, rye, light	0.25	Cup	25.50	93.59	2.14	20.46	3.72	0.35	0.03	0.04	0.14	0.00	0.00	
Flour, rye, med	0.25	Cup	25.50	90.27	2.40	19.76	3.72	0.45	0.05	0.05	0.20	0.00	0.00	
Flour, semolina, enrich	0.25	Cup	41.75	150.30	5.29	30.41	1.63	0.45	0.07	0.06	0.18	0.00	0.00	
Flour, semolina, unenrich	0.25	Cup	41.75	150.30	5.29	30.41	1.63	0.45	0.07	0.06	0.18	0.00	0.00	
Flour, soy, full fat, stirred, raw	0.25	Cup	21.00	91.56	7.25	7.39	2.02	4.34	0.63	0.96	2.45	0.00	1.26	
Flour, soy, low fat, stirred	0.25	Cup	22.00	81.84	10.24	8.35	2.24	1.47	0.21	0.32	0.83	0.00	0.44	
Flour, soy, whole Arrowhead Mills, Inc.	0.25	Cup	23.00	100.00	7.00	9.00	4.00	4.50	1.00	2.50	1.00	0.00	0.00	
Flour, triticale, whole grain	0.25	Cup	32.50	109.85	4.28	23.77	4.75	0.59	0.11	0.05	0.26	0.00	0.00	
Flour, whole wheat	0.25	Cup	30.00	101.70	4.11	21.77	3.66	0.56	0.10	0.07	0.23	0.00	0.14	
Grits, corn, yellow, dry Arrowhead Mills, Inc.	0.25	Cup	39.00	130.00	3.00	30.00	1.00	0.00	0.00	0.00	0.00	0.00		
Grits, soy Heller Seasonings & Ingredients Company	0.25	Cup	39.00	109.20	20.28	11.31		0.39				0.00	0.00	
Millet, ckd	0.5	Cup	87.00	103.53	3.06	20.60	1.13	0.87	0.15	0.16	0.44	0.00	0.13	
Oats, rolled, inst, non-gmo, dry, org Grain Millers, Inc.	0.25	Cup	20.37	85.76	2.85	15.07	2.36	1.41	0.26	0.45	0.51	0.00	0.00	
Oats, Scottish, non-gmo, dry Grain Millers, Inc.	0.25	Cup	29.37	123.65	4.11	21.73	3.41	2.03	0.38	0.65	0.73	0.00	0.00	
Polenta, med American Roland Food Corp.	2	Tablespoon	30.00	80.00	2.00	18.00	2.00	0.00	0.00	0.00	0.00	0.00	0.00	
Quinoa, dry	0.25	Cup	42.50	158.95	5.56	29.28	2.50	2.46	0.25	0.65	1.00	0.00	0.00	0.00
Triticale, grain, dry	0.25	Cup	48.00	161.28	6.26	34.62	8.68	1.00	0.17	0.10	0.44	0.00	0.00	
Wheat, bulgur, dry	0.25	Cup	35.00	119.70	4.30	26.55	6.40	0.47	0.08	0.06	0.19	0.00	0.16	
Wheat, durum, grain	0.25	Cup	48.00	162.72	6.57	34.14	5.99	1.18	0.21	0.16	0.47	0.00	0.00	
Wheat, germ, honey crunch, Kretschmer Quaker Oats	2	Tablespoon	16.90	62.87	4.49	9.83	1.73	1.32	0.23	0.18	0.82	0.00	0.00	0.00

GRAIN PRODUCTS, PREPARED AND BAKED GOODS

Bagels

Food Name	Amount	Measure	Weight (g)	Calories	Protein (g)	Total Carb (g)	Dietary Fiber (g)	Total Fat (g)	Sat Fat (g)	Mono Fat (g)	Poly Fat (g)	Chol (mg)	Vit A (mcg RAE)	Vit D (mcg)
Bagel Chips, onion & garlic, tstd Pepperidge Farm	1	Ounce-weight	28.35	111.38	3.04	18.22	2.02	4.56	1.02	3.04	0.00	0.00	0.00	
Bagel, cinnamon raisin, 4 1/2"	1	Each	118.00	323.32	11.56	65.14	2.71	2.01	0.32	0.21	0.79	0.00	24.78	
Bagel, egg, 4 1/2"	1	Each	110.00	305.80	11.66	58.30	2.53	2.31	0.46	0.46	0.71	26.40	36.30	
Bagel, everything, NY style Thomas'	1	Each	104.00	300.00	11.00	54.00	3.00	4.00	1.00			0.00	0.00	
Bagel, oat bran, 3 1/2"	1	Each	71.00	181.05	7.60	37.84	2.56	0.85	0.14	0.18	0.35	0.00	0.71	
Bagel, oat bran, mini, 2 1/2"	1	Each	26.00	66.30	2.78	13.86	0.94	0.31	0.05	0.06	0.13	0.00	0.26	
Bagel, onion, enrich, w/calc propionate, 3 1/2"	1	Each	71.00	195.25	7.45	37.91	1.63	1.14	0.16	0.09	0.49	0.00	0.00	
Bagel, onion, enrich, w/calc propionate, 4 1/2"	1	Each	110.00	302.50	11.55	58.74	2.53	1.76	0.24	0.14	0.77	0.00	0.00	
Bagel, plain, classic Bruegger's Corporation	1	Each	112.22	296.01	10.81	60.36	3.36	1.87				0.00	0.00	0.00
Bagel, salt, classic Bruegger's Corporation	1	Each	114.69	296.01	10.81	60.36	3.36	1.87				0.00	0.00	0.00
Bagel, sesame, classic Bruegger's Corporation	1	Each	114.30	311.01	10.81	60.36	3.36	1.87				0.00	0.00	0.00
Bagel, sun dried tomato basil Natural Ovens	1	Each	85.00	170.00	6.00	38.00	6.00	2.00	0.00			0.00	0.00	
Bagel, whole grain Natural Ovens	1	Each	85.00	170.00	6.00	37.00	6.00	2.00	0.00			0.00	0.00	

Biscuits

Food Name	Amount	Measure	Weight (g)	Calories	Protein (g)	Total Carb (g)	Dietary Fiber (g)	Total Fat (g)	Sat Fat (g)	Mono Fat (g)	Poly Fat (g)	Chol (mg)	Vit A (mcg RAE)	Vit D (mcg)
Biscuit, buttermilk, bkd f/refrig dough, higher fat, 2 1/2"	1	Each	27.00	93.42	1.81	12.83	0.43	3.97	1.00	2.22	0.53	0.00	0.00	
Biscuit, buttermilk, bkd f/refrig dough, lower fat, 2 1/4"	1	Each	21.00	62.79	1.64	11.63	0.40	1.09	0.27	0.59	0.16	0.00	0.00	

Vit E (mg)	Vit C	Vit B₁-Thia (mg)	Vit B₂-Ribo (mg)	Vit B₃-Nia (mg)	Fol (mcg)	Vit B₆ (mg)	Vita B₁₂ (mcg)	Sodi (mg)	Pota (mg)	Cal (mg)	Phos (mg)	Magn (mg)	Iron (mg)	Zinc (mg)	Caff (mg)	Alco (g)	Sol Fiber (g)	Insol Fiber (g)
0.26	0.00	0.17	0.03	2.50	6.32	0.29	0.00	3.16	114.16	4.35	133.12	44.24	0.78	0.97	0.00	0.00	0.20	1.62
0.04	0.00	0.05	0.01	1.03	1.58	0.17	0.00	0.00	30.02	3.95	38.71	13.83	0.14	0.32	0.00	0.00	0.24	0.71
	0.00	0.23	0.14	1.60	40.00			0.00		0.00			1.44		0.00	0.00		
0.45	0.00	0.10	0.09	1.37	19.20	0.14	0.00	0.32	233.60	17.92	202.24	79.36	2.07	1.80	0.00	0.00	1.18	6.05
0.11	0.00	0.09	0.03	0.20	5.61	0.06	0.00	0.51	59.42	5.36	49.47	17.85	0.46	0.45	0.00	0.00	1.50	2.22
0.20	0.00	0.08	0.03	0.44	4.85	0.07	0.00	0.77	86.70	6.12	52.79	19.13	0.54	0.51	0.00	0.00	0.79	2.93
0.11	0.00	0.33	0.24	2.50	76.40	0.04	0.00	0.42	77.65	7.10	56.78	19.62	1.82	0.45	0.00	0.00	0.58	1.04
0.11	0.00	0.11	0.03	1.38	30.06	0.04	0.00	0.42	77.65	7.10	56.78	19.62	0.51	0.45	0.00	0.00	0.58	1.04
0.41	0.00	0.12	0.24	0.91	72.45	0.10	0.00	2.73	528.15	43.26	103.74	90.09	1.34	0.83	0.00	0.00	0.12	1.90
0.04	0.00	0.08	0.07	0.48	90.20	0.12	0.00	3.96	565.40	41.36	130.46	50.38	1.32	0.26	0.00	0.00	0.13	2.11
	0.00	0.15	0.22	1.60				0.00	380.00	40.00			1.80		0.00	0.00		
0.29	0.00	0.12	0.04	0.93	24.05	0.13	0.00	0.65	151.45	11.38	104.33	49.73	0.85	0.87	0.00	0.00	0.79	3.95
0.25	0.00	0.13	0.06	1.91	13.20	0.10	0.00	1.50	121.50	10.20	103.80	41.40	1.16	0.88	0.00	0.00	0.62	3.04
	0.00							0.00	30.00	0.00			0.36		0.00	0.00		
0.00	0.00	0.24	0.12	1.01	0.00	0.20	0.00	3.90	963.30	124.80	284.70	122.07	3.90	2.07	0.00	0.00		
0.02	0.00	0.09	0.07	1.16	16.53	0.10	0.00	1.74	53.94	2.61	87.00	38.28	0.55	0.79	0.00	0.00	0.61	0.52
	0.00							0.90	78.22	11.61	105.92		0.94		0.00	0.00		
	0.00							1.29	112.78	16.74	152.72		1.35		0.00	0.00		
	0.00							0.00		0.00			0.36		0.00	0.00		
2.07	0.00	0.08	0.17	1.25	20.82	0.09	0.00	8.92	314.50	25.50	174.25	89.25	3.93	1.40	0.00	0.00		
0.43	0.00	0.20	0.06	0.68	35.04	0.06	0.00	2.40	159.36	17.76	171.84	62.40	1.24	1.65	0.00	0.00	1.44	7.24
0.02	0.00	0.08	0.04	1.79	9.45	0.12	0.00	5.95	143.50	12.25	105.00	57.40	0.86	0.68	0.00	0.00	1.09	5.32
0.43	0.00	0.20	0.05	3.23	20.64	0.20	0.00	0.96	206.88	16.32	243.84	69.12	1.69	1.99	0.00	0.00	0.71	5.28
3.42	0.00	0.23	0.12	0.80	102.41	0.08	0.00	1.86	162.92	8.45	170.86	45.97	1.36	2.34	0.00	0.00	0.12	1.61
0.00	0.00	0.22	0.14	2.02				283.50		0.00			1.46		0.00	0.00		
0.37	0.83	0.45	0.33	3.63	130.98	0.07	0.00	379.96	174.64	22.42	118.00	33.04	4.48	1.33	0.00	0.00	0.98	1.73
0.15	0.66	0.59	0.26	3.79	96.80	0.10	0.18	555.50	74.80	14.30	92.40	27.50	4.38	0.85	0.00	0.00	0.91	1.62
	0.00							510.00		100.00			3.60		0.00	0.00		
0.23	0.14	0.24	0.24	2.10	69.58	0.03	0.00	359.97	81.65	8.52	78.10	22.01	2.19	0.64	0.00	0.00	1.20	1.36
0.09	0.05	0.09	0.09	0.77	25.48	0.01	0.00	131.82	29.90	3.12	28.60	8.06	0.80	0.23	0.00	0.00	0.44	0.50
0.21	0.00	0.38	0.22	3.24	75.26	0.04	0.00	379.14	71.71	52.54	68.16	20.59	2.53	0.62	0.00	0.00	0.57	1.06
0.32	0.00	0.59	0.35	5.02	116.60	0.06	0.00	587.40	111.10	81.40	105.60	31.90	3.92	0.97	0.00	0.00	0.88	1.65
0.00	0.14	0.48	0.31	3.96	0.13	0.00	0.00	510.00	80.18	14.35	71.02	0.40	3.33	0.01	0.00	0.00		
0.00	0.14	0.48	0.31	3.96	0.13	0.00	0.00	1471.29	80.31	21.76	71.02	0.40	3.33	0.01	0.00	0.00		
0.00	0.14	0.48	0.31	3.96	0.13	0.00	0.00	510.00	80.18	14.35	71.02	0.40	6.57	0.01	0.00	0.00		
	6.00	0.45		8.00		0.60	1.80	270.00		200.00		120.00	1.08	4.50	0.00	0.00		
	0.00	0.45	0.51	8.00		0.60	1.80	200.00		200.00		120.00	1.08	4.50	0.00	0.00		
0.02	0.00	0.09	0.06	0.83	22.41	0.01	0.00	324.54	42.39	5.40	103.95	3.78	0.70	0.10	0.00	0.00	0.26	0.17
0.01	0.00	0.09	0.05	0.72	17.43	0.01	0.00	304.71	38.85	3.99	97.65	3.57	0.65	0.10	0.00	0.00	0.24	0.16

Food Name	Amount	Measure	Weight (g)	Calories	Protein (g)	Total Carb (g)	Dietary Fiber (g)	Total Fat (g)	Sat Fat (g)	Mono Fat (g)	Poly Fat (g)	Chol (mg)	Vit A (mcg RAE)	Vit D (mcg)
GRAIN PRODUCTS, PREPARED AND BAKED GOODS *(continued)*														
Biscuit, buttermilk, cmrcl bkd, 2 1/2"	1	Each	35.00	127.40	2.17	16.97	0.45	5.77	0.87	2.42	2.17	0.35		
Biscuit, buttermilk, dry mix, svg Martha White	1	Each	41.00	171.38	3.03	26.44		5.94	1.12	3.44	0.57			
Biscuit, buttermilk, prep f/dry mix	1	Ounce-weight	28.35	94.97	2.07	13.72	0.51	3.43	0.79	1.19	1.22	1.13	7.37	
Biscuit, buttermilk, prep f/recipe, 2 1/2"	1	Each	60.00	212.40	4.20	26.76	0.91	9.79	2.60	4.16	2.50	1.80	13.80	
Biscuit, buttermilk, refrig dough, svg PI Grands	1	Each	61.00	194.59	4.15	25.07		8.66	2.35	4.85	0.21			
Biscuit, plain, bkd f/refrig dough, higher fat, 2 1/2"	1	Each	27.00	93.42	1.81	12.83	0.43	3.97	1.00	2.22	0.53	0.00	0.00	
Biscuit, plain, cmrcl bkd, 2 1/2"	1	Each	35.00	127.40	2.17	16.97	0.45	5.77	0.87	2.42	2.17	0.35		
Biscuit, plain, prep f/recipe, 2 1/2"	1	Each	60.00	212.40	4.20	26.76	0.91	9.79	2.60	4.16	2.50	1.80	13.80	
Breads and Rolls														
Bread, 7 grain, slice	1	Piece	26.00	65.00	2.60	12.06	1.66	0.99	0.21	0.40	0.24	0.00	0.00	
Bread, banana, homemade w/margarine, slice	1	Piece	60.00	195.60	2.58	32.76	0.66	6.30	1.34	2.69	1.88	25.80	63.60	
Bread, Boston brown, cnd, slice	1	Piece	45.00	87.75	2.34	19.48	2.11	0.67	0.13	0.09	0.25	0.45	11.25	
Bread, cracked wheat, slice, reg	1	Piece	25.00	65.00	2.17	12.38	1.38	0.98	0.23	0.48	0.17	0.00	0.00	
Bread, cracked wheat, slice, thin	1	Piece	20.00	52.00	1.74	9.90	1.10	0.78	0.18	0.38	0.14	0.00	0.00	
Bread, egg, slice	1	Piece	40.00	114.80	3.80	19.12	0.92	2.40	0.64	0.92	0.44	20.40	25.20	
Bread, focaccia Oroweat	1	Piece	57.00	150.00	4.00	31.00	1.00	1.50	0.00			0.00	0.00	
Bread, French, slice, lrg	1	Piece	96.00	263.04	8.45	49.82	2.88	2.88	0.62	1.17	0.67	0.00	0.00	
Bread, garlic Pepperidge Farm	1	Piece	47.00	160.00	5.00	14.00	1.00	10.00	3.00	4.00	1.50	30.00	0.00	
Bread, Health Nut Oroweat	1	Piece	38.00	100.00	4.00	18.00	2.00	2.00	0.00			0.00	0.00	
Bread, Italian, slice, med	1	Piece	20.00	54.20	1.76	10.00	0.54	0.70	0.17	0.16	0.28	0.00	0.00	
Bread, mixed grain, slice, lrg	1	Piece	32.00	80.00	3.20	14.85	2.05	1.22	0.26	0.49	0.30	0.00	0.00	
Bread, multigrain, Carb Counting Oroweat	1	Piece	27.00	60.00	5.00	9.00	3.00	1.50	0.00			0.00	0.00	
Bread, naan, Tandoori style, original Garden of Eatin'	1	Each	71.00	200.00	7.00	35.00	4.00	4.00	1.00			0.00	0.00	
Bread, oat bran, rducd cal, slice	1	Piece	23.00	46.23	1.84	9.50	2.76	0.74	0.10	0.16	0.38	0.00	0.02	
Bread, oat bran, slice	1	Piece	30.00	70.80	3.12	11.94	1.35	1.32	0.21	0.48	0.51	0.00	0.60	
Bread, oatmeal, slice	1	Piece	27.00	72.63	2.27	13.10	1.08	1.19	0.19	0.43	0.46	0.00	1.35	
Bread, pita, wheat, sml, 4"	1	Each	28.00	74.48	2.74	15.40	2.07	0.73	0.11	0.10	0.30	0.00		
Bread, pita, white, enrich, sml, 4"	1	Each	28.00	77.00	2.55	15.60	0.62	0.34	0.05	0.03	0.15	0.00		
Bread, pumpernickel, slice, thin	1	Piece	20.00	50.00	1.74	9.50	1.30	0.62	0.09	0.19	0.25	0.00	0.00	
Bread, pumpkin, dry quick mix Pillsbury	1	Ounce-weight	28.35	111.68	1.72	22.34	0.64	1.29	0.00			0.00		
Bread, raisin, enrich, slice	1	Piece	26.00	71.24	2.05	13.60	1.12	1.14	0.28	0.60	0.18	0.00	0.00	
Bread, rice bran, slice	1	Piece	27.00	65.61	2.40	11.75	1.32	1.24	0.19	0.45	0.48	0.00	0.01	
Bread, rye, slice	1	Piece	32.00	82.88	2.72	15.46	1.86	1.06	0.20	0.42	0.26	0.00	0.13	
Bread, sourdough, slice, med	1	Piece	64.00	175.36	5.63	33.22	1.92	1.92	0.41	0.78	0.44	0.00	0.00	
Bread, sourdough, slice, med, tstd	1	Piece	59.00	175.82	5.66	33.28	1.95	1.95	0.41	0.78	0.44	0.00	0.00	
Bread, wheat berry, slice	1	Piece	25.00	65.00	2.28	11.80	1.08	1.02	0.22	0.43	0.23	0.00	0.00	
Bread, wheat bran, slice	1	Piece	36.00	89.28	3.17	17.21	1.44	1.22	0.28	0.58	0.23	0.00	0.00	
Bread, wheat free, enrich, Papa's, 1/12 loaf or whole Ener-G Foods	1	Piece	42.00	133.05	1.01	18.99	2.77	5.96	0.46			0.00		
Bread, wheat, rducd calorie, slice	1	Piece	23.00	45.54	2.09	10.03	2.76	0.53	0.08	0.06	0.22	0.00	0.00	
Bread, white, rducd cal, slice	1	Piece	23.00	47.61	2.00	10.19	2.23	0.58	0.13	0.25	0.13	0.00	0.03	
Bread, white, soft, enrich, slice	1	Piece	25.00	66.50	1.91	12.65	0.60	0.82	0.18	0.17	0.34	0.00	0.00	
Bread, whole wheat, slice	1	Piece	28.00	68.88	2.72	12.91	1.93	1.18	0.26	0.47	0.28	0.00	0.04	
Breadsticks, focaccia, 133920, FS Pierre Foods	1	Each	42.53	133.00	3.10	22.70		3.40	0.70			0.03		
Breadsticks, plain, 7 5/8" × 5/8"	1	Each	10.00	41.20	1.20	6.84	0.30	0.95	0.14	0.36	0.36	0.00	0.01	
Breadsticks, plain, 9 1/4" × 3/8"	1	Each	6.00	24.72	0.72	4.10	0.18	0.57	0.08	0.21	0.22	0.00	0.00	
Breadsticks, plain, sml, 4 1/4" long	1	Each	5.00	20.60	0.60	3.42	0.15	0.48	0.07	0.18	0.18	0.00	0.00	
Buns, hamburger	1	Each	43.00	119.97	4.09	21.26	0.90	1.86	0.47	0.48	0.85	0.00	0.00	
Buns, hamburger, mixed grain	1	Each	43.00	113.09	4.13	19.18	1.63	2.58	0.60	1.22	0.50	0.00	0.00	

Vit E (mg)	Vit C	Vit B₁-Thia (mg)	Vit B₂-Ribo (mg)	Vit B₃-Nia (mg)	Fol (mcg)	Vit B₆ (mg)	Vita B₁₂ (mcg)	Sodi (mg)	Pota (mg)	Cal (mg)	Phos (mg)	Magn (mg)	Iron (mg)	Zinc (mg)	Caff (mg)	Alco (g)	Sol Fiber (g)	Insol Fiber (g)
0.46	0.00	0.15	0.10	1.17	24.50	0.02	0.05	368.20	78.40	17.15	150.50	5.95	1.15	0.17	0.00	0.00	0.28	0.18
								504.30		60.68					0.00	0.00		
0.11	0.11	0.10	0.10	0.86	14.74	0.02	0.06	270.74	53.30	52.45	133.24	7.09	0.58	0.18	0.00	0.00	0.31	0.20
0.79	0.12	0.22	0.19	1.77	36.60	0.02	0.04	348.00	72.60	141.00	98.40	10.80	1.75	0.33	0.00	0.00	0.55	0.35
								605.12					1.55		0.00	0.00		
0.02	0.00	0.09	0.06	0.83	22.41	0.01	0.00	324.54	42.39	5.40	103.95	3.78	0.70	0.10	0.00	0.00	0.26	0.17
0.46	0.00	0.15	0.10	1.17	24.50	0.02	0.05	368.20	78.40	17.15	150.50	5.95	1.15	0.17	0.00	0.00	0.28	0.18
0.79	0.12	0.22	0.19	1.77	36.60	0.02	0.04	348.00	72.60	141.00	98.40	10.80	1.75	0.33	0.00	0.00	0.55	0.35
0.09	0.08	0.11	0.09	1.13	30.68	0.09	0.02	126.62	53.04	23.66	45.76	13.78	0.90	0.33	0.00	0.00	0.23	1.43
1.07	1.02	0.10	0.12	0.87	19.80	0.09	0.06	181.20	80.40	12.60	34.80	8.40	0.84	0.21	0.00	0.00		
0.14	0.00	0.01	0.05	0.50	4.95	0.04	0.00	283.95	143.10	31.50	50.40	28.35	0.94	0.22	0.00	0.00		
0.15	0.00	0.09	0.06	0.92	15.25	0.08	0.00	134.50	44.25	10.75	38.25	13.00	0.70	0.31	0.00	0.00	0.20	1.17
0.12	0.00	0.07	0.05	0.73	12.20	0.06	0.00	107.60	35.40	8.60	30.60	10.40	0.56	0.25	0.00	0.00	0.16	0.94
0.10	0.00	0.18	0.17	1.94	42.00	0.03	0.04	196.80	46.00	37.20	42.40	7.60	1.22	0.32	0.00	0.00	0.30	0.62
	0.00	0.30	0.17	2.00	0.00			320.00		0.00			1.80		0.00	0.00		
0.29	0.00	0.50	0.32	4.56	142.08	0.04	0.00	584.64	108.48	72.00	100.80	25.92	2.43	0.84	0.00	0.00	0.92	1.96
	0.00	0.23	0.14	1.60				250.00		0.00			3.60		0.00	0.00		
	0.00	0.12	0.07	1.20	24.00			180.00		20.00			1.08		0.00	0.00		
0.06	0.00	0.09	0.06	0.88	38.20	0.01	0.00	116.80	22.00	15.60	20.60	5.40	0.59	0.17	0.00	0.00	0.17	0.37
0.11	0.10	0.13	0.11	1.40	37.76	0.11	0.02	155.84	65.28	29.12	56.32	16.96	1.11	0.41	0.00	0.00	0.29	1.76
	0.00							140.00		40.00			1.08		0.00	0.00		
	0.00							330.00		20.00			1.80		0.00	0.00		
0.06	0.00	0.08	0.05	0.87	18.63	0.02	0.00	80.73	23.46	13.11	31.97	12.65	0.72	0.24	0.00	0.00	1.71	1.05
0.13	0.00	0.15	0.10	1.45	24.30	0.02	0.00	122.10	44.10	19.50	42.30	10.50	0.94	0.27	0.00	0.00		
0.13	0.00	0.11	0.06	0.85	16.74	0.02	0.01	161.73	38.34	17.82	34.02	9.99	0.73	0.28	0.00	0.00	0.29	0.79
0.17	0.00	0.09	0.02	0.80	9.80	0.07	0.00	148.96	47.60	4.20	50.40	19.32	0.86	0.43	0.00	0.00	0.91	1.16
0.08	0.00	0.17	0.09	1.30	29.96	0.01	0.00	150.08	33.60	24.08	27.16	7.28	0.73	0.24	0.00	0.00	0.27	0.34
0.08	0.00	0.07	0.06	0.62	18.60	0.03	0.00	134.20	41.60	13.60	35.60	10.80	0.57	0.30	0.00	0.00	0.60	0.70
	0.00							163.23		17.18			0.61		0.00	0.00		
0.07	0.03	0.09	0.10	0.90	27.56	0.02	0.00	101.40	59.02	17.16	28.34	6.76	0.75	0.19	0.00	0.00	0.26	0.86
0.18	0.00	0.18	0.08	1.84	23.22	0.07	0.00	118.80	58.05	18.63	48.06	21.60	0.97	0.35	0.00	0.00		
0.11	0.13	0.14	0.11	1.22	35.20	0.02	0.00	211.20	53.12	23.36	40.00	12.80	0.91	0.36	0.00	0.00	0.84	1.02
0.19	0.00	0.33	0.21	3.04	94.72	0.03	0.00	389.76	72.32	48.00	67.20	17.28	1.62	0.56	0.00	0.00	0.61	1.31
0.19	0.00	0.27	0.19	2.74	57.23	0.02	0.00	389.99	71.98	47.79	67.26	17.70	1.62	0.56	0.00	0.00	0.63	1.32
0.07	0.00	0.10	0.07	1.03	22.75	0.02	0.00	132.50	50.25	26.25	37.50	11.50	0.83	0.26	0.00	0.00	0.16	0.92
0.12	0.00	0.14	0.10	1.58	37.80	0.06	0.00	174.96	81.72	26.64	66.60	29.16	1.11	0.49	0.00	0.00		
	0.84	0.05	0.13	0.38	24.23				54.17	58.16			3.09		0.00	0.00		
0.06	0.02	0.10	0.07	0.89	20.93	0.03	0.00	117.53	28.06	18.40	23.46	8.97	0.68	0.26	0.00	0.00	0.17	2.59
0.04	0.12	0.09	0.07	0.84	21.85	0.01	0.06	104.19	17.48	21.62	27.83	5.29	0.73	0.31	0.00	0.00	0.13	2.10
0.06	0.00	0.11	0.08	1.10	27.75	0.02	0.00	170.25	25.00	37.75	24.75	5.75	0.94	0.18	0.00	0.00		
0.09	0.00	0.10	0.06	1.07	14.00	0.05	0.00	147.56	70.56	20.16	64.12	24.08	0.92	0.54	0.00	0.00	0.43	1.51
	1.42							169.70	35.30	29.00			0.54		0.00	0.00		
0.10	0.00	0.06	0.06	0.53	16.20	0.01	0.00	65.70	12.40	2.20	12.10	3.20	0.43	0.09	0.00	0.00	0.12	0.18
0.06	0.00	0.04	0.03	0.32	9.72	0.00	0.00	39.42	7.44	1.32	7.26	1.92	0.26	0.05	0.00	0.00	0.07	0.11
0.05	0.00	0.03	0.03	0.26	8.10	0.00	0.00	32.85	6.20	1.10	6.05	1.60	0.21	0.04	0.00	0.00	0.06	0.09
0.03	0.00	0.17	0.14	1.79	47.73	0.03	0.09	205.97	40.42	59.34	26.66	9.03	1.43	0.28	0.00	0.00	0.26	0.65
0.03	0.00	0.20	0.13	1.92	47.73	0.04	0.00	196.94	68.80	40.85	52.46	18.92	1.70	0.45	0.00	0.00		

Food Name	Amount	Measure	Weight (g)	Calories	Protein (g)	Total Carb (g)	Dietary Fiber (g)	Total Fat (g)	Sat Fat (g)	Mono Fat (g)	Poly Fat (g)	Chol (mg)	Vit A (mcg RAE)	Vit D (mcg)
Buns, hot dog/frankfurter	1	Each	43.00	119.97	4.09	21.26	0.90	1.86	0.47	0.48	0.85	0.00	0.00	
Buns, hot dog/frankfurter, rducd cal	1	Each	43.00	84.28	3.57	18.10	2.67	0.86	0.14	0.23	0.33	0.00	0.00	
Cornbread, 2.5 × 2.5 × 1.5 pce	1	Piece	65.00	151.85	4.03	22.66	1.93	4.93	1.57	2.39	0.54	22.08	30.20	0.39
Cornbread, prep f/dry mix, pce	1	Piece	60.00	188.40	4.32	28.86	1.44	6.00	1.64	3.08	0.73	36.60	26.40	
Croissant, butter, mini	1	Each	28.35	115.10	2.32	12.98	0.74	5.95	3.31	1.57	0.31	18.99	58.40	
Dumpling, gnocchi, potato	1	Cup	188.00	268.21	4.76	33.15	1.75	13.10	8.02	3.70	0.63	35.28	123.39	
Pretzels, soft, parmesan herb Auntie Anne's Incorporated	1	Each	120.00	390.00	11.00	74.00	4.00	5.00	2.50			10.00		
Rolls, dinner, brown & serve, browned	1	Each	28.00	84.00	2.35	14.11	0.84	2.04	0.49	1.04	0.34	0.28	0.01	
Rolls, dinner, egg, 2 1/2"	1	Each	35.00	107.45	3.32	18.20	1.29	2.24	0.55	1.03	0.39	17.50	1.75	
Rolls, dinner, prep f/recipe w/2% milk, 2 1/2"	1	Each	35.00	110.60	2.97	18.69	0.66	2.55	0.63	1.01	0.70	12.25	30.45	
Rolls, dinner, wheat, 1oz each	1	Each	28.35	77.40	2.44	13.04	1.08	1.79	0.42	0.88	0.31	0.00	0.00	
Rolls, French	1	Each	38.00	105.26	3.27	19.08	1.22	1.63	0.37	0.75	0.32	0.00	0.00	
Rolls, hard, 3 1/2"	1	Each	57.00	167.01	5.64	30.04	1.31	2.45	0.35	0.65	0.98	0.00	0.00	
Rolls, onion	1	Each	43.00	129.00	3.61	21.67	1.29	3.14	0.75	1.59	0.52	0.43	0.02	

Bread Crumbs, Croutons, Breading Mixes & Batters

Food Name	Amount	Measure	Weight (g)	Calories	Protein (g)	Total Carb (g)	Dietary Fiber (g)	Total Fat (g)	Sat Fat (g)	Mono Fat (g)	Poly Fat (g)	Chol (mg)	Vit A (mcg RAE)	Vit D (mcg)
Bread Crumbs, plain, grated, dry	1	Tablespoon	6.75	26.66	0.90	4.86	0.30	0.36	0.08	0.07	0.14	0.00	0.00	
Bread Crumbs, seasoned, grated, dry	1	Tablespoon	7.50	28.72	1.06	5.14	0.37	0.41	0.10	0.09	0.17	0.08	0.75	
Cracker Meal	0.25	Cup	28.75	110.11	2.67	23.26	0.75	0.49	0.08	0.05	0.21	0.00	0.00	
Croutons, plain, dry	0.25	Cup	7.50	30.52	0.89	5.52	0.39	0.49	0.12	0.22	0.10	0.00	0.00	
Croutons, seasoned, cubes	0.25	Cup	10.00	46.50	1.09	6.36	0.50	1.83	0.53	0.94	0.24	0.70	0.70	

Crackers

Food Name	Amount	Measure	Weight (g)	Calories	Protein (g)	Total Carb (g)	Dietary Fiber (g)	Total Fat (g)	Sat Fat (g)	Mono Fat (g)	Poly Fat (g)	Chol (mg)	Vit A (mcg RAE)	Vit D (mcg)
Crackers, cheese sandwich	4	Each	28.00	133.56	2.60	17.28	0.53	5.91	1.72	3.15	0.72	0.56	4.76	
Crackers, cheese, 1" square, each	30	Each	30.00	150.90	3.03	17.46	0.72	7.59	2.81	3.63	0.74	3.90	8.70	
Crackers, cheese, cheddar, pkg Frito Lay	1	Each	40.00	210.00	3.00	23.00	1.00	11.00	3.00			5.00	0.00	
Crackers, cheese, cheddar, Goldfish Pepperidge Farm	55	Piece	30.00	140.00	4.00	19.00	1.00	6.00				10.00	0.00	
Crackers, cheese, low sod, gold fish	55	Piece	33.00	165.99	3.33	19.21	0.79	8.35	3.18	3.92	0.81	4.29	5.61	
Crackers, cheese, peanut butter sandwich	4	Each	28.00	138.88	3.47	15.89	0.95	7.04	1.23	3.64	1.43	0.00	0.22	0.00
Crackers, cheese, zesty, svg Snackwell's	1	Ounce-weight	28.35	122.19	2.12	21.83	0.57	2.83	0.63	0.77	0.41	1.13		
Crackers, graham, chocolate coated, 2 1/2" square	2	Each	28.00	135.52	1.62	18.62	0.87	6.50	3.74	2.16	0.29	0.00	1.40	
Crackers, graham, cinnamon, lrg rectangle	2	Each	28.00	118.44	1.93	21.50	0.78	2.83	0.43	1.15	1.07	0.00	0.03	
Crackers, graham, svg Nabisco	1	Ounce-weight	28.35	120.20	1.98	21.60	0.96	2.83	0.44	1.02	0.13	0.00	0.00	
Crackers, matzoh, egg, svg	1	Ounce-weight	28.35	110.85	3.49	22.28	0.79	0.60	0.16	0.17	0.13	23.53	3.69	
Crackers, matzoh, whole wheat, svg	1	Ounce-weight	28.35	99.51	3.71	22.37	3.35	0.43	0.07	0.05	0.19	0.00	0.00	
Crackers, melba toast, plain, rounds	10	Each	30.00	117.00	3.63	22.98	1.89	0.96	0.13	0.23	0.38	0.00	0.00	
Crackers, melba toast, pumpernickel	6	Each	30.00	116.70	3.48	23.22	2.40	1.02	0.12	0.30	0.42	0.00	0.00	
Crackers, milk	3	Each	33.00	150.15	2.51	23.00	0.63	5.21	0.87	2.13	1.89	3.63	5.28	
Crackers, peanut butter sandwich	4	Each	28.00	138.32	3.21	16.34	0.64	6.87	1.37	3.85	1.31	0.00	0.01	
Crackers, Ritz, svg Nabisco	1	Ounce-weight	28.35	139.48	2.04	18.20	0.54	6.49	1.08	4.93	0.48	0.00	0.00	
Crackers, rusk toast	3	Each	30.00	122.10	4.05	21.69	0.60	2.16	0.41	0.83	0.69	23.40	3.60	
Crackers, rye, crispbread	3	Each	30.00	109.80	2.37	24.66	4.95	0.39	0.04	0.05	0.17	0.00	0.00	
Crackers, saltines, low sod, fat free	6	Each	30.00	117.90	3.15	24.69	0.81	0.48	0.07	0.04	0.21	0.00	0.00	
Crackers, saltines, low sod, rounds, lrg	3	Each	30.00	130.20	2.76	21.45	0.90	3.54	0.88	1.93	0.50	0.00	0.00	
Crackers, saltines, original, premium, svg Nabisco	10	Each	30.00	126.00	3.27	21.33	0.78	3.06	0.56	1.76	0.52	0.00	0.00	
Crackers, saltines, unsalted tops	10	Each	30.00	130.20	2.76	21.45	0.90	3.54	0.88	1.93	0.50	0.00	0.00	
Crackers, standard, snack type, rectangle	4	Each	32.00	160.64	2.37	19.52	0.51	8.10	1.21	3.40	3.05	0.00	0.00	
Crackers, Wheat Thins, original Nabisco	16	Each	29.00	136.30	2.41	20.04	0.87	5.80	0.93	2.03	0.36	0.00	0.00	
Crackers, wheat, peanut butter sandwich	4	Each	28.00	138.60	3.78	15.06	1.23	7.48	1.29	3.29	2.48	0.00	0.00	
Crackers, whole wheat	4	Each	32.00	141.76	2.82	21.95	3.36	5.50	1.09	1.88	2.11	0.00	0.00	
Crackers, whole wheat, low sod	7	Each	28.00	124.04	2.46	19.21	2.94	4.82	0.95	1.64	1.85	0.00	0.00	

Vit E (mg)	Vit C	Vit B₁- Thia (mg)	Vit B₂- Ribo (mg)	Vit B₃- Nia (mg)	Fol (mcg)	Vit B₆ (mg)	Vita B₁₂ (mcg)	Sodi (mg)	Pota (mg)	Cal (mg)	Phos (mg)	Magn (mg)	Iron (mg)	Zinc (mg)	Caff (mg)	Alco (g)	Sol Fiber (g)	Insol Fiber (g)
0.03	0.00	0.17	0.14	1.79	47.73	0.03	0.09	205.97	40.42	59.34	26.66	9.03	1.43	0.28	0.00	0.00	0.26	0.65
0.03	0.09	0.17	0.08	2.12	47.73	0.02	0.04	190.06	33.54	25.37	36.12	8.60	1.29	0.29	0.00	0.00		
0.64	0.26	0.12	0.16	0.93	5.54	0.05	0.12	355.80	104.75	70.54	193.21	13.17	0.82	0.38	0.00	0.00		
0.72	0.06	0.15	0.16	1.23	33.00	0.06	0.10	466.80	76.80	43.80	225.60	12.00	1.14	0.38	0.00	0.00	0.79	0.65
0.24	0.06	0.11	0.07	0.62	24.95	0.02	0.05	210.92	33.45	10.49	29.77	4.54	0.58	0.21	0.00	0.00	0.49	0.24
0.31	3.51	0.25	0.19	2.19	10.40	0.19	0.13	141.06	245.15	43.68	79.27	20.74	1.44	0.44	0.00	0.00		
	1.20							780.00		80.00			1.80		0.00	0.00		
0.09	0.03	0.14	0.09	1.13	27.44	0.02	0.02	145.88	37.24	33.32	32.48	6.44	0.88	0.22	0.00	0.00	0.31	0.53
0.13	0.00	0.18	0.18	1.15	64.40	0.02	0.08	190.75	36.40	20.65	35.35	8.75	1.23	0.39	0.00	0.00		
0.34	0.07	0.14	0.14	1.21	31.50	0.02	0.05	145.25	53.20	21.00	44.10	6.65	1.04	0.24	0.00	0.00		
0.10	0.00	0.12	0.08	1.15	17.01	0.02	0.00	96.39	32.60	49.90	29.48	10.21	1.01	0.26	0.00	0.00		
0.11	0.00	0.20	0.11	1.65	42.94	0.01	0.00	231.42	43.32	34.58	31.92	7.60	1.03	0.34	0.00	0.00	0.38	0.84
0.24	0.00	0.27	0.19	2.42	54.15	0.02	0.00	310.08	61.56	54.15	57.00	15.39	1.87	0.54	0.00	0.00	0.48	0.83
0.13	0.04	0.21	0.14	1.73	42.14	0.02	0.03	224.03	57.19	51.17	49.88	9.89	1.35	0.33	0.00	0.00	0.47	0.82
0.00	0.00	0.07	0.03	0.45	7.22	0.01	0.02	49.41	13.23	12.35	11.14	2.90	0.33	0.10	0.00	0.00		
0.02	0.20	0.07	0.03	0.46	8.93	0.01	0.00	131.93	17.32	13.65	13.28	3.45	0.37	0.11	0.00	0.00		
0.12	0.00	0.20	0.13	1.64	39.10	0.01	0.00	8.05	33.06	6.61	29.90	6.90	1.33	0.20	0.00	0.00	0.29	0.46
0.02	0.00	0.04	0.02	0.41	9.90	0.00	0.00	52.35	9.30	5.70	8.62	2.32	0.31	0.06	0.00	0.00		
0.04	0.00	0.06	0.04	0.47	10.50	0.01	0.01	123.80	18.10	9.60	14.00	4.20	0.29	0.10	0.00	0.00		
0.07	0.03	0.12	0.20	1.05	28.00	0.01	0.03	392.28	120.12	71.96	113.68	10.08	0.67	0.18	0.00	0.00	0.21	0.33
0.02	0.00	0.17	0.13	1.40	45.60	0.17	0.14	298.50	43.50	45.30	65.40	10.80	1.43	0.34	0.00	0.00	0.27	0.45
	0.00							390.00		100.00			1.08		0.00	0.00		
	0.00	0.23	0.14	1.60				200.00		20.00			1.44		0.00	0.00		
0.10	0.00	0.19	0.14	1.54	29.37	0.19	0.15	151.14	34.98	49.83	71.94	11.88	1.57	0.37	0.00	0.00		
0.66	0.00	0.16	0.08	1.63	26.32	0.05	0.07	198.80	61.04	14.00	75.04	15.68	0.77	0.29	0.00	0.00		
	0.17	0.07	0.09	1.05	16.16	0.03	0.02	297.67	44.51	12.19	56.70	9.36	0.90	0.43	0.00	0.00		
0.07	0.00	0.04	0.06	0.61	5.60	0.02	0.00	81.48	58.52	16.24	37.52	16.24	1.00	0.27	12.88	0.00		
0.09	0.00	0.07	0.08	1.16	12.88	0.02	0.00	169.40	37.80	6.72	29.12	8.40	1.05	0.22	0.00	0.00	0.23	0.55
	0.00	0.07	0.07	1.07	13.04	0.03		186.83	50.18	22.40	57.27	16.73	1.17	0.55	0.00	0.00		
0.28	0.03	0.22	0.18	1.44	6.80	0.02	0.05	5.95	42.53	11.34	41.96	6.80	0.77	0.21	0.00	0.00	0.30	0.49
	0.00	0.10	0.08	1.53	9.92	0.05	0.00	0.57	89.59	6.52	86.47	37.99	1.32	0.74	0.00	0.00	0.94	2.41
0.13	0.00	0.12	0.08	1.23	37.20	0.03	0.00	248.70	60.60	27.90	58.80	17.70	1.11	0.60	0.00	0.00	0.45	1.44
0.18	0.00	0.12	0.06	1.44	25.50	0.00	0.00	269.70	57.90	23.40	54.90	11.70	1.08	0.42	0.00	0.00	0.54	1.86
0.41	0.07	0.18	0.14	1.46	29.70	0.01	0.02	195.36	37.62	56.76	99.99	7.26	1.18	0.22	0.00	0.00	0.24	0.39
0.58	0.00	0.14	0.07	1.71	24.08	0.04	0.00	201.04	60.20	22.68	76.72	15.40	0.77	0.32	0.00	0.00		
	0.00	0.08	0.09	1.08	17.01	0.01	0.00	220.00	26.37	41.67	85.05	5.67	1.15	0.42	0.00	0.00		
0.16	0.00	0.12	0.12	1.39	26.10	0.01	0.05	75.90	73.50	8.10	45.90	10.80	0.82	0.33	0.00	0.00	0.14	0.46
0.24	0.00	0.07	0.04	0.31	14.10	0.06	0.00	79.20	95.70	9.30	80.70	23.40	0.73	0.72	0.00	0.00	1.09	3.86
0.04	0.00	0.16	0.18	1.71	37.20	0.03	0.00	190.80	34.50	6.60	33.90	7.80	2.32	0.28	0.00	0.00		
0.04	0.00	0.17	0.14	1.57	37.20	0.01	0.00	190.80	217.20	35.70	31.50	8.10	1.62	0.23	0.00	0.00	0.34	0.56
	0.00	0.10	0.13	1.31	25.20	0.01		381.00	29.70	57.90	29.70	6.30	1.56		0.00	0.00		
0.47	0.00	0.17	0.14	1.57	37.20	0.01	0.00	229.80	38.40	35.70	31.50	8.10	1.62	0.23	0.00	0.00	0.35	0.55
0.65	0.00	0.13	0.11	1.29	28.80	0.02	0.00	271.04	42.56	38.40	72.96	8.64	1.15	0.21	0.00	0.00	0.19	0.32
	0.00	0.09	0.09	1.16	12.18	0.03		167.62	56.26	23.20	60.32	15.08	1.07		0.00	0.00		
0.17	0.00	0.11	0.08	1.64	19.60	0.04	0.00	225.96	83.16	47.60	97.16	10.64	0.75	0.23	0.00	0.00	0.27	0.96
0.28	0.00	0.06	0.03	1.45	8.96	0.05	0.00	210.88	95.04	16.00	94.40	31.68	0.98	0.69	0.00	0.00	0.67	2.69
0.24	0.00	0.06	0.03	1.27	7.84	0.05	0.00	69.16	83.16	14.00	82.60	27.72	0.86	0.61	0.00	0.00		

Food Name	Amount	Measure	Weight (g)	Calories	Protein (g)	Total Carb (g)	Dietary Fiber (g)	Total Fat (g)	Sat Fat (g)	Mono Fat (g)	Poly Fat (g)	Chol (mg)	Vit A (mcg RAE)	Vit D (mcg)
GRAIN PRODUCTS, PREPARED AND BAKED GOODS *(continued)*														
Muffins														
English Muffin, cinnamon raisin Oroweat	1	Each	69.00	170.00	5.00	36.00	4.00	1.50	0.00			0.00	0.00	
English Muffin, granola	1	Each	66.00	155.10	6.01	30.56	1.85	1.19	0.15	0.55	0.37	0.00	0.00	
English Muffin, plain Thomas'	1	Each	57.00	131.67	4.96	25.99		0.85	0.17	0.25	0.44		0.00	
English Muffin, raisin cinnamon	1	Each	57.00	138.51	4.27	27.76	1.65	1.54	0.22	0.29	0.78	0.00		
English Muffin, sourdough Oroweat	1	Each	59.00	140.00	5.00	28.00	1.00	1.00	0.00			0.00	0.00	
English Muffin, wheat	1	Each	57.00	127.11	4.96	25.54	2.62	1.14	0.16	0.16	0.48	0.00	0.09	
English Muffin, whole wheat	1	Each	66.00	133.98	5.81	26.66	4.42	1.39	0.22	0.34	0.55	0.00	0.17	
Muffin, banana walnut, fzn, 4oz Krusteaz	1	Each	114.00	430.92	7.18	53.58	1.71	20.75	3.65	6.16	10.94	83.22		
Muffin, blackberry, fzn Krusteaz	1	Each	114.00	419.52	6.84	51.30	1.82	20.75	3.76	6.38	10.49	70.68		
Muffin, blueberry, cmrcl, med, 2" × 2 3/4"	1	Each	57.00	157.89	3.13	27.36	1.48	3.70	0.80	1.12	1.42	17.10	13.11	
Muffin, blueberry, dry mix, svg Martha White	1		40.00	161.60	2.04	30.44		3.52	0.86	1.72	0.42			
Muffin, blueberry, prep f/recipe w/2% milk	1	Each	57.00	162.45	3.70	23.20	1.08	6.16	1.16	1.48	3.07	21.09	21.66	
Muffin, blueberry, toaster, tstd	1	Each	31.00	103.23	1.52	17.58	0.59	3.13	0.48	0.74	1.70	1.55	31.31	
Muffin, corn, prep f/recipe w/2% milk, 2" × 2 3/4"	1	Each	57.00	180.12	4.05	25.19	1.94	7.01	1.32	1.72	3.51	23.94		
Muffin, oat bran, 2 1/4" × 2 1/2"	1	Each	57.00	153.90	3.99	27.53	2.62	4.22	0.62	0.97	2.35	0.00	0.00	
Muffin, plain, prep f/recipe w/2% milk	1	Each	57.00	168.72	3.93	23.60	1.54	6.50	1.23	1.57	3.26	22.23	22.80	
Muffin, whole wheat, low fat, prep f/dry mix, 2 oz each Krusteaz	1	Each	56.70	150.00	3.00	32.00	1.00	1.00	0.00	0.50	0.50	0.00	0.00	
Pancakes, French Toast, and Waffles														
Crepe, chocolate filled	1	Each	78.00	118.58	4.30	15.56	0.66	4.49	1.82	1.65	0.63	56.20	53.92	0.70
French Toast, prep f/recipe w/2% milk	1	Piece	65.00	148.85	5.00	16.25	0.56	7.02	1.77	2.94	1.68	75.40	80.60	
French Toast, rth, fzn	1	Piece	59.00	125.67	4.37	18.94	0.65	3.60	0.91	1.20	0.72	48.38	31.86	
Pancakes, blueberry, prep f/recipe, 6"	1	Each	77.00	170.94	4.70	22.33	0.92	7.08	1.53	1.78	3.21	43.12	38.50	
Pancakes, buttermilk Eggo	1	Each	42.53	99.08	2.55	16.20	0.47	2.84	0.61	1.25	0.91	4.68		
Pancakes, buttermilk, mini, ready to microwave, fzn, svg Krusteaz	1	Each	54.00	116.10	3.62	21.71		1.62	0.24	0.67	0.27			
Pancakes, plain, prep f/complete dry mix, 4"	1	Each	38.00	73.72	1.98	13.95	0.49	0.95	0.19	0.34	0.31	4.56	3.80	
Pancakes, plain, prep f/recipe, 4"	1	Each	38.00	86.26	2.43	10.75	0.56	3.69	0.80	0.94	1.69	22.42	20.52	
Pancakes, plain, prep f/recipe, 6"	1	Each	77.00	174.79	4.93	21.79	1.14	7.47	1.63	1.90	3.42	45.43	41.58	
Pancakes, plain, rth, fzn, 4"	1	Each	36.00	82.44	1.87	15.70	0.65	1.19	0.28	0.43	0.35	3.24	10.44	
Pancakes, potato, prep f/recipe, each	1	Each	76.00	206.72	4.69	21.76	1.52	11.58	2.32	3.52	4.97	72.96	5.32	
Pancakes, whole wheat, prep f/incomplete dry mix, 4"	1	Each	44.00	91.52	3.74	12.94	1.23	2.86	0.77	0.77	1.06	26.84	28.16	
Waffles, homestyle, low fat, fzn Eggo	1	Each	35.00	82.60	2.47	15.45	0.35	1.25	0.32	0.35	0.38	8.75		
Waffles, plain, rth, fzn, 4"	1	Each	35.00	87.85	2.06	13.51	0.77	2.73	0.45	1.10	0.97	11.20	133.70	
Waffles, wildberry, fzn Hungry Jack	1	Each	35.50	100.00	1.50	16.50	0.50	3.00	1.00			0.00		
Pasta														
Couscous, ckd	0.5	Cup	78.50	87.92	2.97	18.23	1.10	0.13	0.03	0.01	0.06	0.00	0.00	
Dish, ravioli, cheese, light, preckd Di Giorno	1	Cup	101.00	280.00	15.00	40.00	2.00	7.00	4.00			40.00		
Dish, tortellini, cheese filled	1	Cup	108.00	331.56	14.58	50.76	2.05	7.81	3.89	2.23	0.50	45.36	41.04	
Pasta, chow mein noodles, ckd Frieda's Specialty Produce	3	Ounce-weight	85.05	249.00	6.75	52.50	1.50	0.75	0.00			11.25	0.00	
Pasta, egg noodles, enrich, ckd	0.5	Cup	80.00	106.40	3.80	19.87	0.88	1.18	0.25	0.34	0.32	26.40	4.80	
Pasta, egg noodles, enrich, ckd w/salt	0.5	Cup	80.00	106.40	3.80	19.87	0.88	1.18	0.25	0.34	0.32	26.40	4.80	
Pasta, egg noodles, spinach, enrich, ckd	0.5	Cup	80.00	105.60	4.03	19.40	1.84	1.25	0.29	0.40	0.28	26.40	8.00	
Pasta, fettuccine noodles, spinach, preckd Di Giorno	3	Ounce-weight	85.05	228.00	9.60	45.60	2.40	1.80	0.00			0.00		
Pasta, macaroni noodles, enrich, dry	0.25	Cup	26.25	97.39	3.36	19.61	0.63	0.42	0.06	0.05	0.17	0.00	0.00	
Pasta, macaroni noodles, unenrich, dry	0.25	Cup	26.25	97.39	3.36	19.61	0.63	0.42	0.06	0.05	0.17	0.00	0.00	

Vit E (mg)	Vit C	Vit B₁-Thia (mg)	Vit B₂-Ribo (mg)	Vit B₃-Nia (mg)	Fol (mcg)	Vit B₆ (mg)	Vita B₁₂ (mcg)	Sodi (mg)	Pota (mg)	Cal (mg)	Phos (mg)	Magn (mg)	Iron (mg)	Zinc (mg)	Caff (mg)	Alco (g)	Sol Fiber (g)	Insol Fiber (g)
	0.00	0.12	0.07	1.20	24.00			220.00		40.00			1.80		0.00	0.00		
0.00	0.00	0.28	0.21	2.36	52.80	0.03	0.00	274.56	102.96	129.36	53.46	27.06	1.99	0.92	0.00	0.00		
0.99	0.06				82.65		0.21	210.33		76.38			1.70		0.00	0.00		
0.18	0.17	0.22	0.17	2.03	63.84	0.04	0.00	254.79	118.56	83.79	39.33	8.55	1.38	0.57	0.00	0.00		
	0.00							250.00		60.00			1.80		0.00	0.00		
0.26	0.00	0.25	0.17	1.91	36.48	0.05	0.00	217.74	106.02	101.46	60.99	21.09	1.64	0.61	0.00	0.00		
0.27	0.00	0.20	0.09	2.25	32.34	0.11	0.00	420.42	138.60	174.90	186.12	46.86	1.62	1.06	0.00	0.00	1.28	3.14
	0.00							427.50	134.52	33.52	169.86		1.48		0.00	0.00		
	0.00							427.50	123.12	33.52	159.60		1.62		0.00	0.00		
0.47	0.63	0.08	0.07	0.63	42.18	0.01	0.33	254.79	70.11	32.49	112.29	9.12	0.92	0.28	0.00	0.00	0.42	1.07
								343.20							0.00	0.00		
0.97	0.85	0.16	0.16	1.26	27.36	0.02	0.08	251.37	70.11	107.73	82.65	9.12	1.29	0.31	0.00	0.00	0.29	0.79
0.30	0.00	0.06	0.09	0.60	18.29	0.01	0.00	157.79	27.28	4.34	59.52	4.65	0.17	0.15	0.00	0.00	0.12	0.47
1.03	0.17	0.17	0.18	1.36	42.75	0.05	0.09	333.45	82.65	147.63	100.89	13.11	1.49	0.35	0.00	0.00	0.13	1.81
0.38	0.00	0.15	0.05	0.24	50.73	0.09	0.01	224.01	288.99	35.91	214.32	89.49	2.39	1.05	0.00	0.00	0.82	1.81
1.03	0.17	0.16	0.17	1.32	29.07	0.02	0.09	266.19	68.97	114.00	87.21	9.69	1.36	0.32	0.00	0.00	0.40	1.14
	0.00							380.00	70.00	70.00	150.00		0.60		0.00	0.00		
0.36	0.48	0.07	0.20	0.46	7.96	0.04	0.27	86.81	126.55	81.07	89.47	12.18	0.68	0.46		0.00		
0.71	0.19	0.13	0.21	1.06	27.95	0.05	0.20	311.35	87.10	65.00	76.05	11.05	1.09	0.44	0.00	0.00		
0.40	0.18	0.16	0.23	1.60	30.68	0.30	0.99	292.05	79.06	63.13	82.01	10.03	1.30	0.46	0.00	0.00		
	1.69	0.15	0.21	1.18	27.72	0.03	0.15	317.24	106.26	158.62	116.27	12.32	1.32	0.41	0.00	0.00	0.20	0.72
0.00	0.60	0.11	0.12	1.47	22.11	0.15	0.44	225.38	43.80	14.88	145.01	7.65	1.32	0.26	0.00	0.00		
								289.98					1.46		0.00	0.00		
0.32	0.08	0.08	0.08	0.65	14.06	0.03	0.08	238.64	66.50	47.88	126.92	7.60	0.59	0.15	0.00	0.00	0.11	0.38
0.36	0.11	0.08	0.11	0.59	14.44	0.02	0.08	166.82	50.16	83.22	60.42	6.08	0.68	0.21	0.00	0.00	0.12	0.44
0.73	0.23	0.15	0.22	1.20	29.26	0.03	0.17	338.03	101.64	168.63	122.43	12.32	1.39	0.43	0.00	0.00	0.25	0.89
0.10	0.11	0.14	0.17	1.44	16.20	0.03	0.06	183.24	26.28	22.32	133.92	5.04	1.25	0.24	0.00	0.00	0.14	0.51
1.52	16.72	0.10	0.13	1.63	17.48	0.29	0.14	386.08	597.36	18.24	84.36	25.08	1.19	0.63	0.00	0.00	0.25	1.27
0.00	0.22	0.09	0.23	1.02	12.76	0.05	0.13	251.68	122.76	110.00	164.12	20.24	1.37	0.46	0.00	0.00	0.22	1.01
	0.00	0.31	0.26	2.60	26.95	0.16	0.55	154.70	50.05	20.30	28.35	23.80	1.94		0.00	0.00		
0.22	0.00	0.16	0.18	1.64	21.35	0.33	0.83	261.80	42.70	77.35	139.65	7.35	1.49	0.19	0.00	0.00	0.17	0.60
	0.00	0.15	0.17	2.00	20.00	0.20	0.60	270.00		10.00			1.80		0.00	0.00		
0.10	0.00	0.04	0.01	0.77	11.77	0.04	0.00	3.92	45.53	6.28	17.27	6.28	0.30	0.20	0.00	0.00	0.31	0.78
	0.00	0.60	0.43	3.00	60.00			400.00	170.00	250.00	250.00		1.80		0.00	0.00		
0.17	0.00	0.34	0.33	2.91	79.92	0.05	0.17	371.52	96.12	164.16	228.96	22.68	1.62	1.10	0.00	0.00		
	0.00							351.00		15.00			2.70		0.00	0.00		
0.13	0.00	0.15	0.06	1.19	51.20	0.03	0.07	5.60	22.40	9.60	55.20	15.20	1.27	0.50	0.00	0.00	0.21	0.67
0.04	0.00	0.15	0.06	1.19	51.20	0.03	0.07	132.00	22.40	9.60	55.20	15.20	1.27	0.50	0.00	0.00	0.24	0.64
0.46	0.00	0.20	0.10	1.18	51.20	0.09	0.11	9.60	29.60	15.20	45.60	19.20	0.87	0.50	0.00	0.00	0.32	1.52
	0.00	0.54	0.31	4.80	72.00			192.00	264.00	48.00	120.00	48.00	2.16		0.00	0.00		
0.02	0.00	0.27	0.11	1.97	72.97	0.03	0.00	1.84	42.52	4.72	39.37	12.60	1.01	0.32	0.00	0.00	0.10	0.53
0.03	0.00	0.02	0.01	0.45	4.72	0.03	0.00	1.84	42.52	4.72	39.37	12.60	0.34	0.32	0.00	0.00	0.10	0.53

Food Name	Amount	Measure	Weight (g)	Calories	Protein (g)	Total Carb (g)	Dietary Fiber (g)	Total Fat (g)	Sat Fat (g)	Mono Fat (g)	Poly Fat (g)	Chol (mg)	Vit A (mcg RAE)	Vit D (mcg)
GRAIN PRODUCTS, PREPARED AND BAKED GOODS *(continued)*														
Pasta, macaroni noodles, veg, enrich, dry	0.25	Cup	21.00	77.07	2.76	15.72	0.90	0.22	0.03	0.03	0.09	0.00	1.68	
Pasta, macaroni noodles, whole wheat, dry	0.25	Cup	26.25	91.35	3.84	19.70	2.18	0.37	0.07	0.05	0.15	0.00	0.00	
Pasta, noodles, cellophane, dehyd	0.25	Cup	35.00	122.85	0.06	30.13	0.18	0.02	0.01	0.00	0.01	0.00	0.00	
Pasta, noodles, fresh refrigerated, as purchased	3	Ounce-weight	85.05	244.94	9.62	46.55	3.32	1.96	0.28	0.23	0.80	62.09	11.91	
Pasta, noodles, fresh refrigerated, ckd	3	Ounce-weight	85.05	111.42	4.38	21.20	1.49	0.89	0.13	0.10	0.36	28.07	5.10	
Pasta, prep f/recipe w/o egg, ckd	3	Ounce-weight	85.05	105.46	3.72	21.37	1.36	0.83	0.12	0.16	0.43	0.00	0.00	
Pasta, ramen noodles, ckd	0.5	Cup	113.50	76.76	1.66	10.10	0.58	3.25	0.83	0.59	1.65	0.11	1.22	0.00
Pasta, ramen noodles, dry, pkg Westbrae Natural	1	Ounce-weight	28.35	96.99	2.98	20.89	2.24	0.37	0.00			0.00	0.00	
Pasta, rice noodle, ckd, cup	0.5	Cup	88.00	95.92	0.80	21.91	0.88	0.18	0.02	0.03	0.02	0.00	0.00	
Pasta, rice noodle, dry	1	Ounce-weight	28.35	103.19	0.97	23.60	0.45	0.16	0.04	0.05	0.04	0.00	0.00	
Pasta, shells, sml, enrich, ckd	0.5	Cup	57.50	81.08	2.74	16.30	0.74	0.38	0.06	0.04	0.16	0.00	0.00	
Pasta, soba noodles, dry	1	Ounce-weight	28.35	95.26	4.08	21.15		0.20	0.04	0.05	0.06	0.00	0.00	
Pasta, somen noodles, dry	1	Ounce-weight	28.35	100.93	3.22	21.01	1.22	0.23	0.03	0.03	0.09	0.00	0.00	0.00
Pasta, spaghetti noodles, enrich, ckd	0.5	Cup	70.00	98.70	3.34	19.84	1.19	0.47	0.06	0.06	0.19	0.00	0.00	
Pasta, spaghetti noodles, enrich, ckd w/salt	0.5	Cup	70.00	98.70	3.34	19.84	1.19	0.47	0.06	0.06	0.19	0.00	0.00	
Pasta, spaghetti noodles, spinach, dry	1	Ounce-weight	28.35	105.46	3.78	21.21	3.01	0.44	0.06	0.05	0.18	0.00	6.52	
Pasta, spaghetti noodles, unenrich, ckd w/salt	0.5	Cup	70.00	98.70	3.34	19.84	1.05	0.47	0.06	0.06	0.19	0.00		
Pasta, spaghetti noodles, unenrich, dry	1	Ounce-weight	28.35	105.18	3.62	21.17	0.68	0.45	0.06	0.05	0.19	0.00	0.00	
Pasta, spaghetti noodles, whole wheat, dry	1	Ounce-weight	28.35	98.66	4.15	21.27	3.60	0.40	0.07	0.06	0.16	0.00	0.00	
Pasta, spinach noodles, fresh refrigerated, as purchased	3	Ounce-weight	85.05	245.79	9.57	47.39	2.81	1.79	0.41	0.56	0.39	62.09	21.26	
Pasta, udon noodles, ckd	3	Ounce-weight	85.05	85.90	2.13	17.27	0.09	0.43					0.00	
Rice														
Bran, rice, crude	1	Tablespoon	7.38	23.32	0.98	3.67	1.55	1.54	0.31	0.56	0.55	0.00	0.00	
Rice, basmati, white, Calif, dry Lundberg Family Foods	0.25	Cup	51.20	182.78	3.92	40.72	0.33	0.63	0.21	0.16	0.23	0.00	0.00	
Rice, brown, med grain, dry	0.25	Cup	47.50	171.95	3.56	36.18	1.62	1.28	0.25	0.46	0.45	0.00	0.00	0.00
Rice, white, long grain, enrich, inst, dry	0.25	Cup	23.75	90.01	1.82	19.86	0.38	0.07	0.02	0.02	0.02	0.00	0.00	
Rice, white, long grain, enrich, parboiled, ckd	0.5	Cup	87.50	99.75	2.00	21.64	0.35	0.24	0.06	0.08	0.06	0.00	0.00	
Rice, white, med grain, ckd	0.5	Cup	93.00	120.90	2.22	26.59	0.28	0.20	0.06	0.06	0.05	0.00	0.00	0.00
Rice, white, med grain, unenrich, dry	0.25	Cup	48.75	175.50	3.22	38.68	0.57	0.28	0.08	0.09	0.08	0.00		
Stuffing and Mixes														
Baking Mix, basic, dairy free Ener-G Foods	0.33	Cup	43.00	150.73	7.25	30.13	4.29	0.10	0.03			0.00	0.00	0.00
Baking Mix, dry, Bisquick	0.33	Cup	40.00	161.60	2.80	24.40	0.72	6.00	1.60	2.48	0.52	0.00	0.00	
Baking Mix, rducd fat, Bisquick	0.33	Cup	40.00	150.00	3.00	28.00	0.50	2.50	0.50			0.00		
Stuffing, cornbread, prep f/dry mix, 6oz pkg	0.5	Cup	100.00	179.00	2.90	21.90	2.90	8.80	1.76	3.86	2.71	0.00	78.00	
Tortillas and Taco/Tostada Shells														
Taco Shells, bkd, lrg, 6 1/2"	1	Each	21.00	98.28	1.51	13.10	1.58	4.75	0.68	1.87	1.78	0.00	0.02	
Tortilla, corn, med, 6", unsalted	1	Each	26.00	57.72	1.48	12.12	1.35	0.65	0.09	0.17	0.29	0.00	0.00	
Tortilla, flour, soft taco, Mission Foods	1	Each	51.00	146.37	4.44	25.30		3.06	0.35	1.41	0.47			
Tortilla, flour, white, enrich, dry mix	0.25	Cup	27.75	112.39	2.68	18.63	0.52	2.95	1.14	1.26	0.42	0.00	0.00	
Tortilla, whole wheat	1	Each	35.00	73.15	2.94	19.98	1.89	0.45	0.08	0.06	0.19	0.00	0.00	0.00
GRANOLA BARS, CEREAL BARS, DIET BARS, SCONES, AND TARTS														
Bar, breakfast, chocolate chip, chewy Carnation	1	Each	35.96	150.00	2.00	24.00	1.00	6.00	2.00			0.00		2.50
Bar, breakfast, peanut butter chocolate chip, chewy Carnation	1	Each	35.96	150.00	3.00	22.00	0.50	5.00	1.50			0.00		2.50

Vit E (mg)	Vit C	Vit B₁-Thia (mg)	Vit B₂-Ribo (mg)	Vit B₃-Nia (mg)	Fol (mcg)	Vit B₆ (mg)	Vita B₁₂ (mcg)	Sodi (mg)	Pota (mg)	Cal (mg)	Phos (mg)	Magn (mg)	Iron (mg)	Zinc (mg)	Caff (mg)	Alco (g)	Sol Fiber (g)	Insol Fiber (g)
0.02	0.00	0.22	0.11	1.54	58.38	0.03	0.00	9.03	59.85	7.14	24.36	9.66	0.90	0.16	0.00	0.00	0.13	0.77
0.03	0.00	0.13	0.04	1.35	14.96	0.06	0.00	2.10	56.44	10.50	67.72	37.54	0.95	0.62	0.00	0.00	0.50	1.68
0.04	0.00	0.05	0.00	0.07	0.70	0.02	0.00	3.50	3.50	8.75	11.20	1.05	0.76	0.15	0.00	0.00		
0.28	0.00	0.60	0.37	2.85	149.69	0.08	0.26	22.11	152.24	12.76	138.63	39.12	2.85	1.04	0.00	0.00	0.52	2.81
0.13	0.00	0.18	0.13	0.84	54.43	0.03	0.12	5.10	20.41	5.10	53.58	15.31	0.97	0.47	0.00	0.00	0.22	1.27
0.13	0.00	0.15	0.13	1.14	36.57	0.02	0.00	62.94	16.16	5.10	34.02	11.91	0.96	0.32	0.00	0.00	0.27	1.09
1.17	0.01	0.01	0.01	0.13	1.57	0.01	0.00	400.95	24.54	6.53	12.10	5.18	0.19	0.09	0.00	0.00	0.09	0.49
	0.00	0.09	0.03	0.60				119.37		0.00					0.00	0.00		
	0.00	0.02	0.01	0.06	2.64	0.01	0.00	16.72	3.52	3.52	17.60	2.64	0.13	0.22	0.00	0.00		
	0.00	0.01	0.01	0.06	0.85	0.01	0.00	51.60	8.50	5.10	43.38	3.40	0.20	0.21	0.00	0.00		
0.04	0.00	0.12	0.06	0.96	44.28	0.02	0.00	0.57	17.82	4.03	31.05	10.35	0.80	0.30	0.00	0.00	0.12	0.63
	0.00	0.13	0.04	0.91	17.01	0.07	0.00	224.53	71.44	9.92	72.01	26.93	0.77	0.48	0.00	0.00		
0.02	0.00	0.03	0.01	0.25	3.97	0.02	0.00	521.64	46.49	6.52	22.68	7.94	0.38	0.13	0.00	0.00		
0.04	0.00	0.14	0.07	1.17	53.90	0.02	0.00	0.70	21.70	4.90	37.80	12.60	0.98	0.37	0.00	0.00	0.55	0.64
0.04	0.00	0.14	0.07	1.17	53.90	0.02	0.00	70.00	21.70	4.90	37.80	12.60	0.98	0.37	0.00	0.00	0.55	0.64
0.18	0.00	0.11	0.06	1.29	13.61	0.09	0.00	10.21	106.60	16.44	94.12	49.33	0.60	0.78	0.00	0.00	0.60	2.41
0.04	0.00	0.02	0.02	0.28	4.90	0.02	0.00	70.00	21.70	4.90	37.80	12.60	0.35	0.37	0.00	0.00	0.48	0.56
0.05	0.00	0.03	0.02	0.48	5.10	0.03	0.00	1.98	45.93	5.10	42.52	13.61	0.37	0.35	0.00	0.00	0.10	0.58
0.04	0.00	0.14	0.04	1.45	16.16	0.06	0.00	2.27	60.95	11.34	73.14	40.54	1.03	0.67	0.00	0.00	0.65	2.95
0.28	0.00	0.52	0.34	2.94	150.54	0.27	0.26	22.96	231.34	36.57	125.87	53.58	2.81	1.19	0.00	0.00	0.43	2.38
	0.00	0.02	0.01	0.09				38.27	5.10	5.95	15.31		0.17		0.00	0.00		
0.36	0.00	0.20	0.02	2.51	4.65	0.30	0.00	0.37	109.59	4.21	123.76	57.64	1.37	0.45	0.00	0.00	0.10	1.45
	0.14							2.51		3.54			0.22		0.00	0.00		
0.30	0.00	0.20	0.02	2.05	9.50	0.24	0.00	1.90	127.30	15.68	125.40	67.93	0.86	0.96	0.00	0.00	0.16	1.46
0.01	0.00	0.15	0.02	1.30	65.31	0.01	0.00	1.43	4.28	4.28	16.15	2.85	1.00	0.23	0.00	0.00	0.10	0.29
0.01	0.00	0.22	0.02	1.23	66.50	0.02	0.00	2.62	32.38	16.62	36.75	10.50	0.99	0.27	0.00	0.00	0.09	0.26
0.04	0.00	0.16	0.02	1.70	53.94	0.04	0.00	0.00	26.97	2.79	34.41	12.09	1.38	0.39	0.00	0.00	0.10	0.18
0.04	0.00	0.03	0.02	0.78	4.39	0.08	0.00	0.49	41.93	4.39	52.65	17.06	0.39	0.56	0.00	0.00	0.14	0.43
0.00	0.00	0.00	0.19	0.06	7.64	0.00	0.04		119.25	59.24	11.77	12.54	1.25	0.13	0.00	0.00		
	0.00	0.20	0.15	1.68				498.80	50.00	60.00			1.40		0.00	0.00		
		0.15	0.10	1.60				460.00	30.00	40.00			1.44		0.00	0.00		
0.85	0.80	0.12	0.09	1.25	97.00	0.04	0.01	455.00	62.00	26.00	34.00	13.00	0.94	0.23	0.00	0.00		
0.35	0.00	0.05	0.01	0.28	27.51	0.06	0.00	77.07	37.59	33.60	52.08	22.05	0.53	0.29	0.00	0.00		
0.04	0.00	0.03	0.02	0.39	29.64	0.06	0.00	2.86	40.04	45.50	81.64	16.90	0.36	0.24	0.00	0.00	0.23	1.12
								248.88		97.41			1.01		0.00	0.00		
0.02	0.00	0.20	0.14	1.61	37.74	0.01	0.00	187.87	27.75	56.89	58.27	5.83	1.96	0.18	0.00	0.00	0.17	0.35
0.43	0.00	0.10	0.02	0.85	8.40	0.07	0.00	171.15	81.55	10.15	81.90	25.55	0.73	0.53	0.00	0.00	0.62	1.27
6.82	15.00	0.37	0.42	5.00	99.97	0.50	1.50	80.00	55.00	500.00	250.00	99.97	4.50	3.70		0.00		
6.82	15.00	0.37	0.42	5.00	99.97	0.50	0.15	85.00	79.80	500.00	250.00	99.97	4.50	3.70		0.00		

Food Name	Amount	Measure	Weight (g)	Calories	Protein (g)	Total Carb (g)	Dietary Fiber (g)	Total Fat (g)	Sat Fat (g)	Mono Fat (g)	Poly Fat (g)	Chol (mg)	Vit A (mcg RAE)	Vit D (mcg)
GRANOLA BARS, CEREAL BARS, DIET BARS, SCONES, AND TARTS *(continued)*														
Bar, cereal, apple cinnamon Nutri Grain	1	Each	37.00	136.16	1.63	26.97	0.78	2.78	0.56	1.85	0.33	0.00	224.96	
Bar, cereal, blueberry Nutri Grain	1	Each	37.00	136.16	1.63	26.97	0.78	2.78	0.56	1.85	0.33	0.00	224.96	
Bar, cereal, blueberry fruit & oatmeal Quaker Oats	1	Each	37.00	135.37	1.56	26.29	0.99	2.90	0.35	0.97	0.22	0.07		0.00
Bar, cereal, chocolate peanut butter Kashi Company	1	Each	78.00	280.00	13.00	50.00	7.00	6.00	3.00			0.00	0.00	
Bar, cereal, honey van yogurt Kashi Company	1	Each	78.00	280.00	11.00	53.00	7.00	4.00	3.00			0.00	0.00	
Bar, chocolate chip, whole grain Kudos	1	Each	37.00	161.69	2.13	25.05	1.33	6.05	3.50	1.94	0.31	50.32	5.55	
Bar, granola, almond, hard	1	Each	23.60	116.82	1.82	14.63	1.13	6.02	2.95	1.83	0.89	0.00	0.47	
Bar, granola, choc chip graham & marshmallow, uncoated, soft	1	Each	28.35	121.05	1.73	20.07	1.13	4.39	2.60	0.83	0.72	0.28	0.57	
Bar, granola, chocolate chip, chocolate coated, soft, 1.25oz	1	Each	35.44	165.14	2.06	22.61	1.20	8.82	5.04	2.75	0.64	1.77	2.48	
Bar, granola, chocolate choc chip, low fat, chewy	1	Each	35.00	127.75	2.59	26.60	1.50	2.45	0.77	1.01	0.46	0.00		
Bar, granola, cookies & cream, chewy Quaker Oats	1	Each	28.00	113.81	1.53	21.93	0.84	2.49	0.46	1.15	0.30	0.03		0.00
Bar, granola, honey nut, low fat, chewy	1	Each	35.00	117.95	2.87	26.60	1.50	2.10	0.28	1.12	0.56	0.00		
Bar, granola, milk chocolate, mini M & M's Kudos	1	Each	28.35	90.00	1.00	17.00	1.00	2.50	1.00			0.00		
Bar, granola, oatmeal raisin, low fat, chewy	1	Each	35.00	117.25	2.62	26.25	1.47	2.10	0.28	1.16	0.52	0.00		
Bar, granola, peanut butter, w/chocolate chips, chewy Quaker Oats	1	Each	28.00	121.94	2.52	18.59	1.20	4.57	1.29	2.27	0.80	0.03		0.00
Bar, granola, raisin, uncoated, soft, 1.5oz each	1	Each	42.53	190.51	3.23	28.24	1.79	7.57	4.07	1.21	1.37	0.43	0.00	
MEALS AND DISHES														
Canned Meals and Dishes														
Beans, baked, vegetarian, cnd Bush's Best	0.5	Cup	130.00	130.00	5.00	24.00	6.00	0.00	0.00	0.00	0.00	0.00		
Beans, baked, w/franks, cnd	0.5	Cup	129.50	183.89	8.74	19.93	8.94	8.51	3.05	3.67	1.09	7.77	5.18	
Beans, baked, w/pork, cnd B & M	0.5	Cup	131.00	180.00	8.00	33.00	7.00	2.00	0.50			3.00	0.00	
Dish, beefaroni, w/tomato sauce, cnd, svg	1	Each	212.63	184.98	8.27	31.23	2.98	2.96	1.19	1.27	0.25	17.01		
Dish, chicken & dumplings, cnd, Sweet Sue, FS Bryan Foods Inc.	1	Cup	240.00	218.40	15.12	22.80	2.64	7.44	1.80	2.95	1.62	36.00	0.00	
Dish, chicken, sweet & sour, w/veg & fruit, cnd Chun King	1	Each	254.00	165.10	5.84	31.75		1.78				22.86	0.00	
Dish, pasta, SpaghettiOs w/meatballs, cnd Franco American	1	Cup	209.00	240.00	11.00	32.00	3.00	8.00	3.50			20.00		1.00
Dish, pasta, SpaghettiOs w/sliced franks Franco American	1	Cup	209.00	230.00	9.00	27.00	5.00	10.00	5.00			20.00		1.00
Dish, pasta, w/meatballs, w/tomato sauce, cnd	1	Each	141.75	146.00	6.13	17.43	3.83	5.78	2.26	2.37	0.32	11.34	26.93	
Dish, pasta, w/sliced franks, w/tomato sauce, cnd, each	1	Each	418.00	434.72	15.47	49.74	3.76	19.23	6.14	7.94	2.50	37.62	25.08	
Dish, ravioli, beef w/tomato & meat sauce, svg Nestle Foods Company	1	Each	244.00	229.36	8.37	36.89	3.66	5.39	2.49	2.00	0.22	14.64		
Dish, ravioli, beef, w/tomato sauce, mini, cnd, svg Nestle Foods Company	1	Each	252.00	239.40	8.79	40.62	3.28	4.74	1.76	2.02	0.18	17.64		
Dish, spaghetti, w/meatballs & tomato sauce, svg Nestle Foods Company	1	Each	240.00	249.60	9.07	34.06	2.16	8.64	3.86	3.67	0.38	21.60		
Hash, beef, corned, cnd Chef-Mate	1	Cup	253.00	485.76	24.24	29.07	6.07	30.33	13.41	14.67	1.11	88.55	0.00	
Hash, beef, corned, cnd, Armour	1	Cup	236.00	497.96	23.84	12.04	1.89	39.41	15.65	17.44	0.83	96.76	0.00	
Pork & Beans, w/tomato sauce, cnd	0.5	Cup	126.50	118.91	6.51	23.65	5.06	1.18	0.33	0.60	0.18	8.86	5.06	

Vit E (mg)	Vit C	Vit B$_1$-Thia (mg)	Vit B$_2$-Ribo (mg)	Vit B$_3$-Nia (mg)	Fol (mcg)	Vit B$_6$ (mg)	Vita B$_{12}$ (mcg)	Sodi (mg)	Pota (mg)	Cal (mg)	Phos (mg)	Magn (mg)	Iron (mg)	Zinc (mg)	Caff (mg)	Alco (g)	Sol Fiber (g)	Insol Fiber (g)
0.00	0.00	0.37	0.41	5.00	39.96	0.52	0.00	109.89	72.89	15.17	38.11	9.99	1.80	1.52	0.00	0.00		
0.00	0.00	0.37	0.41	5.00	39.96	0.52	0.00	109.89	72.89	15.17	38.11	9.99	1.80	1.52	0.00	0.00		
0.04	0.31	0.23	0.51	5.96	119.27	0.60	0.01	118.00	44.15	9.88	33.73	8.41	0.43	0.23	0.00	0.00	0.44	0.55
	0.00		0.03					150.00	130.00	0.00	20.00	8.00	0.36			0.00		
	0.00		0.03	0.40				70.00	90.00	20.00			0.36	0.30	0.00	0.00		
3.99	17.24	0.06	0.07	0.57	4.81	0.04	0.05	103.60	103.23	289.71	76.59	25.90	3.39	0.52		0.00		
0.42	0.00	0.07	0.02	0.14	2.83	0.01	0.00	60.42	64.43	7.55	53.81	19.12	0.59	0.37	0.00	0.00		
0.26	0.00	0.04	0.04	0.28	5.95	0.01	0.00	89.59	77.96	25.23	57.27	20.13	0.73	0.37		0.00		
0.35	0.00	0.03	0.09	0.26	9.21	0.04	0.20	70.88	110.92	36.50	70.52	23.39	0.83	0.46		0.00		
		0.06	0.03	0.39				81.20	86.45	18.20			0.70			0.00		
0.33	0.11	0.06	0.03	0.37	3.74	0.02	0.01	78.30	51.97	7.82	41.70	12.34	0.50	0.31		0.00	0.27	0.57
		0.10	0.04	0.27				84.00	66.50	12.95			0.70		0.00	0.00		
	1.20							105.00		200.00			0.36			0.00		
		0.10	0.03	0.25				77.35	83.30	13.30					0.00	0.00		
0.13	0.14	0.06	0.02	0.91	4.96	0.02	0.00	103.91	70.12	10.22	58.56	16.57	0.54	0.41		0.00	0.29	0.91
0.47	0.00	0.10	0.07	0.47	8.93	0.04	0.08	119.92	153.94	42.95	93.56	30.62	1.04	0.55	0.00	0.00		
	0.00									40.00			0.54		0.00	0.00		
0.60	2.98	0.08	0.07	1.17	38.85	0.06	0.00	556.85	304.32	62.16	134.68	36.26	2.24	2.42	0.00	0.00	5.99	2.95
	0.00							430.00		60.00			2.70		0.00	0.00		
	0.42							801.60		17.01			1.51		0.00	0.00		
								945.60					2.57		0.00	0.00		
	30.23							563.88							0.00	0.00		
	6.00	0.15	0.17	3.00	60.00			990.00		150.00			2.70		0.00	0.00		
	6.00	0.15	0.17	3.00	80.00			930.00		150.00			2.70		0.00	0.00		
0.71	4.25	0.11	0.09	1.86	35.44	0.09	0.32	592.52	233.89	15.59	65.21	19.85	1.32	1.03	0.00	0.00		
								2014.76					3.80		0.00	0.00		
	0.24							1173.64	353.80	19.52			2.42		0.00	0.00		
	0.25							1197.00		22.68			2.42		0.00	0.00		
	0.96							940.80		16.80			1.78		0.00	0.00		
0.33	1.52	0.22	0.30	6.31		0.58	2.45	1593.90	536.36	45.54	240.35	37.95	2.99	7.51	0.00	0.00		
								854.32					2.19		0.00	0.00		
0.13	3.80	0.07	0.06	0.62	18.98	0.08	0.00	552.81	373.18	70.84	146.74	43.01	4.10	6.93	0.00	0.00	3.06	2.00

Food Name	Amount	Measure	Weight (g)	Calories	Protein (g)	Total Carb (g)	Dietary Fiber (g)	Total Fat (g)	Sat Fat (g)	Mono Fat (g)	Poly Fat (g)	Chol (mg)	Vit A (mcg RAE)	Vit D (mcg)
Dry and Prepared Meat Dishes														
Dish, beef, teriyaki, freeze dried, cnd Oregon Freeze Dry, Inc	1	Cup	65.21	260.00	12.00	44.00	3.00	4.00	1.00			15.00		
Dry and Prepared Pasta and Pasta/Rice Dishes														
Dish, cheeseburger macaroni, dry mix, svg General Mills, Inc.	1.5	Ounce-weight	42.53	167.97	4.68	27.34		4.42	1.20			3.83		
Dish, egg noodles, w/creamy alfredo sauce, dry mix, cup Lipton	0.25	Cup	23.25	97.18	3.60	14.51		2.74	1.06	0.90	0.29	26.04		
Dish, macaroni & cheese, all shapes, prep f/dry mix Kraft General Foods, Inc.	1	Cup	196.00	410.00	12.00	49.00	1.00	18.00	4.50			10.00		
Dish, macaroni & cheese, original, deluxe, prep f/mix Kraft General Foods, Inc.	1	Cup	175.00	320.00	14.00	44.00	1.00	10.00	6.00			25.00		
Dish, macaroni & cheese, original, prep f/dry mix Kraft General Foods, Inc.	1	Cup	196.00	410.00	12.00	49.00	1.00	18.00	4.50			10.00		
Dish, pad Thai, w/rice noodles, vegetarian, rth Fantastic Foods Fast Naturals	1	Each	201.00	350.00	15.00	51.00	3.00	11.00	2.50			0.00		
Dish, pasta, oriental stir fry, dry Pasta Roni	2	Ounce-weight	56.70	198.22	6.98	39.59	2.08	1.87	0.31	0.77	0.67	0.05		0.00
Dish, rice & pasta, flvrd, dry	0.25	Cup	40.75	149.96	3.82	30.70	0.76	1.00	0.18	0.26	0.40	0.82	0.00	
Dish, risotto, three cheese, meal in a cup, dry The Spice Hunter, Inc. Meals In A Cup	1	Each	63.40	234.30	7.19	45.60	1.13	2.95	1.78	0.66	0.08	9.13		0.06
Dish, spaghetti, w/meat sauce, freeze dried, sml pouch Oregon Freeze Dry, Inc	1	Each	79.38	340.00	17.00	46.00	3.00	10.00	4.50			25.00		
Dish, Thai lemon grass, w/rice noodles, vegetarian, rth Fantastic Foods Fast Naturals	1	Each	201.00	300.00	7.00	48.00	3.00	10.00	3.50			0.00		
Dish, tortellini, spinach	1	Cup	122.00	232.23	11.64	25.26	1.10	8.98	3.29	3.38	1.33	158.17	138.28	
Dish, tuna noodle casserole, creamy, Tuna Helper	1	Cup	138.00	300.00	14.00	30.00	1.70	14.00				5.00		
Dry and Prepared Rice/Grain Dishes														
Dish, pilaf, black beans & rice, Mediterranean, dry Near East	2	Ounce-weight	56.70	185.79	6.30	41.62	4.47	0.73	0.13	0.21	0.35	0.00		0.00
Dish, rice pilaf, long grain & wild, dry Rice A Roni	2	Ounce-weight	56.70	190.80	4.64	43.07	1.67	0.50	0.12	0.17	0.13	0.00		0.00
Dish, rice, broccoli cheese flvr, dry Uncle Ben's Inc.	2	Ounce-weight	56.70	200.50	5.60	41.70	1.70	1.90	1.10			4.50		
Dish, rice, fried, Oriental style, dry Uncle Ben's Inc.	2	Ounce-weight	56.70	190.00	4.00	43.00	1.00	0.50	0.00			0.00		
Dish, rice, paella, dry Uncle Ben's Inc.	2	Ounce-weight	56.70	190.00	5.00	43.00	1.00	0.50	0.00			0.00		
Dish, rice, risotto mushroom herb, seasoned, dry Uncle Ben's Inc.	2	Ounce-weight	56.70	192.50	6.20	40.40	0.80	0.80	0.20			2.20	0.00	
Dry and Prepared Vegetable and Bean Dishes														
Dish, falafel, dry Fantastic Foods International Dish	0.25	Cup	35.00	120.00	7.00	21.00	6.00	2.00	0.00			0.00	0.00	
Frozen/Refrigerated Breakfasts														
Burrito, breakfast, ham & cheese flvr, fzn	1	Each	99.00	211.86	9.60	27.82	1.39	6.93	1.99	2.08	1.80	192.06	0.00	
Burrito, breakfast, original w/scrambled eggs Swanson's Great Starts	1	Each	99.00	200.00	8.00	25.00	2.00	8.00	3.00			60.00		
Frozen/Refrigerated Children's Meals														
Frozen/Refrigerated Dinners														
Dinner, beef, pot roast, yankee, ckd f/fzn Banquet	1	Each	266.50	230.00	14.00	20.00	4.00	10.00	4.00			60.00		
Dinner, beef, sliced, w/gravy mashed potatoes & peas, fzn Banquet	1	Each	255.00	270.30	26.39	18.79	4.08	10.05	4.33	4.95	0.76	71.40		

Vit E (mg)	Vit C	Vit B₁-Thia (mg)	Vit B₂-Ribo (mg)	Vit B₃-Nia (mg)	Fol (mcg)	Vit B₆ (mg)	Vita B₁₂ (mcg)	Sodi (mg)	Pota (mg)	Cal (mg)	Phos (mg)	Magn (mg)	Iron (mg)	Zinc (mg)	Caff (mg)	Alco (g)	Sol Fiber (g)	Insol Fiber (g)
	6.00							910.00		40.00			1.44		0.00	0.00		
								863.26							0.00	0.00		
								411.52		29.53			0.70		0.00	0.00		
	0.00	0.38	0.34	3.00	60.00			750.00	340.00	100.00	300.00	40.00	2.70		0.00	0.00		
	0.00	0.38	0.26	3.00	60.00			730.00	190.00	200.00	450.00	40.00	1.80		0.00	0.00		
	0.00	0.38	0.34	3.00	60.00			750.00	340.00	100.00	300.00	40.00	2.70		0.00	0.00		
	2.40							690.00		60.00			1.80		0.00	0.00		
0.09	0.61	0.36	0.18	2.53	82.18	0.08	0.05	987.97	163.89	23.69	85.04	27.55	1.64	0.71	0.00	0.00	0.85	1.23
0.06	0.24	0.31	0.11	2.86	84.76	0.06	0.08	760.40	85.16	18.74	64.39	16.30	1.62	0.50	0.00	0.00		
0.00	0.33	0.04	0.14	1.09	0.00	0.01	0.00	521.60	82.74	89.99	6.03	1.30	0.63	0.03	0.00	0.00		
	0.00	0.15	0.26	5.00				990.00		60.00			3.60		0.00	0.00		
	4.80							690.00		40.00			1.44		0.00	0.00		
0.86	1.01	0.24	0.37	1.85	34.80	0.10	0.48	252.02	138.44	143.34	167.54	23.70	2.42	0.98	0.00	0.00		
				6.00											0.00	0.00		
0.00	0.21	0.08	0.06	0.91	7.43	0.13	0.66	659.07	321.98	45.46	62.68	13.80	1.54	0.49	0.00	0.00	1.36	3.11
0.00	1.01	0.19	0.11	1.76	66.88	0.18	0.00	837.22	230.61	23.72	88.90	25.70	1.76	0.68	0.00	0.00	0.53	1.14
	2.40							759.00		68.70			1.44		0.00	0.00		
								560.00		35.10			1.80		0.00	0.00		
								550.00		34.10			2.16		0.00	0.00		
	3.60							848.80		33.90			0.54		0.00	0.00		
	1.20							370.00		40.00			2.70		0.00	0.00		
								404.91					3.17		0.00	0.00		
	2.40							510.00		80.00			1.44		0.00	0.00		
	3.60							1130.00		40.00			1.80		0.00	0.00		
	7.65							742.05		45.90			3.75		0.00	0.00		

Food Name	Amount	Measure	Weight (g)	Calories	Protein (g)	Total Carb (g)	Dietary Fiber (g)	Total Fat (g)	Sat Fat (g)	Mono Fat (g)	Poly Fat (g)	Chol (mg)	Vit A (mcg RAE)	Vit D (mcg)
MEALS AND DISHES *(continued)*														
Dinner, cannelloni, cheese, w/tomato sauce, low cal, fzn	1	Each	259.00	298.42	21.86	24.20	1.48	12.45	7.01	3.43	1.24	41.68	143.42	
Dinner, chicken & noodles, ckd Marie Callender's (Frozen)	1	Each	368.60	520.00	21.00	42.00	5.00	30.00	11.00			80.00		
Dinner, chicken, alfredo, w/broccoli, fzn Healthy Choice	1	Each	326.00	300.00	25.00	34.00	2.00	7.00	3.00			50.00		
Dinner, chicken, fingers, ckd Banquet	1	Each	201.30	740.00	22.00	67.00	6.00	43.00	11.00			70.00	0.00	
Dinner, chicken, fried, w/mashed potatoes & corn, fzn Banquet	1	Each	228.00	469.68	21.45	35.09	2.05	27.04	9.25	15.35	2.44	88.92	0.00	
Dinner, chicken, parmigiana, ckd f/fzn Banquet	1	Each	269.00	320.00	10.00	29.00	3.00	18.00	7.00			50.00		
Dinner, chicken, teriyaki, w/oriental veg, fzn The Budget Gourmet-Light & Healthy	1	Each	311.00	317.22	18.66	52.25	4.04	3.73	0.62	0.91	1.60	24.88	43.54	
Dinner, chicken, teriyaki, w/rice medley veg & compote, fzn Healthy Choice	1	Each	312.00	268.32	17.07	37.10	2.81	5.62	3.00	2.15	0.47	43.68		
Dinner, chow mein, chicken, w/rice, low cal, fzn	1	Each	319.00	289.65	19.01	38.22	1.95	6.28	1.76	2.39	1.44	47.05	31.01	
Dinner, enchilada, beef Van de Kamp's	1	Each	340.00	400.00	16.00	54.00		14.00				40.00		
Dinner, enchilada, cheese, ckd f/fzn Banquet	1	Each	312.00	360.00	12.00	56.00	8.00	10.00	4.00			20.00		
Dinner, enchilada, cheese, fzn	1	Each	284.00	586.74	24.46	67.16	13.78	26.20	14.12	8.40	2.12	60.92	190.99	
Dinner, enchilada, chicken, w/sauce rice corn & compote, fzn Healthy Choice	1	Each	320.00	297.60	12.99	45.98	4.16	6.72	3.10	2.59	1.02	38.40		
Dinner, fettuccine, w/broccoli & chicken, ckd f/fzn Marie Callender's (Frozen)	1	Each	368.60	710.00	26.00	53.00	6.00	43.00	17.00			85.00		
Dinner, green pepper, stuffed, fzn	1	Each	397.00	410.38	18.23	38.94	5.03	21.34	6.13	8.26	4.78	49.04	161.62	
Dinner, lasagna, extra cheese, ckd f/fzn Marie Callender's (Frozen)	1	Each	425.30	590.00	27.00	61.00	7.00	27.00	13.00			50.00		
Dinner, lasagna, w/cheese & meat, low cal, fzn	1	Each	340.00	388.82	24.27	41.32		14.40	6.67	5.50	0.84	54.81	284.47	
Dinner, lasagna, w/meat sauce, ckd f/fzn Marie Callender's (Frozen)	1	Each	425.30	629.99	29.01	59.00	3.01	30.99	15.01			75.00		
Dinner, macaroni & cheese, ckd f/fzn Banquet	1	Each	340.20	420.00	15.00	57.00	5.00	14.00	8.00			20.00	0.00	
Dinner, meatballs, swedish, ckd Marie Callender's (Frozen)	1	Each	354.40	520.00	28.00	44.00	3.00	26.00	12.00			65.00		
Dinner, meatloaf, ckd f/fzn Banquet	1	Each	269.00	280.00	12.00	23.00	3.00	16.00	6.00			60.00		
Dinner, meatloaf, extra helping, w/sauce potato carrot, fzn Banquet	1	Each	453.00	611.55	29.08	33.57	6.34	40.05	15.49	17.30	7.25	113.25		
Dinner, salisbury steak, w/red potato & veg, fzn The Budget Gourmet-Light & Healthy	1	Each	311.00	261.24	18.35	33.90	7.15	5.91	2.02	1.75	0.94	43.54	71.53	
Dinner, shrimp & vegetables, fzn Healthy Choice	1	Each	335.00	270.00	15.00	39.00	6.00	6.00	3.00			50.00		
Dinner, spaghetti, w/meat sauce & garlic bread, ckd f/fzn Marie Callender's (Frozen)	1	Each	482.00	670.00	27.00	85.00	9.00	25.00	11.00			35.00		
Dinner, steak, chicken fried, ckd Banquet	1	Each	283.50	420.00	15.00	39.00	4.00	23.00	12.00			35.00		
Dinner, stir fry, chicken & veg, oriental, fzn Healthy Choice	1	Each	337.00	360.00	19.00	57.00	5.00	6.00	2.00			25.00		
Dinner, stroganoff, beef, fzn Healthy Choice	1	Each	312.00	320.00	22.00	40.00	7.00	8.00	3.00			60.00		
Dinner, tuna & noodles, homestyle, ckd Marie Callender's (Frozen)	1	Each	340.20	600.00	18.00	52.00	5.00	35.00	18.00			90.00		
Dinner, turkey, breast meat, honey rstd, ckd f/fzn Banquet	1	Each	255.20	270.00	11.00	29.00	4.00	12.00	2.50			30.00		

Vit E (mg)	Vit C	Vit B$_1$-Thia (mg)	Vit B$_2$-Ribo (mg)	Vit B$_3$-Nia (mg)	Fol (mcg)	Vit B$_6$ (mg)	Vita B$_{12}$ (mcg)	Sodi (mg)	Pota (mg)	Cal (mg)	Phos (mg)	Magn (mg)	Iron (mg)	Zinc (mg)	Caff (mg)	Alco (g)	Sol Fiber (g)	Insol Fiber (g)
1.26	4.08	0.16	0.29	1.67	19.27	0.13	0.42	1221.21	226.17	268.66	262.00	29.77	1.58	1.67	0.00	0.00		
	9.00							1320.00		100.00			2.70		0.00	0.00		
	12.00							530.00		100.00			1.80		0.00	0.00		
	0.00							1070.00		40.00			2.70		0.00	0.00		
	1.37							1500.24		38.76			1.37		0.00	0.00		
	30.00							900.00		60.00			1.80		0.00	0.00		
	44.47							674.87							0.00	0.00		
	12.17							602.16	424.32	37.44	224.64		1.09		0.00	0.00		
0.49	20.04	0.21	0.19	5.66	29.29	0.34	0.12	1068.62	336.03	44.44	158.58	36.60	2.55	1.83	0.00	0.00		
								1480.00	700.00						0.00	0.00		
	2.40							1500.00		200.00			1.80		0.00	0.00		
4.27	17.84	0.27	0.38	2.72	155.85	0.43	0.47	1751.57	786.54	566.69	594.95	96.07	3.46	3.06	0.00	0.00		
	18.24							563.20	384.00	134.40	236.80		0.77		0.00	0.00		
	9.00							910.00		150.00			2.70		0.00	0.00		
2.26	67.82	0.21	0.25	5.35	44.23	0.58	1.62	1216.57	811.23	149.01	203.21	65.22	7.30	3.72	0.00	0.00		
	0.00							1230.00		800.00			2.70		0.00	0.00		
3.45	12.54	0.29	0.39	5.07	28.26	0.32	0.88	839.53	758.98	264.77	306.61	64.04	3.82	3.70	0.00	0.00		
	0.00							1230.00		500.00			2.70		0.00	0.00		
	0.00							1330.00		150.00			1.44		0.00	0.00		
	0.00							1020.00		40.00			2.70		0.00	0.00		
	0.00	0.21	0.31	6.90				1020.00	900.00	40.00			1.80		0.00	0.00		
	7.70							1943.37		77.01			3.94		0.00	0.00		
	51.00							494.49					3.05		0.00	0.00		
	30.00							580.00		150.00			1.80		0.00	0.00		
	0.00							1160.00		150.00			2.70		0.00	0.00		
	0.00							1200.00		100.00			1.80		0.00	0.00		
	4.80							600.00		40.00			2.70		0.00	0.00		
	12.00							600.00		60.00			1.80		0.00	0.00		
	0.00							1570.00		100.00			2.70		0.00	0.00		
	0.00							1310.00		60.00			1.80		0.00	0.00		

Food Name	Amount	Measure	Weight (g)	Calories	Protein (g)	Total Carb (g)	Dietary Fiber (g)	Total Fat (g)	Sat Fat (g)	Mono Fat (g)	Poly Fat (g)	Chol (mg)	Vit A (mcg RAE)	Vit D (mcg)
MEALS AND DISHES (continued)														
Dinner, turkey, breast, w/potatoes & veg, homestyle, fzn Stouffer's	1	Each	453.60	460.00	24.00	55.00	7.00	16.00	5.00			60.00		
Dinner, turkey, w/gravy & dressing, extra helping, ckd Banquet Hearty Ones	1	Each	481.95	620.00	28.00	54.00	10.00	32.00	8.00			80.00	0.00	
Dinner, turkey, w/stuffing & dessert, extra lrg, fzn	1	Each	524.00	565.24	33.74	67.93	8.36	18.11	6.10	6.69	3.90	104.59	103.56	
Dinner, veal parmigiana, w/spaghetti & veg, homestyle, fzn Stouffer's	1	Each	496.10	530.00	27.00	66.00	7.00	17.00	4.50			60.00		
Dish, teriyaki stir fry, w/chicken & pasta, fzn Everyday Foods Lean Cuisine	1	Each	283.50	290.00	18.00	45.00	4.00	4.00	1.00	1.00	1.50	20.00		
Frozen/Refrigerated Dishes														
Burrito, beef bean cheese	1	Each	101.50	165.44	7.29	19.84	2.45	6.65	3.57	2.23	0.51	61.91	75.11	
Corn Dog	1	Each	175.00	460.25	16.80	55.79		18.90	5.16	9.11	3.50	78.75	59.50	
Dinner, beef, pot roast, w/whipped potatoes, homestyle, fzn Lean Cuisine	1	Each	255.00	206.55	17.34	22.44	3.57	5.35	1.31	2.28	0.81	38.25	48.45	
Dinner, cheese spinach manicotti, w/broccoli & carrots, fzn Hearty Portions Lean Cuisine	1	Each	439.40	350.00	19.00	50.00	6.00	8.00	3.00	2.50	1.50	40.00		
Dinner, chicken, piccata, w/cheese rice & peppers, fzn Cafe Classics Lean Cuisine	1	Each	255.00	300.00	14.00	41.00	2.00	9.00	2.50	2.00	1.50	30.00		
Dinner, Italian meatballs & rigatoni pasta, w/veg, fzn Hearty Portions Lean Cuisine	1	Each	435.90	440.00	25.00	64.00	7.00	9.00	3.50	4.00	1.00	35.00		
Dinner, salisbury steak, w/macaroni & cheese, fzn Cafe Classics Lean Cuisine	1	Each	272.00	386.24	22.58	26.38		21.22	8.00	7.94	1.85	62.56	0.00	
Dish, beef & broccoli, w/rice, skillet, fzn Stouffer's Skillet Sensations	0.5	Each	354.40	320.00	17.00	51.00	3.00	5.00	2.00			30.00		
Dish, beef macaroni, fzn, svg Healthy Choice	1	Each	226.80	199.58	13.36	31.62	4.31	2.11	0.63	1.13	0.32	13.61	52.16	
Dish, beef, pepper steak, oriental, fzn La Choy	1	Cup	246.00	103.81	9.99	12.47	3.69	2.36	0.59			12.30		
Dish, beef, stroganoff, skillet, fzn Stouffer's Skillet Sensations	0.25	Each	283.50	340.00	19.00	38.00	4.00	12.00	3.50			35.00		
Dish, cannelloni, cheese, fzn Everyday Foods Lean Cuisine	1	Each	258.70	220.00	21.00	27.00	3.00	3.50	2.00	1.00	0.50	15.00		
Dish, casserole, macaroni & beef, w/tomato sauce Swanson	1	Each	284.00	270.00	18.00	39.00	2.00	5.00	5.00	0.00	0.00	35.00		
Dish, cheese ravioli, fzn Everyday Foods Lean Cuisine	1	Each	241.00	260.00	12.00	38.00	4.00	7.00	3.50	1.50	0.50	35.00		1.53
Dish, chicken & noodles, escalloped, fzn Stouffer's	1	Each	283.00	418.84	16.98	31.41		25.19	5.95	6.95	12.29	76.41	0.00	
Dish, chicken & rice, stir fry, fzn, Lunch Express Lean Cuisine	1	Each	255.00	270.30	11.73	39.52	5.86	7.39	0.93	3.47	2.02	25.50	262.65	
Dish, chicken & vegetables, w/vermicelli, fzn Cafe Classics Lean Cuisine	1	Each	297.00	252.45	18.71	32.08	5.05	5.64	1.03	2.13	1.38	23.76		
Dish, chicken a l'orange, w/broccoli & rice, fzn Cafe Classics Lean Cuisine	1	Each	255.00	267.75	24.48	38.50		1.78	0.42	0.50	0.41	45.90		
Dish, chicken alfredo, fettuccine fzn, Lunch Express Lean Cuisine	1	Each	272.00	372.64	19.04	32.64	3.81	18.50	6.99	6.26	2.39	57.12		
Dish, chicken, ala king, fzn Stouffer's	1	Each	326.00	370.00	21.00	47.00	2.00	11.00	4.00			45.00		
Dish, chicken, carbonara, pasta w/cheese sauce, fzn Cafe Classics Lean Cuisine	1	Each	255.00	280.00	17.00	36.00	4.00	7.00	1.50	2.00	2.50	30.00		
Dish, chicken, marsala, w/veg, fzn Healthy Choice	1	Each	326.00	240.00	20.00	32.00	3.00	4.00	2.00			30.00		
Dish, chicken, rstd, w/garlic sauce pasta & veg, fzn, fs Tyson Food Service	1	Each	255.00	214.20	16.93	21.52	3.57	6.71	1.30	2.35	2.14	28.05		

Vit E (mg)	Vit C	Vit B₁-Thia (mg)	Vit B₂-Ribo (mg)	Vit B₃-Nia (mg)	Fol (mcg)	Vit B₆ (mg)	Vita B₁₂ (mcg)	Sodi (mg)	Pota (mg)	Cal (mg)	Phos (mg)	Magn (mg)	Iron (mg)	Zinc (mg)	Caff (mg)	Alco (g)	Sol Fiber (g)	Insol Fiber (g)
	9.00							1620.00	480.00	100.00			2.70		0.00	0.00		
	0.00	0.41	0.31	4.50		0.31		2250.00	605.80	60.00	289.00		1.44		0.00	0.00		
2.41	21.04	0.39	0.39	8.20	69.92	0.60	0.49	1893.74	792.08	104.88	361.95	75.98	3.80	3.87	0.00	0.00		
	27.00							1130.00	1040.00	200.00			3.60		0.00	0.00		
	0.00							590.00	610.00	40.00			1.08		0.00	0.00		
0.41	2.54	0.15	0.36	1.93	37.55	0.11	0.55	495.32	205.03	64.96	70.03	25.37	1.87	1.18	0.00	0.00		
0.70	0.00	0.28	0.70	4.16	103.25	0.09	0.44	973.00	262.50	101.50	166.25	17.50	6.18	1.31	0.00	0.00		
								494.70							0.00	0.00		
	9.00							840.00	910.00	400.00			1.80		0.00	0.00		
	12.00							690.00	290.00	100.00			0.72		0.00	0.00		
	24.00							820.00	1150.00	200.00			3.60		0.00	0.00		
	1.21							1014.56	616.12	195.84			2.28		0.00	0.00		
	9.00							1250.00	637.00	60.00			1.44		0.00	0.00		
1.59	54.89	0.26	0.15	2.94	99.79	0.18	0.11	419.58	344.74	43.09	127.01	34.02	2.56	1.15	0.00	0.00		
	7.33							969.24		23.91			0.49		0.00	0.00		
	2.40							1090.00		150.00			2.70		0.00	0.00		
	6.00	0.12	0.26	1.60		0.14	0.00	550.00	440.00	350.00		36.00	0.72	1.60	0.00	0.00		
	12.00							1060.00		60.00			2.70		0.00	0.00		
	4.80	0.06	0.26	1.20	48.00	0.20	0.30	590.00	450.00	150.00	168.00	42.00	1.44	1.50	0.00	0.00		
	0.00							1211.24	329.42	116.03			1.13		0.00	0.00		
	23.71							632.40							0.00	0.00		
	14.55							582.12	647.82	103.95			1.34		0.00	0.00		
	18.10							359.55	430.00	20.00			0.36	1.00	0.00	0.00		
	24.21							587.52		146.88					0.00	0.00		
	6.00	0.12	0.12	1.81				1300.00	450.00	100.00			0.36		0.00	0.00		
	12.00							690.00	710.00	150.00			1.44		0.00	0.00		
	3.60							440.00		40.00			0.72		0.00	0.00		
								466.65					1.56		0.00	0.00		

Food Name	Amount	Measure	Weight (g)	Calories	Protein (g)	Total Carb (g)	Dietary Fiber (g)	Total Fat (g)	Sat Fat (g)	Mono Fat (g)	Poly Fat (g)	Chol (mg)	Vit A (mcg RAE)	Vit D (mcg)
MEALS AND DISHES (*continued*)														
Dish, chicken, teriyaki, w/rice, bowl, fzn Healthy Choice	1	Each	269.00	270.00	17.00	41.00	4.00	4.00	1.00			30.00		
Dish, chili, w/beans, fzn Stouffer's	1	Each	248.10	290.00	19.00	29.00	6.00	11.00	4.00			45.00		
Dish, chow mein, beef, bi-pack, fzn La Choy	1	Cup	247.00	104.98	9.24	14.87	3.46	1.73	0.82			12.35		
Dish, chow mein, chicken, fzn La Choy	1	Each	250.00	91.25	5.32	11.40	2.10	3.65	0.95			8.75		
Dish, chow mein, shrimp, bi-pack, fzn La Choy	1	Each	141.75	35.15	2.27	6.01	1.70	0.61	0.00			17.58		
Dish, enchilada, beef, fzn Ortega	1	Each	265.78	360.00	12.00	49.00	5.00	13.00	5.00			25.00		
Dish, enchilada, cheese	1	Each	163.00	319.48	9.63	28.54		18.84	10.59	6.31	0.82	44.01	99.43	
Dish, green peppers, stuffed w/beef, w/tomato sauce, fzn Stouffer's	0.5	Each	219.50	188.77	7.90	20.85	5.27	8.12	2.72	3.75	0.53	21.95	0.00	
Dish, inari, svg Hissho Sushi	1	Each	113.00	250.00	7.00	33.00	0.00	8.00	1.00			0.00	0.00	
Dish, lasagna, bake, fzn Stouffer's	1	Each	326.00	450.00	25.00	51.00	4.00	16.00	7.00			45.00		
Dish, lasagna, Italian sausage, fzn The Budget Gourmet	1	Each	298.00	455.94	20.56	39.93	2.98	23.84	8.17	9.77	2.00	47.68		
Dish, lasagna, w/meat sauce, fzn, svg Stouffer's	1	Each	215.00	277.35	18.71	26.45	3.23	10.75	4.71	3.48	0.56	40.85	0.00	
Dish, macaroni & beef, w/tomato sauce, fzn Everyday Foods Lean Cuisine	1	Each	283.00	249.04	13.87	36.51	3.40	5.38	1.64	2.06	0.70	22.64		
Dish, macaroni & beef, w/tomato sauce, fzn, Weight Watchers	1	Each	269.00	282.45	15.60	44.65	6.73	4.57	1.58	1.77	0.61	13.45		
Dish, macaroni & cheese, fzn Stouffer's Family Style Favorites	5	Ounce-weight	226.80	380.00	16.00	40.00	2.00	17.00	8.00			35.00		
Dish, manicotti, cheese, fzn Stouffer's	1	Each	255.20	360.00	19.00	34.00	4.00	16.00	9.00			40.00		
Dish, meatballs w/pasta, Swedish, fzn Everyday Foods Lean Cuisine	1	Each	258.00	276.06	21.67	31.22	2.58	7.22	2.42	2.34	1.04	46.44	0.00	0.22
Dish, meatloaf, beef, homestyle, rtb, fzn, 4 oz, FS Travis Meats	1	Each	113.40	335.90	16.54	4.08	0.62	28.15	11.48	12.14	1.05	68.89		
Dish, noodles romanoff, fzn Stouffer's	1	Each	340.20	490.00	17.00	53.00	5.00	23.00	6.00			55.00		
Dish, pasta, w/chicken wine & mushroom sauce, low fat The Budget Gourmet	1	Each	241.00	280.00	13.00	41.00	4.00	7.00	2.00			25.00		
Dish, pea & potato curry	5	Ounce-weight	141.75	201.29	3.26	17.72	4.39	15.31					0.00	
Dish, penne pasta, w/tomato basil sauce, fzn Everyday Foods Lean Cuisine	1	Each	283.50	260.00	9.00	47.00	5.00	3.50	0.50	1.50	0.50	0.00		
Dish, penne pasta, w/tomato Italian sausage & sauce, low fat The Budget Gourmet	1	Each	226.00	270.00	10.00	46.00	3.00	6.00	1.50			10.00		
Dish, pot pie, beef, fzn	1	Each	198.00	449.46	13.27	44.15	2.18	24.35	8.51	9.68	2.67	37.62	51.48	
Dish, pot pie, chicken Swanson	1	Each	198.00	410.00	10.00	43.00	2.00	22.00	9.00			25.00		
Dish, pot pie, chicken, fzn	1	Each	217.00	483.91	13.04	42.71	1.74	29.10	9.67	12.48	4.49	41.23	256.06	
Dish, pot pie, chicken, fzn Stouffer's	1	Each	283.00	571.66	23.21	36.51	3.11	37.07	10.73	12.37	10.44	76.41		
Dish, pot pie, turkey, ckd f/fzn Banquet	1	Each	198.00	370.00	10.00	38.00	3.00	20.00	8.00			45.00		
Dish, potatoes, scalloped, fzn Stouffer's Family Style Favorites	5	Ounce-weight	141.75	140.00	4.00	19.00	2.00	5.00	1.50			3.00	0.00	
Dish, rice bowl, beef & broccoli, spicy Uncle Ben's Inc.	1	Each	340.20	370.00	21.00	62.00	5.00	4.50	1.50			25.00		
Dish, rice bowl, chicken, Szechuan Uncle Ben's Inc.	1	Each	340.20	360.00	23.00	58.00	3.00	4.00	1.00			35.00		
Dish, rice bowl, southwest style black bean & veg Uncle Ben's Inc.	1	Each	340.20	360.00	11.00	68.00	10.00	4.50	1.00			0.00		
Dish, rice bowl, teriyaki stir fry veg Uncle Ben's Inc.	1	Each	340.20	360.00	8.00	74.00	4.00	3.00	0.50			0.00		
Dish, rice pilaf, wild, w/veg The Budget Gourmet	1	Each	226.00	340.00	6.00	44.00	2.00	13.00	3.00			10.00		
Dish, rice, w/broccoli, fzn Green Giant's Rice & Vegetable Combos	1	Each	283.00	320.00	8.00	44.00	2.00	12.00	3.50			15.00		

Vit E (mg)	Vit C	Vit B$_1$-Thia (mg)	Vit B$_2$-Ribo (mg)	Vit B$_3$-Nia (mg)	Fol (mcg)	Vit B$_6$ (mg)	Vita B$_{12}$ (mcg)	Sodi (mg)	Pota (mg)	Cal (mg)	Phos (mg)	Magn (mg)	Iron (mg)	Zinc (mg)	Caff (mg)	Alco (g)	Sol Fiber (g)	Insol Fiber (g)
	12.00							570.00		20.00			1.08		0.00	0.00		
	3.60	0.10	0.10	1.20				1000.00	610.00	80.00			3.60		0.00	0.00		
	11.07							755.82		29.64			0.62		0.00	0.00		
	4.15							865.00		42.75			0.68		0.00	0.00		
	13.24							547.16		1.83			2.37		0.00	0.00		
	9.00							1460.00		150.00			1.80		0.00	0.00		
1.47	0.98	0.08	0.42	1.91	65.20	0.39	0.75	784.03	239.61	324.37	133.66	50.53	1.32	2.51	0.00	0.00		
	86.48							577.28	369.66	19.98			1.08		0.00	0.00		
	0.00							703.00		120.00			1.08		0.00	0.00	0.00	0.00
	2.40							1110.00	440.00	200.00			2.70		0.00	0.00		
								902.94		315.88			2.68		0.00	0.00		
	2.60							735.30	411.59	230.05			1.17		0.00	0.00		
	157.35							563.17	638.87	39.93			2.18		0.00	0.00		
	27.44							492.27					5.68		0.00	0.00		
	0.00							1020.00	220.00	350.00			0.72		0.00	0.00		
	4.80							850.00	525.00	450.00			1.08		0.00	0.00		
0.34	0.00	0.59	0.52	4.98	31.89	0.31	1.01	562.44	598.56	206.40	206.40	43.86	2.06	3.69	0.00	0.00		
	6.00	0.11	0.15	2.82				280.60	308.10	18.00	158.30		2.52	3.07	0.00	0.00		
	0.00	0.10	0.10	0.70				1260.00	140.00	150.00			1.44		0.00	0.00		
	1.20							670.00		60.00			1.44		0.00	0.00		
	8.51	0.07	0.06	1.70	18.43		0.00	524.48	378.47	39.69		24.10	1.28	0.57	0.00	0.00		
	6.00							390.00	520.00	60.00			1.80		0.00	0.00		
	2.40							410.00		40.00			2.70		0.00	0.00		
								736.56							0.00	Alco		
	1.20							780.00		20.00			1.80		0.00	0.00		
3.84	1.52	0.25	0.36	4.13	41.23	0.20	0.15	857.15	256.06	32.55	119.35	23.87	2.06	1.02	0.00	0.00		
	0.00							942.39		101.88			3.00		0.00	0.00		
	0.00							850.00		40.00			1.08		0.00	0.00		
	0.00							560.00	231.00	100.00			0.00		0.00	0.00		
								1550.00							0.00	0.00		
								1800.00							0.00	0.00		
								1250.00							0.00	0.00		
								1360.00							0.00	0.00		
	2.40							700.00		40.00			0.36		0.00	0.00		
	18.00							1000.00		150.00			3.60		0.00	0.00		

Food Name	Amount	Measure	Weight (g)	Calories	Protein (g)	Total Carb (g)	Dietary Fiber (g)	Total Fat (g)	Sat Fat (g)	Mono Fat (g)	Poly Fat (g)	Chol (mg)	Vit A (mcg RAE)	Vit D (mcg)
Dish, rigatoni, w/cream sauce broccoli & chicken, low fat The Budget Gourmet	1	Each	226.00	260.00	9.00	40.00	2.00	6.00	2.00			15.00		
Dish, spaghetti, w/meat sauce, fzn Everyday Foods Lean Cuisine	1	Each	326.00	312.96	14.34	50.53	5.54	5.87	1.35	2.28	1.32	13.04		
Dish, spaghetti, w/meatballs, fzn, 12.6oz Stouffer's	1	Each	357.20	390.00	19.00	49.00	5.00	13.00	4.00			30.00		
Dish, steak, salisbury The Budget Gourmet	1	Each	241.00	350.00	15.00	23.00	2.00	23.00	9.00			55.00		
Dish, stir fry, vegetable szechuan, fzn mix Green Giant's Create-A-Meal	1	Cup	114.00	85.50	3.42	11.40	2.28	2.85	0.28			0.00		
Dish, stroganoff, beef, homestyle, fzn Stouffer's	1	Each	276.40	370.00	21.00	32.00	3.00	17.00	7.00			65.00		
Dish, tuna noodle casserole, fzn Healthy Choice	1	Each	255.00	240.00	16.00	33.00	4.00	5.00	2.00			25.00	0.00	
Dish, turkey, w/gravy & mashed potato, ckd Marie Callender's (Frozen)	5	Ounce-weight	141.75	167.57	12.43	9.73	1.08	8.65	3.24			37.84	0.00	
Dish, vegetable lasagna, fzn Everyday Foods Lean Cuisine	1	Each	298.00	260.00	17.00	33.00	4.00	7.00	3.50	2.00	1.00	20.00		

Frozen/Refrigerated Dinners/Dishes—Vegetarian

Food Name	Amount	Measure	Weight (g)	Calories	Protein (g)	Total Carb (g)	Dietary Fiber (g)	Total Fat (g)	Sat Fat (g)	Mono Fat (g)	Poly Fat (g)	Chol (mg)	Vit A (mcg RAE)	Vit D (mcg)
Dish, lasagna, garden vegetable, fzn Amy's Kitchen Inc	1	Each	291.00	290.00	13.00	41.00	5.00	9.00	4.00			20.00		
Dish, lasagna, tofu vegetable, fzn Amy's Kitchen Inc	1	Each	269.00	300.00	13.00	41.00	6.00	10.00	1.50			0.00		
Dish, meatloaf, meatless, w/gravy, slice Gardenburger Inc.	1	Piece	142.00	130.00	12.00	12.00	4.00	3.50	1.00			0.00		
Dish, pasta primavera, fzn Amy's Kitchen Inc	1	Each	255.00	300.00	15.00	37.00	3.00	11.00	6.00			45.00		
Dish, pot pie, vegetarian	1	Each	227.00	509.75	14.49	40.72	5.23	32.45	8.56	12.40	9.62	19.54	453.50	0.20
Dish, quiche, spinach, vegetarian	5	Ounce-weight	141.75	340.16	11.16	16.36	1.22	25.89	12.00	8.81	3.43	156.84	300.14	
Dish, ravioli, cheese, w/sauce, fzn Amy's Kitchen Inc	1	Each	227.00	340.00	15.00	43.00	3.00	12.00	5.00			25.00		
Dish, tamale pie, vgtrn, Mexican, fzn Amy's Kitchen Inc	1	Each	227.00	150.00	5.00	27.00	4.00	3.00	0.00			0.00		

Homemade and Generic Meals and Dishes

Food Name	Amount	Measure	Weight (g)	Calories	Protein (g)	Total Carb (g)	Dietary Fiber (g)	Total Fat (g)	Sat Fat (g)	Mono Fat (g)	Poly Fat (g)	Chol (mg)	Vit A (mcg RAE)	Vit D (mcg)
Beef, round steak, lean, fried, med	3	Ounce-weight	85.05	197.18	28.86	0.00	0.00	8.19	2.66	3.01	1.35	83.25	0.00	0.26
Burrito, bean & cheese	1	Each	93.00	188.79	7.53	27.48		5.85	3.42	1.24	0.89	13.95	49.29	
Burrito, beef	1	Each	110.00	261.80	13.30	29.26	0.79	10.41	5.23	3.70	0.43	31.90	6.60	
Burrito, beef & cheese, w/chili peppers	1	Each	152.00	316.16	20.46	31.86		12.39	5.20	4.97	1.11	85.12	98.80	
Burrito, meat & bean	1	Each	115.50	254.10	11.24	33.01	2.49	8.91	4.16	3.51	0.61	24.25	16.17	
Chimichanga, beef	1	Each	174.00	424.56	19.61	42.80	2.00	19.68	8.51	8.06	1.14	8.70	6.96	
Chimichanga, beef & cheese	1	Each	183.00	442.86	20.06	39.33		23.44	11.18	9.43	0.73	51.24	131.76	
Dish, beef burgundy	1	Cup	244.00	291.29	35.05	8.91	1.42	11.79	3.37	4.14	2.36	94.24	2.72	0.73
Dish, beef curry	1	Cup	236.00	435.94	27.08	13.12	2.66	31.35	7.02	14.46	7.38	69.49	286.41	
Dish, chicken curry	1	Cup	236.00	293.82	27.45	10.35	2.15	16.09	3.33	7.01	4.35	84.25	157.24	
Dish, chicken, kiev	1	Each	258.00	642.55	73.33	10.02	0.34	32.62	15.83	10.51	3.71	283.15	208.26	
Dish, chicken, kung pao	1	Cup	162.00	431.21	28.81	11.39	2.23	30.61	5.19	13.94	9.69	64.39	31.44	
Dish, chicken, parmigiana	1	Piece	182.00	319.50	28.47	15.52	1.14	15.63	5.31	4.86	4.04	137.12	118.16	
Dish, chop suey, beef, w/o noodles	1	Cup	220.00	271.46	22.13	12.35	2.74	15.08	3.70	6.50	3.49	50.36	99.34	
Dish, chow mein, pork, w/noodles	1	Cup	220.00	447.94	21.96	31.03	3.73	27.02	4.85	7.72	12.80	47.76	10.07	
Dish, curried shrimp	1	Cup	236.00	297.67	27.52	13.60	0.38	14.33	3.97	5.74	3.51	176.76	168.93	
Dish, egg foo yung patty	1	Each	86.00	113.23	6.44	3.32	0.61	8.38	1.95	3.37	2.11	185.46	84.75	
Dish, egg roll, chicken	1	Each	64.00	103.31	3.93	9.39	0.62	5.51	1.23	2.67	1.18	38.01	17.32	
Dish, egg roll, meat	1	Each	64.00	113.07	4.95	9.26	0.68	6.21	1.44	2.98	1.32	37.07	14.62	
Dish, egg roll, shrimp	1	Each	64.00	104.09	3.51	9.87	0.72	5.63	1.17	2.69	1.35	39.50	16.17	
Dish, egg roll, w/o meat	1	Each	64.00	100.82	2.54	9.82	0.82	5.81	1.23	2.86	1.33	30.16	14.83	

Vit E (mg)	Vit C	Vit B1-Thia (mg)	Vit B2-Ribo (mg)	Vit B3-Nia (mg)	Fol (mcg)	Vit B6 (mg)	Vita B12 (mcg)	Sodi (mg)	Pota (mg)	Cal (mg)	Phos (mg)	Magn (mg)	Iron (mg)	Zinc (mg)	Caff (mg)	Alco (g)	Sol Fiber (g)	Insol Fiber (g)
	2.40							480.00		100.00			1.44		0.00	0.00		
	34.88	0.30	0.34	4.00				609.62	580.00	80.00			2.12		0.00	0.00		
	4.80	0.00	0.10	1.40				850.00	500.00	60.00			1.80		0.00	0.00		
	6.00							1440.00		80.00			1.80		0.00	0.00		
	13.68						0.00	763.80		22.80			0.62		0.00	0.00		
	0.00	0.00	0.10	1.10		0.14		950.00	570.00	40.00			1.44		0.00			
	0.00							580.00		150.00			1.44		0.00	0.00		
	0.00							594.59		32.43			0.19		0.00	0.00		
	4.80	0.10	0.20	0.30				580.00	540.00	350.00			1.08		0.00	0.00		
	36.00							720.00		250.00			2.70		0.00	0.00		
	21.00							630.00		100.00			4.50		0.00	0.00		
	2.40							520.00		80.00			0.72		0.00	0.00		
	18.00							670.00		300.00			1.80		0.00	0.00		
4.23	9.90	0.82	0.44	5.17	57.81	0.41	1.01	486.42	377.80	68.10	262.50	32.45	2.96	1.08	0.00	0.00		
1.73	5.32	0.18	0.39	1.13	56.19	0.13	0.39	110.79	275.35	245.08	210.26	40.33	2.17	1.32	0.00	0.00		
	1.20							580.00		250.00			2.70		0.00	0.00		
	6.00							590.00		40.00			1.80		0.00	0.00		
0.12	0.00	0.10	0.26	4.22	9.93	0.48	3.01	62.63	418.34	6.50	238.99	29.02	2.96	4.60	0.00	0.00	0.00	0.00
	0.84	0.11	0.35	1.79	37.20	0.12	0.45	583.11	248.31	106.95	90.21	39.99	1.13	0.82	0.00	0.00		
0.55	0.55	0.12	0.46	3.22	64.90	0.15	0.98	745.80	369.60	41.80	86.90	40.70	3.05	2.37	0.00	0.00		
	1.82	0.30	0.62	4.16	69.92	0.18	1.03	1045.76	332.88	110.96	158.08	34.96	3.91	3.95	0.00	0.00		
0.69	0.92	0.27	0.42	2.70	57.75	0.18	0.87	667.59	328.02	53.13	70.45	41.58	2.45	1.92	0.00	0.00		
	4.70	0.49	0.64	5.78	83.52	0.28	1.51	910.02	586.38	62.64	123.54	62.64	4.54	4.96	0.00	0.00		
	2.75	0.38	0.86	4.67	91.50	0.22	1.30	957.09	203.13	237.90	186.66	60.39	3.84	3.37	0.00	0.00		
1.06	4.29	0.19	0.49	6.73	22.67	0.45	4.11	114.34	844.29	28.83	377.18	53.47	4.89	8.01	0.00	0.00		0.55
5.88	24.59	0.18	0.34	5.42	20.33	0.48	3.05	801.64	977.87	43.96	291.86	59.00	4.23	6.06	0.00	0.00		
3.13	18.43	0.13	0.23	10.28	20.29	0.50	0.30	629.18	625.75	43.71	251.43	51.21	2.07	2.15	0.00	0.00		
1.54	0.00	0.25	0.35	32.00	14.18	1.37	0.87	454.23	622.71	62.79	558.18	72.82	3.27	2.51	0.00	0.00		
3.90	7.51	0.15	0.15	13.23	42.56	0.59	0.26	906.76	428.26	49.47	263.04	63.13	1.96	1.50	0.00	0.20		
2.41	8.65	0.18	0.34	8.47	16.56	0.37	0.43	640.93	470.87	198.03	316.95	45.23	2.31	2.38	0.00	0.00		
2.03	23.42	0.18	0.25	4.20	42.01	0.41	1.96	923.87	556.38	37.50	238.00	41.54	2.91	3.48	0.00	0.00		
2.68	20.23	0.78	0.43	6.24	41.75	0.42	0.42	848.19	488.91	44.86	248.95	52.85	3.30	2.56	0.00	0.00		
2.43	3.68	0.12	0.29	3.16	11.25	0.17	1.36	342.25	443.11	229.28	367.00	60.21	3.02	1.80	0.00	0.00		
1.22	4.81	0.04	0.26	0.43	29.52	0.09	0.37	317.36	117.32	31.31	93.02	11.59	1.04	0.70	0.00	0.00		
0.73	2.35	0.08	0.11	1.06	10.97	0.05	0.08	163.87	73.20	15.15	40.95	7.73	0.85	0.33	0.00	0.00		
0.80	2.14	0.16	0.12	1.28	9.92	0.10	0.12	273.51	124.24	15.15	56.83	10.03	0.83	0.46	0.00	0.00		
0.85	2.32	0.08	0.10	0.91	9.96	0.05	0.11	292.53	99.77	17.09	46.71	9.81	0.90	0.29	0.00	0.00		
0.85	2.89	0.08	0.11	0.80	13.36	0.05	0.06	274.22	96.61	14.34	38.03	9.07	0.81	0.25	0.00	0.00		

Food Name	Amount	Measure	Weight (g)	Calories	Protein (g)	Total Carb (g)	Dietary Fiber (g)	Total Fat (g)	Sat Fat (g)	Mono Fat (g)	Poly Fat (g)	Chol (mg)	Vit A (mcg RAE)	Vit D (mcg)
Dish, eggplant, parmesan casserole	1	Cup	198.00	319.43	14.47	17.21	3.16	22.16	9.22	7.83	3.90	55.02	133.32	
Dish, enchilada, beef & cheese	1	Each	192.00	322.56	11.92	30.47		17.64	9.05	6.15	1.39	40.32	97.92	
Dish, enchirito, beef, bean & cheese	1	Each	193.00	343.54	17.89	33.79		16.08	7.95	6.52	0.33	50.18	88.78	
Dish, fajitas, beef	1	Each	223.00	399.44	22.62	35.67	3.21	18.15	5.53	7.57	3.47	45.08	21.55	
Dish, fajitas, chicken	1	Each	223.00	363.16	20.01	44.27	5.11	11.98	2.25	5.53	3.12	39.30	36.03	
Dish, goulash, beef	1	Cup	249.00	270.26	33.08	6.98	0.95	11.62	3.24	4.32	2.47	84.38	15.47	0.37
Dish, grape leaves, stuffed w/beef & rice	6	Each	126.00	301.63	10.26	14.26	4.00	23.25	5.42	13.82	2.14	30.50	404.29	
Dish, grape leaves, stuffed w/lamb & rice	6	Each	126.00	333.01	10.54	14.97	4.24	26.41	6.70	15.25	2.76	32.19	435.09	
Dish, jambalaya, shrimp	1	Cup	243.00	310.48	27.21	27.95	1.37	9.39	1.82	3.77	2.85	180.73	104.78	
Dish, knish, cheese	1	Each	60.00	208.17	6.46	18.69	0.64	11.80	2.79	5.33	2.92	55.97	118.65	
Dish, knish, meat	1	Each	50.00	175.27	6.63	12.89	0.56	10.64	2.63	4.88	2.28	52.37	83.27	
Dish, knish, potato	1	Each	61.00	215.09	4.73	20.80	0.92	12.49	2.61	5.78	3.27	59.10	120.78	
Dish, lamb curry	1	Cup	236.00	256.44	28.33	3.36	1.02	13.87	3.94	4.93	3.36	89.07	0.88	0.24
Dish, lo Mein, veg, vegetarian	5	Ounce-weight	141.75	95.79	4.35	19.19	2.66	0.55	0.09	0.06	0.22	0.00	46.00	
Dish, lo mein, w/pork	5	Ounce-weight	141.75	200.43	13.91	14.82	1.89	9.68	1.84	2.79	4.28	29.83	4.42	
Dish, macaroni & cheese, cnd, svg	1	Each	252.00	206.64	8.52	29.03	1.26	6.20	2.22	1.51	0.76	15.12		
Dish, pot pie, greek meat, 8"	1	Each	417.00	947.13	33.95	72.63	4.84	57.39	13.49	25.62	14.23	66.11	475.69	
Dish, quiche, cheese, w/o meat	5	Ounce-weight	141.75	420.33	12.45	19.73	0.57	32.57	15.86	10.87	3.85	178.81	241.84	
Dish, quiche, lorraine	1	Piece	176.00	526.35	14.93	25.04	0.73	40.87	18.85	14.34	5.19	221.04	275.87	1.07
Dish, rice pilaf	1	Cup	206.00	260.88	4.36	44.65	1.32	6.87	1.35	3.24	1.91	0.00	58.47	
Dish, spaghetti, w/tomato sauce & cheese, prep f/recipe	1	Cup	250.00	260.00	8.75	37.00		8.75	2.00			7.50		
Dish, spring roll, fresh	1	Each	64.00	113.07	4.95	9.26	0.68	6.21	1.44	2.98	1.32	37.07	14.62	
Dish, spring roll, meat	1	Each	64.00	113.07	4.95	9.26	0.68	6.21	1.44	2.98	1.32	37.07	14.62	
Dish, sweet & sour pork, w/rice	1	Cup	244.00	270.40	13.13	40.18	1.45	6.30	1.63	2.39	1.72	28.36	11.79	
Dish, turkey & noodles, w/gravy	1	Cup	224.00	303.95	19.73	27.11	1.19	12.28	3.43	4.92	2.79	77.77	29.96	
Dish, turkey & stuffing	1	Cup	200.00	273.46	34.64	18.94	0.80	5.44	1.39	1.71	1.30	104.66	19.09	
Dish, vegetables, w/pasta & cream sauce	1	Cup	162.00	180.71	7.87	20.73	1.26	7.54	2.26	3.03	1.78	6.81	272.09	
Dish, vegetables, w/pasta, New England, ckd	1	Cup	190.00	195.57	6.07	28.13		7.30	1.38	3.26	2.15	0.00	421.20	
Dish, wonton, meat filled, fried	3	Each	57.00	163.90	8.70	14.38	0.68	7.63	2.49	3.56	0.84	60.30	18.22	
Dish, ziti, w/meat, prep f/recipe	5	Ounce-weight	141.75	226.81	13.33	23.07		9.00	4.64	3.00	0.49	33.70	69.85	
Sandwich, bacon egg	1	Each	177.00	392.87	20.53	27.02	1.13	21.82	6.75	9.16	3.55	417.88	223.26	
Sushi, w/veg & fish	3	Ounce-weight	85.05	118.67	4.57	23.90	0.98	0.35	0.09	0.08	0.11	5.75	35.48	
Sushi, w/veg, rolled in seaweed	3	Ounce-weight	85.05	99.47	1.89	22.21	0.45	0.21	0.06	0.06	0.06	0.00	16.85	
Sushi, w/veg, w/o fish	3	Ounce-weight	85.05	123.03	2.63	27.33	1.14	0.24	0.06	0.06	0.08	0.00	39.05	
Taco, sml	1	Each	171.00	369.36	20.66	26.73		20.55	11.37	6.58	0.96	56.43	107.73	
Tostada, bean & cheese	1	Each	144.00	223.20	9.60	26.52		9.86	5.37	3.05	0.75	30.24	44.64	
Tostada, beef bean & cheese	1	Each	225.00	333.00	16.09	29.66		16.94	11.48	3.51	0.60	74.25	101.25	

Pizza

Food Name	Amount	Measure	Weight (g)	Calories	Protein (g)	Total Carb (g)	Dietary Fiber (g)	Total Fat (g)	Sat Fat (g)	Mono Fat (g)	Poly Fat (g)	Chol (mg)	Vit A (mcg RAE)	Vit D (mcg)
Pizza, bagel, cheese & pepperoni, fzn Ore-Ida	2	Piece	22.00	52.50	2.75	6.00	0.75	2.00	0.75			3.75		
Pizza, cheese, fzn Jeno's Crisp 'n Tasty	0.5	Each	97.50	230.00	9.50	26.00	1.00	9.50	3.00			10.00	0.00	
Pizza, combination, fzn Totino's Family Size	0.25	Each	125.00	310.00	11.00	29.00	2.00	17.00	3.50			10.00	0.00	
Pizza, combination, w/sausage & pepperoni, fzn Jeno's Crisp 'n Tasty	0.5	Each	99.00	245.52	8.41	25.84	1.39	12.08	2.85	5.96	1.53	12.87	0.00	
Pizza, combination, w/sausage & pepperoni, fzn Totino's Party Pizza	0.5	Each	152.00	384.56	14.14	36.02		20.37	4.42	10.31	2.48	12.16	0.00	
Pizza, deluxe, 1/4 ea, fzn Celeste	1	Piece	158.00	378.00	15.50	29.30	3.10	22.10				20.00		
Pizza, deluxe, French bread, fzn Lean Cuisine	1	Each	173.60	290.00	16.00	43.00	3.00	6.00	2.50	2.00	1.00	25.00		
Pizza, deluxe, two cheese sausage pepperoni & onion, fzn 1/5 Red Baron Pizza	1	Piece	129.00	336.69	12.00	31.99		17.80	6.27	6.90	2.27	24.51	0.00	

Vit E (mg)	Vit C	Vit B₁-Thia (mg)	Vit B₂-Ribo (mg)	Vit B₃-Nia (mg)	Fol (mcg)	Vit B₆ (mg)	Vita B₁₂ (mcg)	Sodi (mg)	Pota (mg)	Cal (mg)	Phos (mg)	Magn (mg)	Iron (mg)	Zinc (mg)	Caff (mg)	Alco (g)	Sol Fiber (g)	Insol Fiber (g)
2.62	8.10	0.14	0.25	1.63	23.52	0.19	0.45	683.97	447.44	366.34	281.40	37.52	1.30	1.52	0.00	0.00		
1.54	1.34	0.10	0.40	2.52	67.20	0.27	1.02	1319.04	574.08	228.48	167.04	82.56	3.07	2.69	0.00	0.00		
1.54	4.63	0.17	0.69	2.99	94.57	0.21	1.62	1250.64	559.70	218.09	223.88	71.41	2.39	2.76	0.00	0.00		
1.74	26.81	0.39	0.30	5.40	22.99	0.38	2.06	316.35	478.71	84.22	238.25	37.58	3.76	3.52	0.00	0.00		
1.71	36.83	0.43	0.33	6.12	41.80	0.38	0.10	343.02	533.62	100.80	188.31	48.17	3.32	1.65	0.00	0.00		
1.83	8.74	0.15	0.31	5.74	21.27	0.46	3.25	225.45	698.37	18.08	336.17	45.56	3.58	5.26	0.00	0.00		
2.66	10.33	0.09	0.21	2.91	29.68	0.22	0.71	87.70	279.92	120.68	107.12	45.53	2.38	2.02	0.00	0.00		
2.78	9.04	0.11	0.20	3.51	33.04	0.22	0.76	84.30	245.67	132.61	112.78	47.54	2.38	1.97	0.00	0.00		
2.34	16.87	0.29	0.10	4.77	12.15	0.22	1.18	370.06	439.32	103.94	300.25	63.59	4.39	1.73	0.00	0.00		
1.58	0.03	0.16	0.20	1.28	10.65	0.04	0.18	203.65	61.65	24.71	75.29	7.84	1.32	0.37	0.00	0.00		
1.21	0.36	0.11	0.16	1.50	8.28	0.05	0.32	106.64	88.39	12.24	61.46	8.47	1.24	1.01	0.00	0.00		
1.71	0.94	0.17	0.18	1.48	10.37	0.07	0.13	140.22	95.50	16.07	60.01	10.07	1.34	0.37	0.00	0.00		
1.20	1.35	0.09	0.28	8.06	27.52	0.20	2.89	323.18	496.10	36.39	283.81	40.02	2.97	6.63	0.00	0.00		
0.25	8.52	0.16	0.17	1.99	34.08	0.14	0.00	399.45	273.82	32.91	78.19	23.10	1.44	0.66	0.00	0.00		
1.46	8.06	0.29	0.19	3.55	37.54	0.25	0.18	100.55	235.12	20.68	132.68	29.96	1.47	1.30	0.00	0.14		
	0.00	0.25	0.29	2.98		0.09	0.38	1060.92	211.68	88.20	118.44	22.68	2.27	1.13	0.00	0.00		
6.53	15.04	0.67	0.60	8.82	42.42	0.49	2.38	1032.70	750.68	45.14	355.32	62.37	6.48	4.68	0.00	0.00		
1.59	0.50	0.17	0.41	1.19	16.22	0.07	0.43	146.84	171.09	249.14	235.69	20.15	1.46	1.30	0.00	0.00		
2.02	0.63	0.26	0.49	2.01	19.26	0.10	0.61	220.69	239.29	231.09	261.32	23.95	1.88	1.50	0.00	0.00		
1.07	0.94	0.26	0.03	2.49	7.66	0.12	0.01	151.07	110.94	25.47	76.04	19.08	2.34	0.77	0.00	0.00		
2.75	12.50	0.25	0.18	2.25	8.00	0.20	0.00		407.50	80.00	135.00	26.00	2.25	1.30	0.00	0.00		
0.80	2.14	0.16	0.12	1.28	9.92	0.10	0.12	273.51	124.24	15.15	56.83	10.03	0.83	0.46	0.00	0.00		
0.80	2.14	0.16	0.12	1.28	9.92	0.10	0.12	273.51	124.24	15.15	56.83	10.03	0.83	0.46	0.00	0.00		
0.84	14.42	0.53	0.16	3.81	9.91	0.38	0.26	617.95	310.90	28.25	142.48	34.56	1.99	1.46	0.00	0.00		
0.48	0.18	0.23	0.20	5.04	11.36	0.17	0.20	590.31	144.70	25.47	155.39	31.58	2.38	1.67	0.00	0.00		
0.61	2.92	0.23	0.31	13.11	28.69	0.45	0.36	510.90	402.72	42.53	293.10	47.49	2.28	2.54	0.00	0.00		
0.33	17.95	0.17	0.23	1.35	27.91	0.14	0.25	442.65	261.18	163.36	150.07	28.70	1.21	0.81	0.00	0.00		
1.76	39.59	0.24	0.15	2.13	47.57	0.19	0.01	125.53	307.31	43.11	99.22	35.15	1.83	0.83	0.00	0.00		
0.55	0.48	0.26	0.18	1.89	8.41	0.12	0.19	29.61	152.89	13.37	89.36	11.69	1.21	0.97	0.00	0.00		
0.67	8.36	0.14	0.19	2.43	11.48	0.14	0.57	226.31	266.00	156.46	172.90	29.13	1.78	1.92	0.00	0.00		
1.72	0.23	0.38	0.71	2.93	52.07	0.20	1.11	780.94	276.70	136.82	283.36	28.60	3.08	1.85	0.00	0.00		
0.32	2.04	0.14	0.04	1.52	7.85	0.08	0.17	47.60	111.83	12.87	55.84	13.70	1.19	0.43	0.00	0.04		
0.07	1.30	0.11	0.02	1.02	5.50	0.08	0.00	2.50	54.10	11.02	32.61	11.00	0.85	0.38	0.00	0.04		
0.10	2.11	0.15	0.03	1.34	8.14	0.07	0.00	45.26	86.63	12.65	43.01	12.32	1.31	0.46	0.00	0.04		
1.88	2.22	0.15	0.44	3.21	68.40	0.24	1.04	801.99	473.67	220.59	203.49	70.11	2.41	3.93	0.00	0.00		
1.15	1.30	0.10	0.33	1.32	43.20	0.16	0.69	542.88	403.20	210.24	116.64	59.04	1.89	1.90	0.00	0.00		
1.80	4.05	0.09	0.50	2.86	85.50	0.25	1.12	870.75	490.50	189.00	173.25	67.50	2.45	3.17	0.00	0.00		
	2.25							162.50	37.50	25.00			0.36		0.00	0.00		
	0.00							430.00		175.00			0.72		0.00	0.00		
	0.00							720.00		150.00			1.80		0.00	0.00		
								619.74		83.16					0.00	0.00		
						0.00		1041.20		209.76			2.66		0.00	0.00		
3.00									352.00		357.00	38.00	3.00		0.00	0.00		
	6.00							550.00	440.00	150.00			1.80		0.00	0.00		
								704.34		147.06			2.54		0.00	0.00		

Food Name	Amount	Measure	Weight (g)	Calories	Protein (g)	Total Carb (g)	Dietary Fiber (g)	Total Fat (g)	Sat Fat (g)	Mono Fat (g)	Poly Fat (g)	Chol (mg)	Vit A (mcg RAE)	Vit D (mcg)
MEALS AND DISHES *(continued)*														
Pizza, deluxe, w/sausage & pepperoni, French bread, fzn, svg Stouffer's	1	Each	175.00	428.75	16.10	44.45	3.50	20.65	6.37	8.72	2.52	33.25		
Pizza, hamburger, roll, fzn Totino's Pizza Rolls	1	Each	85.00	231.20	9.35	26.44		9.78	2.98	6.80	0.00		0.00	
Pizza, pepperoni & sausage, original, fzn, 1/5 of 12" Tombstone	1	Piece	125.00	327.50	14.38	30.62	2.12	16.38	6.09	5.62	2.30	31.25		
Pizza, pepperoni & sausage, original, fzn, svg Tombstone	1	Each	118.00	317.42	13.33	27.26	1.65	17.23	6.30	5.82	2.41	31.86		
Pizza, pepperoni, deep dish, for one, fzn, Pappalo's	1	Each	199.00	525.36	22.69	64.68	3.18	19.50	7.34	7.26	1.89	37.81	0.00	
Pizza, pepperoni, deep dish, singles, premium, fzn Red Baron Pizza	1	Each	168.00	480.48	15.96	47.88		25.03	8.20	10.77	2.79	28.56	0.00	
Pizza, pepperoni, fzn Jeno's Crisp 'n Tasty	1	Each	192.00	516.48	18.62	45.89	3.07	28.80	6.47	14.53	3.90	23.04	0.00	
Pizza, pepperoni, original, fzn, 1/4 of 12" JK Original	1	Piece	122.00	323.30	15.01	29.52		16.10	6.22	5.23	2.07	40.26		
Pizza, pepperoni, original, fzn, 12" or pce Tombstone	1	Piece	113.00	311.88	14.46	28.25		15.71	6.00	5.31	2.05	31.64		
Pizza, pepperoni, roll, fzn Totino's Pizza Rolls	1	Each	141.00	384.93	14.38	39.48	2.26	18.89	4.99	9.24	2.21	31.02	0.00	
Pizza, pepperoni, w/Italian style pastry crust, fzn Tony's Pizza Service	0.25	Each	104.75	307.97	11.31	27.55		16.97	5.79	6.89	1.96	24.09	0.00	
Pizza, sausage & mushroom, original, fzn, 1/8 of 12" Tombstone	1	Piece	132.00	306.24	14.39	31.15		13.73	5.07	4.44	2.09	26.40		
Pizza, sausage & pepperoni, fzn, 12" or 1/4 pce JK Great Combinations	1	Piece	137.00	347.98	17.40	30.14		17.54	6.60	6.12	2.27	43.84		
Pizza, sausage mushroom, 1/4 ea, fzn Celeste	1	Piece	177.00	387.00	16.90	29.40	1.47	22.40				15.00		
Pizza, sausage, for one, fzn Celeste	1	Each	213.00	571.00	22.60	48.80	4.20	31.70	10.00	7.00	3.00	20.00		
Pizza, sausage, roll, fzn Totino's Pizza Rolls	1	Each	141.00	351.09	14.10	40.18	2.82	14.95	3.45	7.18	2.17	23.97	0.00	
Pizza, supreme, w/sausage mushroom & pepperoni, fzn Red Baron Pizza	0.125	Each	85.75	216.95	8.58	20.07		11.40	3.84	4.52	1.56	14.58	0.00	
Pizza, taco, w/Mexican sausage taco sauce corn crust, fzn Tony's Pizza Service	0.25	Each	116.75	331.57	10.86	32.46		17.63	5.87	6.75	2.64	21.02		
Pizza, vegetable, 1/2 less fat, for one, fzn Tombstone	1	Each	206.00	360.00	21.00	48.00	5.00	9.00	4.00			10.00		
Pizza, vegetable, rising crust, fzn, 12" or 1/6 pce Di Giorno	1	Piece	159.00	310.00	15.00	41.00	3.00	10.00	5.00			20.00		
MEATS														
Beef														
Beef, average of all cuts, ckd, 1/4" trim	3	Ounce-weight	85.05	259.40	22.06	0.00	0.00	18.32	7.26	7.84	0.66	74.84	0.00	
Beef, average of all cuts, ckd, prime, 1/2" trim	3	Ounce-weight	85.05	344.45	19.90	0.00	0.00	28.76	11.92	12.89	1.09	78.25	0.00	
Beef, average of all cuts, lean, ckd, 1/4" trim	3	Ounce-weight	85.05	183.71	25.16	0.00	0.00	8.43	3.22	3.55	0.29	73.14	0.00	
Beef, average of all cuts, lean, ckd, prime, 1/4" trim	3	Ounce-weight	85.05	204.97	24.70	0.00	0.00	11.04	4.42	4.68	0.39	69.74	0.00	
Beef, average of all cuts, lean, ckd, select, 0" trim	3	Ounce-weight	85.05	170.95	25.42	0.00	0.00	6.88	2.63	2.89	0.24	73.14	0.00	
Beef, average of all cuts, lean, raw, choice, 1/4" trim	4	Ounce-weight	113.40	170.10	23.56	0.00	0.00	7.73	2.90	3.27	0.31	66.91	0.00	
Beef, bottom round roast, lean, brsd, 0" trim	3	Ounce-weight	85.05	182.01	28.92	0.00	0.00	6.52	2.28	2.75	0.24	88.45	0.00	
Beef, brisket, corned, cured, ckd	3	Ounce-weight	85.05	213.48	15.45	0.40	0.00	16.14	5.39	7.84	0.57	83.35	0.00	
Beef, chuck arm pot roast, lean, brsd, choice, 1/8" trim	3	Ounce-weight	85.05	190.51	29.53	0.00	0.00	7.12	2.70	3.03	0.25	68.89	0.00	

Vit E (mg)	Vit C	Vit B₁-Thia (mg)	Vit B₂-Ribo (mg)	Vit B₃-Nia (mg)	Fol (mcg)	Vit B₆ (mg)	Vita B₁₂ (mcg)	Sodi (mg)	Pota (mg)	Cal (mg)	Phos (mg)	Magn (mg)	Iron (mg)	Zinc (mg)	Caff (mg)	Alco (g)	Sol Fiber (g)	Insol Fiber (g)
	29.93							840.00	159.64	231.00			2.71		0.00	0.00		
		0.00						417.35							0.00	0.00		
								790.00		178.75					0.00	0.00		
								728.06		184.08					0.00	0.00		
								983.06		248.75			3.60		0.00	0.00		
								888.72		152.88			3.46		0.00	0.00		
	0.00							1221.12		203.52			1.44		0.00	0.00		
								612.44		220.82					0.00	0.00		
								551.44		202.27					0.00	0.00		
								865.74		102.93					0.00	0.00		
								632.69		163.41			2.12		0.00	0.00		
								718.08		200.64					0.00	0.00		
								708.29		224.68					0.00	0.00		
3.00									361.00		407.00	45.00		3.00	0.00	0.00		
4.00	0.00	0.30	0.77	2.85	109.00	0.23	2.00	1363.00	456.00	371.00	505.00	60.00	2.28	0.00	0.00	0.00		
								631.68		101.52					0.00	0.00		
								465.62		140.63			1.44		0.00	0.00		
								573.24		142.44			1.93		0.00	0.00		
	1.20							860.00	500.00	350.00			1.80		0.00	0.00		
	3.60							830.00	290.00	250.00			1.06		0.00	0.00		
0.17	0.00	0.07	0.18	3.10	5.95	0.28	2.08	52.73	266.21	8.51	172.65	18.71	2.23	4.98	0.00	0.00	0.00	0.00
0.20	0.00	0.06	0.17	2.77	5.95	0.25	1.96	48.48	228.78	8.51	152.24	16.16	2.08	4.29	0.00	0.00	0.00	0.00
0.12	0.00	0.09	0.20	3.51	6.80	0.31	2.25	56.98	306.18	7.65	198.17	22.11	2.54	5.89	0.00	0.00	0.00	0.00
0.15	0.00	0.09	0.21	4.05	7.65	0.35	2.40	56.98	338.50	6.80	193.06	23.81	2.42	5.67	0.00	0.00	0.00	0.00
0.09	0.00	0.08	0.20	3.40	6.80	0.30	2.25	56.13	301.08	6.80	196.47	22.11	2.54	5.78	0.00	0.00	0.00	0.00
0.15	0.00	0.12	0.20	4.08	7.94	0.50	3.69	71.44	403.70	6.80	225.67	24.95	2.42	4.90	0.00	0.00	0.00	0.00
0.38	0.00	0.07	0.16	5.20	9.36	0.39	1.60	37.42	236.44	5.95	182.01	19.56	2.41	4.95	0.00	0.00	0.00	0.00
0.14	0.00	0.02	0.14	2.58	5.10	0.20	1.39	964.47	123.32	6.80	106.31	10.21	1.58	3.90	0.00	0.00	0.00	0.00
0.39	0.00	0.06	0.20	4.46	10.21	0.29	2.29	47.63	233.89	12.76	181.16	19.56	2.59	6.97	0.00	0.00	0.00	0.00

Food Name	Amount	Measure	Weight (g)	Calories	Protein (g)	Total Carb (g)	Dietary Fiber (g)	Total Fat (g)	Sat Fat (g)	Mono Fat (g)	Poly Fat (g)	Chol (mg)	Vit A (mcg RAE)	Vit D (mcg)
Beef, chuck blade roast, brsd, 1/4" trim	3	Ounce-weight	85.05	293.42	22.60	0.00	0.00	21.85	8.70	9.44	0.78	88.45	0.00	0.26
Beef, chuck clod roast, lean, rstd, choice, 1/4" trim	3	Ounce-weight	85.05	151.39	22.20	0.00	0.00	6.30	2.02	3.32	0.25	65.49	0.00	
Beef, chuck tender steak, lean, brld, choice, 0" trim	3	Ounce-weight	85.05	136.93	21.89	0.00	0.00	4.84	1.45	2.30	0.34	55.28	0.00	
Beef, chuck, ground, extra lean, raw Maverick Ranch Naturalite	4	Ounce-weight	113.40	130.00	22.00	0.00	0.00	5.00	2.00	2.00	0.50	60.00	0.00	
Beef, corned, cured, cnd, slices, 3/4oz each	3	Ounce-weight	85.05	212.63	23.05	0.00	0.00	12.70	5.26	5.07	0.54	73.14	0.00	
Beef, cube steak, homestyle, fzn, 3oz, FS Travis Meats	3	Ounce-weight	85.05	283.97	13.79	0.00	0.00	25.21	10.28	10.90	0.92	61.88	0.00	
Beef, fajita style, flame brld, fzn, 9974, FS Pierre Foods Lean Magic	3	Ounce-weight	85.05	152.29	18.46	4.15		6.92	2.77					
Beef, flank steak, london broil, lean, brld, 0" trim	3	Ounce-weight	85.05	158.19	23.72	0.00	0.00	6.29	2.61	2.48	0.25	41.67	0.00	
Beef, ground, extra lean, raw Maverick Ranch Naturalite	4	Ounce-weight	113.40	130.00	22.00	0.00	0.00	4.50	1.50	2.00	0.50	60.00	0.00	
Beef, ground, hamburger patty, brld, 10% fat	3	Ounce-weight	85.05	184.56	22.21	0.00	0.00	9.98	3.94	4.21	0.36	72.29	0.00	
Beef, ground, hamburger patty, brld, 15% fat	3	Ounce-weight	85.05	212.63	22.05	0.00	0.00	13.17	5.01	5.67	0.41	76.55	0.00	
Beef, ground, hamburger patty, brld, 20% fat	3	Ounce-weight	85.05	230.49	21.90	0.00	0.00	15.16	5.75	6.72	0.44	77.40	0.00	
Beef, ground, hamburger, bkd, 15% fat	3	Ounce-weight	85.05	204.12	22.05	0.00	0.00	12.21	4.65	5.26	0.38	77.40	0.00	
Beef, ground, hamburger, bkd, 20% fat	3	Ounce-weight	85.05	216.03	21.48	0.00	0.00	13.75	5.92	6.09	0.40	76.55	0.00	
Beef, ground, hamburger, pan browned, 10% fat	3	Ounce-weight	85.05	195.62	24.20	0.00	0.00	10.24	4.06	4.32	0.37	75.69	0.00	
Beef, ground, hamburger, pan browned, 15% fat	3	Ounce-weight	85.05	217.73	23.58	0.00	0.00	13.01	4.93	5.61	0.41	76.55	0.00	
Beef, ground, hamburger, pan browned, 20% fat	3	Ounce-weight	85.05	231.34	22.96	0.00	0.00	14.76	6.36	6.55	0.43	75.69	0.00	
Beef, ground, hamburger, pan browned, 5% fat	3	Ounce-weight	85.05	164.15	24.81	0.00	0.00	6.45	2.93	2.67	0.32	75.69	0.00	
Beef, jerky, lrg pce	1	Each	19.80	81.18	6.57	2.18	0.36	5.07	2.15	2.24	0.20	9.50	0.00	
Beef, jerky, teriyaki, California style Snackmasters	1	Ounce-weight	28.35	81.00	13.16	5.07	0.00	1.01	0.00			20.25	0.00	
Beef, patty, salisbury shape, fzn, 3oz, FS Travis Meats	1	Each	85.00	196.50	14.05	3.00	1.40	14.47	5.88	6.23	0.57	39.42		
Beef, porterhouse steak, brld, select, 1/4" trim	3	Ounce-weight	85.05	264.51	19.96	0.00	0.00	19.84	8.05	8.79	0.85	56.13	0.00	
Beef, rib pot roast, lean, brld, choice, 1/4" trim	3	Ounce-weight	85.05	204.12	21.41	0.00	0.00	12.46	5.09	5.04	0.47	64.64	0.00	
Beef, rib pot roast, rstd, select, 1/8" trim	3	Ounce-weight	85.05	283.22	19.90	0.00	0.00	21.98	8.86	9.41	0.77	71.44	0.00	
Beef, rib steak, lean, brld, select, 1/8" trim	3	Ounce-weight	85.05	159.89	26.25	0.00	0.00	5.29	2.01	2.11	0.19	49.33	0.00	
Beef, ribs, w/bbq sauce	3	Ounce-weight	85.05	147.86	17.98	2.48	0.23	6.75	2.57	2.90	0.34	51.89	8.00	
Beef, roast, lean, rstd	3	Ounce-weight	85.05	168.57	24.11	0.00	0.00	7.27	2.77	3.02	0.23	65.59	0.00	0.26
Beef, roast, rstd	3	Ounce-weight	85.05	226.97	21.91	0.00	0.00	14.81	5.85	6.30	0.53	67.50	0.00	0.26
Beef, round eye roast, lean, raw, select, 1/8" trim	4	Ounce-weight	113.40	134.95	25.30	0.00	0.00	2.97	1.02	1.25	0.13	40.82	0.00	
Beef, round eye roast, lean, rstd, 0" trim	3	Ounce-weight	85.05	137.78	24.95	0.00	0.00	3.48	1.21	1.46	0.13	46.78	0.00	
Beef, round roast, brld, choice, 1/4" trim	3	Ounce-weight	85.05	204.12	23.26	0.00	0.00	11.58	4.39	4.97	0.46	68.04	0.00	
Beef, round tip roast, lean, rstd, choice, 1/4" trim	3	Ounce-weight	85.05	159.89	24.42	0.00	0.00	6.21	2.17	2.47	0.25	68.89	0.00	
Beef, sandwich steak, formed & thinly sliced, raw, 14oz pkg	4	Ounce-weight	113.40	350.41	18.71	0.00	0.00	30.62	13.08	12.51	0.55	80.51	0.00	
Beef, sirloin strip steak, brld, 1/8" trim	3	Ounce-weight	85.05	224.53	22.49	0.00	0.00	14.27	5.62	5.95	0.53	74.84	0.00	

Vit E (mg)	Vit C	Vit B$_1$-Thia (mg)	Vit B$_2$-Ribo (mg)	Vit B$_3$-Nia (mg)	Fol (mcg)	Vit B$_6$ (mg)	Vita B$_{12}$ (mcg)	Sodi (mg)	Pota (mg)	Cal (mg)	Phos (mg)	Magn (mg)	Iron (mg)	Zinc (mg)	Caff (mg)	Alco (g)	Sol Fiber (g)	Insol Fiber (g)
0.17	0.00	0.06	0.20	2.06	4.25	0.22	1.94	54.43	196.47	11.06	170.10	16.16	2.64	7.08	0.00	0.00	0.00	0.00
0.14	0.00	0.07	0.21	2.92	7.65	0.23	2.54	60.39	313.83	5.95	181.16	18.71	2.60	5.43	0.00	0.00	0.00	0.00
0.14	0.00	0.09	0.19	3.07	6.80	0.27	2.87	62.09	249.20	6.80	199.02	19.56	2.57	6.66	0.00	0.00	0.00	0.00
	0.00			5.00			2.40	65.00		0.00			1.80	4.50	0.00	0.00	0.00	0.00
0.13	0.00	0.02	0.13	2.07	7.65	0.11	1.38	855.60	115.67	10.21	94.41	11.91	1.77	3.04	0.00	0.00	0.00	0.00
	0.00	0.07	0.12	2.35				42.53	210.12	6.30	126.97		1.44	2.62	0.00	0.00	0.00	0.00
	0.23							405.18		29.53			2.49		0.00	0.00		
0.32	0.00	0.06	0.12	6.79	7.65	0.51	1.36	48.48	297.68	15.31	184.56	19.56	1.48	4.33	0.00	0.00	0.00	0.00
	0.00			5.00			2.70	65.00		0.00			1.80	4.50	0.00	0.00	0.00	0.00
0.35	0.00	0.04	0.15	4.81	6.80	0.34	2.18	57.83	283.22	11.06	171.80	18.71	2.30	5.42	0.00	0.00	0.00	0.00
0.38	0.00	0.04	0.15	4.57	7.65	0.32	2.25	61.24	270.46	15.31	168.40	17.86	2.21	5.37	0.00	0.00	0.00	0.00
0.40	0.00	0.04	0.15	4.34	8.51	0.31	2.32	63.79	258.55	20.41	165.00	17.01	2.11	5.32	0.00	0.00	0.00	0.00
0.37	0.00	0.03	0.15	4.19	5.10	0.29	2.12	54.43	243.24	15.31	158.19	17.01	2.33	5.49	0.00	0.00	0.00	0.00
0.38	0.00	0.04	0.14	3.94	5.95	0.28	2.11	56.98	230.49	19.56	152.24	16.16	2.19	5.31	0.00	0.00	0.00	0.00
0.37	0.00	0.04	0.16	5.79	6.80	0.36	2.30	73.99	368.27	13.61	212.63	22.96	2.62	5.82	0.00	0.00	0.00	0.00
0.40	0.00	0.04	0.16	5.37	8.51	0.36	2.37	75.69	346.15	18.71	202.42	21.26	2.49	5.63	0.00	0.00	0.00	0.00
0.41	0.00	0.04	0.16	4.96	9.36	0.36	2.43	77.40	323.19	23.81	192.21	19.56	2.36	5.44	0.00	0.00	0.00	0.00
0.34	0.00	0.04	0.17	6.20	5.95	0.36	2.25	72.29	390.38	7.65	223.68	23.81	2.75	6.00	0.00	0.00	0.00	0.00
0.10	0.00	0.03	0.03	0.34	26.53	0.03	0.20	438.17	118.21	3.96	80.59	10.10	1.08	1.60	0.00	0.00		
	0.00							648.00		0.00			1.82		0.00	0.00	0.00	0.00
	1.20	0.19	0.14	3.12				224.50	333.60	33.00	148.30		1.98	4.58	0.00	0.00		
0.18	0.00	0.08	0.18	3.35	5.95	0.29	1.80	53.58	221.13	6.80	153.94	17.01	2.33	3.60	0.00	0.00	0.00	0.00
0.18	0.00	0.07	0.16	2.70	5.95	0.22	2.82	61.24	316.39	7.65	184.56	19.56	2.19	5.34	0.00	0.00	0.00	0.00
0.19	0.00	0.06	0.16	3.18	6.80	0.20	2.02	55.28	254.30	7.65	149.69	17.01	2.03	5.09	0.00	0.00	0.00	0.00
0.34	0.00	0.07	0.14	7.67	8.51	0.58	1.25	56.13	347.85	18.71	215.18	22.96	1.62	4.84	0.00	0.00	0.00	0.00
0.31	1.29	0.05	0.13	2.62	5.80	0.20	2.19	204.45	295.12	11.56	149.69	19.91	2.09	4.12	0.00	0.00		
0.12	0.00	0.08	0.19	3.42	6.86	0.29	2.17	57.07	321.29	5.23	190.65	22.31	2.19	5.50	0.00	0.00		0.00
0.16	0.00	0.07	0.17	3.07	6.06	0.27	2.04	53.43	289.67	6.18	172.55	19.64	1.98	4.79	0.00	0.00		0.00
0.32	0.00	0.10	0.16	7.53	14.74	0.74	1.47	70.31	412.78	24.95	248.35	28.35	2.18	5.06	0.00	0.00	0.00	0.00
0.31	0.00	0.06	0.14	4.48	8.51	0.33	1.38	32.32	203.27	5.10	156.49	16.16	2.08	4.26	0.00	0.00	0.00	0.00
0.16	0.00	0.08	0.18	3.39	7.65	0.32	2.56	51.88	333.40	5.10	202.42	21.26	2.15	3.67	0.00	0.00	0.00	0.00
0.12	0.00	0.09	0.23	3.18	6.80	0.34	2.46	55.28	328.29	4.25	205.82	22.96	2.50	6.01	0.00	0.00	0.00	0.00
0.24	0.00	0.04	0.18	5.20	7.94	0.28	3.08	77.11	264.22	13.61	150.82	18.14	2.11	4.11	0.00	0.00	0.00	0.00
0.39	0.00	0.06	0.11	5.98	6.80	0.47	1.33	45.93	278.96	16.16	173.50	18.71	1.44	4.04	0.00	0.00	0.00	0.00

MEATS (continued)

Food Name	Amount	Measure	Weight (g)	Calories	Protein (g)	Total Carb (g)	Dietary Fiber (g)	Total Fat (g)	Sat Fat (g)	Mono Fat (g)	Poly Fat (g)	Chol (mg)	Vit A (mcg RAE)	Vit D (mcg)
Beef, sirloin strip steak, lean, brld, choice, 1/8" trim	3	Ounce-weight	85.05	170.95	24.80	0.00	0.00	7.19	2.74	2.87	0.26	67.19	0.00	
Beef, snack stick, smkd	1	Each	19.80	108.90	4.26	1.07		9.82	4.12	4.05	0.88	26.33	2.57	
Beef, steak, country fried, fzn, 1965, FS Pierre Foods	3	Ounce-weight	85.05	319.50	15.00	12.15		23.25	6.60			47.46		
Beef, taco filling, fzn Ortega	0.33	Cup	55.28	100.00	7.00	4.00	1.00	6.00	2.50			20.00		
Beef, T-bone steak, brld, choice, 1/4" trim	3	Ounce-weight	85.05	273.86	19.38	0.00	0.00	21.22	8.29	9.59	0.75	57.83	0.00	
Beef, tenderloin, filet mignon, brld, choice, 1/8" trim	3	Ounce-weight	85.05	232.19	22.48	0.00	0.00	15.12	5.95	6.30	0.56	79.10	0.00	
Beef, tenderloin, filet mignon, lean, rstd, 1/4" trim	3	Ounce-weight	85.05	188.81	23.57	0.00	0.00	9.76	3.68	3.81	0.44	70.59	0.00	
Beef, tenderloin, filet mignon, raw, choice, 1/8" trim	4	Ounce-weight	113.40	278.96	22.48	0.00	0.00	20.28	8.18	8.68	0.77	73.71	0.00	
Beef, top round steak, brld, choice, 1/8" trim	3	Ounce-weight	85.05	190.51	26.11	0.00	0.00	8.73	3.32	3.72	0.34	56.13	0.00	
Beef, top sirloin steak, lean, brld, choice, 1/8" trim	3	Ounce-weight	85.05	159.04	25.10	0.00	0.00	5.72	2.18	2.28	0.20	53.58	0.00	
Beef, tri-tip roast, loin, lean, rstd, 0" trim	3	Ounce-weight	85.05	154.79	22.75	0.00	0.00	7.09	2.64	3.58	0.23	60.39	0.00	
Beef, whole rib, rstd, select, 1/8" trim	3	Ounce-weight	85.05	280.67	19.65	0.00	0.00	21.80	8.78	9.36	0.77	71.44	0.00	

Game Meats

Food Name	Amount	Measure	Weight (g)	Calories	Protein (g)	Total Carb (g)	Dietary Fiber (g)	Total Fat (g)	Sat Fat (g)	Mono Fat (g)	Poly Fat (g)	Chol (mg)	Vit A (mcg RAE)	Vit D (mcg)
Buffalo, burger/patty, extra lean, raw Maverick Ranch	4	Ounce-weight	113.40	140.00	24.00	0.00	0.00	4.00	1.50			55.00	0.00	
Deer, ground, pan brld	3	Ounce-weight	85.05	159.04	22.50	0.00	0.00	6.99	3.40	1.65	0.38	83.35	0.00	
Deer, top round steak, lean, 1" thick, brld	3	Ounce-weight	85.05	129.28	26.77	0.00	0.00	1.63	0.88	0.35	0.10	72.29	0.00	
Elk, rstd	3	Ounce-weight	85.05	124.17	25.68	0.00	0.00	1.62	0.60	0.41	0.34	62.09	0.00	
Rabbit, stewed, domestic	3	Ounce-weight	85.05	175.20	25.84	0.00	0.00	7.15	2.13	1.93	1.39	73.14	0.00	

Goat
Lamb

Food Name	Amount	Measure	Weight (g)	Calories	Protein (g)	Total Carb (g)	Dietary Fiber (g)	Total Fat (g)	Sat Fat (g)	Mono Fat (g)	Poly Fat (g)	Chol (mg)	Vit A (mcg RAE)	Vit D (mcg)
Lamb, average of all cuts, lean, raw, choice, 1/4" trim	4	Ounce-weight	113.40	151.96	23.01	0.00	0.00	5.95	2.13	2.39	0.54	73.71	0.00	
Lamb, average of all cuts, raw, choice, 1/4" trim	4	Ounce-weight	113.40	302.78	19.14	0.00	0.00	24.48	10.74	10.05	1.93	81.65	0.00	
Lamb, average of all cuts, raw, choice, 1/8" trim	4	Ounce-weight	113.40	275.56	19.89	0.00	0.00	21.16	9.15	8.68	1.68	79.38	0.00	

Lunchmeats and Sausages

Food Name	Amount	Measure	Weight (g)	Calories	Protein (g)	Total Carb (g)	Dietary Fiber (g)	Total Fat (g)	Sat Fat (g)	Mono Fat (g)	Poly Fat (g)	Chol (mg)	Vit A (mcg RAE)	Vit D (mcg)
Frank, beef Oscar Mayer	1	Each	45.00	147.15	5.11	1.06	0.00	13.62	5.61	6.63	0.61	25.20	0.00	0.27
Frank, beef, fat free Oscar Mayer	1	Each	50.00	39.00	6.60	2.55	0.00	0.25	0.11	0.10	0.02	15.00	0.00	
Frank, turkey & chicken Louis Rich	1	Each	45.00	84.60	5.04	2.38	0.00	6.07	1.73	2.50	1.42	41.40	0.00	
Frank, turkey chicken & cheese, svg Louis Rich	1	Each	45.00	90.45	5.71	2.29	0.00	6.52	2.34	2.80	1.34	42.30	0.00	0.00
Frankfurter, beef, 10 per lb, 5" × 3/4"	1	Each	45.00	148.50	5.06	1.83	0.00	13.31	5.26	6.44	0.53	23.85	0.00	0.40
Frankfurter, cheese, w/pork & beef, smokies	1	Each	43.00	140.61	6.06	0.65	0.00	12.47	4.52	5.89	1.30	29.24	20.21	0.12
Frankfurter, chicken	1	Each	45.00	115.65	5.82	3.06	0.00	8.77	2.49	3.82	1.82	45.45	17.55	0.00
Frankfurter, turkey	1	Each	45.00	101.70	6.43	0.67	0.00	7.96	2.65	2.51	2.25	48.15	0.00	
Hot Dog, beef, bunsize Ball Park	1	Each	56.00	180.00	6.00	3.00	0.00	16.00	7.00			35.00	0.00	
Hot Dog, fat free Oscar Mayer	1	Each	50.00	36.50	6.30	2.15	0.00	0.30	0.10	0.10	0.06	14.50	0.00	
Hot Dog, pork & turkey, Little Wieners Oscar Mayer	6	Each	54.00	167.94	5.89	1.24	0.00	15.50	6.02	7.74	1.44	29.70	0.00	0.71
Hot Dog, pork turkey beef, light Oscar Mayer	1	Each	57.00	110.58	6.90	1.60	0.00	8.49	2.96	3.85	1.17	35.34	0.00	
Lunchmeat Loaf, beef, slice, 4" × 4" × 3/32"	1	Piece	28.35	87.32	4.08	0.82	0.00	7.43	3.17	3.46	0.24	18.14	0.00	
Lunchmeat Loaf, corned beef, jellied, slice, 4" × 4" × 3/32"	1	Piece	28.35	43.38	6.49	0.00	0.00	1.73	0.74	0.76	0.09	13.32	0.00	

Vit E (mg)	Vit C	Vit B₁-Thia (mg)	Vit B₂-Ribo (mg)	Vit B₃-Nia (mg)	Fol (mcg)	Vit B₆ (mg)	Vita B₁₂ (mcg)	Sodi (mg)	Pota (mg)	Cal (mg)	Phos (mg)	Magn (mg)	Iron (mg)	Zinc (mg)	Caff (mg)	Alco (g)	Sol Fiber (g)	Insol Fiber (g)
0.35	0.00	0.07	0.13	7.32	8.51	0.52	1.55	51.03	307.88	13.61	192.21	21.26	1.68	4.65	0.00	0.00	0.00	0.00
0.06	1.35	0.03	0.09	0.90	0.00	0.04	0.20	293.04	50.89	13.46	35.64	4.16	0.67	0.48	0.00	0.00		
	0.02							320.85	177.45	13.95			2.31		0.00	0.00		
	1.20							290.00		40.00			0.72		0.00	0.00		
0.19	0.00	0.08	0.18	3.29	5.95	0.28	1.79	57.83	233.89	6.80	153.94	17.86	2.56	3.56	0.00	0.00	0.00	0.00
0.40	0.00	0.06	0.10	6.10	6.80	0.45	1.48	44.23	270.46	14.46	166.70	17.86	1.50	3.97	0.00	0.00	0.00	0.00
0.13	0.00	0.09	0.26	2.90	7.65	0.25	2.30	51.88	332.55	5.95	203.27	22.96	3.14	4.07	0.00	0.00	0.00	0.00
0.46	0.00	0.06	0.10	7.25	12.47	0.61	1.25	56.70	343.60	28.35	200.72	22.68	1.62	3.97	0.00	0.00	0.00	0.00
0.37	0.00	0.05	0.15	4.72	8.51	0.34	1.56	34.02	210.92	5.95	159.04	17.01	2.16	4.33	0.00	0.00	0.00	0.00
0.33	0.00	0.06	0.11	6.61	7.65	0.47	1.39	51.88	313.83	14.46	196.47	21.26	1.71	4.75	0.00	0.00	0.00	0.00
0.32	0.00	0.06	0.12	6.51	7.65	0.49	1.30	46.78	289.17	14.46	179.46	19.56	1.44	4.19	0.00	0.00	0.00	0.00
0.19	0.00	0.06	0.15	2.99	5.95	0.20	2.19	55.28	263.66	9.36	153.09	17.01	2.05	4.74	0.00	0.00	0.00	0.00
	0.00							50.00		0.00			2.70	3.75	0.00	0.00	0.00	0.00
0.58	0.00	0.43	0.28	7.87	6.80	0.40	1.97	66.34	309.58	11.91	193.91	20.41	2.85	4.42	0.00	0.00	0.00	0.00
0.54	0.00	0.21	0.43	7.14	8.51	0.60	1.93	38.27	320.64	3.40	231.34	25.52	3.60	3.12	0.00	0.00	0.00	0.00
0.02	0.00				7.65		5.53	51.88	278.96	4.25	153.09	20.41	3.09	2.69	0.00	0.00	0.00	0.00
0.37	0.00	0.05	0.14	6.09	7.65	0.29	5.54	31.47	255.15	17.01	192.21	17.01	2.02	2.02	0.00	0.00	0.00	0.00
0.24	0.00	0.15	0.26	6.80	26.08	0.18	2.97	74.84	317.52	11.34	214.33	29.48	2.01	4.60	0.00	0.00	0.00	0.00
0.24	0.00	0.14	0.25	6.92	20.41	0.15	2.71	65.77	260.82	13.61	181.44	24.95	1.78	3.78	0.00	0.00	0.00	0.00
0.24	0.00	0.14	0.25	6.88	21.55	0.16	2.77	66.91	271.03	13.61	188.24	24.95	1.84	3.99	0.00	0.00	0.00	0.00
	0.00	0.02	0.04	1.03	2.70	0.03	0.73	461.25	58.50	4.50	63.00	5.85	0.60	0.99	0.00	0.00	0.00	0.00
	0.00							463.50	233.50	10.00	64.50	9.50	0.98	1.20	0.00	0.00	0.00	0.00
	0.00							511.20	72.00	58.95	66.15	10.35	0.98	0.84	0.00	0.00	0.00	0.00
	0.00							481.50	71.10	109.35	91.80	9.90	0.95	0.81	0.00	0.81	0.00	0.00
0.09	0.00	0.02	0.07	1.07	2.25	0.04	0.77	513.00	70.20	6.30	72.00	6.30	0.68	1.11	0.00	0.00	0.00	0.00
0.00	0.00	0.11	0.07	1.25	1.29	0.06	0.74	465.26	88.58	24.94	76.54	5.59	0.46	0.97	0.00	0.00	0.00	0.00
0.10	0.00	0.03	0.05	1.39	1.80	0.14	0.11	616.50	37.80	42.75	48.15	4.50	0.90	0.47	0.00	0.00	0.00	0.00
0.28	0.00	0.02	0.08	1.86	3.60	0.10	0.13	641.70	80.55	47.70	60.30	6.30	0.83	1.40	0.00	0.00	0.00	0.00
	3.60							620.00	460.00	0.00			0.72		0.00	0.00	0.00	0.00
	0.00							487.00	235.50	7.50	81.00	10.50	0.46	0.60	0.00	0.00	0.00	0.00
	0.00	0.14	0.09	1.44	1.10	0.07	0.68	561.06	85.86	7.02	52.38	7.02	0.55	0.99	0.00	0.00	0.00	0.00
	0.00							590.52	226.29	21.66	96.33	9.69	0.73	1.01	0.00	0.00	0.00	0.00
0.06	0.00	0.03	0.06	1.04	1.42	0.06	1.10	376.77	58.97	3.12	33.74	3.97	0.66	0.72	0.00	0.00	0.00	0.00
0.05	0.00	0.00	0.03	0.50	2.27	0.03	0.36	270.18	28.63	3.12	20.70	3.12	0.58	1.16	0.00	0.00	0.00	0.00

Food Name	Amount	Measure	Weight (g)	Calories	Protein (g)	Total Carb (g)	Dietary Fiber (g)	Total Fat (g)	Sat Fat (g)	Mono Fat (g)	Poly Fat (g)	Chol (mg)	Vit A (mcg RAE)	Vit D (mcg)
MEATS *(continued)*														
Lunchmeat Loaf, ham & cheese Oscar Mayer	1	Ounce-weight	28.35	66.34	3.93	1.06	0.00	5.16	1.86	2.35	0.51	17.58	0.00	0.29
Lunchmeat Loaf, ham & cheese, slice, 4" × 4" × 3/32"	1	Piece	28.35	68.32	3.86	1.14	0.00	5.30	1.98	2.44	0.57	16.44	0.00	0.31
Lunchmeat Loaf, honey, w/pork & beef, slice, 4" × 4" × 3/32"	1	Piece	28.35	35.44	4.47	1.51	0.00	1.26	0.40	0.57	0.13	9.64	0.00	0.26
Lunchmeat Loaf, luxury, w/pork, slice, 4" × 4" × 3/32"	1	Piece	28.35	39.98	5.22	1.39	0.00	1.36	0.45	0.66	0.14	10.20	0.00	0.20
Lunchmeat Loaf, olive, w/chicken pork & turkey Oscar Mayer	1	Ounce-weight	28.35	74.56	2.80	1.95	0.00	6.18	1.99	3.16	0.75	20.13	0.00	
Lunchmeat Loaf, peppered, w/pork & beef, slice, 4" × 4" × 3/32"	1	Piece	28.35	41.96	4.90	1.30	0.00	1.81	0.65	0.85	0.14	13.04	0.00	0.23
Lunchmeat Loaf, pickle pimiento, w/chicken Oscar Mayer	1	Ounce-weight	28.35	76.26	2.72	2.58	0.00	6.13	1.98	2.96	0.80	22.68	0.00	
Lunchmeat Loaf, pickle pimiento, w/pork, slice, 4" × 4" × 3/32"	1	Piece	28.35	63.79	3.18	2.40	0.17	4.52	1.50	2.00	0.80	16.44	25.80	0.31
Lunchmeat Loaf, pork & beef, Dutch brand, slice, 4" × 4" × 3/32"	1	Piece	28.35	77.40	3.40	1.11	0.06	6.49	2.58	2.86	0.87	17.01	13.32	0.28
Lunchmeat Loaf, spiced Oscar Mayer	1	Ounce-weight	28.35	66.34	3.83	1.98	0.00	4.79	1.52	2.10	0.79	18.99	0.00	
Lunchmeat Loaf, turkey, light meat, slice	1	Ounce-weight	28.35	41.67	5.30	0.15	0.00	2.05	0.57	0.71	0.49	12.19	0.00	
Lunchmeat Spread, chicken salad, rts, cnd Libby's Spreadables	1	Ounce-weight	28.35	41.11	1.39	2.87		2.66	0.55	0.83	1.02	7.37	0.00	
Lunchmeat Spread, chicken, cnd	2	Tablespoon	26.00	41.08	4.68	1.05	0.08	4.57	0.84	1.25	0.61	14.56	7.80	
Lunchmeat Spread, ham & cheese	2	Tablespoon	30.00	73.50	4.85	0.68	0.00	5.56	2.59	2.12	0.41	18.30	27.30	
Lunchmeat Spread, pork & beef	2	Tablespoon	30.00	70.50	2.30	3.58	0.06	5.20	1.79	2.29	0.77	11.40	7.80	
Lunchmeat Spread, pork chicken & beef, svg Oscar Mayer	1	Ounce-weight	28.35	67.19	1.85	4.37	0.09	4.71	1.63	2.04	0.71	12.76		
Lunchmeat Spread, poultry salad	2	Tablespoon	26.00	52.00	3.03	1.93	0.00	3.52	0.90	0.85	1.62	7.80	10.92	
Lunchmeat Spread, tuna salad	0.5	Cup	127.00	237.49	20.37	11.96	0.00	11.75	1.96	3.67	5.24	16.51	30.48	
Lunchmeat, beef, thin slice	1	Ounce-weight	28.35	42.24	5.42	0.25	0.00	2.02	0.83	0.88	0.10	19.84	0.00	
Lunchmeat, bologna, beef & pork, 4" × 1/8" slice	1	Piece	23.00	70.84	3.50	1.26	0.00	5.65	2.14	2.42	0.26	13.80	5.75	0.18
Lunchmeat, bologna, beef, 4" × 1/8" slice	1	Piece	32.00	100.48	3.29	1.27	0.00	9.02	3.56	3.91	0.25	17.92	4.16	
Lunchmeat, bologna, beef, light Oscar Mayer	1	Ounce-weight	28.35	56.70	3.33	1.59	0.00	4.11	1.65	2.03	0.13	12.47	0.00	
Lunchmeat, bologna, beef Oscar Mayer	1	Ounce-weight	28.35	89.59	3.13	0.70	0.00	8.25	3.63	4.30	0.31	18.14	0.00	0.23
Lunchmeat, bologna, pork, 4" × 1/8" slice	1	Piece	23.00	56.81	3.52	0.17	0.00	4.57	1.58	2.25	0.49	13.57	0.00	0.32
Lunchmeat, bologna, ring, Wisconsin made, svg Oscar Mayer	1	Ounce-weight	28.35	88.74	3.35	0.74	0.00	8.05	3.16	3.99	0.56	17.58	0.00	0.28
Lunchmeat, bologna, turkey	1	Ounce-weight	28.35	59.25	3.24	1.32	0.14	4.55	1.24	1.94	1.10	21.26	2.55	0.00
Lunchmeat, bologna, turkey Louis Rich	1	Ounce-weight	28.35	52.16	3.21	1.38	0.00	3.74	1.07	1.51	1.02	18.99	0.00	
Lunchmeat, chicken breast, classic, bkd/grilled Louis Rich	1	Ounce-weight	28.35	27.78	5.58	1.05	0.00	0.14	0.04	0.05	0.03	14.74	0.00	
Lunchmeat, chicken breast, honey glazed, slice Oscar Mayer	1	Ounce-weight	28.35	30.90	5.63	1.11	0.00	0.43	0.11	0.16	0.06	15.03	0.00	
Lunchmeat, chicken breast, oven rstd, deluxe Louis Rich	1	Ounce-weight	28.35	28.63	5.19	0.71	0.00	0.57	0.15	0.23	0.09	13.89	0.00	
Lunchmeat, chicken breast, oven rstd, fat free, slice Oscar Mayer	1	Ounce-weight	28.35	24.10	5.19	0.48	0.00	0.17	0.05	0.04	0.02	12.47	0.00	
Lunchmeat, chicken breast, oven rstd, resealable Healthy Choice	1	Ounce-weight	28.35	35.44	5.06	1.01	0.00	1.01	0.51			15.19	0.00	
Lunchmeat, chicken, light & dark meat, smkd, sliced, pkg Carl Buddig & Company	1	Ounce-weight	28.35	46.78	5.07	0.20	0.00	2.86	0.74	1.53	0.60	15.03		
Lunchmeat, chicken, white, oven rstd Louis Rich	1	Ounce-weight	28.35	36.29	4.82	0.65	0.00	1.59	0.41	0.66	0.28	16.73	0.00	
Lunchmeat, ham, chpd, w/natural juices Oscar Mayer	1	Ounce-weight	28.35	51.03	4.62	1.04	0.00	3.16	1.15	1.65	0.36	16.73	0.00	

Vit E (mg)	Vit C	Vit B₁-Thia (mg)	Vit B₂-Ribo (mg)	Vit B₃-Nia (mg)	Fol (mcg)	Vit B₆ (mg)	Vita B₁₂ (mcg)	Sodi (mg)	Pota (mg)	Cal (mg)	Phos (mg)	Magn (mg)	Iron (mg)	Zinc (mg)	Caff (mg)	Alco (g)	Sol Fiber (g)	Insol Fiber (g)
0.00	0.00	0.16	0.05	0.98	0.85	0.07	0.21	330.84	75.13	18.99	76.55	5.39	0.24	0.52	0.00	0.00	0.00	0.00
0.08	0.00	0.17	0.06	0.98	0.85	0.08	0.23	306.18	83.35	16.44	71.72	4.54	0.26	0.56	0.00	0.00	0.00	0.00
0.06	0.00	0.14	0.07	0.89	2.27	0.10	0.30	374.22	97.24	4.82	40.54	4.82	0.38	0.68	0.00	0.00	0.00	0.00
0.06	0.00	0.20	0.08	0.98	0.56	0.09	0.39	347.29	106.88	10.20	52.45	5.67	0.30	0.86	0.00	0.00	0.00	0.00
	0.00							373.65	52.73	31.47	37.42	7.65	0.50	0.29	0.00	0.00	0.00	0.00
0.06	0.00	0.11	0.09	0.87	0.57	0.08	0.56	431.77	111.70	15.31	48.20	5.67	0.30	0.92	0.00	0.00	0.00	0.00
	0.00							361.46	49.33	31.19	42.53	8.22	0.62	0.33	0.00	0.00	0.00	0.00
0.12	2.21	0.14	0.04	0.97	4.54	0.09	0.22	369.68	89.58	30.90	40.54	5.96	0.38	0.54	0.00	0.00		
0.01	0.43	0.06	0.04	0.91	3.40	0.09	0.45	299.09	61.24	1.98	36.85	4.54	0.05	0.58	0.00	0.00		
	0.00							347.57	76.54	30.90	55.28	6.80	0.38	0.55	0.00	0.00	0.00	0.00
0.04	0.00	0.03	0.06	1.98	1.13	0.09	0.07	138.63	71.16	11.34	51.88	4.54	0.36	0.44	0.00	0.00	0.00	0.00
								132.68							0.00	0.00		
0.09	0.00	0.00	0.03	0.71	0.78	0.04	0.03	187.72	27.56	4.16	23.14	3.12	0.23	0.30				
	0.00	0.09	0.07	0.64	0.90	0.04	0.22	359.10	48.60	65.10	148.50	5.40	0.23	0.68	0.00	0.00	0.00	0.00
0.52	0.00	0.05	0.04	0.52	0.60	0.04	0.34	303.90	33.00	3.60	17.70	2.40	0.23	0.31	0.00	0.00		
	0.00							232.75	33.45	7.65	19.56	3.40	0.23	0.25	0.00	0.00		
0.57	0.26	0.00	0.02	0.43	1.30	0.03	0.10	98.02	47.58	2.60	8.58	2.60	0.16	0.27	0.00	0.00	0.00	0.00
1.20	2.79	0.05	0.09	8.52	10.16	0.09	1.52	510.54	226.06	21.59	226.06	24.13	1.27	0.72	0.00	0.00	0.00	0.00
0.05	0.00	0.02	0.05	1.21	3.12	0.10	0.73	400.59	121.62	3.12	47.63	5.39	0.59	1.13	0.00	0.00	0.00	0.00
0.00	0.18	0.05	0.04	0.58	1.38	0.07	0.42	169.28	72.45	19.55	37.49	3.91	0.28	0.53	0.00	0.00	0.00	0.00
0.11	4.86	0.01	0.03	0.80	2.88	0.05	0.41	345.60	55.04	9.92	55.04	4.48	0.35	2.91	0.00	0.00	0.00	0.00
	0.00				3.69			326.31	44.23	3.69	50.46	3.97	0.35	0.54	0.00	0.00	0.00	0.00
	0.00	0.02	0.03	0.69	3.69	0.05	0.41	334.25	47.63	3.40	30.90	3.97	0.39	0.58	0.00	0.00	0.00	0.00
0.06	0.00	0.12	0.04	0.90	1.15	0.06	0.21	272.32	64.63	2.53	31.97	3.22	0.18	0.47	0.00	0.00	0.00	0.00
	0.00	0.08	0.04	0.75		0.04	0.36	234.45	39.41	4.25	30.05	4.25	0.33	0.53	0.00	0.00		0.00
0.13	3.77	0.02	0.02	0.74	2.55	0.07	0.06	354.94	38.28	34.87	32.32	4.54	0.85	0.37	0.00	0.00		
	0.00				1.70			305.33	43.09	35.15	55.57	6.24	0.46	0.53	0.00	0.00	0.00	0.00
	0.00							323.76	82.50	2.27	79.95	9.07	0.37	0.25	0.00	0.00	0.00	0.00
	0.00				1.13			407.67	93.27	2.83	81.93	10.21	0.32	0.20	0.00	0.00	0.00	0.00
	0.00							336.80	75.13	1.98	75.41	6.80	0.32	0.21	0.00	0.00	0.00	0.00
	0.00							352.11	89.59	3.40	72.58	10.21	0.38	0.17	0.00	0.00	0.00	0.00
	0.00							243.00		0.00			0.00		0.00	0.00	0.00	0.00
		0.02	0.07	1.91				270.46	72.58	35.15				0.44	0.00	0.00	0.00	0.00
	0.00							339.07	85.62	4.82	70.31	6.80	0.45	0.32	0.00	0.00	0.00	0.00
	0.00				0.85			354.09	73.71	2.55	62.09	6.52	0.37	0.64	0.00	0.00	0.00	0.00

Food Name	Amount	Measure	Weight (g)	Calories	Protein (g)	Total Carb (g)	Dietary Fiber (g)	Total Fat (g)	Sat Fat (g)	Mono Fat (g)	Poly Fat (g)	Chol (mg)	Vit A (mcg RAE)	Vit D (mcg)
MEATS *(continued)*														
Lunchmeat, ham, reg, 11% fat, sliced, 6 1/4" × 4" × 1/16"	1	Piece	28.35	46.21	4.71	1.09	0.37	2.44	0.83	1.23	0.22	16.16	0.00	0.00
Lunchmeat, ham, smkd, 40% water add, fat free, slice	1	Ounce-weight	28.35	20.41	4.14	0.54	0.00	0.20	0.06	0.08	0.04	10.77	0.00	
Lunchmeat, ham, smkd, ckd, w/water add, slice Oscar Mayer	1	Ounce-weight	28.35	28.07	4.71	0.03	0.00	1.02	0.35	0.47	0.10	13.61	0.00	
Lunchmeat, olive, w/pork, slice, 4" × 4" × 3/32"	1	Piece	28.35	66.62	3.34	2.61	0.00	4.68	1.66	2.23	0.55	10.78	17.01	0.31
Lunchmeat, pork, cnd, slice, 4.25" × 4.25" × 1/16"	1	Piece	21.00	70.14	2.63	0.44	0.00	6.36	2.26	3.00	0.75	13.02	0.00	
Lunchmeat, turkey breast & white meat, oven rstd Louis Rich	1	Ounce-weight	28.35	28.07	4.85	0.92	0.00	0.57	0.13	0.16	0.12	11.62	0.00	
Lunchmeat, turkey breast, oven rstd, fat free, slice Louis Rich	1	Ounce-weight	28.35	23.81	4.25	1.28	0.00	0.20	0.06	0.06	0.04	9.07	0.00	
Lunchmeat, turkey breast, oven rstd, fat free Louis Rich	1	Ounce-weight	28.35	25.52	5.42	0.54	0.00	0.20	0.06	0.06	0.04	11.34	0.00	
Lunchmeat, turkey breast, smkd, fat free, slice Oscar Mayer	1	Ounce-weight	28.35	22.68	4.23	1.02	0.00	0.17	0.05	0.04	0.03	8.79	0.00	
Lunchmeat, turkey ham, cured thigh meat, slice	1	Ounce-weight	28.35	35.72	4.96	0.58	0.06	1.37	0.44	0.54	0.38	20.41	1.98	
Lunchmeat, turkey, light & dark meat, smkd, sliced, pkg Carl Buddig & Company	1	Ounce-weight	28.35	45.36	4.96	0.51	0.00	2.58	0.88	0.94	0.77	16.16		
Pastrami, beef, cured, 1 oz slice	1	Ounce-weight	28.35	41.39	6.18	0.54	0.14	1.65	0.76	0.59	0.05	19.28	9.36	
Pastrami, beef, smkd, chpd, pressed, ckd, pkg Carl Buddig & Company	1	Ounce-weight	28.35	39.97	5.56	0.28	0.00	1.84	0.85	0.91	0.09	18.43		
Pastrami, turkey, slices	1	Ounce-weight	28.35	34.87	4.62	1.04	0.03	1.23	0.34	0.42	0.32	19.28	1.14	
Salami, cotto, beef, slice Oscar Mayer	1	Ounce-weight	28.35	58.40	4.02	0.54	0.00	4.45	1.91	1.96	0.22	23.53		
Salami, hard, slice Oscar Mayer	1	Ounce-weight	28.35	104.33	7.34	0.47	0.00	8.14	3.12	4.22	0.80	27.50	1.28	0.44
Sausage, beef, smokies Oscar Mayer	1	Each	43.00	127.28	5.27	0.84	0.00	11.46	4.84	5.50	0.39	26.66	0.00	
Sausage, bockwurst, pork veal milk & eggs, raw	1	Each	65.00	180.70	7.09	0.32	0.00	16.82	6.73	8.58	1.51	60.45	0.00	0.19
Sausage, Italian, pork, link, ckd, 4 per lb	1	Each	83.00	285.52	15.87	3.54	0.08	22.67	7.91	9.92	2.72	47.31	8.30	
Sausage, knockwurst/knackwurst, beef & pork, link, 4" long	1	Each	68.00	208.76	7.55	2.18	0.00	18.84	6.94	8.71	1.99	40.80	0.00	
Sausage, Polish, pork, each, 10" × 1 1/4"	1	Each	227.00	740.02	32.01	3.70	0.00	65.19	23.45	30.69	6.99	158.90	0.00	
Sausage, pork & beef, smkd, link, w/nonfat dry milk, lrg, 4"	1	Each	68.00	212.84	9.03	1.31	0.00	18.77	6.61	8.60	2.05	44.20	0.00	
Sausage, pork, smkd, link, lrg, 4" × 1 1/8"	1	Each	68.00	264.52	15.10	1.43	0.00	21.56	7.70	9.95	2.56	46.24	0.00	
Sausage, smokies, links Oscar Mayer	1	Each	43.00	129.86	5.33	0.73	0.00	11.74	4.03	5.66	1.20	27.09	0.00	
Sausage, thuringer cervelat, beef, summer style, slice Oscar Mayer	1	Each	23.00	71.07	3.36	0.44	0.00	6.21	2.71	2.97	0.26	18.40		0.23
Sausage, Vienna, beef & pork, drained, 4oz can	1	Piece	16.00	36.80	1.68	0.42	0.00	3.10	1.14	1.54	0.21	13.92	0.00	
Pork and Ham														
Bacon, cured, raw, med slices, 20/lb	1	Piece	22.67	103.83	2.63	0.15	0.00	10.21	3.40	4.54	1.09	15.42	2.49	
Canadian Bacon, cured, grilled f/6oz pkg	2	Piece	46.33	85.71	11.23	0.63	0.00	3.91	1.32	1.87	0.38	26.87	0.00	
Canadian Bacon, cured, unheated, 6/6oz pkg	2	Piece	56.70	89.02	11.70	0.95	0.00	3.95	1.26	1.79	0.36	28.35	0.00	
Pork, avg of retail cuts, leg shoulder & loin, lean, ckd	3	Ounce-weight	85.05	180.31	24.89	0.00	0.00	8.22	2.90	3.70	0.64	73.14	1.70	
Pork, chop, center loin, lean, brsd	3	Ounce-weight	85.05	171.80	25.33	0.00	0.00	7.07	2.61	3.16	0.54	72.29	1.70	
Pork, chop, center rib loin, lean, brsd	3	Ounce-weight	85.05	179.46	23.77	0.00	0.00	8.62	3.37	4.12	0.62	60.39	1.70	
Pork, chop, center rib loin, w/bone, brsd	3	Ounce-weight	85.05	212.63	22.68	0.00	0.00	12.82	4.97	5.84	1.08	62.09	1.70	
Pork, chop, sirloin, lean, brsd	3	Ounce-weight	85.05	148.84	22.96	0.00	0.00	5.61	1.99	2.47	0.48	68.89	1.70	
Pork, chop, sirloin, w/bone, brsd	3	Ounce-weight	85.05	208.37	21.57	0.00	0.00	12.85	4.73	5.58	1.19	69.74	1.70	

Vit E (mg)	Vit C	Vit B₁-Thia (mg)	Vit B₂-Ribo (mg)	Vit B₃-Nia (mg)	Fol (mcg)	Vit B₆ (mg)	Vita B₁₂ (mcg)	Sodi (mg)	Pota (mg)	Cal (mg)	Phos (mg)	Magn (mg)	Iron (mg)	Zinc (mg)	Caff (mg)	Alco (g)	Sol Fiber (g)	Insol Fiber (g)
0.02	1.13	0.18	0.05	0.82	1.98	0.09	0.12	369.68	81.36	6.80	43.38	6.24	0.29	0.38	0.00	0.00		
	0.00							307.31	66.34	3.12	55.85	7.65	0.26	0.44	0.00	0.00	0.00	0.00
	0.00							344.17	75.98	2.84	66.06	8.79	0.37	0.51	0.00	0.00	0.00	0.00
0.07	0.00	0.08	0.08	0.52	0.56	0.06	0.36	420.72	84.20	30.90	36.01	5.38	0.16	0.39	0.00	0.00	0.00	0.00
0.05	0.21	0.08	0.04	0.66	1.26	0.05	0.19	270.69	45.15	1.26	17.22	2.10	0.15	0.31	0.00	0.00	0.00	0.00
	0.00				1.70			273.86	62.94	1.70	71.16	6.24	0.28	0.27	0.00	0.00	0.00	0.00
	0.00							337.93	58.12	3.12	65.77	7.65	0.31	0.24	0.00	0.00	0.00	0.00
	0.00							333.68	75.98	4.82	80.80	8.22	0.31	0.27	0.00	0.00	0.00	0.00
	0.00							310.43	61.80	2.83	68.89	8.50	0.22	0.24	0.00	0.00	0.00	0.00
0.18	0.00	0.01	0.04	0.60	1.98	0.06	0.06	315.82	81.36	2.27	83.35	6.24	0.66	0.74	0.00	0.00		
		0.05	0.09	1.66				310.72	93.27	17.01			0.52		0.00	0.00	0.00	0.00
0.14	0.37	0.02	0.05	1.21	1.98	0.08	0.52	250.90	66.62	2.84	49.61	5.39	0.63	1.39	0.00	0.00		
		0.03	0.07	1.16				299.38	103.48	4.82			0.69		0.00	0.00	0.00	0.00
0.06	4.57	0.02	0.07	1.00	1.42	0.08	0.07	278.12	97.81	3.12	56.70	3.97	1.19	0.61	0.00	0.00		
	0.00							371.10	58.68	1.98	63.50	4.82	0.77	0.59	0.00	0.00	0.00	0.00
	0.00	0.16	0.07	1.43	0.85	0.13	0.54	560.20	100.93	3.40	51.03	5.95	0.51	0.89	0.00	0.00	0.00	0.00
	0.00				4.73			415.81	74.39	4.73	98.90	6.45	0.75	1.27	0.00	0.00	0.00	0.00
0.06	0.00	0.14	0.14	2.97	4.55	0.20	0.48	323.05	148.20	26.65	105.30	11.05	0.75	1.16	0.00	0.00	0.00	0.00
0.21	0.08	0.52	0.19	3.46	4.15	0.27	1.08	1001.81	252.32	17.43	141.10	14.94	1.19	1.98	0.00	0.00		
0.39	0.00	0.23	0.10	1.86	1.36	0.12	0.80	632.40	135.32	7.48	66.64	7.48	0.45	1.13	0.00	0.00	0.00	0.00
0.52	2.27	1.14	0.34	7.82	4.54	0.43	2.22	1988.52	537.99	27.24	308.72	31.78	3.27	4.38	0.00	0.00	0.00	0.00
	0.00	0.13	0.15	1.93	1.36	0.12	1.07	797.64	194.48	27.88	93.16	10.88	1.00	1.33	0.00	0.00	0.00	0.00
0.17	1.36	0.48	0.18	3.08	3.40	0.24	1.11	1020.00	228.48	20.40	110.16	12.92	0.79	1.92	0.00	0.00	0.00	0.00
	0.00							433.01	77.40	4.30	103.20	7.31	0.50	0.90	0.00	0.00	0.00	0.00
	0.00	0.03	0.08	0.99	1.15	0.06	1.27	327.52	53.59	1.84	27.83	3.45	0.57	0.54	0.00	0.00	0.00	0.00
0.04	0.00	0.01	0.02	0.26	0.64	0.02	0.16	155.04	16.16	1.60	7.84	1.12	0.14	0.26	0.00	0.00	0.00	0.00
0.06	0.00	0.06	0.03	0.87	0.45	0.05	0.16	188.84	47.15	1.36	42.62	2.72	0.11	0.27	0.00	0.00	0.00	0.00
0.16	0.00	0.38	0.09	3.20	1.85	0.21	0.36	716.26	180.69	4.63	137.14	9.73	0.38	0.79	0.00	0.00	0.00	0.00
0.12	0.00	0.43	0.10	3.53	2.27	0.22	0.38	798.90	195.05	4.54	137.78	9.64	0.39	0.79	0.00	0.00	0.00	0.00
0.15	0.26	0.72	0.29	4.40	0.85	0.37	0.64	50.18	318.94	17.86	201.57	22.11	0.94	2.53	0.00	0.00	0.00	0.00
0.18	0.85	0.70	0.19	4.13	2.55	0.34	0.43	52.73	312.13	19.56	153.94	17.01	0.96	1.92	0.00	0.00	0.00	0.00
0.18	0.26	0.47	0.22	3.84	3.40	0.28	0.37	34.87	344.45	4.25	147.14	16.16	0.84	1.84	0.00	0.00	0.00	0.00
0.31	0.26	0.50	0.20	4.20	1.70	0.27	0.45	34.02	329.14	21.26	150.54	15.31	0.77	1.71	0.00	0.00	0.00	0.00
0.35	0.77	0.59	0.24	3.36	2.55	0.38	0.48	39.12	302.78	11.06	154.79	18.71	0.94	2.02	0.00	0.00	0.00	0.00
0.31	0.68	0.56	0.22	3.23	2.55	0.35	0.48	43.38	276.41	15.31	147.99	16.16	1.00	2.08	0.00	0.00	0.00	0.00

Food Name	Amount	Measure	Weight (g)	Calories	Protein (g)	Total Carb (g)	Dietary Fiber (g)	Total Fat (g)	Sat Fat (g)	Mono Fat (g)	Poly Fat (g)	Chol (mg)	Vit A (mcg RAE)	Vit D (mcg)
MEATS *(continued)*														
Pork, cured ham, ckd, w/wtr add, slice Oscar Mayer	3	Ounce-weight	85.05	88.45	14.12	1.03	0.00	3.15	1.07	1.47	0.30	39.97	0.00	
Pork, cured ham, extra lean, 4% fat, cnd, unheated, cup	3	Ounce-weight	85.05	102.06	15.73	0.00	0.00	3.88	1.28	1.88	0.33	32.32	0.00	
Pork, cured ham, reg, 13% fat, cnd, rstd, cup	3	Ounce-weight	85.05	192.21	17.46	0.36	0.00	12.93	4.29	6.01	1.51	52.73	0.00	
Pork, cured ham, whole, rstd, cup	3	Ounce-weight	85.05	206.67	18.35	0.00	0.00	14.26	5.09	6.70	1.54	52.73	0.00	
Pork, ground, ckd	3	Ounce-weight	85.05	252.60	21.85	0.00	0.00	17.66	6.57	7.87	1.59	79.95	1.70	0.26
Pork, ribs, spareribs, brsd, each	3	Ounce-weight	85.05	337.65	24.72	0.00	0.00	25.77	9.46	11.46	2.32	102.91	2.55	
Pork, roast, center loin, rstd	3	Ounce-weight	85.05	199.02	22.38	0.00	0.00	11.45	4.30	5.01	1.00	68.04	1.70	
Pork, roast, center rib loin, lean, rstd	3	Ounce-weight	85.05	182.01	24.50	0.00	0.00	8.62	3.01	3.82	0.72	70.59	1.70	
Pork, roast, sirloin, lean, w/bone, rstd	3	Ounce-weight	85.05	183.71	24.50	0.00	0.00	8.75	3.08	3.84	0.74	73.14	1.70	
Pork, roast, sirloin, rstd	3	Ounce-weight	85.05	176.05	24.24	0.00	0.00	8.02	2.91	3.50	0.72	73.14	1.70	0.26
Pork, sweet & sour	3	Ounce-weight	85.05	87.00	5.65	9.44	0.59	3.11	0.80	1.19	0.85	14.50	6.03	0.26
Pork, tenderloin, lean, chop, brld	3	Ounce-weight	85.05	159.04	25.87	0.00	0.00	5.38	1.91	2.19	0.48	79.95	1.70	
Pork, tenderloin, rstd	3	Ounce-weight	85.05	147.14	23.65	0.00	0.00	5.15	1.82	2.09	0.46	67.19	1.70	0.26
Veal														
Veal, avg of all cuts, ckd	3	Ounce-weight	85.05	196.47	25.60	0.00	0.00	9.69	3.64	3.74	0.68	96.96	0.00	
Veal, sirloin roast, lean, brsd	3	Ounce-weight	85.05	173.50	28.88	0.00	0.00	5.54	1.55	1.98	0.49	96.11	0.00	
Variety Meats and By-Products														
Beef, heart, ckd	3	Ounce-weight	85.05	140.33	24.22	0.13	0.00	4.02	1.19	0.86	0.84	180.31	0.00	
Beef, liver, brsd	3	Ounce-weight	85.05	162.45	24.73	4.36	0.00	4.47	1.44	0.55	0.54	336.80	8030.42	
Beef, liver, fried	3	Ounce-weight	85.05	148.84	22.56	4.39	0.00	3.98	1.27	0.56	0.49	324.04	6586.27	
Chicken, liver, avg, simmered, chpd, cup	3	Ounce-weight	85.05	142.03	20.80	0.74	0.00	5.54	1.75	1.20	1.08	478.83	3385.84	
Goose, liver, raw	1	Each	94.00	125.02	15.39	5.94	0.00	4.02	1.49	0.76	0.24	484.10	8750.46	
Pate, liver, unspecified, cnd	1	Tablespoon	13.00	41.47	1.85	0.19	0.00	3.64	1.24	1.61	0.41	33.15	128.83	
MEAT SUBSTITUTES, SOY TOFU AND VEGETABLE														
Bacon Substitute, vegetarian, strips	3	Each	15.00	46.50	1.60	0.95	0.39	4.43	0.69	1.06	2.32	0.00	0.60	
Beef Substitute, vegetarian, ground round, Italian Yves Veggie Cuisine	0.33	Cup	55.00	60.00	10.00	4.00	3.00	0.00	0.00	0.00	0.00	0.00	0.00	
Beef Substitute, vegetarian, Burger Crumbles, svg Morningstar Farms	0.5	Cup	55.00	115.50	11.08	3.31	2.53	6.46	1.63	2.31	2.46	0.00	0.00	
Beef Substitute, vegetarian, meatballs Gardenburger Inc.	6	Piece	85.00	110.00	12.00	8.00	4.00	4.50	1.00			0.00	0.00	
Burger Substitute, vegetarian, black bean, spicy Morningstar Farms	1	Each	78.00	114.66	11.79	15.20	4.76	0.78	0.18	0.25	0.35	0.78		
Burger Substitute, vegetarian, Diner Deluxe Gardenburger Inc.	1	Each	71.00	110.00	12.00	6.00	4.00	5.00	0.50			0.00		
Burger Substitute, vegetarian, flame grilled Gardenburger Inc.	1	Each	71.00	120.00	14.00	7.00	4.00	4.00	0.00			0.00	0.00	
Burger Substitute, vegetarian, fzn Morningstar Better 'N Burger	1	Each	85.00	90.95	13.91	7.53	4.25	0.54	0.10	0.28	0.15	0.00	0.00	
Burger Substitute, vegetarian, garden vegan Gardenburger Inc.	1	Each	71.00	90.00	10.00	12.00	2.00	0.00	0.00	0.00	0.00	0.00	0.00	
Burger Substitute, vegetarian, garden veggie, fzn Morningstar Farms	1	Each	67.00	119.26	11.21	10.20	4.02	3.77	0.54	1.07	2.16	0.67	134.00	
Burger Substitute, vegetarian, Harvest Burger, original, fzn Green Giant	1	Each	90.00	137.70	18.00	7.02	5.67	4.14	1.02	2.13	0.27	0.00	0.00	
Burger Substitute, vegetarian, roasted garlic Boca Foods Company	1	Each	71.00	100.00	14.00	7.00	5.00	2.00	0.50			3.00	0.00	
Burger Substitute, vegetarian, savory portabella Gardenburger Inc.	1	Each	71.00	120.00	6.00	18.00	4.00	2.50	1.00			20.00		
Burger Substitute, vegetarian, soy	1	Each	70.00	125.30	12.54	9.38	3.22	4.18	0.50	0.77	1.65	0.00	0.00	

Vit E (mg)	Vit C	Vit B₁-Thia (mg)	Vit B₂-Ribo (mg)	Vit B₃-Nia (mg)	Fol (mcg)	Vit B₆ (mg)	Vita B₁₂ (mcg)	Sodi (mg)	Pota (mg)	Cal (mg)	Phos (mg)	Magn (mg)	Iron (mg)	Zinc (mg)	Caff (mg)	Alco (g)	Sol Fiber (g)	Insol Fiber (g)
	0.00							1146.47	240.69	8.51	203.27	26.37	1.26	1.58	0.00	0.00	0.00	0.00
0.14	0.00	0.71	0.20	4.51	5.10	0.38	0.70	1067.38	309.58	5.10	190.51	14.46	0.80	1.64	0.00	0.00	0.00	0.00
0.34	11.91	0.70	0.22	4.51	4.25	0.26	0.90	800.32	303.63	6.80	206.67	14.46	1.17	2.13	0.00	0.00	0.00	0.00
0.31	0.00	0.51	0.19	3.79	2.55	0.32	0.54	1009.54	243.24	5.95	182.01	16.16	0.74	1.97	0.00	0.00	0.00	0.00
0.18	0.60	0.60	0.19	3.58	5.10	0.33	0.46	62.09	307.88	18.71	192.21	20.41	1.10	2.73	0.00	0.00	0.00	0.00
0.29	0.00	0.35	0.32	4.66	3.40	0.30	0.92	79.10	272.16	39.97	221.98	20.41	1.57	3.91	0.00	0.00	0.00	0.00
0.28	0.77	0.73	0.22	4.44	3.40	0.30	0.48	53.58	299.38	22.96	182.86	17.01	0.84	1.72	0.00	0.00	0.00	0.00
0.35	0.34	0.54	0.27	4.55	7.65	0.34	0.47	42.53	308.73	5.10	188.81	20.41	0.85	2.41	0.00	0.00	0.00	0.00
0.40	0.26	0.68	0.28	4.72	5.10	0.36	0.66	53.58	311.28	17.01	193.91	21.26	0.95	2.19	0.00	0.00	0.00	0.00
0.16	0.85	0.75	0.32	4.32	4.25	0.40	0.64	47.63	341.90	13.61	214.33	22.11	1.00	2.13	0.00	0.00	0.00	0.00
0.41	7.37	0.21	0.08	1.37	3.88	0.16	0.13	315.56	145.16	10.50	55.89	12.94	0.54	0.55	0.00	0.00		
0.41	0.85	0.84	0.33	4.37	5.10	0.45	0.85	55.28	383.58	4.25	250.90	30.62	1.22	2.51	0.00	0.00	0.00	0.00
0.16	0.34	0.79	0.33	3.97	5.10	0.35	0.47	46.78	368.27	5.10	218.58	22.96	1.23	2.21	0.00	0.00	0.00	0.00
0.34	0.00	0.05	0.27	6.78	12.76	0.26	1.34	73.99	276.41	18.71	203.27	22.11	0.98	4.05	0.00	0.00	0.00	0.00
0.37	0.00	0.05	0.32	6.00	13.61	0.32	1.35	68.89	288.32	16.16	220.28	24.66	1.05	4.04	0.00	0.00	0.00	0.00
0.25	0.00	0.09	1.03	5.68	4.25	0.21	9.19	50.18	186.26	4.25	216.03	17.86	5.43	2.44	0.00	0.00	0.00	0.00
0.43	1.62	0.16	2.91	14.91	215.18	0.86	60.03	67.19	299.38	5.10	422.70	17.86	5.56	4.51	0.00	0.00	0.00	0.00
0.39	0.60	0.15	2.91	14.86	221.13	0.87	70.70	65.49	298.53	5.10	412.49	18.71	5.25	4.45	0.00	0.00	0.00	0.00
0.70	23.73	0.25	1.70	9.39	491.59	0.64	14.33	64.64	223.68	9.36	344.45	21.26	9.89	3.38	0.00	0.00	0.00	0.00
1.35	4.23	0.53	0.84	6.11	693.72	0.71	50.76	131.60	216.20	40.42	245.34	22.56	28.70	2.89	0.00	0.00	0.00	0.00
	0.26	0.00	0.08	0.43	7.80	0.01	0.42	90.61	17.94	9.10	26.00	1.69	0.71	0.37	0.00	0.00	0.00	0.00
1.04	0.00	0.66	0.07	1.13	6.30	0.07	0.00	219.75	25.50	3.45	10.50	2.85	0.36	0.06	0.00	0.00	0.29	0.11
	0.00	0.23	0.14	3.00		0.20	1.50	270.00	240.00	40.00			2.70	3.00	0.00	0.00		
0.35	0.00	4.96	0.18	1.49		0.27	2.18	238.15	89.10	39.60	86.90	1.10	3.20	0.82	0.00	0.00		
	0.00							400.00		60.00			1.80		0.00	0.00		
0.36	0.00	8.06	0.14	0.00		0.21	0.07	499.20	269.10	56.16	149.76	43.68	1.84	0.93	0.00	0.00		
	0.00							380.00		80.00			1.44		0.00	0.00		
	0.00							300.00		0.00			0.00		0.00	0.00		
0.01	0.00	0.26	0.55	4.11	245.65	0.20	0.00	382.50	433.50	86.70	181.05	16.15	2.90	0.75	0.00	0.00		
	0.00							230.00		40.00			4.50		0.00	0.00		
0.55	0.00	6.47	0.10	0.00	58.96	0.00	0.00	381.90	179.56	48.24	123.95	29.48	1.21	0.58	0.00	0.00		
1.56	0.00	0.31	0.20	6.30	21.60	0.39	0.00	411.30	432.00	101.70	225.00	70.20	3.85	8.07	0.00	0.00		
	1.20							400.00		100.00			1.80		0.00	0.00		
	0.00							370.00		100.00			0.36		0.00	0.00	4.00	0.00
1.21	0.00	0.63	0.42	7.00	54.60	0.84	1.68	385.00	126.00	20.30	240.80	12.60	1.47	1.26	0.00	0.00		

Food Name	Amount	Measure	Weight (g)	Calories	Protein (g)	Total Carb (g)	Dietary Fiber (g)	Total Fat (g)	Sat Fat (g)	Mono Fat (g)	Poly Fat (g)	Chol (mg)	Vit A (mcg RAE)	Vit D (mcg)
MEAT SUBSTITUTES, SOY TOFU AND VEGETABLE *(continued)*														
Burger Substitute, vegetarian, vegan, fzn Morningstar Better 'N Burger	1	Each	85.00	90.95	13.91	7.53	4.25	0.54	0.10	0.28	0.15	0.00	0.00	
Chicken Substitute, vegetarian, Chik Patties, fzn Morningstar Farms	1	Each	71.00	148.18	9.51	13.65	2.83	6.17	0.86	1.60	3.61	0.58	0.00	
Hot Dog Substitute, vegetarian Morningstar Farms	1	Each	45.00	111.60	10.39	3.70	2.74	6.16	0.89	1.95	3.31	0.45	0.00	
Hot Dog Substitute, vegetarian	1	Each	51.00	102.00	10.20	4.08	2.35	5.10	0.81	1.24	2.64	0.00	0.00	
Hot Dog Substitute, vegetarian, Big Franks, cnd Loma Linda	1	Each	51.00	118.32	12.12	1.51	1.32	7.08	0.81	1.52	3.69	0.00		
Meat Extender	1	Cup	88.00	275.44	33.54	33.72	15.40	2.61	0.37	0.57	1.46	0.00	1.76	
Meat Substitute, vegetarian, prot, pces, Quorn Myco Marlow Foods Limited	3	Ounce-weight	85.05	67.04	10.21	5.40	4.20	2.40	0.40			0.00	0.00	
Sausage Substitute, vegetarian, breakfast links, fzn Morningstar Farms	1	Each	22.50	32.11	4.48	1.22	0.72	1.03	0.18	0.27	0.53	0.67	0.00	
Sausage Substitute, vegetarian, breakfast patty, fzn Morningstar Farms	1	Each	38.00	79.42	9.92	3.72	1.98	2.77	0.51	0.69	1.32	0.76	0.00	
Tempeh	0.5	Cup	83.00	160.19	15.39	7.79		8.96	1.85	2.49	3.17	0.00	0.00	
Tofu, fermented & salted, block	3	Ounce-weight	85.05	98.66	6.93	4.38	0.23	6.80	0.98	1.50	3.84	0.00	6.80	
Tofu, firm, silken, light, slice Mori-Nu	3	Ounce-weight	85.05	31.47	5.36	0.93	0.00	0.68	0.11	0.11	0.38	0.00	0.00	
Tofu, firm, silken, slice Mori-Nu	3	Ounce-weight	85.05	52.73	5.87	2.05	0.08	2.30	0.34	0.46	1.27	0.00	0.00	
Tofu, fried, each pce	3	Ounce-weight	85.05	230.49	14.62	8.93	3.32	17.16	2.48	3.79	9.69	0.00	0.85	
Tofu, soft, silken, slice Mori-Nu	3	Ounce-weight	85.05	46.78	4.08	2.47	0.08	2.30	0.30	0.45	1.32	0.00	0.00	
NUTS, SEEDS, AND PRODUCTS														
Almond Butter, unsalted	2	Tablespoon	32.00	202.56	4.83	6.79	1.18	18.91	1.79	12.28	3.97	0.00	0.00	
Cashew Butter, plain, unsalted	2	Tablespoon	32.00	187.84	5.62	8.82	0.64	15.82	3.12	9.32	2.68	0.00	0.00	
Coconut, creamed f/dry	2	Tablespoon	30.00	205.20	1.59	6.46	4.29	20.72	18.38	0.88	0.23	0.00	0.00	
Coconut, dried, flaked, swtnd, pkg	2	Tablespoon	9.25	43.85	0.30	4.40	0.40	2.97	2.64	0.13	0.03	0.00	0.00	
Coconut, dried, unswtnd	2	Tablespoon	9.25	61.05	0.64	2.19	1.51	5.97	5.29	0.25	0.07	0.00	0.00	
Coconut, milk, cnd	2	Tablespoon	28.25	55.65	0.57	0.79	0.32	6.03	5.34	0.26	0.07	0.00	0.00	
Coconut, milk, fzn	2	Tablespoon	30.00	60.60	0.48	1.67	0.67	6.24	5.53	0.27	0.07	0.00	0.00	
Coconut, tstd f/dried	2	Tablespoon	9.25	54.76	0.49	4.11	0.59	4.35	3.86	0.18	0.05	0.00	0.00	
Nuts, acorns, raw	1	Ounce-weight	28.35	109.71	1.75	11.56		6.77	0.88	4.28	1.30	0.00	0.57	
Nuts, almonds	0.25	Cup	35.50	205.19	7.55	7.01	4.19	17.97	1.37	11.42	4.33	0.00	0.09	
Nuts, almonds, dry rstd, salted, whole	22	Each	28.35	169.25	6.27	5.47	3.35	14.98	1.14	9.54	3.58	0.00	0.02	
Nuts, almonds, oil rstd, salted	22	Each	28.35	172.08	6.02	5.01	2.98	15.64	1.19	9.87	3.84	0.00	0.02	
Nuts, almonds, oil rstd, whole, blanched Blue Diamond Growers	0.25	Cup	35.50	217.61	7.35	5.08		20.41				0.00		
Nuts, Brazil, dried, lrg	6	Each	28.35	185.98	4.06	3.48	2.13	18.83	4.29	6.96	5.83	0.00	0.00	
Nuts, butternuts, dried	0.25	Cup	30.00	183.60	7.47	3.62	1.41	17.09	0.39	3.13	12.82	0.00	1.80	
Nuts, cashews, dry rstd, salted	0.25	Cup	34.25	196.59	5.24	11.20	1.03	15.88	3.14	9.36	2.68	0.00	0.00	
Nuts, cashews, dry rstd, unsalted	0.25	Cup	34.25	196.59	5.24	11.20	1.03	15.88	3.14	9.36	2.68	0.00	0.00	
Nuts, cashews, oil rstd, salted	0.25	Cup	32.50	188.83	5.47	9.80	1.07	15.52	2.75	8.43	2.77	0.00	0.00	
Nuts, cashews, oil rstd, unsalted	0.25	Cup	32.50	188.50	5.47	9.71	1.07	15.52	2.75	8.43	2.77	0.00	0.00	
Nuts, chestnuts, Chinese, dried	1	Ounce-weight	28.35	102.91	1.94	22.61	0.64	0.51	0.08	0.26	0.13	0.00	4.54	
Nuts, chestnuts, European, rstd, cup	0.25	Cup	35.75	87.59	1.13	18.94	1.82	0.79	0.14	0.27	0.31	0.00	0.36	
Nuts, chestnuts, Japanese, ckd	1	Ounce-weight	28.35	15.88	0.24	3.58	0.10	0.06	0.01	0.03	0.02	0.00	0.28	
Nuts, hazelnuts, chpd	0.25	Cup	28.75	180.55	4.30	4.80	2.79	17.47	1.28	13.13	2.28	0.00	0.29	
Nuts, macadamia, dried	11	Each	28.35	203.55	2.24	3.92	2.44	21.48	3.42	16.69	0.43	0.00	0.00	
Nuts, mixed, w/o peanuts, oil rstd, salted	0.25	Cup	36.00	221.40	5.59	8.02	1.98	20.22	3.28	11.93	4.12	0.00	0.14	
Nuts, mixed, w/o peanuts, oil rstd, unsalted	0.25	Cup	36.00	221.40	5.59	8.02	1.98	20.22	3.28	11.93	4.12	0.00	0.36	
Nuts, mixed, w/peanuts, dry rstd, salted	0.25	Cup	34.25	203.44	5.93	8.69	3.08	17.63	2.36	10.75	3.69	0.00	0.09	
Nuts, mixed, w/peanuts, dry rstd, unsalted	0.25	Cup	34.25	203.44	5.93	8.69	3.08	17.63	2.36	10.75	3.69	0.00	0.34	
Nuts, mixed, w/peanuts, oil rstd, salted	0.25	Cup	35.50	219.03	5.95	7.60	3.19	20.00	3.10	11.25	4.72	0.00	0.13	
Nuts, mixed, w/peanuts, oil rstd, unsalted	0.25	Cup	35.50	219.03	5.95	7.60	3.51	20.00	3.10	11.25	4.72	0.00	0.35	

Vit E (mg)	Vit C	Vit B₁-Thia (mg)	Vit B₂-Ribo (mg)	Vit B₃-Nia (mg)	Fol (mcg)	Vit B₆ (mg)	Vita B₁₂ (mcg)	Sodi (mg)	Pota (mg)	Cal (mg)	Phos (mg)	Magn (mg)	Iron (mg)	Zinc (mg)	Caff (mg)	Alco (g)	Sol Fiber (g)	Insol Fiber (g)
0.01	0.00	0.26	0.55	4.11	245.65	0.20	0.00	382.50	433.50	86.70	181.05	16.15	2.90	0.75	0.00	0.00		
	0.00	1.39	0.23	2.26		0.18	2.47	513.90	173.88	23.93	124.25		2.31	0.58	0.00	0.00		
1.26	0.00	0.14	0.02	0.00		0.01	0.01	430.65	49.95	17.10	42.30	3.60	0.61	0.38	0.00	0.00		
0.98	0.00	0.56	0.61	8.16	39.78	0.50	1.22	219.30	76.50	16.83	175.44	9.18	0.92	0.61	0.00	0.00		
		0.28	0.68	5.78		0.67	2.94	223.89	60.69	10.20	84.66		0.99	1.20	0.00	0.00		
0.44	0.00	0.62	0.78	19.38	174.24	1.18	5.28	8.80	1673.76	179.52	562.32	190.08	10.55	1.94	0.00	0.00		
	0.00							170.10		3.00			1.00		0.00	0.00		
	0.00	2.72	0.08	1.25		0.19	1.16	177.68	22.95	4.52	32.40		0.89	0.17	0.00	0.00		
0.30	0.00	5.38	0.13	1.84		0.19	1.50	259.16	101.84	18.24	106.40	1.14	1.92	0.37	0.00	0.00		
0.02	0.00	0.07	0.29	2.19	19.92	0.18	0.07	7.47	341.96	92.13	220.78	67.23	2.25	0.95	0.00	0.00		
0.02	0.17	0.13	0.09	0.32	24.66	0.08	0.00	2443.49	63.79	39.12	62.09	44.23	1.68	1.33	0.00	0.00	0.11	0.12
0.05	0.00	0.03	0.02	0.09		0.08	0.00	72.29	53.58	30.62	68.89	8.51	0.64	0.28	0.00	0.00	0.00	0.00
0.16	0.00	0.08	0.03	0.21		0.01	0.00	30.62	165.00	27.22	76.55	22.96	0.88	0.52	0.00	0.00		
0.03	0.00	0.14	0.04	0.09	22.96	0.08	0.00	13.61	124.17	316.39	244.09	51.03	4.14	1.69	0.00	0.00	1.59	1.73
0.17	0.00	0.08	0.03	0.25		0.01	0.00	4.25	153.09	26.37	52.73	24.66	0.70	0.45	0.00	0.00		
6.50	0.22	0.04	0.20	0.92	20.80	0.02	0.00	3.52	242.56	86.40	167.36	96.96	1.18	0.98	0.00	0.00		
0.50	0.00	0.10	0.06	0.52	21.76	0.08	0.00	4.80	174.72	13.76	146.24	82.56	1.60	1.66	0.00	0.00	0.36	0.28
0.41	0.45	0.02	0.03	0.18	2.70	0.09	0.00	11.10	165.30	7.80	62.70	27.60	1.01	0.61	0.00	0.00		
0.04	0.00	0.00	0.00	0.03	0.74	0.02	0.00	23.68	29.23	1.30	9.25	4.44	0.17	0.16	0.00	0.00	0.04	0.35
0.04	0.14	0.01	0.01	0.06	0.83	0.03	0.00	3.42	50.23	2.41	19.06	8.33	0.31	0.19	0.00	0.00	0.12	1.39
0.18	0.28	0.01	0.00	0.18	3.95	0.01	0.00	3.67	62.15	5.08	27.12	12.99	0.93	0.16	0.00	0.00		
0.20	0.33	0.01	0.00	0.20	4.20	0.01	0.00	3.60	69.60	1.20	17.70	9.60	0.24	0.18	0.00	0.00		
0.09	0.14	0.01	0.01	0.06	0.83	0.03	0.00	3.42	51.25	2.50	19.52	8.51	0.31	0.19	0.00	0.00	0.06	0.53
	0.00	0.03	0.04	0.52	24.66	0.15	0.00	0.00	152.81	11.62	22.40	17.58	0.23	0.14	0.00	0.00		
9.18	0.00	0.08	0.28	1.40	10.29	0.05	0.00	0.35	258.44	88.04	168.27	97.62	1.53	1.20	0.00	0.00	0.51	3.68
7.37	0.00	0.02	0.25	1.10	9.36	0.04	0.00	96.11	211.49	75.41	138.63	81.08	1.28	1.00	0.00	0.00	0.37	2.98
7.36	0.00	0.03	0.22	1.04	7.65	0.04	0.00	96.11	198.17	82.50	132.11	77.68	1.04	0.87	0.00	0.00	0.33	2.65
		0.27	0.50	1.51			0.00	0.00	205.90	81.65			1.74		0.00	0.00		
1.62	0.20	0.17	0.01	0.08	6.24	0.03	0.00	0.85	186.83	45.36	205.54	106.60	0.69	1.15	0.00	0.00		
1.05	0.96	0.11	0.04	0.31	19.80	0.17	0.00	0.30	126.30	15.90	133.80	71.10	1.21	0.94	0.00	0.00		
0.32	0.00	0.07	0.07	0.48	23.63	0.09	0.00	219.20	193.51	15.41	167.82	89.05	2.05	1.92	0.00	0.00	0.55	0.48
0.32	0.00	0.07	0.07	0.48	23.63	0.09	0.00	5.48	193.51	15.41	167.82	89.05	2.05	1.92	0.00	0.00	0.55	0.48
0.30	0.10	0.12	0.08	0.56	8.13	0.11	0.00	100.10	205.40	13.98	172.58	88.73	1.97	1.74	0.00	0.00	0.56	0.51
0.30	0.10	0.12	0.08	0.56	8.13	0.11	0.00	4.23	205.40	13.98	172.58	88.73	1.97	1.74	0.00	0.00	0.56	0.51
0.26	16.58	0.08	0.09	0.37	31.18	0.19	0.00	1.42	205.82	8.22	43.94	38.84	0.65	0.40	0.00	0.00		
0.18	9.30	0.08	0.06	0.48	25.03	0.18	0.00	0.72	211.64	10.37	38.25	11.80	0.32	0.20	0.00	0.00	0.45	1.37
0.03	2.69	0.04	0.02	0.15	4.82	0.03	0.00	1.42	33.74	3.12	7.37	5.10	0.15	0.11	0.00	0.00		
4.32	1.81	0.18	0.03	0.52	32.49	0.16	0.00	1.42	195.50	32.77	83.37	46.86	1.35	0.71	0.00	0.00	0.89	1.90
0.15	0.34	0.34	0.05	0.70	3.12	0.08	0.00	1.42	104.33	24.10	53.30	36.86	1.05	0.37	0.00	0.00	0.88	1.56
2.95	0.18	0.18	0.18	0.71	20.16	0.06	0.00	110.16	195.84	38.16	161.64	90.36	0.92	1.68	0.00	0.00		
2.16	0.18	0.18	0.18	0.71	20.16	0.06	0.00	3.96	195.84	38.16	161.64	90.36	0.92	1.68	0.00	0.00		
3.74	0.14	0.07	0.07	1.61	17.12	0.10	0.00	229.13	204.47	23.97	148.99	77.06	1.27	1.30	0.00	0.00		
2.05	0.14	0.07	0.07	1.61	17.12	0.10	0.00	4.11	204.47	23.97	148.99	77.06	1.27	1.30	0.00	0.00		
2.56	0.18	0.18	0.08	1.80	29.46	0.08	0.00	148.74	206.25	38.34	164.72	83.42	1.14	1.80	0.00	0.00		
2.13	0.18	0.18	0.08	1.80	29.46	0.08	0.00	3.90	206.25	38.34	164.72	83.42	1.14	1.80	0.00	0.00		

Food Name	Amount	Measure	Weight (g)	Calories	Protein (g)	Total Carb (g)	Dietary Fiber (g)	Total Fat (g)	Sat Fat (g)	Mono Fat (g)	Poly Fat (g)	Chol (mg)	Vit A (mcg RAE)	Vit D (mcg)
NUTS, SEEDS, AND PRODUCTS (*continued*)														
Nuts, peanuts, dry rstd, salted, each	30	Each	30.00	175.50	7.10	6.45	2.40	14.90	2.07	7.39	4.71	0.00	0.00	
Nuts, peanuts, dry rstd, unsalted	30	Each	30.00	175.50	7.10	6.45	2.40	14.90	2.07	7.39	4.71	0.00	0.00	
Nuts, peanuts, oil rstd, salted, each	30	Each	27.00	161.73	7.57	4.12	2.54	14.17	2.34	7.00	4.12	0.00	0.00	
Nuts, peanuts, oil rstd, unsalted, each	32	Each	28.00	162.68	7.38	5.30	1.93	13.80	1.91	6.85	4.36	0.00	0.00	
Nuts, peanuts, raw	0.25	Cup	36.50	206.96	9.42	5.89	3.10	17.97	2.49	8.92	5.68	0.00	0.00	
Nuts, peanuts, Spanish, raw	0.25	Cup	36.50	208.05	9.55	5.78	3.47	18.10	2.79	8.15	6.28	0.00	0.00	
Nuts, pecans, chpd	0.25	Cup	29.75	205.57	2.73	4.13	2.86	21.41	1.83	12.14	6.43	0.00	0.89	
Nuts, pecans, dry rstd, salted	1	Ounce-weight	28.35	201.28	2.69	3.85	2.66	21.05	1.78	12.46	5.83	0.00	1.98	
Nuts, pecans, dry rstd, unsalted	1	Ounce-weight	28.35	201.28	2.69	3.85	2.66	21.05	1.78	12.46	5.83	0.00	1.98	
Nuts, pine, pinon/pinyon, dried	10	Each	1.00	6.29	0.12	0.19	0.11	0.61	0.09	0.23	0.26	0.00	0.01	
Nuts, pistachio, dry rstd, salted	0.25	Cup	32.00	181.76	6.83	8.57	3.30	14.71	1.77	7.75	4.45	0.00	4.17	
Nuts, pistachio, dry rstd, unsalted	0.25	Cup	32.00	182.72	6.83	8.85	3.30	14.71	1.77	7.75	4.45	0.00	4.17	
Nuts, walnuts, English, dried, chpd	0.25	Cup	30.00	196.20	4.57	4.11	2.01	19.56	1.84	2.68	14.15	0.00	0.30	
Peanut Butter, chunky	2	Tablespoon	32.00	188.48	7.70	6.90	2.56	15.98	2.59	7.86	4.74	0.00	0.00	0.00
Peanut Butter, chunky, unsalted	2	Tablespoon	32.00	188.48	7.70	6.90	2.56	15.98	2.59	7.86	4.74	0.00	0.00	
Peanut Butter, creamy, unsalted	2	Tablespoon	32.00	188.16	8.03	6.26	1.92	16.12	3.29	7.59	4.44	0.00	0.00	
Peanut Butter, natural, creamy, rducd fat The J.M. Smucker Co.	2	Tablespoon	35.00	200.00	9.00	12.00	2.00	12.00	2.00			0.00	0.00	
Seeds, flax/linseed, ground, Canada Flax Council of Canada	1	Tablespoon	8.00	36.00	1.68	2.72	2.24	3.36		0.94	1.01		0.08	
Seeds, sunflower, kernels, dry rstd, salted	0.25	Cup	32.00	186.24	6.19	7.70	2.88	15.94	1.67	3.04	10.53	0.00	0.15	
Seeds, sunflower, kernels, dry rstd, unsalted	0.25	Cup	32.00	186.24	6.19	7.70	3.55	15.94	1.67	3.04	10.53	0.00	0.15	
Seeds, sunflower, oil rstd, salted	0.25	Cup	33.75	199.80	6.77	7.73	3.58	17.31	2.38	2.72	11.58	0.00	0.16	
Tahini, f/raw & stone ground kernels	2	Tablespoon	30.00	171.00	5.34	7.86	2.79	14.40	2.02	5.44	6.31	0.00	0.90	
POULTRY														
Chicken—BBQ, Breaded, Fried, Glazed, Grilled, Raw														
Chicken, breast, teriyaki	3	Ounce-weight	85.05	118.19	17.77	4.43	0.27	2.43	0.62	0.71	0.60	54.59	9.99	
Chicken, broiler/fryer, breast, w/o skin, fried	3	Ounce-weight	85.05	159.04	28.44	0.43	0.00	4.01	1.10	1.46	0.91	77.40	5.95	
Chicken, broiler/fryer, breast, w/o skin, rstd, each or cup	3	Ounce-weight	85.05	140.33	26.38	0.00	0.00	3.04	0.86	1.05	0.65	72.29	5.10	
Chicken, broiler/fryer, breast, w/o skin, stwd	3	Ounce-weight	85.05	128.43	24.65	0.00	0.00	2.58	0.72	0.88	0.56	65.49	5.10	
Chicken, broiler/fryer, breast, w/skin, rstd	3	Ounce-weight	85.05	167.55	25.34	0.00	0.00	6.62	1.86	2.58	1.41	71.44	22.96	
Chicken, broiler/fryer, breast, w/skin, stwd	3	Ounce-weight	85.05	156.49	23.30	0.00	0.00	6.31	1.77	2.47	1.34	63.79	20.41	
Chicken, broiler/fryer, dark meat, w/o skin, fried, cup	3	Ounce-weight	85.05	203.27	24.66	2.20	0.00	9.88	2.65	3.67	2.36	81.65	20.41	
Chicken, broiler/fryer, dark meat, w/o skin, rstd	3	Ounce-weight	85.05	174.35	23.28	0.00	0.00	8.28	2.26	3.03	1.92	79.10	18.71	
Chicken, broiler/fryer, dark meat, w/o skin, stwd	3	Ounce-weight	85.05	163.30	22.09	0.00	0.00	7.64	2.08	2.77	1.78	74.84	17.86	
Chicken, broiler/fryer, dark meat, w/skin, rstd	3	Ounce-weight	85.05	215.18	22.09	0.00	0.00	13.42	3.72	5.26	2.97	77.40	51.03	
Chicken, broiler/fryer, dark meat, w/skin, stwd	3	Ounce-weight	85.05	198.17	19.99	0.00	0.00	12.47	3.45	4.89	2.76	69.74	47.63	
Chicken, broiler/fryer, leg, w/o skin, rstd, each or cup	3	Ounce-weight	85.05	162.45	22.99	0.00	0.00	7.17	1.95	2.59	1.68	79.95	16.16	
Chicken, broiler/fryer, leg, w/o skin, stwd, each or cup	3	Ounce-weight	85.05	157.34	22.33	0.00	0.00	6.86	1.87	2.49	1.60	75.69	15.31	
Chicken, broiler/fryer, leg, w/skin, rstd, each or cup	3	Ounce-weight	85.05	197.32	22.08	0.00	0.00	11.45	3.16	4.46	2.55	78.25	33.17	
Chicken, broiler/fryer, leg, w/skin, stwd, each or cup	3	Ounce-weight	85.05	187.11	20.56	0.00	0.00	10.99	3.04	4.29	2.44	71.44	30.62	

Vit E (mg)	Vit C	Vit B$_1$-Thia (mg)	Vit B$_2$-Ribo (mg)	Vit B$_3$-Nia (mg)	Fol (mcg)	Vit B$_6$ (mg)	Vita B$_{12}$ (mcg)	Sodi (mg)	Pota (mg)	Cal (mg)	Phos (mg)	Magn (mg)	Iron (mg)	Zinc (mg)	Caff (mg)	Alco (g)	Sol Fiber (g)	Insol Fiber (g)
2.34	0.00	0.13	0.03	4.06	43.50	0.08	0.00	243.90	197.40	16.20	107.40	52.80	0.68	0.99	0.00	0.00	0.67	1.73
2.08	0.00	0.13	0.03	4.06	43.50	0.08	0.00	1.80	197.40	16.20	107.40	52.80	0.68	0.99	0.00	0.00		
1.87	0.22	0.03	0.03	3.73	32.40	0.13	0.00	86.40	196.02	16.47	107.19	47.52	0.41	0.88	0.00	0.00	0.07	2.47
1.93	0.00	0.07	0.03	3.99	35.28	0.07	0.00	1.68	190.96	24.64	144.76	51.80	0.51	1.86	0.00	0.00	0.53	1.40
3.04	0.00	0.23	0.05	4.40	87.60	0.12	0.00	6.57	257.33	33.58	137.24	61.32	1.67	1.19	0.00	0.00	0.86	2.24
2.70	0.00	0.24	0.05	5.82	87.60	0.12	0.00	8.03	271.56	38.69	141.62	68.62	1.42	0.78	0.00	0.00	0.97	2.49
0.42	0.33	0.20	0.04	0.35	6.55	0.06	0.00	0.00	121.98	20.83	82.41	36.00	0.75	1.35	0.00	0.00	0.88	1.97
0.37	0.20	0.13	0.03	0.33	4.54	0.06	0.00	108.58	120.20	20.41	83.07	37.42	0.79	1.44	0.00	0.00	0.64	2.02
0.37	0.20	0.13	0.03	0.33	4.54	0.06	0.00	0.28	120.20	20.41	83.07	37.42	0.79	1.44	0.00	0.00	0.64	2.02
0.04	0.02	0.01	0.00	0.04	0.58	0.00	0.00	0.72	6.28	0.08	0.35	2.34	0.03	0.04	0.00	0.00	0.02	0.09
0.62	0.73	0.27	0.05	0.45	16.01	0.41	0.00	129.60	333.44	35.21	155.20	38.40	1.34	0.73	0.00	0.00	0.09	3.21
0.62	0.73	0.27	0.05	0.45	16.01	0.41	0.00	3.21	333.44	35.21	155.20	38.40	1.34	0.73	0.00	0.00	0.09	3.21
0.21	0.39	0.10	0.05	0.34	29.40	0.16	0.00	0.60	132.30	29.40	103.80	47.40	0.87	0.93	0.00	0.00	0.66	1.35
2.02	0.00	0.03	0.04	4.38	29.44	0.13	0.00	155.52	238.40	14.40	102.08	51.20	0.61	0.89	0.00	0.00	0.72	1.84
2.02	0.00	0.03	0.04	4.38	29.44	0.13	0.00	5.44	238.40	14.40	102.08	51.20	0.61	0.89	0.00	0.00	0.72	1.84
2.88	0.00	0.02	0.03	4.29	23.68	0.17	0.00	5.44	207.68	13.76	114.56	49.28	0.60	0.93	0.00	0.00	0.54	1.38
	0.00			5.00	24.00	0.12	0.00	120.00		0.00		60.00	0.72	0.90	0.00	0.00		
0.03		0.06	0.02	0.35		0.06	0.04	3.68	60.00	20.00	52.00	28.00	0.80	0.16	0.00	0.00	0.56	1.68
8.35	0.45	0.03	0.07	2.25	75.84	0.26	0.00	131.20	272.00	22.40	369.60	41.28	1.22	1.70	0.00	0.00	0.92	1.96
8.35	0.45	0.03	0.07	2.25	75.84	0.26	0.00	0.96	272.00	22.40	369.60	41.28	1.22	1.70	0.00	0.00	1.14	2.42
12.26	0.37	0.11	0.09	1.40	78.97	0.27	0.00	138.38	163.01	29.36	384.41	42.86	1.44	1.76	0.00	0.00	1.15	2.43
0.66	0.00	0.38	0.15	1.78	29.40	0.04	0.00	22.20	124.20	126.00	225.60	28.80	0.75	1.39	0.00	0.00		
0.23	2.11	0.05	0.13	5.82	8.06	0.31	0.19	1118.49	205.16	18.01	131.93	23.44	1.14	1.31	0.00	0.56		
0.36	0.00	0.07	0.11	12.57	3.40	0.54	0.31	67.19	234.74	13.61	209.22	26.37	0.97	0.92	0.00	0.00	0.00	0.00
0.23	0.00	0.06	0.10	11.66	3.40	0.51	0.29	62.94	217.73	12.76	193.91	24.66	0.88	0.85	0.00	0.00	0.00	0.00
0.23	0.00	0.04	0.10	7.20	2.55	0.28	0.20	53.58	159.04	11.06	140.33	20.41	0.75	0.82	0.00	0.00	0.00	0.00
0.23	0.00	0.06	0.10	10.81	3.40	0.48	0.27	60.39	208.37	11.91	182.01	22.96	0.91	0.87	0.00	0.00	0.00	0.00
0.23	0.00	0.03	0.10	6.64	2.55	0.25	0.18	52.73	151.39	11.06	132.68	18.71	0.78	0.82	0.00	0.00	0.00	0.00
0.49	0.00	0.08	0.21	6.01	7.65	0.31	0.28	82.50	215.18	15.31	159.04	21.26	1.27	2.47	0.00	0.00	0.00	0.00
0.23	0.00	0.06	0.19	5.57	6.80	0.31	0.27	79.10	204.12	12.76	152.24	19.56	1.13	2.38	0.00	0.00	0.00	0.00
0.23	0.00	0.05	0.17	4.03	5.95	0.18	0.19	62.94	153.94	11.91	121.62	17.01	1.16	2.26	0.00	0.00	0.00	0.00
0.48	0.00	0.06	0.18	5.41	5.95	0.26	0.25	73.99	187.11	12.76	142.88	18.71	1.16	2.12	0.00	0.00	0.00	0.00
0.51	0.00	0.04	0.15	3.84	5.10	0.14	0.17	59.54	141.18	11.91	113.12	15.31	1.11	1.92	0.00	0.00	0.00	0.00
0.23	0.00	0.06	0.20	5.37	6.80	0.31	0.27	77.40	205.82	10.21	155.64	20.41	1.11	2.43	0.00	0.00	0.00	0.00
0.23	0.00	0.05	0.18	4.08	6.80	0.18	0.20	66.34	161.60	9.36	126.72	17.86	1.19	2.36	0.00	0.00	0.00	0.00
0.23	0.00	0.06	0.18	5.27	5.95	0.28	0.26	73.99	191.36	10.21	147.99	19.56	1.13	2.21	0.00	0.00	0.00	0.00
0.23	0.00	0.05	0.16	3.90	5.10	0.15	0.17	62.09	149.69	9.36	118.22	17.01	1.15	2.07	0.00	0.00	0.00	0.00

Food Name	Amount	Measure	Weight (g)	Calories	Protein (g)	Total Carb (g)	Dietary Fiber (g)	Total Fat (g)	Sat Fat (g)	Mono Fat (g)	Poly Fat (g)	Chol (mg)	Vit A (mcg RAE)	Vit D (mcg)
POULTRY *(continued)*														
Chicken, broiler/fryer, light meat, w/o skin, fried, cup	3	Ounce-weight	85.05	163.30	27.91	0.36	0.00	4.71	1.29	1.68	1.07	76.55	7.65	
Chicken, broiler/fryer, light meat, w/skin, stwd	3	Ounce-weight	85.05	170.95	22.23	0.00	0.00	8.48	2.38	3.33	1.80	62.94	24.66	
Chicken, broiler/fryer, thigh, w/o skin, fried	3	Ounce-weight	85.05	185.41	23.97	1.00	0.00	8.76	2.36	3.25	2.07	86.75	17.86	
Chicken, broiler/fryer, thigh, w/o skin, rstd	3	Ounce-weight	85.05	177.75	22.06	0.00	0.00	9.25	2.58	3.53	2.11	80.80	17.01	
Chicken, broiler/fryer, thigh, w/o skin, stwd	3	Ounce-weight	85.05	165.85	21.26	0.00	0.00	8.33	2.30	3.15	1.91	76.55	16.16	
Chicken, broiler/fryer, thigh, w/skin, rstd	3	Ounce-weight	85.05	210.07	21.31	0.00	0.00	13.17	3.68	5.23	2.91	79.10	40.82	
Chicken, broiler/fryer, thigh, w/skin, stwd	3	Ounce-weight	85.05	197.32	19.78	0.00	0.00	12.54	3.50	4.97	2.76	71.44	37.42	
Chicken, broiler/fryer, whole, w/skin, rstd, each or cup	3	Ounce-weight	85.05	203.27	23.22	0.00	0.00	11.57	3.22	4.54	2.53	74.84	39.97	
Chicken, broiler/fryer, whole, w/skin, stwd, each or cup	3	Ounce-weight	85.05	186.26	20.99	0.00	0.00	10.68	2.98	4.19	2.33	66.34	35.72	
Chicken, broiler/fryer, wing, w/o skin, fried	3	Ounce-weight	85.05	179.46	25.64	0.00	0.00	7.78	2.13	2.62	1.76	71.44	15.31	
Chicken, broiler/fryer, wing, w/o skin, rstd	3	Ounce-weight	85.05	172.65	25.91	0.00	0.00	6.91	1.92	2.22	1.51	72.29	15.31	
Chicken, broiler/fryer, wing, w/o skin, stwd	3	Ounce-weight	85.05	153.94	23.12	0.00	0.00	6.11	1.70	1.96	1.34	62.94	13.61	
Chicken, broiler/fryer, wing, w/skin, rstd, each or cup	3	Ounce-weight	85.05	246.65	22.84	0.00	0.00	16.55	4.64	6.50	3.52	71.44	39.97	
Chicken, broiler/fryer, wing, w/skin, stwd	3	Ounce-weight	85.05	211.77	19.37	0.00	0.00	14.31	4.01	5.61	3.04	59.54	34.02	
Chicken, nuggets, brd, fzn, 1598, FS Pierre Foods	1	Each	17.00	50.00	3.10	2.60		3.00	0.60					
Chicken, patty, southern fried, w/o bone, ckd f/fzn Banquet	1	Each	63.79	190.00	8.00	10.00	1.00	13.00	3.00			25.00	0.00	
Chicken, w/o skin, w/broth, can	3	Ounce-weight	85.05	140.33	18.52	0.00	0.00	6.76	1.87	2.68	1.49	52.73	28.92	
Dish, chicken patty, breaded strips Swanson	1	Each	150.00	340.00	11.00	31.00	3.00	19.00	3.50			30.00		
Turkey														
Bacon, turkey, svg Louis Rich	1	Ounce-weight	28.35	70.88	4.27	0.47	0.00	5.75	1.50	2.13	1.34	25.52	0.00	
Turkey, breast, prebasted, w/skin, rstd	3	Ounce-weight	85.05	107.16	18.85	0.00	0.00	2.94	0.83	0.97	0.71	35.72	0.00	
Turkey, fryer/roaster, dark meat, w/o skin, raw	4	Ounce-weight	113.40	125.87	23.20	0.00	0.00	3.03	1.02	0.69	0.91	91.85	0.00	
Turkey, fryer/roaster, leg, w/skin, raw	4	Ounce-weight	113.40	133.81	22.83	0.00	0.00	4.05	1.25	1.22	1.10	98.66	1.13	
Turkey, fryer/roaster, light meat, w/o skin, raw	4	Ounce-weight	113.40	122.47	27.42	0.00	0.00	0.56	0.18	0.10	0.15	74.84	0.00	
Turkey, fryer/roaster, whole, w/o skin, raw	4	Ounce-weight	113.40	124.74	25.31	0.00	0.00	1.79	0.60	0.40	0.53	82.78	0.00	
Turkey, fryer/roaster, wing, w/o skin, rstd	3	Ounce-weight	85.05	138.63	26.24	0.00	0.00	2.93	0.94	0.51	0.78	86.75	0.00	
Turkey, ground, 8% fat, raw	4	Ounce-weight	113.40	168.97	19.80	0.00	0.00	9.37	2.55	3.52	2.27	89.59	2.27	
Turkey, ham, dark meat, USDA, smkd, fzn, svg	3	Ounce-weight	85.05	100.36	13.86	2.64	0.00	3.40	1.02	1.14	0.74	54.43	13.61	
Turkey, hen, back, w/skin, raw	4	Ounce-weight	113.40	247.21	19.86	0.00	0.00	18.06	5.00	6.94	4.41	77.11	2.27	
Turkey, light & dark meat, diced, seasoned	3	Ounce-weight	85.05	117.37	15.90	0.85	0.00	5.10	1.49	1.68	1.30	46.78	0.00	
Turkey, nuggets, brd, svg Louis Rich	3	Piece	84.00	231.84	12.02	12.94	0.42	14.70	2.85	6.88	4.61	33.60	0.00	
Turkey, sticks, brd, batter fried, 2.25oz each	1	Each	63.79	177.97	9.06	10.84	0.34	10.78	2.79	4.41	2.80	40.83	7.65	
Turkey, thigh, prebasted, w/skin, w/o bone, rstd	3	Ounce-weight	85.05	133.53	15.99	0.00	0.00	7.26	2.25	2.15	2.00	52.73	0.00	

Vit E (mg)	Vit C	Vit B₁-Thia (mg)	Vit B₂-Ribo (mg)	Vit B₃-Nia (mg)	Fol (mcg)	Vit B₆ (mg)	Vita B₁₂ (mcg)	Sodi (mg)	Pota (mg)	Cal (mg)	Phos (mg)	Magn (mg)	Iron (mg)	Zinc (mg)	Caff (mg)	Alco (g)	Sol Fiber (g)	Insol Fiber (g)
0.26	0.00	0.06	0.11	11.37	3.40	0.54	0.31	68.89	223.68	13.61	196.47	24.66	0.97	1.08	0.00	0.00	0.00	0.00
0.22	0.00	0.03	0.10	5.90	2.55	0.23	0.17	53.58	142.03	11.06	124.17	17.01	0.83	0.97	0.00	0.00	0.00	0.00
0.49	0.00	0.07	0.22	6.06	7.65	0.32	0.28	80.80	220.28	11.06	169.25	22.11	1.24	2.37	0.00	0.00	0.00	0.00
0.23	0.00	0.06	0.20	5.55	6.80	0.30	0.26	74.84	202.42	10.21	155.64	20.41	1.11	2.19	0.00	0.00	0.00	0.00
0.23	0.00	0.05	0.19	4.42	5.95	0.18	0.18	63.79	155.64	9.36	126.72	17.86	1.21	2.19	0.00	0.00	0.00	0.00
0.23	0.00	0.06	0.18	5.41	5.95	0.26	0.25	71.44	188.81	10.21	147.99	18.71	1.14	2.01	0.00	0.00	0.00	0.00
0.23	0.00	0.05	0.16	4.16	5.10	0.14	0.16	60.39	144.59	9.36	118.22	16.16	1.17	1.91	0.00	0.00	0.00	0.00
0.23	0.00	0.05	0.14	7.22	4.25	0.34	0.26	69.74	189.66	12.76	154.79	19.56	1.07	1.65	0.00	0.00	0.00	0.00
0.23	0.00	0.04	0.13	4.76	4.25	0.19	0.17	56.98	141.18	11.06	118.22	16.16	0.99	1.50	0.00	0.00	0.00	0.00
0.26	0.00	0.04	0.11	6.16	3.40	0.50	0.29	77.40	176.90	12.76	139.48	17.86	0.97	1.80	0.00	0.00	0.00	0.00
0.23	0.00	0.04	0.11	6.22	3.40	0.50	0.29	78.25	178.61	13.61	141.18	17.86	0.99	1.82	0.00	0.00	0.00	0.00
0.23	0.00	0.04	0.09	4.42	2.55	0.27	0.19	62.09	130.13	11.06	113.97	15.31	0.95	1.72	0.00	0.00	0.00	0.00
0.23	0.00	0.04	0.11	5.65	2.55	0.36	0.25	69.74	156.49	12.76	128.43	16.16	1.08	1.55	0.00	0.00	0.00	0.00
0.23	0.00	0.03	0.09	3.93	2.55	0.19	0.15	56.98	118.22	10.21	102.91	13.61	0.96	1.39	0.00	0.00	0.00	0.00
	0.00							98.80		5.90			0.42		0.00	0.00		
	1.20	0.08	0.03	2.88				430.00	135.00	0.00	117.00		0.72		0.00	0.00		
0.22	1.70	0.01	0.11	5.38	3.40	0.30	0.25	427.80	117.37	11.91	94.41	10.21	1.34	1.20	0.00	0.00	0.00	0.00
	6.00							560.00		20.00			1.44		0.00	0.00		
	0.00			2.27				343.89	58.97	11.34	56.42	5.39	0.41	0.71	0.00	0.00	0.00	0.00
	0.00	0.05	0.11	7.71	4.25	0.27	0.27	337.65	210.92	7.65	182.01	17.86	0.56	1.30	0.00	0.00	0.00	0.00
0.73	0.00	0.06	0.23	3.35	12.47	0.42	0.46	78.25	276.70	14.74	193.91	24.95	1.88	3.02	0.00	0.00	0.00	0.00
0.73	0.00	0.05	0.23	2.97	11.34	0.40	0.45	78.25	278.96	12.47	190.51	23.81	1.97	3.29	0.00	0.00	0.00	0.00
0.10	0.00	0.04	0.13	6.52	9.07	0.65	0.52	58.97	312.98	11.34	222.26	29.48	1.38	1.58	0.00	0.00	0.00	0.00
0.39	0.00	0.05	0.18	4.94	10.21	0.53	0.50	69.17	294.84	13.61	208.66	27.22	1.63	2.30	0.00	0.00	0.00	0.00
0.08	0.00	0.03	0.14	3.51	5.95	0.50	0.35	66.34	173.50	22.11	147.99	18.71	1.51	3.26	0.00	0.00	0.00	0.00
0.40	0.00	0.06	0.15	3.96	7.94	0.40	0.39	106.60	264.22	14.74	176.90	21.55	1.42	2.19	0.00	0.00	0.00	0.00
	0.00	0.20	0.23	3.50		0.05	0.68	773.10	215.18	5.95	245.79	13.61	0.85	1.79	0.00	0.00	0.00	0.00
0.72	0.00	0.07	0.20	2.69	10.21	0.31	0.40	69.17	261.95	20.41	173.50	20.41	2.02	2.87	0.00	0.00	0.00	0.00
	0.00	0.03	0.09	4.08	4.25	0.24	0.20	722.93	263.66	0.85	204.12	14.46	1.53	1.72	0.00	0.00	0.00	0.00
	0.00							570.36	147.84	7.56	165.48	17.64	0.73	1.54	0.00	0.00		
1.28	0.00	0.06	0.11	1.34	18.50	0.13	0.15	534.56	165.85	8.93	149.27	9.57	1.40	0.93	0.00	0.00		
0.82	0.00	0.07	0.22	2.05	5.10	0.20	0.20	371.67	204.97	6.80	145.44	14.46	1.28	3.50	0.00	0.00	0.00	0.00

Food Name	Amount	Measure	Weight (g)	Calories	Protein (g)	Total Carb (g)	Dietary Fiber (g)	Total Fat (g)	Sat Fat (g)	Mono Fat (g)	Poly Fat (g)	Chol (mg)	Vit A (mcg RAE)	Vit D (mcg)
Duck, Emu, Ostrich and Other														
Cornish Game Hen, whole, w/o skin, rstd	3	Ounce-weight	85.05	113.97	19.82	0.00	0.00	3.29	0.84	1.05	0.80	90.15	17.01	
Cornish Game Hen, whole, w/skin, rstd	3	Ounce-weight	85.05	221.13	18.94	0.00	0.00	15.49	4.30	6.80	3.06	111.42	27.22	
Dove, whole, ckd	3	Ounce-weight	85.05	186.26	20.33	0.00	0.00	11.06	3.18	4.65	2.32	98.66	23.81	
Duck, breast, w/o skin, raw, wild	4	Ounce-weight	113.40	139.48	22.51	0.00	0.00	4.82	1.50	1.37	0.66	87.32	18.14	
Duck, domesticated, whole, rstd	3	Ounce-weight	85.05	286.62	16.15	0.00	0.00	24.11	8.22	10.97	3.10	71.44	53.63	
Duck, whole, w/o skin, rstd, domesticated	3	Ounce-weight	85.05	170.95	19.97	0.00	0.00	9.53	3.55	3.15	1.22	75.69	19.56	
Duck, whole, w/skin, rstd, domesticated	3	Ounce-weight	85.05	286.62	16.15	0.00	0.00	24.11	8.22	10.97	3.10	71.44	53.58	
Duckling, white pekin, breast, w/o skin, brld, cup	3	Ounce-weight	85.05	119.07	23.47	0.00	0.00	2.13	0.49	0.74	0.32	121.62		
Emu, ground, brld	3	Ounce-weight	85.05	138.63	24.18	0.00	0.00	3.95	1.06	1.66	0.58	73.99	0.00	
Goose, whole, w/o skin, raw	4	Ounce-weight	113.40	182.57	25.80	0.00	0.00	8.09	3.16	2.10	1.02	95.26	13.61	
Goose, whole, w/o skin, rstd	3	Ounce-weight	85.05	202.42	24.64	0.00	0.00	10.78	3.88	3.69	1.31	81.65	10.21	
Guinea Hen, whole, w/skin, raw	4	Ounce-weight	113.40	179.17	26.54	0.00	0.00	7.31	2.01	2.76	1.60	83.92	31.75	
Ostrich, ground, brld	3	Ounce-weight	85.05	148.84	22.24	0.00	0.00	6.01	1.52	1.83	0.63	70.59	0.00	
SALAD DRESSINGS, DIPS, AND MAYONNAISE														
Dips														
Dip, avocado Kraft General Foods, Inc.	2	Tablespoon	32.00	60.00	1.00	4.00	0.00	4.00	3.00			0.00	0.00	
Dip, baba ganoush, all natural, low fat, dry mix Casbah	0.5	Tablespoon	7.00	35.00	1.00	4.00	0.00	1.50	0.00			0.00	0.00	
Dip, bean, black Old El Paso	2	Tablespoon	30.00	25.00	1.00	5.00	1.00	0.00	0.00	0.00	0.00	0.00	0.00	
Dip, bean, black, mild Guiltless Gourmet	2	Tablespoon	30.00	30.00	2.00	5.00	1.00	0.00	0.00	0.00	0.00	0.00	0.00	
Dip, hummus, original, dry mix Fantastic Foods International Dish	2	Tablespoon	19.00	80.00	3.00	11.00	1.00	3.00	0.50			0.00	0.00	
Dip, jalapeno Old El Paso	2	Tablespoon	29.00	30.00	1.00	4.00	2.00	1.00	0.00			3.00	0.00	
Dip, ranch Kraft General Foods, Inc.	2	Tablespoon	31.00	60.00	1.00	3.00	0.00	4.50	3.00			0.00	0.00	
Guacamole, Rancho Grande, zesty, fzn JR Simplot	2	Tablespoon	30.00	40.00	0.00	3.00	1.00	3.50	0.50			0.00	5.00	
Guacamole, svg	1	Each	21.00	35.00	0.00	2.00	1.00	3.00	0.00			0.00	0.00	
Guacamole, w/tomatoes	2	Tablespoon	29.13	34.15	0.47	2.03	1.10	3.05	0.48	1.90	0.40	0.00	8.05	0.00
Mayonnaise														
Mayonnaise, light Kraft General Foods, Inc.	1	Tablespoon	15.00	50.10	0.09	1.28	0.02	4.94	0.75			5.25		
Mayonnaise, rducd fat, Just 2 Good!, jar Best Foods	1	Tablespoon	15.00	25.00	0.00	2.00	0.00	2.00	0.50			0.00	0.00	
Mayonnaise, soybean oil	1	Tablespoon	13.80	98.95	0.15	0.54	0.00	10.79	1.64	2.70	5.89	5.24	11.18	
Mayonnaise, soybean oil, unsalted	1	Tablespoon	13.80	98.95	0.15	0.37	0.00	10.96	1.63	3.13	5.12	8.14	11.59	0.04
Salad Dressings-Lower Calorie/Fat/Sodium/Cholest														
Dip, hummus, low fat, dry mix Casbah	2	Tablespoon	15.00	75.00	3.00	7.50	1.50	3.00	0.00			0.00	0.00	
Salad Dressing, blue cheese, low cal	2	Tablespoon	30.00	29.70	1.53	0.87	0.00	2.16	0.77	0.53	0.73	0.30	0.05	
Salad Dressing, French, diet, 5cal/tsp	2	Tablespoon	32.60	75.63	0.18	9.54	0.36	4.39	0.36	1.92	1.64	0.00	8.80	
Salad Dressing, honey dijon, fat free Kraft General Foods, Inc.	2	Tablespoon	34.00	45.00	0.00	10.00	1.00	0.00	0.00	0.00	0.00	0.00	0.00	
Salad Dressing, Italian, diet, 2cal/tsp, cmrcl	2	Tablespoon	30.00	22.50	0.14	1.37	0.00	1.91	0.14	0.66	0.51	1.80	0.30	
Salad Dressing, ranch, fat free	1	Ounce-weight	28.35	33.74	0.08	7.51	0.03	0.55	0.12	0.11	0.20	1.98	0.28	
Salad Dressing, ranch, fat free Kraft General Foods, Inc.	2	Tablespoon	35.00	48.30	0.24	10.71	0.21	0.35	0.07			0.35		
Salad Dressing, thousand island, diet, 10cal/tsp	2	Tablespoon	30.60	62.42	0.27	6.79	0.40	4.03	0.22	1.98	0.83	0.31	4.90	
Salad Dressing, vinaigrette, raspberry, f at free Seven Seas	2	Tablespoon	34.00	30.00	0.00	7.00	0.00	0.00	0.00	0.00	0.00	0.00	0.00	

Vit E (mg)	Vit C	Vit B_1-Thia (mg)	Vit B_2-Ribo (mg)	Vit B_3-Nia (mg)	Fol (mcg)	Vit B_6 (mg)	Vita B_{12} (mcg)	Sodi (mg)	Pota (mg)	Cal (mg)	Phos (mg)	Magn (mg)	Iron (mg)	Zinc (mg)	Caff (mg)	Alco (g)	Sol Fiber (g)	Insol Fiber (g)
0.20	0.51	0.06	0.19	5.34	1.70	0.30	0.26	53.58	212.63	11.06	126.72	16.16	0.65	1.30	0.00	0.00	0.00	0.00
0.31	0.43	0.06	0.17	5.02	1.70	0.26	0.24	54.43	208.37	11.06	124.17	15.31	0.77	1.27	0.00	0.00	0.00	0.00
0.05	2.47	0.24	0.30	6.46	5.10	0.48	0.35	48.48	217.73	14.46	282.37	22.11	5.03	3.26	0.00	0.00	0.00	0.00
0.33	7.03	0.47	0.35	3.91	28.35	0.71	0.86	64.64	303.91	3.40	210.92	24.95	5.11	0.84	0.00	0.00	0.00	0.00
0.60	0.00	0.15	0.23	4.10	5.10	0.15	0.26	50.18	173.50	9.36	132.68	13.61	2.30	1.58	0.00	0.00	0.00	0.00
0.60	0.00	0.22	0.40	4.34	8.51	0.21	0.34	55.28	214.33	10.21	172.65	17.01	2.30	2.21	0.00	0.00	0.00	0.00
0.60	0.00	0.15	0.23	4.10	5.10	0.15	0.26	50.18	173.50	9.36	132.68	13.61	2.30	1.58	0.00	0.00	0.00	0.00
	2.72		8.80	8.80				89.30		7.65			3.82		0.00	0.00	0.00	
0.20	0.00	0.27	0.46	7.59	7.65	0.71	7.25	55.28	318.94	6.80	228.78	24.66	4.26	3.88	0.00	0.00	0.00	0.00
1.30	8.16	0.15	0.43	4.85	35.15	0.73	0.56	98.66	476.28	14.74	353.81	27.22	2.91	2.65	0.00	0.00	0.00	0.00
1.32	0.00	0.08	0.33	3.47	10.21	0.40	0.42	64.64	329.99	11.91	262.80	21.26	2.44	2.70	0.00	0.00	0.00	0.00
0.34	1.47	0.07	0.12	8.69	5.67	0.43	0.39	75.98	218.86	12.47	173.50	24.95	0.95	1.28	0.00	0.00	0.00	0.00
0.20	0.00	0.18	0.23	5.58	11.91	0.43	4.88	68.04	274.71	6.80	190.51	19.56	2.92	3.68	0.00	0.00	0.00	0.00
	0.00							240.00	25.00	0.00	0.00			0.00	0.00	0.00	0.00	0.00
	1.20							100.00		0.00				0.36	0.00	0.00	0.00	0.00
	0.00							280.00		0.00				0.36	0.00	0.00		
	1.20							100.00		20.00				0.36	0.00	0.00		
	0.00							280.00		20.00			1.44		0.00	0.00		
	0.00							125.00		0.00				0.36	0.00	0.00		
	0.00							210.00	20.00	0.00					0.00	0.00	0.00	0.00
	3.60							110.00		0.00				0.36	0.00	0.00		
	0.00							100.00		0.00				0.00	0.00	0.00		
0.29	3.53	0.03	0.03	0.42	13.66	0.06	0.00	2.62	136.98	3.08	10.26	8.68	0.24	0.09	0.00	0.00		
0.57	0.05							119.55	7.80	0.90	8.70		0.03		0.00	0.00		
	0.00							130.00		0.00			0.00		0.00	0.00	0.00	0.00
0.72	0.00	0.00	0.00	0.00	1.10	0.08	0.04	78.38	4.69	2.48	3.86	0.14	0.07	0.02	0.00	0.00	0.00	0.00
2.87	0.00	0.00	0.00	0.00	1.06	0.08	0.04	4.14	4.69	2.48	3.86		0.07		0.00	0.00		
	0.00							240.00		0.00				0.54	0.00	0.00		
0.08	0.09	0.01	0.03	0.02	0.90	0.01	0.07	360.00	1.50	26.70	24.90	2.10	0.15	0.08	0.00	0.00	0.00	0.00
0.10	0.00	0.01	0.02	0.15	0.65	0.02	0.00	262.10	34.88	3.59	5.22	2.61	0.28	0.07	0.00	0.00		
	0.00							330.00	35.00	0.00	20.00		0.00		0.00	0.00		
0.06	0.00	0.00	0.00	0.00	0.00	0.02	0.00	409.80	25.50	2.70	3.30	1.20	0.20	0.06	0.00	0.00	0.00	0.00
0.05	0.00	0.01	0.01	0.00	1.70	0.01	0.00	214.04	31.47	14.17	32.04	2.27	0.30	0.11	0.00	0.00		
	0.03							353.85	30.80	9.10	27.65		0.02		0.00	0.00		
0.31	0.00	0.01	0.01	0.13	0.00	0.00	0.00	254.29	61.81	4.90	4.28	2.14	0.29	0.06	0.00	0.00		
	0.00							320.00	15.00	0.00	0.00				0.00	0.00	0.00	0.00

Food Name	Amount	Measure	Weight (g)	Calories	Protein (g)	Total Carb (g)	Dietary Fiber (g)	Total Fat (g)	Sat Fat (g)	Mono Fat (g)	Poly Fat (g)	Chol (mg)	Vit A (mcg RAE)	Vit D (mcg)
SALAD DRESSINGS, DIPS, AND MAYONNAISE *(continued)*														
Salad Dressings-Regular														
Salad Dressing, blue cheese, cmrcl	2	Tablespoon	30.60	154.22	1.47	2.26	0.00	16.00	3.03	3.76	8.51	5.20	20.50	0.09
Salad Dressing, caesar	2	Tablespoon	29.40	155.23	0.35	0.91	0.03	16.96	2.58	3.97	9.66	0.59	0.59	
Salad Dressing, French, cmrcl	2	Tablespoon	31.20	142.58	0.24	4.86	0.00	13.98	1.76	2.63	6.56	0.00	7.18	
Salad Dressing, honey dijon Kraft General Foods, Inc.	2	Tablespoon	31.00	110.00	0.00	6.00	0.00	10.00	1.50			0.00	0.00	
Salad Dressing, Italian, cmrcl	2	Tablespoon	29.40	85.55	0.11	3.07	0.00	8.34	1.31	1.85	3.80	0.00	0.59	
Salad Dressing, ranch Kraft General Foods, Inc.	2	Tablespoon	29.00	147.90	0.41	1.33	0.09	15.57	2.38			8.12		
Salad Dressing, ranch, cmrcl	1	Ounce-weight	28.35	137.21	0.29	1.90	0.20	14.57	2.28	3.23	8.03	9.36	2.83	0.02
Salad Dressing, sesame seed	2	Tablespoon	30.60	135.56	0.95	2.63	0.30	13.83	1.90	3.64	7.68	0.00	0.61	
Salad Dressing, sweet and sour	2	Tablespoon	32.00	4.80	0.03	1.18	0.00	0.00	0.00	0.00	0.00	0.00	0.00	
Salad Dressing, thousand island Kraft General Foods, Inc.	2	Tablespoon	31.00	110.00	0.00	5.00	0.00	10.00	1.50			10.00	0.00	
Salad Dressing, vinaigrette, herb Seven Seas	2	Tablespoon	30.00	140.00	0.00	1.00	0.00	15.00	2.00			0.00	0.00	
Salad Dressing, vinegar & oil, prep f/recipe	2	Tablespoon	31.20	140.09	0.00	0.78	0.00	15.63	2.84	4.62	7.52	0.00	0.00	
SALADS														
Cole Slaw, prep f/recipe	0.5	Cup	60.00	41.40	0.77	7.45	0.90	1.57	0.23	0.42	0.81	4.80	31.80	
Salad, bean, three	0.5	Cup	75.00	70.05	2.17	7.45	2.66	3.79	0.55	0.85	2.19	0.00	5.79	
Salad, fruit, w/ight syrup, cnd, not drained, cup	0.5	Cup	126.00	73.08	0.43	19.08	1.26	0.09	0.01	0.02	0.04	0.00	26.46	
Salad, fruit, w/juice, cnd, not drained, cup	0.5	Cup	124.50	62.25	0.63	16.25	1.25	0.04	0.00	0.01	0.01	0.00	37.35	
Salad, macaroni, elbow, classic, FS Orval Kent Food Company	0.5	Cup	106.00	196.86	3.03	24.99	1.51	9.09	1.51			7.57		
Salad, potato, prep f/recipe	0.5	Cup	125.00	178.75	3.35	13.96	1.62	10.25	1.79	3.10	4.67	85.00	40.00	
Salad, seafood	0.5	Cup	104.00	163.88	12.88	2.28	0.35	11.46	1.59	7.98	1.18	65.76	17.21	
Salad, tabouli/tabbouleh	0.5	Cup	80.00	99.56	1.31	8.02	1.87	7.50	1.02	5.41	0.69	0.00	17.14	
SANDWICHES														
Cheeseburger, reg, w/condiments	1	Each	113.00	294.93	15.96	26.53		14.15	6.31	5.35	1.09	37.29	85.88	
Pizza, pocket, pepperoni, fzn Chef America, Inc.	1	Each	128.00	367.36	13.57	38.66		17.66	6.63	6.35	2.00	40.96		
Sandwich, bbq beef, w/bun	1	Each	186.00	357.53	18.26	36.33	2.38	14.78	5.03	6.59	1.43	46.44	36.28	
Sandwich, bbq pork, w/bun	1	Each	186.00	321.95	22.76	34.36	2.25	9.57	2.80	4.37	1.42	50.65	35.49	
Sandwich, breakfast, egg cheese, w/biscuit, preckd, fzn Sunny Fresh	1	Each	99.23	224.26	9.89	24.64	0.00	8.89	2.36	1.14	3.68	111.14		
Sandwich, breakfast, egg ham cheese, w/biscuit, preckd, fzn Sunny Fresh	1	Each	120.40	243.21	12.24	25.21	0.12	9.70	2.63	1.23	3.77	114.38		
Sandwich, chicken, bbq	1	Each	119.00	251.42	20.53	26.85	1.32	6.19	1.58	2.40	1.40	50.10	14.22	
Sandwich, chicken, fillet, plain	1	Each	182.00	515.06	24.12	38.69		29.45	8.53	10.41	8.38	60.06	30.94	
Sandwich, egg patty cheese, vegetarian, w/English muffin Morningstar Farms	1	Each	171.00	277.88	30.01	32.71	7.01	2.99				3.69		
Sandwich, fajita beef, w/cheese, w/pita	1	Each	207.00	292.45	19.36	28.05	2.49	11.37	4.42	3.21	2.69	39.39	70.09	
Sandwich, fish, w/tartar sauce	1	Each	158.00	431.34	16.94	41.02	0.40	22.77	5.23	7.69	8.25	55.30	33.18	
Sandwich, ham cheese, grilled	1	Each	141.00	380.90	20.57	29.77	1.19	19.59	7.91	7.86	2.42	54.15	98.97	
Sandwich, ham cheese, pocket, fzn Chef America, Inc.	1	Each	128.00	340.48	14.85	38.40		14.21	5.79	4.42	1.48	49.92	0.00	
Sandwich, meatball, w/mozzarella, pocket, fzn Chef America, Inc.	1	Each	128.00	320.00	13.00	41.00	2.00	11.00	5.00			35.00	0.00	
Sandwich, meatball, w/mozzarella, pocket, fzn Chef America, Inc.	1	Each	128.00	300.00	13.00	44.00	2.00	7.00	3.50			30.00	0.00	

Vit E (mg)	Vit C	Vit B₁-Thia (mg)	Vit B₂-Ribo (mg)	Vit B₃-Nia (mg)	Fol (mcg)	Vit B₆ (mg)	Vita B₁₂ (mcg)	Sodi (mg)	Pota (mg)	Cal (mg)	Phos (mg)	Magn (mg)	Iron (mg)	Zinc (mg)	Caff (mg)	Alco (g)	Sol Fiber (g)	Insol Fiber (g)
1.84	0.61	0.00	0.03	0.03	8.57	0.01	0.08	334.76	11.32	24.79	22.64	0.00	0.06	0.08	0.00	0.00	0.00	0.00
1.54	0.00	0.00	0.00	0.01	0.88	0.00	0.01	316.93	8.53	7.06	5.59	0.59	0.05	0.03	0.00	0.00		
1.56	0.00	0.01	0.02	0.06	0.00	0.00	0.04	260.83	20.90	7.49	5.93	1.56	0.25	0.09	0.00	0.00	0.00	0.00
	0.00							210.00	35.00	0.00	0.00		0.00		0.00	0.00	0.00	0.00
1.47	0.00	0.00	0.01	0.00	0.00	0.02	0.00	486.28	14.11	2.06	2.65	0.88	0.19	0.04	0.00	0.00	0.00	0.00
	0.06							287.10	14.21	8.41	26.39		0.05		0.00	0.00		
1.34	0.96	0.03	0.02	0.00	1.13	0.01	0.09	231.34	17.58	8.79	45.64	1.42	0.18	0.11	0.00	0.00		
1.53	0.00	0.00	0.00	0.00	0.00	0.00	0.00	306.00	48.04	5.81	11.32	0.00	0.18	0.03	0.00	0.00		
0.82	2.59	0.00	0.00	0.02	0.64	0.00	0.00	66.56	10.56	1.28	0.96	0.96	0.01	0.01	0.00	0.00		
	0.00							310.00	40.00	0.00	0.00		0.00		0.00	0.00	0.00	0.00
	0.00							250.00	10.00	0.00	0.00		0.00		0.00	0.00	0.00	0.00
1.44	0.00	0.00	0.00	0.00	0.00	0.00	0.00	0.31	2.50	0.00	0.00	0.00	0.00	0.00	0.00	0.00	0.00	0.00
0.06	19.62	0.04	0.04	0.16	16.20	0.08	0.00	13.80	108.60	27.00	19.20	6.00	0.35	0.12	0.00	0.00		
0.87	2.02	0.04	0.05	0.22	28.00	0.02	0.01	260.09	123.26	17.64	37.82	13.74	0.74	0.29	0.00	0.00		
0.82	3.15	0.02	0.03	0.46	3.78	0.04	0.00	7.56	103.32	8.82	11.34	6.30	0.37	0.09	0.00	0.00		
0.75	4.11	0.01	0.02	0.44	3.74	0.03	0.00	6.23	144.42	13.70	17.43	9.96	0.31	0.17	0.00	0.00	0.61	0.63
								560.29							0.00	0.00		
2.32	12.50	0.10	0.07	1.12	8.75	0.18	0.00	661.25	317.50	23.75	65.00	18.75	0.81	0.38	0.00	0.00		
2.00	6.19	0.04	0.05	1.18	15.67	0.09	0.92	176.13	251.49	46.22	141.39	27.12	0.99	1.65	0.00	0.00		
1.08	14.25	0.04	0.03	0.57	15.54	0.06	0.00	399.53	122.78	14.49	31.78	17.79	0.62	0.24	0.00	0.00		
0.53	1.92	0.25	0.23	3.72	54.24	0.11	0.94	615.85	222.61	110.74	176.28	20.34	2.43	2.09	0.00	0.00		
								675.84			280.32		3.16		0.00	0.00		
1.28	5.84	0.29	0.27	5.73	21.75	0.23	1.52	1008.14	367.68	92.42	149.28	35.53	3.63	3.16	0.00	0.00		
1.25	5.70	0.76	0.37	5.65	19.71	0.34	0.45	947.67	426.09	94.40	197.79	39.16	2.89	2.21	0.00	0.00		
1.98	0.00	0.24	0.30	2.02	11.91	0.04	0.27	564.62	39.69	101.21	49.62	2.98	2.25	0.30	0.00	0.00	0.00	0.00
2.41	0.12	0.24	0.31	2.02	12.04	0.04	0.29	724.81	46.96	105.95	54.18	3.61	2.44	0.33	0.00	0.00		
0.43	0.85	0.28	0.28	7.25	21.20	0.30	0.19	422.13	217.40	65.86	159.11	28.39	2.33	1.51	0.00	0.00		
	8.92	0.33	0.24	6.81	100.10	0.20	0.38	957.32	353.08	60.06	232.96	34.58	4.68	1.87	0.00	0.00		
	0.00	5.30	1.06	7.83		0.10	1.32	1051.14	354.14	283.35	579.69		6.05	2.77	0.00	0.00		
1.46	33.41	0.34	0.30	4.16	36.85	0.42	1.66	777.86	464.05	182.39	251.77	38.55	2.54	2.72	0.00	0.00		
0.87	2.84	0.33	0.22	3.40	85.32	0.11	1.07	614.62	339.70	83.74	211.72	33.18	2.61	1.00	0.00	0.00		
1.11	0.01	0.71	0.44	5.01	16.41	0.27	0.81	1464.85	337.38	233.26	342.97	32.40	2.41	2.47	0.00	0.00		
								665.60		250.88			2.61		0.00	0.00		
	0.00							660.00		250.00			3.60		0.00	0.00		
	0.00							600.00		300.00			3.60		0.00	0.00		

Food Name	Amount	Measure	Weight (g)	Calories	Protein (g)	Total Carb (g)	Dietary Fiber (g)	Total Fat (g)	Sat Fat (g)	Mono Fat (g)	Poly Fat (g)	Chol (mg)	Vit A (mcg RAE)	Vit D (mcg)
SANDWICHES *(continued)*														
Sandwich, philly steak cheese, pocket, fzn Chef America, Inc.	1	Each	128.00	350.00	12.00	40.00	2.00	16.00	7.00			45.00	0.00	
Sandwich, philly steak cheese, pocket, fzn Chef America, Inc.	1	Each	128.00	290.00	12.00	43.00	2.00	7.00	3.00			30.00	0.00	
Sandwich, roast beef, plain	1	Each	139.00	346.11	21.50	33.44		13.76	3.61	6.80	1.71	51.43	11.12	
Sandwich, roast beef, w/cheese	1	Each	176.00	473.44	32.23	45.37		18.00	9.03	3.66	3.50	77.44	58.08	
Sandwich, sausage, w/biscuit, fzn, Jimmy Dean, FS Travis Meats	1	Each	48.00	192.48	4.75	11.57	0.72	14.11	4.31			15.84		
Sandwich, steak	1	Each	204.00	459.00	30.33	51.96		14.08	3.81	5.34	3.35	73.44	20.40	
Sandwich, submarine, w/cold cuts	1	Each	228.00	456.00	21.84	51.05	1.70	18.63	6.81	8.23	2.28	36.48	70.68	
Sandwich, submarine, w/roast beef	1	Each	216.00	410.40	28.64	44.30		12.96	7.09	1.84	2.61	73.44	30.24	
Sandwich, submarine, w/tuna salad	1	Each	256.00	583.68	29.70	55.37		27.98	5.33	13.40	7.30	48.64	46.08	
SAUCES AND GRAVIES														
Gravies														
Gravy, au jus, dry mix	1	Teaspoon	3.00	9.39	0.28	1.42		0.29	0.06	0.14	0.01	0.12	0.03	
Gravy, beef, can	0.25	Cup	58.25	30.87	2.18	2.80	0.23	1.37	0.67	0.56	0.05	1.75	0.58	
Gravy, beef, hearty, jar Pepperidge Farm	0.25	Cup	60.00	25.80	1.80	3.72		0.42	0.14	0.15	0.04	3.00	0.00	
Gravy, brown, dry mix	1	Tablespoon	6.00	22.02	0.64	3.56	0.12	0.58	0.20	0.27	0.02	0.18	0.48	
Gravy, brown, dry mix, 16oz pkg Trio	1	Tablespoon	6.00	24.36	0.63	3.47	0.21	0.89	0.26	0.16	0.46	0.00	0.00	
Gravy, brown, homestyle, savory, cnd Heinz	0.25	Cup	60.00	24.60	0.90	3.41		0.78	0.32	0.28	0.04	2.40		
Gravy, chicken, can	0.25	Cup	59.50	47.01	1.15	3.22	0.24	3.40	0.84	1.52	0.89	1.19	0.60	
Gravy, chicken, dry pkt	1	Tablespoon	8.00	30.48	0.90	4.97		0.78	0.23	0.37	0.15	1.52	3.04	
Gravy, country, dry mix, 22oz pkg Trio	1	Tablespoon	8.00	34.64	0.73	5.19	0.72	1.22	0.32	0.14	0.54	0.48	0.00	
Gravy, mushroom, dry mix, svg, makes 1 cup prep	1	Each	21.30	69.86	2.13	13.77	1.02	0.85	0.50	0.28	0.03	0.64	0.01	
Gravy, pork, dry mix, svg	1	Each	6.70	24.59	0.59	4.26	0.16	0.58	0.29	0.26	0.03	0.67	2.28	
Gravy, southern, dry mix Trio	1	Tablespoon	10.00	48.10	0.25	6.05	0.00	2.55	0.56	0.30	1.19	0.20		
Gravy, turkey, dry mix, svg	1	Each	7.00	25.69	0.73	4.56		0.50	0.14	0.18	0.15	0.98	0.56	
Sauces														
Marinade, cooking sauce, teriyaki S & W	1	Tablespoon	18.00	25.00	1.00	5.00	0.00	0.00	0.00	0.00	0.00	0.00	0.00	
Sauce, alfredo, dry mix Corn Products International	2	Tablespoon	15.00	61.80	2.22	7.13		2.72	1.61	1.01	0.09	5.40		
Sauce, bearnaise, dehyd, svg, makes 1 cup prep	1	Each	16.50	59.73	2.32	9.86	0.10	1.49	0.22	0.64	0.56	0.17	0.17	
Sauce, cheese, cheddar, basic, rts Chef-Mate	0.25	Cup	62.00	81.84	1.80	8.02	0.00	4.70	1.57			6.20		
Sauce, cheese, cheddar, inst, dry mix, FS Custom Food Products Superb	2	Tablespoon	14.20	60.07	1.13	8.02	0.62	2.60	1.51	0.95	0.14	3.83		
Sauce, cheese, dry mix, 2lb pkg Nestle Foods Company	2	Tablespoon	12.00	53.52	0.89	7.31	0.00	2.30	0.78	0.88	0.63	2.28		
Sauce, cheese, nacho, dry mix, 2lb pkg Nestle Foods Company	2	Tablespoon	12.00	51.36	1.07	7.57	0.07	1.86	0.80	0.54	0.42	2.04		
Sauce, cheese, nacho, rts, pkg Ortega	0.25	Cup	63.00	127.89	5.24	4.02	0.44	10.10	5.80			28.98		
Sauce, creole, rts, pkg Chef-Mate	0.25	Cup	62.00	24.80	0.92	3.71	0.81	0.69	0.07	0.23	0.29	0.00		
Sauce, curry, dehyd, pkt	1	Each	35.40	151.16	3.31	17.93	0.46	8.18	1.21	3.51	3.08	0.35	1.76	
Sauce, enchilada, rts Ortega	2	Tablespoon	30.00	15.00	0.44	2.01	0.30	0.59	0.09	0.17	0.28	0.00		
Sauce, fish, rts	2	Tablespoon	36.00	12.60	1.82	1.31	0.00	0.00	0.00	0.00	0.00	0.00	1.44	
Sauce, hoisin, rts	2	Tablespoon	32.00	70.40	1.06	14.11	0.90	1.08	0.18	0.31	0.54	0.96	0.10	
Sauce, hollandaise, prep f/recipe	2	Tablespoon	20.00	85.44	1.00	0.26	–	9.09	5.13	2.78	0.50	89.99	96.94	
Sauce, lemon, rts, pkg Chef-Mate	2	Tablespoon	32.00	42.88	0.07	10.21	0.00	0.19	0.02	0.05	0.09	0.00	0.00	
Sauce, marinara Di Giorno	0.5	Cup	127.00	70.00	2.00	15.00	2.00	0.00	0.00	0.00	0.00	0.00	25.00	
Sauce, mole poblano, prep f/recipe	2	Tablespoon	30.30	49.69	1.07	3.92	1.27	3.32		1.46	0.86	0.28	45.45	

Vit E (mg)	Vit C	Vit B₁-Thia (mg)	Vit B₂-Ribo (mg)	Vit B₃-Nia (mg)	Fol (mcg)	Vit B₆ (mg)	Vita B₁₂ (mcg)	Sodi (mg)	Pota (mg)	Cal (mg)	Phos (mg)	Magn (mg)	Iron (mg)	Zinc (mg)	Caff (mg)	Alco (g)	Sol Fiber (g)	Insol Fiber (g)
	0.00							630.00		250.00			2.70		0.00	0.00		
	0.00							560.00		250.00			3.60		0.00	0.00		
0.19	2.08	0.38	0.31	5.87	56.99	0.26	1.22	792.30	315.53	54.21	239.08	30.58	4.23	3.39	0.00	0.00		
	0.00	0.39	0.46	5.90	63.36	0.33	2.06	1633.28	344.96	183.04	401.28	40.48	5.05	5.37	0.00	0.00		
								440.64		37.92			0.79		0.00	0.00		
	5.51	0.41	0.37	7.30	89.76	0.37	1.57	797.64	524.28	91.80	297.84	48.96	5.16	4.53	0.00	0.00		
	12.31	1.00	0.80	5.49	86.64	0.14	1.09	1650.72	394.44	189.24	287.28	68.40	2.51	2.58	0.00	0.00		
	5.62	0.41	0.41	5.96	71.28	0.32	1.81	844.56	330.48	41.04	192.24	66.96	2.81	4.38	0.00	0.00		
	3.58	0.46	0.33	11.34	102.40	0.23	1.61	1292.80	335.36	74.24	220.16	79.36	2.64	1.87	0.00	0.00		
0.01	0.03	0.01	0.01	0.12	2.43	0.01	0.01	347.64	8.37	4.20	4.59	1.68	0.28	0.02	0.00	0.00		
0.01	0.00	0.02	0.02	0.38	1.16	0.01	0.06	326.20	47.18	3.49	17.47	1.16	0.41	0.58	0.00	0.00		
								378.60							0.00	0.00		
0.02	0.02	0.01	0.02	0.22	1.86	0.01	0.04	290.58	15.72	7.92	12.18	2.04	0.10	0.07	0.00	0.00		
0.04	0.00	0.00	0.00	0.01	1.56	0.00	0.00	261.78	0.84	2.16	7.32	0.48	0.11	0.04	0.00	0.00		
								351.60							0.00	0.00		
0.08	0.00	0.01	0.03	0.26	1.19	0.01	0.06	343.32	64.86	11.90	17.26	1.19	0.28	0.48	0.00	0.00		
0.02	0.05	0.02	0.05	0.32	10.00	0.02	0.04	332.16	32.32	11.68	19.92	3.20	0.11	0.11	0.00	0.00		
0.07	0.00	0.01	0.02	0.10	0.80	0.00	0.01	204.72	11.12	5.20	8.88	1.12	0.10	0.05	0.00	0.00		
0.03	1.49	0.04	0.09	0.79	6.60	0.02	0.15	1401.54	55.81	48.99	43.24	7.24	0.21	0.33	0.00	0.00		
0.02	0.09	0.01	0.02	0.15	2.08	0.01	0.03	358.85	15.75	9.31	12.60	2.28	0.26	0.07	0.00	0.00		
0.43	0.07	0.00	0.01	0.01	0.30	0.00	0.02	290.00	13.80	7.50	6.60	1.40	0.06	0.03	0.00	0.00	0.00	0.00
0.01	0.01	0.01	0.03	0.19	5.74	0.01	0.04	307.44	29.96	10.22	17.78	3.08	0.23	0.09	0.00	0.00		
	3.00							480.00	40.00	0.00			0.00		0.00	0.00	0.00	0.00
								730.20							0.00	0.00		
0.05	0.33	0.02	0.03	0.10	2.15	0.01	0.07	559.35	48.18	27.23	24.42	4.62	0.08	0.12	0.00	0.00		
1.24	0.56	0.00	0.04	0.04	1.86	0.01	0.06	471.20	16.12	45.88	50.84	3.72	0.18	0.33	0.00	0.00	0.00	0.00
0.33	0.14	0.03	0.10	0.34	19.03	0.03	0.07	685.15	60.78	40.47	40.19	5.11	0.07	0.16	0.00	0.00		
0.28	0.00	0.03	0.08	0.29	16.08	0.02	0.06	309.60	51.36	21.96	33.96	4.32	0.09	0.13	0.00	0.00	0.00	0.00
0.28	0.29	0.03	0.08	0.29	16.08	0.02	0.06	338.40	51.36	20.04	33.96	4.32	0.09	0.13	0.00	0.00		
0.26	0.44	0.00	0.08	0.02	3.15	0.01	0.09	579.60	20.16	180.81	105.21	6.30	0.15	0.65	0.00	0.00		
0.61	0.00	0.03	0.02	0.53	8.68	0.07	0.00	339.14	187.24	34.72	17.36	8.68	0.31	0.10	0.00	0.00		
	0.71	0.04	0.08	0.29	3.19	0.01	0.14	1444.32	124.61	62.66	52.75	14.51	1.10	0.31	0.00	0.00		
0.00	2.13	0.02	0.01	0.32	2.40	0.04	0.00	77.40	83.40	7.20	10.50	5.10	0.31	0.06	0.00	0.00		
0.00	0.18	0.00	0.02	0.83	18.36	0.14	0.17	2779.20	103.68	15.48	2.52	63.00	0.28	0.07	0.00	0.00	0.00	0.00
0.09	0.13	0.00	0.07	0.37	7.36	0.02	0.00	516.80	38.08	10.24	12.16	7.68	0.32	0.10	0.00	0.00		
0.32	0.85	0.01	0.04	0.01	8.49	0.02	0.18	77.83	9.79	9.88	28.88	0.82	0.21	0.18	0.00	0.00		
0.01	2.75	0.00	0.00	0.01	0.32	0.00	0.00	2.56	6.40	1.28	1.28	0.64	0.12	0.01	0.00	0.00	0.00	0.00
	0.00	0.09	0.10	1.60	0.00		0.00	220.00	400.00	40.00	20.00		0.72		0.00	0.00		
0.44	0.00	0.01	0.00	0.50	8.48	0.08	0.01	40.60	98.78	7.27	24.85	9.70	0.56	0.14	0.00	0.00		

Food Name	Amount	Measure	Weight (g)	Calories	Protein (g)	Total Carb (g)	Dietary Fiber (g)	Total Fat (g)	Sat Fat (g)	Mono Fat (g)	Poly Fat (g)	Chol (mg)	Vit A (mcg RAE)	Vit D (mcg)
SAUCES AND GRAVIES *(continued)*														
Sauce, mushroom, dehyd, svg, makes 1 cup prep	1	Each	22.70	79.22	3.26	12.42		2.16	0.32	0.93	0.81	0.00	0.00	
Sauce, oyster, rts	2	Tablespoon	8.00	4.08	0.11	0.87	0.02	0.02	0.00	0.01	0.01	0.00	0.00	
Sauce, pasta, fresh mushroom, jar Prego	0.5	Cup	122.80	120.00	2.00	21.00	3.00	3.50	1.50			0.00		
Sauce, pasta, marinara, jar Prego	0.5	Cup	122.80	90.00	2.00	10.00	3.00	5.00	1.50			0.00		
Sauce, pasta, pesto, dry mix Knorr	2	Teaspoon	5.00	15.00	1.00	3.00	0.00	0.00	0.00	0.00	0.00	0.00		
Sauce, pasta, smooth, traditional, jar, Old World Style Ragu	0.5	Cup	125.00	80.00	1.88	12.11	2.62	2.62	0.36	0.55	1.29	0.00	32.50	
Sauce, pepper/hot, rts	1	Teaspoon	4.70	0.52	0.02	0.08	0.01	0.02	0.00	0.00	0.01	0.00	0.38	
Sauce, pizza, traditional, all natural, Prince Heinz	1	Ounce-weight	28.35	12.23	0.55	2.27	0.62	0.10	0.02	0.06	0.02	0.29	10.66	
Sauce, plum, rts	2	Tablespoon	38.13	70.15	0.34	16.32	0.27	0.40	0.06	0.09	0.22	0.00	0.76	
Salsa, rts	2	Tablespoon	32.38	8.74	0.50	2.03	0.52	0.05	0.01	0.01	0.04	0.00	4.86	
Sauce, sofrito, prep f/recipe, tbsp	2	Tablespoon	29.80	70.63	3.81	1.63	0.51	5.42						
Sauce, sour cream, dehyd, svg	1	Ounce-weight	28.35	145.16	4.45	13.69		8.89	4.45	3.03	1.00	22.68	20.42	
Sauce, spaghetti, w/meat, cnd Del Monte Foods	0.5	Cup	125.00	60.00	3.00	14.00	3.00	1.00	0.00			0.00		
Sauce, spaghetti/marinara, rts	0.5	Cup	125.00	92.50	2.44	14.09	0.50	2.97	0.41	0.95	1.18	0.00	33.75	
Sauce, sweet & sour, dehyd, svg	1	Ounce-weight	28.35	110.28	0.27	27.24	0.54	0.03	0.00	0.00	0.03	0.00	0.00	
Sauce, szechuan, rts Chef-Mate	2	Tablespoon	32.00	41.60	0.46	5.84	0.10	1.82	0.24	0.53	0.88	0.00		
Sauce, teriyaki, rts Chef-Mate	2	Tablespoon	32.00	41.60	0.30	7.48	0.00	1.16	0.12	0.34	0.56	0.00	0.00	
Sauce, white, thick, prep f/recipe	2	Tablespoon	31.25	58.12	1.25	3.63	0.09	4.32	1.07	1.83	1.22	1.88	36.56	
Tomato Paste, 6oz can	0.25	Cup	65.50	53.71	2.84	12.38	2.95	0.31	0.07	0.04	0.15	0.00	49.78	
Tomato Sauce, cnd	0.5	Cup	122.50	39.20	1.61	9.02	1.84	0.29	0.04	0.04	0.12	0.00	20.83	
SNACK FOODS-CHIPS, PRETZELS, POPCORN														
Cheese Puffs, white cheddar, svg Season's Enterprises, Ltd.	1	Each	30.00	180.00	3.00	13.00	2.00	13.00	3.00			5.00	0.00	
Chips, bagel	5	Piece	70.00	298.18	6.18	52.41	4.25	7.33	1.26	2.08	3.45	0.00		
Chips, corn cones, plain, extruded	1	Ounce-weight	28.35	144.58	1.64	17.83	0.31	7.63	6.45	0.48	0.22	0.00	4.54	
Chips, corn, bbq flvr, extruded, 7oz bag	1	Ounce-weight	28.35	148.27	1.98	15.93	1.47	9.27	1.27	2.68	4.58	0.00	8.79	
Chips, corn, plain, extruded, 7oz bag	1	Ounce-weight	28.35	152.81	1.87	16.13	1.39	9.47	1.29	2.74	4.67	0.00	1.42	
Chips, potato, bbq flvr, 7 oz bag	1	Ounce-weight	28.35	139.20	2.18	14.97	1.25	9.19	2.29	1.85	4.64	0.00	3.12	
Chips, potato, bkd	1	Ounce-weight	28.35	132.96	1.42	20.25	1.37	5.15	0.76	2.81	1.20	0.00	0.00	
Chips, potato, cheese flvr, f/dried potato, can	1	Ounce-weight	28.35	156.21	1.98	14.35	0.96	10.49	2.71	2.02	5.29	1.13	0.28	
Chips, potato, fat free, Wow! Lays	1	Ounce-weight	28.35	75.00	2.00	18.00	1.00	0.00	0.00	0.00	0.00	0.00	0.00	
Chips, potato, Kettle, lightly salted Season's Enterprises, Ltd.	1	Ounce-weight	28.35	140.00	2.00	17.00	1.00	8.00	1.50			0.00	0.00	
Chips, potato, plain, bag	1	Ounce-weight	28.35	151.96	1.98	15.00	1.28	9.81	3.11	2.79	3.45	0.00	0.00	
Chips, potato, plain, unsalt, w/part hydrog soy oil, bag	1	Ounce-weight	28.35	151.96	1.98	15.00	1.36	9.81	1.54	5.10	2.60	0.00	0.00	
Chips, potato, plain, w/part hydrog soy oil, bag	1	Ounce-weight	28.35	151.96	1.98	15.00	1.36	9.81	1.54	5.10	2.60	0.00	0.00	
Chips, potato, rducd fat, unsalted	1	Ounce-weight	28.35	138.06	2.01	19.22	1.73	5.90	1.18	1.36	3.10	0.00	0.00	
Chips, potato, sour cream & onion flvr, bag	1	Ounce-weight	28.35	150.54	2.30	14.60	1.47	9.61	2.52	1.74	4.94	1.98	3.97	
Chips, taro	1	Ounce-weight	28.35	141.18	0.65	19.31	2.04	7.06	1.82	1.26	3.65	0.00	1.98	
Chips, tortilla, blue corn, Blue Chips Garden of Eatin'	1	Ounce-weight	28.35	140.00	2.00	18.00	2.00	7.00	0.50			0.00	0.00	
Chips, tortilla, nacho flvr, rducd fat, bag	1	Ounce-weight	28.35	126.16	2.47	20.30	1.36	4.31	0.82	2.54	0.60	0.85	6.80	
Chips, tortilla, nacho, made w/enrich masa flour	1	Ounce-weight	28.35	141.18	2.21	17.69	1.50	7.26	1.39	4.28	1.00	0.85	6.80	
Chips, tortilla, plain, bag	1	Ounce-weight	28.35	142.03	1.98	17.83	1.84	7.43	1.43	4.38	1.03	0.00	1.13	
Chips, tortilla, ranch flvr, bag	1	Ounce-weight	28.35	138.91	2.15	18.31	1.11	6.75	1.29	3.99	0.94	0.28	4.25	
Chips, tortilla, taco flvr, bag	1	Ounce-weight	28.35	136.08	2.24	17.89	1.50	6.86	1.31	4.05	0.95	1.42	12.76	

Vit E (mg)	Vit C	Vit B$_1$-Thia (mg)	Vit B$_2$-Ribo (mg)	Vit B$_3$-Nia (mg)	Fol (mcg)	Vit B$_6$ (mg)	Vita B$_{12}$ (mcg)	Sodi (mg)	Pota (mg)	Cal (mg)	Phos (mg)	Magn (mg)	Iron (mg)	Zinc (mg)	Caff (mg)	Alco (g)	Sol Fiber (g)	Insol Fiber (g)
0.00	0.00	0.02	0.11	1.04	6.13	0.02	0.00	1414.21	98.29	2.04	30.19	4.09	0.23	0.20	0.00	0.00		
0.00	0.01	0.00	0.01	0.12	1.20	0.00	0.03	218.64	4.32	2.56	1.76	0.32	0.01	0.01	0.00	0.00		
	2.40							560.00		20.00			1.08		0.00	0.00		
	2.40							550.00		40.00			0.72		0.00	0.00		
	0.00							490.00		0.00			0.00		0.00	0.00	0.00	0.00
								756.25					1.02		0.00	0.00		
0.01	3.52	0.00	0.00	0.01	0.28	0.01	0.00	124.22	6.77	0.38	0.52	0.23	0.02	0.01	0.00	0.00		
	1.73	0.02	0.04	0.43				134.17	113.90	3.54	14.54	5.35	0.16	0.07	0.00	0.00		
0.08	0.19	0.01	0.03	0.39	2.29	0.03	0.00	205.11	98.74	4.57	8.39	4.57	0.55	0.07	0.00	0.00		
0.38	0.62	0.01	0.01	0.02	1.29	0.06	0.00	194.25	96.15	8.74	10.04	4.86	0.15	0.12	0.00	0.00		
	6.08	0.08	0.06	0.87	12.81	0.11		341.21	119.50	5.96	41.42	7.45	0.28	0.42	0.00	0.00		
	0.13	0.03	0.13	0.13	1.13	0.03	0.10	357.21	146.00	102.90	33.44	5.96	0.19	0.52	0.00	0.00		
	9.00							720.00		40.00			1.44		0.00	0.00		
2.55	3.88	0.03	0.08	4.90	13.75	0.22	0.00	601.25	470.00	33.75	45.00	26.25	1.06	0.68	0.00	0.00		
0.00	0.00	0.00	0.03	0.30	0.84	0.15	0.00	291.99	24.66	15.30	17.01	3.39	0.60	0.03	0.00	0.00		
0.14	0.51	0.00	0.01	0.19	1.28	0.02	0.24	436.16	25.60	3.52	11.84	3.20	0.24	0.04	0.00	0.00		
0.05		0.00	0.01	0.19	0.96	0.01	0.00	318.72	16.00	2.56	6.72	2.56	0.18	0.03	0.00	0.00	0.00	0.00
0.12	0.22	0.03	0.06	0.18	3.44	0.01	0.08	116.56	46.56	34.69	30.00	4.38	0.16	0.12	0.00	0.00		
2.82	14.34	0.04	0.11	2.01	7.86	0.13	0.00	517.45	664.17	23.58	54.37	27.51	1.94	0.41	0.00	0.00	0.76	2.18
2.55	8.58	0.02	0.08	1.20	11.03	0.12	0.00	641.90	405.48	15.93	31.85	19.60	1.25	0.25	0.00	0.00		
	0.00							270.00		40.00			0.36		0.00	0.00		
1.70	0.00	0.14	0.12	1.61	46.04	0.16	0.00	418.90	167.42	8.94	144.62	39.22	1.38	0.89	0.00	0.00		
0.54	0.00	0.09	0.07	0.40	0.85	0.01	0.00	289.74	22.96	0.85	12.47	3.12	0.72	0.06	0.00	0.00		
0.38	0.48	0.02	0.06	0.46	11.06	0.07	0.00	216.31	66.91	37.14	58.68	21.83	0.43	0.30	0.00	0.00		
0.39	0.00	0.01	0.04	0.33	5.67	0.07	0.00	178.60	40.26	36.00	52.45	21.55	0.38	0.36	0.00	0.00		
1.42	9.61	0.06	0.06	1.33	23.53	0.18	0.00	212.62	357.49	14.17	52.73	21.26	0.55	0.26	0.00	0.00		
0.61	0.00	0.09	0.02	1.16	0.00	0.14	0.00	259.97	204.40	35.44	77.68	12.19	0.24	0.12	0.00	0.00		
1.38	2.41	0.05	0.04	0.74	5.10	0.15	0.00	214.04	108.01	31.18	46.21	15.03	0.45	0.18	0.00	0.00		
	6.00	0.02	0.04	0.27				200.00	76.00	0.00	44.00		0.36	0.40	0.00	0.00		
	18.00							80.00		0.00			0.36		0.00	Alco		
2.58	8.82	0.05	0.06	1.09	12.76	0.19	0.00	168.40	361.46	6.80	46.78	18.99	0.46	0.31	0.00	0.00		
1.38	8.82	0.05	0.06	1.09	12.76	0.19	0.00	2.27	361.46	6.80	46.78	18.99	0.46	0.31	0.00	0.00		
1.38	8.82	0.05	0.06	1.09	12.76	0.19	0.00	168.40	361.46	6.80	46.78	18.99	0.46	0.31	0.00	0.00		
1.55	7.29	0.06	0.08	1.98	2.83	0.19	0.00	2.27	494.42	5.95	54.72	25.23	0.39	0.28	0.00	0.00		
1.38	10.57	0.06	0.06	1.14	17.58	0.19	0.28	177.19	377.34	20.41	49.90	20.98	0.45	0.27	0.00	0.00		
3.21	1.42	0.05	0.01	0.14	5.67	0.12	0.00	96.96	214.04	17.01	37.14	23.81	0.34	0.10	0.00	0.00		
	0.00							60.00		20.00			0.36		0.00	0.00		
0.23	0.06	0.07	0.08	0.11	7.37	0.07	0.00	284.35	77.11	45.08	90.15	27.50	0.46		0.00	0.00		
	0.51	0.11	0.10	1.13	36.85	0.09	0.02	200.72	61.24	41.67	69.17	23.25	1.05	0.34	0.00	0.00		
1.00	0.00	0.02	0.06	0.36	2.83	0.09	0.00	149.69	55.85	43.66	58.12	24.95	0.43	0.43	0.00	0.00		
0.39	0.26	0.03	0.07	0.42	4.82	0.06	0.00	173.50	69.17	39.97	67.76	25.23	0.42	0.35	0.00	0.00		
0.39	0.26	0.07	0.06	0.57	5.95	0.09	0.00	223.11	61.52	43.94	67.76	24.95	0.58	0.36	0.00	0.00		

Food Name	Amount	Measure	Weight (g)	Calories	Protein (g)	Total Carb (g)	Dietary Fiber (g)	Total Fat (g)	Sat Fat (g)	Mono Fat (g)	Poly Fat (g)	Chol (mg)	Vit A (mcg RAE)	Vit D (mcg)
SNACK FOODS-CHIPS, PRETZELS, POPCORN (continued)														
Chips, tortilla, w/cinnamon & sugar	1	Ounce-weight	28.35	153.94	1.87	16.49	0.86	9.36	4.73	3.08	1.08	10.21	1.42	
Corn Nuts, bbq flvr	1	Ounce-weight	28.35	123.61	2.55	20.33	2.38	4.05	0.73	2.09	0.92	0.00	4.82	
Corn Nuts, plain	1	Ounce-weight	28.35	126.44	2.41	20.37	1.96	4.43	0.69	2.68	0.87	0.00	0.00	
Fruit Leather, roll, sml	1	Each	14.00	51.94	0.01	12.00	0.46	0.42	0.09	0.21	0.08	0.00	0.84	
Popcorn, air popped	1	Cup	8.00	30.56	0.96	6.23	1.21	0.34	0.05	0.09	0.15	0.00	0.80	
Popcorn, caramel coated, w/o peanuts	1	Ounce-weight	28.35	122.19	1.08	22.42	1.47	3.63	1.02	0.81	1.27	1.42	0.57	
Popcorn, cheese flvrd	1	Cup	11.00	57.86	1.02	5.68	1.09	3.65	0.70	1.07	1.69	1.21	4.18	
Popcorn, oil popped	1	Cup	11.00	55.00	0.99	6.29	1.10	3.09	0.54	0.90	1.48	0.00	0.88	
Popcorn, white, oil popped	1	Cup	11.00	55.00	0.99	6.29	1.10	3.09	0.54	0.90	1.48	0.00	0.11	
Pork Skins, bbq flvr	1	Ounce-weight	28.35	152.52	16.41	0.45		9.02	3.28	4.26	0.98	32.60	18.43	
Pretzels, hard	10	Each	60.00	228.60	5.46	47.52	1.92	2.10	0.46	0.82	0.74	0.00	0.00	
Pretzels, hard, unsalted, w/unenrich flour	5	Each	30.00	114.30	2.73	23.76	0.84	1.05	0.23	0.41	0.37	0.00	0.00	
Pretzels, hard, whole wheat	1	Ounce-weight	28.35	102.63	3.15	23.02	2.18	0.74	0.16	0.29	0.24	0.00	0.00	
Rice Cake, brown rice & buckwheat, salted	1	Each	9.00	34.20	0.81	7.21	0.34	0.32	0.06	0.10	0.10	0.00	0.00	
Rice Cake, brown rice & multigrain, unsalted	1	Each	9.00	34.83	0.77	7.21	0.38	0.32	0.05	0.11	0.13	0.00	0.00	
Rice Cake, brown rice, plain, unsalted	1	Each	9.00	34.83	0.74	7.34	0.38	0.25	0.05	0.09	0.09	0.00	0.00	
Rice Krispies Treats, square, single svg Kellogg's Company	1	Each	37.00	153.18	1.26	29.79	0.22	3.33	0.52	0.93	1.89	0.00	119.88	
Snack Mix, Chex, traditional Ralston Foods	0.66	Cup	30.00	130.00	3.00	22.00	1.00	3.50	1.00			0.00	0.00	
Snack Mix, oriental, rice based	1	Ounce-weight	28.35	143.45	4.90	14.64	3.74	7.25	1.08	2.80	3.01	0.00	0.00	
Trail Mix, regular	0.25	Cup	37.50	173.25	5.18	16.84	1.92	11.02	2.09	4.70	3.62	0.00	0.38	
Trail Mix, w/chocolate chips salted nuts & seeds	0.25	Cup	36.25	175.45	5.15	16.28	2.02	11.56	2.21	4.91	4.10	1.45	0.73	
SOUPS, STEWS AND CHILIS														
Canned/Frozen/Prepared Soups, Stews and Chilis														
Beans, chili style, med, cnd Bush's Best	0.5	Cup	130.00	120.00	6.00	20.00	6.00	1.00	0.50			0.00		
Bouillon/Broth, beef, cond, prep w/water, can	1	Cup	240.00	16.80	2.74	0.10	0.00	0.53	0.26	0.22	0.02	0.00	0.00	
Broth, chicken, prep f/cnd w/water, cmrcl	1	Cup	244.00	39.04	4.93	0.93	0.00	1.39	0.39	0.59	0.27	0.00	0.00	
Chili, con carne	1	Cup	253.00	255.53	24.62	21.94		8.27	3.43	3.41	0.53	134.09	83.49	
Chili, con carne, w/beans, cnd, svg	1	Cup	222.00	268.62	15.74	25.37	8.66	11.68	3.86	4.76	0.95	28.86		
Chili, mild vegetarian, w/soy protein, low fat, cnd Health Valley Foods	1	Cup	245.00	160.00	14.00	30.00	11.00	1.00	0.00			0.00		
Chili, vegetarian lentil, w/soy protein, low fat, cnd Health Valley Foods	1	Cup	245.00	160.00	15.00	28.00	11.00	1.00	0.00			0.00		
Chili, vegetarian, w/beans, cnd	1	Cup	247.00	205.01	11.93	38.01	9.88	0.69	0.12	0.07	0.40	0.00		
Chili, w/beans, classic, cnd	1	Cup	247.00	323.57	17.22	29.22	7.41	16.33	6.69	6.89	1.11	41.99		
Chili, w/beans, cnd	1	Cup	256.00	286.72	14.62	30.49	11.26	14.05	6.02	5.97	0.93	43.52	43.52	
Chili, w/beans, cnd Chef-Mate	1	Cup	253.00	412.39	17.74	29.04	11.13	25.02	10.93	10.75	1.40	55.66		
Chili, w/beans, dynamite, cnd Hormel Foods Corporation	1	Cup	247.00	333.45	18.28	30.73	8.15	15.36	5.66	6.79	0.91	44.46		
Chili, w/black beans, spicy, vegetarian, fat free, cnd Health Valley Foods	1	Cup	245.00	160.00	13.00	28.00	12.00	1.00	0.00			0.00		
Chowder, clam, Manhattan style, chunky, rts, can	1	Cup	240.00	134.40	7.25	18.82	2.88	3.38	2.11	0.98	0.12	14.40	168.00	
Chowder, clam, New England, prep f/cnd w/milk, cmrcl	1	Cup	248.00	163.68	9.47	16.62	1.49	6.60	2.95	2.26	1.09	22.32	57.04	
Chowder, clam, New England, prep f/cnd w/water, cmrcl	1	Cup	244.00	95.16	4.81	12.42	1.46	2.88	0.41	1.22	1.10	4.88	2.44	
Soup, beef barley, 99% fat free, rts, cnd Progresso Healthy Classics	8	Ounce-weight	226.80	129.28	11.57	16.10	3.41	1.54	0.66	0.68	0.21	18.14	95.26	
Soup, beef mushroom, cond, cmrcl, can	1	Cup	251.00	153.11	11.55	13.05	0.50	6.02	3.01	2.51	0.25	12.55	0.00	

Vit E (mg)	Vit C	Vit B₁-Thia (mg)	Vit B₂-Ribo (mg)	Vit B₃-Nia (mg)	Fol (mcg)	Vit B₆ (mg)	Vita B₁₂ (mcg)	Sodi (mg)	Pota (mg)	Cal (mg)	Phos (mg)	Magn (mg)	Iron (mg)	Zinc (mg)	Caff (mg)	Alco (g)	Sol Fiber (g)	Insol Fiber (g)
	2.07	0.05	0.11	1.02	1.98	0.05	0.44	114.25	20.41	22.11	8.50	5.10	0.76	0.15	0.00	0.00		
0.28	0.11	0.10	0.04	0.43	0.00	0.06	0.00	276.70	81.08	4.82	80.23	30.90	0.48	0.53	0.00	0.00		
0.56	0.00	0.01	0.04	0.48	0.00	0.07	0.00	155.64	78.81	2.55	77.96	32.04	0.47	0.50	0.00	0.00		
0.08	16.80	0.01	0.00	0.01	0.56	0.04	0.00	44.38	41.16	4.48	4.34	2.80	0.14	0.03	0.00	0.00		
0.02	0.00	0.02	0.02	0.15	1.84	0.02	0.00	0.32	24.08	0.80	24.00	10.48	0.21	0.27	0.00	0.00		
0.34	0.00	0.02	0.02	0.62	1.42	0.01	0.00	58.40	30.90	12.19	23.53	9.92	0.49	0.16	0.00	0.00		
0.01	0.06	0.01	0.03	0.16	1.21	0.03	0.06	97.79	28.71	12.43	39.71	10.01	0.25	0.22	0.00	0.00		
0.55	0.03	0.01	0.01	0.17	1.87	0.02	0.00	97.24	24.75	1.10	27.50	11.88	0.30	0.29	0.00	0.00		
0.03	0.03	0.01	0.01	0.17	1.87	0.02	0.00	97.24	24.75	1.10	27.50	11.88	0.30	0.29	0.00	0.00		
	0.43	0.03	0.12	0.95	8.79	0.05	0.04	756.09	51.03	12.19	62.37	0.00	0.29	0.20	0.00	0.00		
0.22	0.00	0.28	0.38	3.16	102.60	0.06	0.00	1029.00	87.60	21.60	67.80	21.00	2.60	0.52	0.00	0.00		
0.06	0.00	0.05	0.03	0.58	24.90	0.03	0.00	86.70	43.80	10.80	33.90	10.50	0.50	0.26	0.00	0.00		
0.07	0.28	0.12	0.09	1.85	15.31	0.08	0.00	57.55	121.90	7.94	35.44	8.50	0.77	0.18	0.00	0.00		
.01	0.00	0.01	0.01	0.73	1.89	0.01	0.00	10.44	26.91	0.99	34.20	13.59	0.10	0.23	0.00	0.00		
0.01	0.00	0.01	0.02	0.59	1.80	0.01	0.00	0.36	26.46	1.89	33.30	12.33	0.18	0.23	0.00	0.00		
0.11	0.00	0.01	0.02	0.70	1.89	0.02	0.00	2.34	26.10	0.99	32.40	11.79	0.14	0.27	0.00	0.00		
0.00	0.00	0.47	0.51	6.03	40.33	0.33	0.00	129.87	14.43	1.11	15.54	4.81	0.47	0.19	0.00	0.00		
	0.60	0.30	0.03	3.00	60.00	0.30	0.90	280.00		0.00			4.50		0.00	0.00		
1.59	0.09	0.09	0.04	0.87	10.77	0.02	0.00	117.09	92.99	15.31	74.28	33.45	0.69	0.76	0.00	0.00		
1.34	0.52	0.18	0.08	1.76	26.62	0.11	0.00	85.88	256.88	29.25	129.38	59.25	1.15	1.21	0.00	0.00		
3.88	0.47	0.15	0.08	1.60	23.56	0.10	0.00	43.86	234.90	39.51	140.29	58.36	1.23	1.14	2.18	0.00		
	1.20							480.00		20.00			1.44		0.00	0.00		
0.00	0.00	0.00	0.05	1.87	4.80	0.02	0.17	782.40	129.60	14.40	31.20	4.80	0.41	0.00	0.00	0.00	0.00	0.00
0.05	0.00	0.01	0.07	3.35	4.88	0.02	0.24	775.92	209.84	9.76	73.20	2.44	0.51	0.24	0.00	0.00	0.00	0.00
1.62	1.52	0.13	1.14	2.48	45.54	0.33	1.14	1006.94	690.69	68.31	197.34	45.54	5.19	3.57	0.00	0.00		
0.29	3.11	0.12	0.22	2.16	57.72	0.28	1.44	941.28	608.28	84.36	215.34	64.38	5.79	2.31	0.00	0.00		
	12.00							390.00		40.00			5.40		0.00	0.00		
	9.00							390.00		40.00			3.60		0.00	0.00		
	1.24							778.05	802.75	96.33		81.51	3.46	1.73	0.00	0.00		
	2.47							824.98	785.46	91.39		64.22	3.95	2.72	0.00	0.00		
1.46	4.35	0.12	0.27	0.92	58.88	0.34	0.00	1336.32	934.40	120.32	394.24	115.20	8.78	5.12	0.00	0.00		
1.21	0.76	0.11	0.20	3.48		0.23	1.44	1171.39	511.06	88.55	166.98	45.54	4.83	3.87	0.00	0.00		
	2.96							862.03	778.05	103.74		69.16	4.45	2.72	0.00	0.00		
	12.00							320.00		40.00			3.60		0.00	0.00		
1.61	12.24	0.06	0.06	1.85	9.60	0.26	7.92	1000.80	384.00	67.20	84.00	19.20	2.64	1.68	0.00	0.00		
0.45	3.47	0.07	0.24	1.03	9.92	0.13	10.24	992.00	300.08	186.00	156.24	22.32	1.49	0.79	0.00	0.00		
0.24	1.95	0.02	0.04	0.96	4.88	0.08	8.00	915.00	146.40	43.92	53.68	7.32	1.49	0.76	0.00	0.00		
								496.69					1.48		0.00	0.00		
	0.00	0.05	0.15	2.26	17.57	0.10	0.40	1940.23	316.26	10.04	72.79	17.57	1.76	2.76	0.00	0.00		

Food Name	Amount	Measure	Weight (g)	Calories	Protein (g)	Total Carb (g)	Dietary Fiber (g)	Total Fat (g)	Sat Fat (g)	Mono Fat (g)	Poly Fat (g)	Chol (mg)	Vit A (mcg RAE)	Vit D (mcg)
Soup, beef noodle, cond, cmrcl, can	1	Cup	251.00	168.17	9.66	17.97	1.51	6.17	2.28	2.48	0.98	10.04	27.61	
Soup, beef, w/country veg, chunky, rts, cnd	8	Ounce-weight	226.80	142.88	11.56	14.97		4.08	1.22	1.01	1.16	22.68	204.12	
Soup, black bean, cond, cnd, cmrcl	0.5	Cup	128.50	116.93	6.21	19.81	8.74	1.70	0.44	0.62	0.53	0.00	28.27	
Soup, broccoli cheese, cond, cmrcl, can	4	Ounce-weight	113.40	98.66	2.38	8.73	2.04	6.01	1.81	2.27	1.93	4.54	74.84	
Soup, chicken gumbo, cond, cmrcl, can	0.5	Cup	125.50	56.47	2.64	8.37	2.01	1.43	0.33	0.65	0.35	3.76	6.27	
Soup, chicken mushroom, prep f/cnd w/water, cmrcl	1	Cup	244.00	131.76	4.39	9.27	0.24	9.15	2.39	4.03	2.32	9.76	56.12	
Soup, chicken noodle, chunky, rts, can	8	Ounce-weight	226.80	106.60	7.26	12.93		2.95	0.73	1.13	0.59	22.68	122.47	
Soup, chicken rice, chunky, rts, cnd	1	Cup	240.00	127.20	12.26	12.98	0.96	3.19	0.96	1.44	0.67	12.00	292.80	
Soup, chicken vegetable, cond, cnd, cmrcl	0.5	Cup	123.00	75.03	3.62	8.62	0.86	2.85	0.85	1.28	0.60	8.61	134.07	
Soup, crab, rts, can	1	Cup	244.00	75.64	5.49	10.30	0.73	1.51	0.39	0.68	0.39	9.76	24.40	
Soup, cream of asparagus, cond, cnd, cmrcl	0.5	Cup	125.50	86.59	2.28	10.69	0.50	4.09	1.03	0.94	1.83	5.02	32.63	
Soup, cream of asparagus, prep f/cnd w/water, cmrcl	1	Cup	244.00	85.40	2.29	10.69	0.49	4.10	1.05	0.95	1.85	4.88	36.60	
Soup, cream of celery, prep f/cnd w/milk, cmrcl	1	Cup	248.00	163.68	5.68	14.53	0.74	9.70	3.94	2.46	2.65	32.24	114.08	
Soup, cream of celery, prep f/cnd w/water, cmrcl	1	Cup	244.00	90.28	1.66	8.83	0.73	5.59	1.42	1.29	2.51	14.64	56.12	
Soup, cream of chicken, prep f/cnd w/milk, cmrcl	1	Cup	248.00	190.96	7.46	14.98	0.25	11.46	4.64	4.46	1.64	27.28	178.56	
Soup, cream of mushroom, prep f/cnd w/water, cmrcl	1	Cup	244.00	129.32	2.32	9.30	0.49	8.98	2.44	1.71	4.22	2.44	14.64	
Soup, cream of onion, cond, cnd, cmrcl	0.5	Cup	125.50	110.44	2.76	13.05	0.50	5.27	1.47	2.10	1.46	15.06	35.14	
Soup, cream of potato, prep w/milk	1	Cup	248.00	148.80	5.78	17.16	0.50	6.45	3.77	1.74	0.57	22.32	52.08	
Soup, cream of shrimp, prep f/cnd w/milk, cmrcl	1	Cup	248.00	163.68	6.82	13.91	0.25	9.30	5.78	2.68	0.35	34.72	62.00	
Soup, lentil, rts, cnd Progresso Healthy Classics	1	Cup	242.00	125.84	7.79	20.30	5.57	1.50	0.27	0.82	0.24	0.00		
Soup, minestrone, chunky, rts, can	1	Cup	240.00	127.20	5.11	20.74	5.76	2.81	1.49	0.91	0.26	4.80	213.60	
Soup, onion, cond, cnd, cmrcl	0.5	Cup	123.00	56.58	3.76	8.22	0.86	1.75	0.26	0.75	0.65	0.00	3.69	
Soup, split pea, w/ham, chunky, rducd fat & sod, rts, cnd	8	Ounce-weight	226.80	172.37	11.80	25.63		2.49	0.68	0.91	0.45	13.61	297.11	
Soup, tomato rice, prep f/cnd w/water, cmrcl	1	Cup	247.00	118.56	2.10	21.93	1.48	2.72	0.52	0.59	1.36	2.47	34.58	
Soup, tomato, prep f/cnd w/milk, cmrcl	1	Cup	248.00	161.20	6.10	22.30	2.73	6.00	2.90	1.61	1.12	17.36	64.48	
Soup, tomato, prep f/cnd w/water, cmrcl	1	Cup	244.00	85.40	2.05	16.59	0.49	1.93	0.37	0.44	0.95	0.00	24.40	
Soup, turkey noodle, cond, cnd, cmrcl	0.5	Cup	125.50	69.02	3.90	8.63	0.75	2.00	0.55	0.80	0.49	5.02	16.31	
Soup, turkey vegetable, cond, cnd, cmrcl	0.5	Cup	123.00	73.80	3.10	8.67	0.62	3.04	0.90	1.33	0.68	1.23	130.38	
Soup, vegetable beef, prep f/cnd w/water, cmrcl	1	Cup	244.00	78.08	5.59	10.17	0.49	1.90	0.85	0.81	0.12	4.88	95.16	
Soup, vegetable, vegetarian, cond, cnd, cmrcl	0.5	Cup	123.00	72.57	2.12	12.03	0.62	1.94	0.30	0.84	0.73	0.00	174.66	
Soup, won ton	1	Cup	241.00	181.69	14.08	14.28	0.90	7.03	2.26	3.01	0.98	52.95	56.01	
Stew, beef, cnd Chef-Mate	1	Cup	252.00	191.52	15.02	18.93	3.28	6.15	2.27	2.50	0.32	32.76	154.98	
Stew, beef, hearty, family size, ckd f/fzn Banquet	1	Cup	245.70	170.00	10.00	18.00	4.00	7.00	3.00			30.00		

Dry and Prepared Soups and Chilis

Food Name	Amount	Measure	Weight (g)	Calories	Protein (g)	Total Carb (g)	Dietary Fiber (g)	Total Fat (g)	Sat Fat (g)	Mono Fat (g)	Poly Fat (g)	Chol (mg)	Vit A (mcg RAE)	Vit D (mcg)
Soup, beefy mushroom, dry mix Lipton Recipe Secrets	1.5	Tablespoon	11.00	32.78	0.85	6.62	0.11	0.38	0.05			0.22		
Soup, beefy onion, dry mix Lipton Recipe Secrets	1	Tablespoon	8.00	25.12	0.52	4.68	0.35	0.63	0.14			0.00	0.00	
Soup, broccoli cheese & rice, dry mix Uncle Ben's Inc.	1	Ounce-weight	28.35	101.90	4.20	16.74	0.70	2.00	1.10			4.20		

Vit E (mg)	Vit C	Vit B₁-Thia (mg)	Vit B₂-Ribo (mg)	Vit B₃-Nia (mg)	Fol (mcg)	Vit B₆ (mg)	Vita B₁₂ (mcg)	Sodi (mg)	Pota (mg)	Cal (mg)	Phos (mg)	Magn (mg)	Iron (mg)	Zinc (mg)	Caff (mg)	Alco (g)	Sol Fiber (g)	Insol Fiber (g)
2.51	0.75	0.14	0.12	2.13	37.65	0.08	0.40	1905.09	198.29	30.12	92.87	12.55	2.21	3.09	0.00	0.00		
								809.68					2.02		0.00	0.00		
0.46	0.26	0.05	0.05	0.53	25.70	0.09	0.00	1246.45	321.25	44.97	96.37	42.40	1.93	1.41	0.00	0.00		
0.82	2.27	0.02	0.04	0.28	45.36	0.07	0.02	774.52	234.74	46.49	47.63	14.74	0.34	0.29	0.00	0.00		
0.45	5.02	0.25	0.38	0.67	6.27	0.06	0.03	955.05	75.30	23.84	25.10	3.76	0.89	0.38	0.00	0.00		
1.22	0.00	0.02	0.11	1.63	0.00	0.05	0.05	941.84	153.72	29.28	26.84	9.76	0.88	0.98	0.00	0.00		
								816.48					1.11		0.00	0.00		
0.58	3.84	0.02	0.10	4.10	4.80	0.05	0.31	888.00	108.00	33.60	72.00	9.60	1.87	0.96	0.00	0.00		
0.31	0.98	0.04	0.06	1.23	4.92	0.05	0.12	948.33	154.98	17.22	40.59	6.15	0.87	0.37	0.00	0.00		
0.24	0.00	0.20	0.07	1.34	14.64	0.12	0.20	1234.64	326.96	65.88	87.84	14.64	1.22	1.46	0.00	0.00		
0.61	2.76	0.05	0.08	0.78	23.84	0.01	0.05	981.41	173.19	28.86	38.90	3.76	0.80	0.88	0.00	0.00		
0.66	2.68	0.05	0.08	0.78	21.96	0.01	0.05	980.88	173.24	29.28	39.04	4.88	0.81	0.88	0.00	0.00		
0.97	1.49	0.07	0.25	0.44	7.44	0.06	0.50	1009.36	310.00	186.00	151.28	22.32	0.69	0.20	0.00	0.00		
0.90	0.24	0.03	0.05	0.33	2.44	0.01	0.24	949.16	122.00	39.04	36.60	7.32	0.63	0.15	0.00	0.00		
0.25	1.24	0.07	0.26	0.92	7.44	0.07	0.55	1046.56	272.80	181.04	151.28	17.36	0.67	0.67	0.00	0.00		
0.95	0.98	0.05	0.09	0.72	4.88	0.01	0.05	880.84	100.04	46.36	48.80	4.88	0.51	0.59	0.00	0.00		
0.54	1.25	0.05	0.08	0.50	7.53	0.03	0.05	953.80	122.99	33.88	37.65	6.27	0.63	0.15	0.00	0.00		
0.10	1.24	0.08	0.24	0.64	9.92	0.09	0.50	1061.44	322.40	166.16	161.20	17.36	0.55	0.67	0.00	0.00		
0.99	1.24	0.06	0.23	0.53	9.92	0.45	1.04	1036.64	248.00	163.68	146.32	22.32	0.60	0.79	0.00	0.00		
0.58	0.97	0.11	0.09	0.70	101.64	0.16	0.00	442.86	336.38	41.14	128.26	41.14	2.66	1.04	0.00	0.00		
1.61	4.80	0.06	0.12	1.18	52.80	0.24	0.00	864.00	612.00	60.00	110.40	14.40	1.78	1.44	0.00	0.00		
0.27	1.23	0.03	0.02	0.60	14.76	0.05	0.00	1057.80	68.88	27.06	11.07	2.46	0.68	0.62	0.00	0.00		
	9.53							777.92					2.09		0.00	0.00		
2.45	14.82	0.06	0.05	1.05	14.82	0.08	0.00	815.10	330.98	22.23	34.58	4.94	0.79	0.52	0.00	0.00		
1.24	67.70	0.13	0.25	1.52	17.36	0.16	0.45	744.00	448.88	158.72	148.80	22.32	1.81	0.30	0.00	0.00		
2.32	66.37	0.09	0.05	1.42	14.64	0.11	0.00	695.40	263.52	12.20	34.16	7.32	1.76	0.24	0.00	0.00		
0.18	0.13	0.07	0.06	1.40	18.82	0.04	0.16	815.75	75.30	11.29	47.69	5.02	0.94	0.58	0.00	Alco		
0.42	0.00	0.03	0.04	1.01	4.92	0.05	0.17	908.97	175.89	17.22	40.59	3.69	0.76	0.62	0.00	0.00		
0.37	2.44	0.04	0.05	1.03	9.76	0.08	0.32	790.56	173.24	17.08	41.48	4.88	1.12	1.54	0.00	0.00		
1.44	1.48	0.05	0.05	0.92	11.07	0.06	0.00	826.56	210.33	20.91	34.44	7.38	1.08	0.47	0.00	0.00		
0.39	3.36	0.41	0.26	4.60	18.85	0.20	0.40	542.88	316.10	31.07	152.50	20.62	1.76	1.12	0.00	0.00		
0.56	2.52	0.18	0.25	3.10		0.30	0.55	1186.92	388.08	63.00	158.76	35.28	1.59	2.49	0.00	0.00		
	3.60							1120.00		20.00			1.44		0.00	0.00		
	0.16	0.00	0.01	0.08	0.00			645.15		10.78			0.10		0.00	0.00		
	0.66	0.01	0.02	0.12	0.00			606.56		11.20			0.12		0.00	0.00		
	9.00							605.10		89.30			0.18		0.00	0.00		

Food Name	Amount	Measure	Weight (g)	Calories	Protein (g)	Total Carb (g)	Dietary Fiber (g)	Total Fat (g)	Sat Fat (g)	Mono Fat (g)	Poly Fat (g)	Chol (mg)	Vit A (mcg RAE)	Vit D (mcg)
SOUPS, STEWS AND CHILIS *(continued)*														
Soup, chicken, supreme, hearty, in a cup, dry Lipton Cup-A-Soup	1	Each	100.00	429.00	5.02	64.87	3.10	17.86	6.62			3.00		
Soup, cream of vegetable, dehyd, svg, makes 1 cup prep	1	Each	23.60	105.26	1.89	12.30	0.71	5.69	1.42	2.53	1.48	0.47	141.60	
Soup, noodle, giggle, dry mix, svg Lipton Soup Secrets	1	Each	19.00	73.53	2.52	11.46	0.42	2.13	0.69			17.86		
Soup, noodle, ring shape, dry mix, svg Lipton Soup Secrets	1	Each	17.00	65.96	2.20	9.91	0.36	1.98	0.64			15.64		
Soup, onion mushroom, dry mix Lipton Recipe Secrets	1	Ounce-weight	28.35	91.29	2.38	16.30	0.91	2.24	0.31			0.00	0.00	
Soup, ramen noodle, chicken flvr, dry, Cup Of Noodles Nissin Foods	1	Each	64.00	296.32	5.57	36.80		14.08	6.25				19.84	
Soup, tomato vegetable, prep f/dry pkt w/water	1	Cup	253.00	55.66	2.00	10.22	0.51	0.86	0.38	0.30	0.08	0.00	10.12	
Homemade/Generic Soups and Chilis														
Soup, cheese, cond, cnd, cmrcl	0.5	Cup	218.50	264.38	9.22	17.90	1.75	17.81	11.34	5.05	0.50	50.25	159.50	
Soup, cheese, prep w/water, cmrcl, can	1	Cup	247.00	155.61	5.41	10.52	0.99	10.47	6.67	2.96	0.30	29.64	296.40	
Stew, chicken, w/potatoes veg gravy	1	Cup	252.00	290.68	24.36	15.14	1.97	14.31	4.03	5.73	3.12	87.42	384.25	
SPICES, FLAVORS, AND SEASONINGS														
Basil, fresh, leaves	1	Each	0.50	0.14	0.01	0.02	0.02	0.00	0.00	0.00	0.00	0.00	1.32	0.00
Cilantro, leaves, fresh	0.25	Cup	4.00	0.92	0.09	0.15	0.11	0.02	0.00	0.01	0.00	0.00	13.48	
Cream of Tartar	1	Teaspoon	3.00	7.74	0.00	1.84	0.01	0.00	0.00	0.00	0.00	0.00	0.00	
Curry, pwd	1	Teaspoon	2.00	6.48	0.24	1.16	0.68	0.28	0.04	0.12	0.04	0.00	0.96	0.00
Flavor, vanilla extract	1	Teaspoon	4.33	12.47	0.00	0.52	0.00	0.00	0.00	0.00	0.00	0.00	0.00	
Garlic Salt McCormick & Co., Inc.	0.25	Teaspoon	0.90	0.00	0.00	0.00	0.00	0.00	0.00	0.00	0.00	0.00		
Ginger Root, fresh, slices, 2"	5	Piece	11.00	8.80	0.20	1.95	0.22	0.08	0.02	0.02	0.02	0.00	0.00	
Marjoram, dried	1	Teaspoon	0.60	1.63	0.08	0.36	0.24	0.04	0.00	0.01	0.03	0.00	2.42	0.00
Salt Substitute Morton International Incorporated	0.25	Teaspoon	1.20	0.10	0.00	0.02		0.00	0.00	0.00	0.00			
Salt, table	0.25	Teaspoon	1.50	0.00	0.00	0.00	0.00	0.00	0.00	0.00	0.00	0.00	0.00	
Tenderizer, unseasoned McCormick & Co., Inc.	0.25	Teaspoon	1.10	0.00	0.00	0.00	0.00	0.00	0.00	0.00	0.00	0.00		
SPORTS BARS AND DRINKS														
Bar, energy, apple cinnamon Power Bar	1	Each	65.00	230.00	10.00	45.00	3.00	2.50	0.50	1.50	0.50	0.00	0.00	
Bar, energy, apricot Clif Bar Inc	1	Each	68.00	221.78	8.55	43.15	5.35	2.29	0.35			0.04		
Bar, energy, caramel nut blast Balance Bar Co Gold	1	Each	50.00	200.00	15.00	23.00	1.00	7.00	4.00			0.00		2.00
Bar, energy, choc dipped strawberry Experimental & Applied Sciences Myoplex Carb Sense	1	Each	70.00	250.00	30.00	23.00	2.00	6.00	4.00			5.00		
Bar, energy, chocolate Balance Bar Co	1	Each	50.00	200.00	14.00	22.00	1.00	6.00	3.50			3.00		2.00
Bar, energy, chocolate Power Bar	1	Each	65.00	240.00	7.00	45.00	4.00	4.00	1.00			0.00	0.00	
Bar, energy, chocolate Power Bar	1	Each	65.00	230.00	10.00	45.00	3.00	2.00	0.50	0.50	1.00	0.00	0.00	
Bar, energy, chocolate almond fudge Clif Bar Inc	1	Each	68.00	230.80	10.43	38.43	5.23	4.80	0.93			0.07		
Bar, energy, chocolate celebration Balance Bar Co Oasis	1	Each	48.00	180.00	9.00	26.00	0.75	3.50	2.50			0.00	109.41	
Bar, energy, chocolate chip peanut crunch Clif Bar Inc	1	Each	68.00	241.40	11.82	38.64	5.36	5.43	1.06			0.05		
Bar, energy, chocolate crisp, uncoated Balance Bar Co Outdoor	1	Each	50.00	200.00	14.00	22.00	0.75	6.00	3.00			3.00		

Vit E (mg)	Vit C	Vit B1-Thia (mg)	Vit B2-Ribo (mg)	Vit B3-Nia (mg)	Fol (mcg)	Vit B6 (mg)	Vita B12 (mcg)	Sodi (mg)	Pota (mg)	Cal (mg)	Phos (mg)	Magn (mg)	Iron (mg)	Zinc (mg)	Caff (mg)	Alco (g)	Sol Fiber (g)	Insol Fiber (g)
	0.60	0.27	0.25	2.83	0.00			3023.00		109.00			0.89		0.00	0.00		
0.57	3.92	1.22	0.11	0.52	7.08	0.02	0.12	1169.85	96.29	31.62	53.81	11.33	0.61	0.38	0.00	0.00		
	0.06	0.26	0.10	1.29	25.27			736.06		3.61			0.65		0.00	0.00		
	0.07	0.23	0.09	1.12	21.76			724.03		3.40			0.56		0.00	0.00		
	1.47	0.60	0.06	0.85	0.00			1773.86		28.63			0.34		0.00	0.00		
								1433.60					2.18		0.00	0.00		
0.35	6.07	0.06	0.05	0.79	10.12	0.05	0.00	1146.09	103.73	7.59	30.36	20.24	0.63	0.18	0.00	0.00		
1.22	0.00	0.03	0.23	0.68	6.55	0.04	0.00	1632.19	262.20	242.53	231.61	6.55	1.27	1.09	0.00	0.00		
	0.00	0.02	0.14	0.40	4.94	0.02	0.00	958.36	153.14	140.79	135.85	4.94	0.74	0.64	0.00	0.00		
0.46	12.21	0.14	0.20	9.02	18.05	0.45	0.24	112.64	631.89	32.36	220.79	42.02	1.86	1.91	0.00	0.00		
0.00	0.09	0.00	0.00	0.00	0.32	0.00	0.00	0.02	2.31	0.77	0.35	0.41	0.02	0.00	0.00	0.00		
0.10	1.08	0.00	0.01	0.04	2.48	0.01	0.00	1.84	20.84	2.68	1.92	1.04	0.07	0.02	0.00	0.00		
0.00	0.00	0.00	0.00	0.00	0.00	0.00	0.00	1.56	495.00	0.24	0.15	0.06	0.11	0.01	0.00	0.00		
0.44	0.24	0.00	0.00	0.08	3.08	0.04	0.00	1.04	30.84	9.56	6.96	5.08	0.60	0.08	0.00	0.00		
0.00	0.00	0.00	0.00	0.00	0.00	0.00	0.00	0.35	6.41	0.43	0.26	0.52	0.00	0.00	0.00	1.47	0.00	0.00
								242.00							0.00	0.00	0.00	0.00
0.03	0.55	0.00	0.00	0.08	1.21	0.02	0.00	1.43	45.65	1.76	3.74	4.73	0.07	0.04	0.00	0.00		
0.01	0.31	0.00	0.00	0.02	1.64	0.01	0.00	0.46	9.13	11.94	1.84	2.08	0.50	0.02	0.00	0.00		
							0.00	0.12	603.60	6.60	5.40	0.01			0.00	0.00		
0.00	0.00	0.00	0.00	0.00	0.00	0.00	0.00	581.37	0.12	0.36	0.00	0.02	0.00	0.00	0.00	0.00	0.00	0.00
								400.00							0.00	0.00	0.00	0.00
18.35	60.00	1.50	1.70	20.00	400.00	2.00	6.00	90.00	110.00	300.00	350.00	140.00	6.30	5.25	0.00	0.00		
20.32	67.10	0.40	0.28	3.49	82.60	0.42	0.98	70.83	274.61	273.99	287.20	109.39	4.94	3.19	0.00	0.00		
13.64	60.00	0.60	0.51	9.00	80.00	6.00	1.20	90.00	160.00	100.00	100.00	40.00	3.60	3.00		0.00		
4.77	18.00	0.45	0.51	6.00	120.00	0.60	2.40	190.00	70.00	300.00	300.00	40.00	6.30	5.25		0.00		
13.64	60.00	0.60	0.51	9.00	80.00	0.60	1.20	230.00	180.00	100.00	100.00	40.00	3.60	3.00		0.00		
18.34	60.00	0.75	0.85	10.00	200.00	1.00	3.00	80.00		150.00	150.00	60.00	2.70	2.25		0.00		
18.35	60.00	1.50	1.70	20.00	400.00	2.00	6.00	90.00	145.00	300.00	350.00	140.00	6.30	5.25	15.00	0.00		
20.76	65.67	0.39	0.31	3.63	84.62	0.43	0.98	139.30	231.80	278.00	304.10	128.30	5.74	3.71	0.01	0.00		
4.77	6.00	0.53	0.60	7.00	140.00	0.70	2.10	230.00	300.00	350.00	250.00	140.00	6.30	5.25		0.00		
20.34	65.88	0.40	0.30	6.09	94.58	0.41	0.98	274.24	304.60	265.12	297.40	111.09	5.37	3.51		0.00		
	120.00							160.00	160.00	100.00			3.60			0.00		

SPORTS BARS AND DRINKS *(continued)*

Food Name	Amount	Measure	Weight (g)	Calories	Protein (g)	Total Carb (g)	Dietary Fiber (g)	Total Fat (g)	Sat Fat (g)	Mono Fat (g)	Poly Fat (g)	Chol (mg)	Vit A (mcg RAE)	Vit D (mcg)
Bar, energy, chocolate fudge Experimental & Applied Sciences Myoplex Lite	1	Each	56.00	190.00	15.00	27.00	1.00	4.00	3.00			10.00		5.00
Bar, energy, chocolate fudge brownie Power Bar	1	Each	78.00	290.00	24.00	38.00	4.00	5.00	4.00			5.00	0.00	
Bar, energy, chocolate peanut butter Balance Bar Co Gold	1	Each	50.00	210.00	15.00	22.00	0.75	7.00	4.00			0.00	131.26	
Bar, energy, chocolate peanut butter Power Bar	1	Each	78.00	290.00	24.00	38.00	3.00	5.00	3.50			5.00	0.00	
Bar, energy, chocolate peanut crisp Balance Bar Co Oasis	1	Each	48.00	190.00	9.00	25.00	0.75	5.00	2.50			0.00	109.41	
Bar, energy, chocolate raspberry fudge Balance Bar Co	1	Each	50.00	200.00	14.00	22.00	1.00	6.00	3.50			3.00		2.00
Bar, energy, chocolate raspberry truffle Power Bar	1	Each	53.00	180.00	10.00	28.00	3.00	4.00	3.00			0.00	0.00	
Bar, energy, cookies & cream Clif Bar Inc	1	Each	68.00	224.80	10.42	39.25	5.26	3.73	1.45			0.06		
Bar, energy, cranberry apple cherry Clif Bar Inc	1	Each	68.00	220.20	8.19	43.94	5.06	1.94	0.30			0.04		
Bar, energy, fresh wild berry Experimental & Applied Sciences Results for Women	1	Each	55.00	190.00	11.00	28.00	4.00	6.00	2.00			0.00		
Bar, energy, honey nut, plus ginseng Balance Bar Co	1	Each	50.00	200.00	14.00	22.00	0.75	6.00	3.50			3.00		2.00
Bar, energy, honey peanut Balance Bar Co	1	Each	50.00	200.00	14.00	22.00	1.00	6.00	3.50			3.00		2.00
Bar, energy, mocha Power Bar	1	Each	65.00	230.00	10.00	45.00	3.00	2.50	1.00	1.00	0.50	0.00	0.00	
Bar, energy, nutz over chocolate Clif Bar Inc Luna Bar	1	Each	48.00	173.48	9.63	25.25	1.69	4.38	2.74			0.03		
Bar, energy, oatmeal raisin Balance Bar Co Oasis	1	Each	48.00	180.00	8.00	29.00	0.75	3.00	2.00			0.00	109.41	
Bar, energy, oatmeal raisin Power Bar	1	Each	65.00	230.00	10.00	45.00	3.00	2.50	0.50	1.00	1.00	0.00	0.00	
Bar, energy, peanut butter Clif Bar Inc	1	Each	68.00	239.63	12.28	38.26	4.96	5.11	0.77			0.05		
Bar, energy, peanut butter honey, Tiger's Milk Weider Nutrition Company	1	Each	35.00	150.00	6.00	18.00	1.00	6.00	1.00			0.00		1.50
Bar, energy, peanut caramel crisp Experimental & Applied Sciences Myoplex Lite	1	Each	54.00	180.00	15.00	26.00	1.00	4.50	3.00			5.00		
Bar, energy, rocky road Balance Bar Co Gold	1	Each	50.00	210.00	15.00	22.00	1.00	7.00	4.00			0.00	131.26	
Bar, energy, s'mores Clif Bar Inc Luna Bar	1	Each	48.00	178.03	9.86	26.32	2.08	4.33	3.01			0.03		
Bar, energy, tstd nuts & cranberries Clif Bar Inc Luna Bar	1	Each	48.00	167.23	9.86	25.53	1.35	3.33	0.50			0.03		
Bar, energy, yogurt honey peanut Balance Bar Co	1	Each	50.00	200.00	14.00	22.00	1.00	6.00	3.00			3.00		2.00
Carbohydrate Gel, chocolate, pkt Power Bar	1	Each	41.00	120.00	0.00	28.00	0.00	1.50	1.00			0.00	0.00	
Drink, Anabolic Activator III, chocolate, pwd, scoop Optimum Nutrition	2	Each	57.00	180.00	26.00	15.00	1.00	1.50	1.00			15.00		5.00
Drink, carbohydrate, Carbo Pump, pwd, scoop Optimum Nutrition	2.5	Each	85.05	320.00	0.00	80.00		0.00	0.00	0.00	0.00			
Drink, creatine, HP, lemon lime, pwd, scoop Experimental & Applied Sciences Phosphagen	1	Each	43.00	140.00	0.00	34.00	0.00	0.00	0.00	0.00	0.00		0.00	
Drink, energy, w/caff & vit B complex	1	Cup	240.00	103.20	0.94	26.33	0.00	0.00	0.00	0.00	0.00	0.00	0.00	

Vit E (mg)	Vit C	Vit B₁- Thia (mg)	Vit B₂- Ribo (mg)	Vit B₃- Nia (mg)	Fol (mcg)	Vit B₆ (mg)	Vita B₁₂ (mcg)	Sodi (mg)	Pota (mg)	Cal (mg)	Phos (mg)	Magn (mg)	Iron (mg)	Zinc (mg)	Caff (mg)	Alco (g)	Sol Fiber (g)	Insol Fiber (g)
6.82	30.00	0.75	0.85	10.00	200.00	1.00	3.00	150.00	150.00	300.00	250.00	160.00	7.20	5.25		0.00		
18.34	60.00	1.50	1.70	20.00	400.00	2.00	6.00	150.00		300.00	350.00	140.00	6.30	5.25		0.00		
13.64	60.00	0.38	0.43	5.00	100.00	0.50	1.50	125.00	125.00	100.00	150.00	40.00	4.50	3.75		0.00		
18.34	60.00	1.50	1.70	20.00	400.00	2.00	6.00	290.00		300.00	350.00	140.00	6.30	5.25		0.00		
4.77	6.00	0.53	0.60	7.00	140.00	0.70	2.10	270.00	290.00	350.00	250.00	140.00	6.30	5.25		0.00		
13.64	60.00	0.60	0.51	9.00	80.00	0.60	1.20	150.00	190.00	100.00	100.00	40.00	3.60	3.00		0.00		
18.34	60.00	0.75	0.85	10.00	200.00	1.00	6.00	100.00		500.00	150.00	100.00	4.50	3.75		0.00		
20.26	66.15	0.35	0.27	3.45	85.13	0.43	0.98	179.00	211.90	278.60	266.50	102.60	5.23	3.21	0.00	0.00		
20.32	66.77	0.36	0.27	3.46	82.02	0.40	0.98	132.10	234.70	267.40	272.20	99.11	4.71	3.06	0.00	0.00		
4.09	21.00	0.45	0.51	5.00	120.00	0.50	1.50	150.00	170.00	300.00	250.00	40.00	6.30	5.25	0.00	0.00		
13.64	60.00	0.60	0.51	9.00	80.00	0.60	1.20	220.00	125.00	100.00	100.00	40.00	3.60	3.00		0.00		
13.64	60.00	0.60	0.51	9.00	80.00	0.60	1.20	220.00	115.00	100.00	100.00	40.00	3.60	3.00		0.00		
18.35	60.00	1.50	1.70	20.00	400.00	2.00	6.00	90.00	145.00	300.00	350.00	140.00	6.30	5.25	20.00	0.00		
18.10	58.91	1.72	1.69	20.79	416.10	2.41	5.88	213.13	153.73	446.20	422.12	17.01	7.96	5.46		0.00		
4.77	60.00	0.53	0.60	7.00	140.00	0.70	2.10	220.00	250.00	350.00	250.00	140.00	6.30	5.25	0.00	0.00		
18.35	60.00	1.50	1.70	20.00	400.00	2.00	6.00	120.00	180.00	300.00	350.00	140.00	6.30	5.25	0.00	0.00		
20.36	65.83	0.40	0.30	6.25	96.24	0.42	0.98	289.03	300.58	268.34	305.03	113.70	5.31	3.57	0.00	0.00		
	6.00	1.28	0.60	3.00		0.60	1.50	70.00		300.00	100.00	100.00	2.70		0.00	0.00		
6.82	30.00	0.75	0.85	10.00	200.00	1.00	3.00	240.00	200.00	250.00	250.00	100.00	5.40	3.75	0.00	0.00		
13.64	60.00	0.38	0.43	5.00	100.00	0.50	1.50	80.00	140.00	100.00	150.00	40.00	4.50	3.75		0.00		
13.76	45.03	1.32	1.28	15.14	321.58	1.84	4.48	183.03	125.88	346.53	343.24	11.27	6.75	4.27	0.00	0.00		
18.35	58.72	1.70	1.68	19.67	412.78	2.39	5.82	189.06	142.95	447.89	436.10	23.63	7.54	5.61	0.00	0.00		
13.64	60.00	0.60	0.51	9.00	80.00	0.60	1.20	220.00	130.00	100.00	100.00	40.00	3.60	3.00	0.00	0.00		
2.77	9.00							50.00	40.00	0.00			0.00		25.00	0.00	0.00	0.00
9.24	30.00	0.75	0.85		200.00	1.00	3.00	240.00	490.00	250.00	250.00	100.00	4.50	3.75		0.00		
															0.00	0.00		
	0.00							95.00	80.00	0.00	200.00	60.00	0.00		0.00	0.00	0.00	0.00
0.00	0.00	0.00	0.01	18.81	0.00	4.70	4.70	187.20	273.60	196.80	24.00	26.40	0.36	0.05	74.40	0.00	0.00	0.00

Food Name	Amount	Measure	Weight (g)	Calories	Protein (g)	Total Carb (g)	Dietary Fiber (g)	Total Fat (g)	Sat Fat (g)	Mono Fat (g)	Poly Fat (g)	Chol (mg)	Vit A (mcg RAE)	Vit D (mcg)
SPORTS BARS AND DRINKS (continued)														
Drink, protein, muscle building mix, natural, choc pwd scoop Optimum Nutrition Pro-Complex	2	Each	70.00	270.00	54.00	7.00		2.50	1.50			75.00		5.00
Drink, protein, Simply Protein, whey, chocolate, pwd, scoop Experimental & Applied Sciences Simply Protein	2	Each	28.35	115.00	20.00	4.00	1.00	2.00	1.00			45.00	0.00	0.00
Drink, protein, whey, 100%, natural, vanilla, pwd, scoop Optimum Nutrition	1	Each	31.40	120.00	22.00	5.00	0.75	1.50	0.50			15.00		
Drink, protein, whey, Precision Protein, choc, pwd, scoop Experimental & Applied Sciences	1	Each	25.50	100.00	20.00	2.50		1.00	0.50			15.00	0.00	0.00
Drink, thermogenic, straw kiwi, rtd Experimental & Applied Sciences Results for Women	1	Each	236.00	0.00	0.00	0.00	0.00	0.00	0.00	0.00	0.00	0.00	0.00	
Drink, weight gain, Mighty One 3000, chocolate, pwd, scoop Optimum Nutrition	1	Each	56.00	210.00	5.25	46.25		0.50	0.25			8.75		1.25
Sports Drink, fruit flvr, low cal	1	Cup	240.00	26.40	0.00	7.20	0.00	0.00	0.00	0.00	0.00	0.00	0.00	
Sports Drink, tropical punch, btld Thirst Quencher	1	Cup	240.90	60.22	0.00	15.18	0.00	0.00	0.00	0.00	0.00	0.00	0.00	0.00
Supplement Drink, chocolate, prep w/2% milk Balance Bar Co Total Balance	1	Cup	290.00	280.00	22.00	33.00	1.00	10.40	4.00			24.00		5.00
SUPPLEMENTAL FOODS AND FORMULAS														
Protein, whey, isolate, vanilla, pwd, svg Visical, LLC	1	Ounce-weight	28.35	101.25	24.30	0.00	0.00	0.00	0.00	0.00	0.00	5.06		
Medical Nutritionals														
Bar, supplement, chocolate crunch Mead Johnson	1	Each	44.00	190.00	4.00	29.00	1.00	7.00	3.50			5.00		1.50
Custard, supplement, vanilla, rts Hormel HealthLabs	1	Each	118.00	140.00	7.00	22.00	2.00	3.50	2.00			2.50		
Fiber, supplement, Opti-Fiber, pwd Optimum Nutrition	1	Teaspoon	5.60	15.00	0.00	4.00	4.00	0.00	0.00	0.00	0.00			
Formula, chocolate, rtu	1	Cup	259.79	366.30	13.41	51.65	0.00	11.74	1.56	2.97	7.21	5.20	387.09	2.58
Formula, light, chocolate supreme, rtu Ross Laboratories	1	Cup	253.87	200.00	10.00	33.00	0.00	3.00	0.31	1.90	0.57	5.00		2.50
Supplement Drink, Hi Protein, vanilla, rtu Mead Johnson	1	Cup	255.50	240.00	15.00	33.00	0.00	6.00	0.50			10.00		3.75
Supplement Drink, vanilla, rtu Mead Johnson	1	Cup	255.50	240.00	10.00	41.00	0.00	4.00	0.50			5.00		2.50
Soy Nutritionals														
Bar, soy milk, vegetarian Galaxy Nutritional Foods	1	Each	41.00	140.00	7.00	23.00		2.00	1.50			0.00		
Bar, soy, cafe mocha Genisoy Products	1	Each	61.50	220.00	14.00	34.00	1.00	3.50	2.50			0.00		2.50
Bar, soy, cookies n cream Genisoy Products	1	Each	61.50	220.00	14.00	33.00	2.00	4.00	3.00			0.00		2.50
Bar, soy, hi prot, chocolate peanut butter Max Muscle	1	Each	56.70	234.00	19.00	20.20	0.00	8.00	3.00			3.00		
Drink, soy, Opti-Soy 50, natural, chocolate, pwd, scoop Optimum Nutrition	1	Each	35.00	130.00	14.00	16.00	1.00	1.00						
SWEETENERS AND SWEET SUBSTITUTES														
Jams and Jellies														
Fruit Butter, apple	1	Tablespoon	18.00	31.14	0.07	7.70	0.27	0.00	0.00	0.00	0.00	0.00	0.18	
Fruit Spread, strawberry, All-Fruit, Polaner's B&G Foods, Inc.	1	Tablespoon	18.00	41.58	0.13	10.26		0.00	0.00	0.00	0.00			

Vit E (mg)	Vit C	Vit B₁-Thia (mg)	Vit B₂-Ribo (mg)	Vit B₃-Nia (mg)	Fol (mcg)	Vit B₆ (mg)	Vita B₁₂ (mcg)	Sodi (mg)	Pota (mg)	Cal (mg)	Phos (mg)	Magn (mg)	Iron (mg)	Zinc (mg)	Caff (mg)	Alco (g)	Sol Fiber (g)	Insol Fiber (g)
10.07	30.00	0.85		10.00	200.00	1.00	7.50	420.00	200.00	243.00			0.64			0.00		
								60.00	200.00	160.00			0.40			0.00		
								75.00	200.00	138.00			0.80			0.00		
		0.00				1.00		50.00	80.00	50.00		100.00					0.00	
	0.00							10.00	33.00	0.00			0.00		206.00	0.00	0.00	0.00
1.69	7.50	0.19	0.21	2.50	50.00	0.25	0.75	205.00	417.50	125.00		25.50	1.38	0.92	0.00	0.00		
0.00	15.12	0.00	0.00	0.00	0.00	0.00	0.00	84.00	24.00	0.00	21.60	2.40	0.12	0.05	0.00	0.00	0.00	0.00
0.00	0.00	0.01	0.00	0.00	0.00	0.00	0.00	96.36	26.50	0.00	21.68	2.41	0.12	0.05	0.00	0.00	0.00	0.00
13.64	60.00	0.45	0.77	5.00	100.00	0.60	2.40	408.00	840.00	700.00	400.00	160.00	2.70	5.25		0.00		
								40.50	263.25	111.38	53.66				0.00	0.00	0.00	0.00
2.05	9.00	0.23	0.23	3.00	60.00	0.30	0.90	90.00	105.00	150.00	150.00	60.00	1.08	2.30		0.00		
	2.40							260.00		250.00			0.00			0.00	0.00	
	100.00														0.00	0.00		
3.48	30.92	0.39	0.44	5.15	103.92	0.51	1.56	246.80	454.63	205.23	205.23	103.92	4.65	3.92	0.00	0.00	0.00	0.00
3.41	30.00	0.38	0.43	5.00	100.00	0.50	1.50	200.00	370.00	250.00	250.00	100.00	4.50	3.80		0.00	0.00	0.00
13.64	60.00	0.38	0.43	5.00	140.00	0.70	2.10	170.00	380.00	330.00	310.00	105.00	4.50	4.50	0.00	0.00	0.00	0.00
13.64	60.00	0.38	0.43	5.00	140.00	0.70	2.10	130.00	400.00	300.00	250.00	100.00	3.60	4.50	0.00	0.00	0.00	0.00
								140.00	25.00	400.00	250.00				0.00	0.00		
13.64	15.00	0.38	0.43	5.00	100.00	0.50	1.50	150.00	250.00	250.00	250.00	100.00	4.50	3.75		0.00		
3.41	15.00	0.38	0.43	5.00	100.00	0.50	1.50	160.00	260.00	250.00	250.00	100.00	4.50	3.75		0.00		
								162.00								0.00	0.00	0.00
40.27	60.00				200.00						310.00		5.00			0.00		
0.00	0.18	0.00	0.00	0.01	0.18	0.01	0.00	2.70	16.38	2.52	1.26	0.90	0.06	0.01	0.00	0.00		
								3.60								0.00	0.00	

Food Name	Amount	Measure	Weight (g)	Calories	Protein (g)	Total Carb (g)	Dietary Fiber (g)	Total Fat (g)	Sat Fat (g)	Mono Fat (g)	Poly Fat (g)	Chol (mg)	Vit A (mcg RAE)	Vit D (mcg)
SWEETENERS AND SWEET SUBSTITUTES *(continued)*														
Jam	1	Tablespoon	20.00	55.60	0.07	13.77	0.22	0.01	0.00	0.01	0.00	0.00	0.00	
Jam, concord grape The J.M. Smucker Co.	1	Tablespoon	20.00	50.00	0.00	13.00	0.00	0.00	0.00	0.00	0.00	0.00	0.00	
Jam, rducd sug	1	Tablespoon	20.00	36.30	0.21	8.89	0.50	0.14	0.01	0.01	0.05	0.00	0.21	
Jam, strawberry The J.M. Smucker Co.	1	Tablespoon	20.00	50.00	0.00	13.00	0.00	0.00	0.00	0.00	0.00	0.00	0.00	
Jam/Preserves, any flvr, w/sod sacc, dietetic	1	Tablespoon	14.00	18.48	0.04	7.50	0.35	0.04	0.00	0.01	0.02	0.00	0.00	
Jelly	1	Tablespoon	19.00	50.54	0.03	13.29	0.19	0.00	0.00	0.00	0.00	0.00	0.05	
Jelly, rducd sug, prep f/recipe	1	Tablespoon	19.00	34.01	0.06	8.76	0.15	0.01	0.00	0.00	0.00	0.00	0.03	
Marmalade, orange	1	Tablespoon	20.00	49.20	0.06	13.26	0.14	0.00	0.00	0.00	0.00	0.00	0.60	
Preserves, strawberry The J.M. Smucker Co.	1	Tablespoon	20.00	50.00	0.00	13.00	0.00	0.00	0.00	0.00	0.00	0.00	0.00	
Sugars, Sugar Substitutes, and Syrups														
Honey, amber light Pure Sweet Honey Farm Incorporated	1	Tablespoon	21.00	63.84	0.15	17.01	0.00	0.00	0.00	0.00	0.00	0.00	0.00	0.00
Honey, strained/extracted	1	Tablespoon	21.19	64.41	0.06	17.46	0.04	0.00	0.00	0.00	0.00	0.00	0.00	
Molasses	1	Tablespoon	20.50	59.45	0.00	15.32	0.00	0.02	0.00	0.01	0.01	0.00	0.00	
Molasses, blackstrap	1	Tablespoon	20.50	48.17	0.00	12.46	0.00	0.00	0.00	0.00	0.00	0.00	0.00	
Sugar Substitute, Sweet 'N Low, granular Brooklyn Premium Corp.	1	Teaspoon	4.00	0.00	0.00	4.00	0.00	0.00	0.00	0.00	0.00	0.00	0.00	
Sugar, brown, packed	1	Teaspoon	4.60	17.34	0.00	4.47	0.00	0.00	0.00	0.00	0.00	0.00	0.00	
Sugar, confectioners/powdered, unsftd	1	Teaspoon	2.50	9.72	0.00	2.49	0.00	0.00	0.00	0.00	0.00	0.00	0.00	
Sugar, white, granulated, cubed	1	Each	2.50	9.68	0.00	2.50	0.00	0.00	0.00	0.00	0.00	0.00	0.00	
Syrup, corn, dark	2	Tablespoon	41.00	117.26	0.00	31.82	0.00	0.00	0.00	0.00	0.00	0.00	0.00	0.00
Syrup, maple	2	Tablespoon	40.00	104.40	0.00	26.84	0.00	0.08	0.01	0.03	0.04	0.00	0.00	
Syrup, pancake, w/2% maple	2	Tablespoon	39.40	104.41	0.00	27.42	0.00	0.04	0.01	0.01	0.03	0.00	0.00	
VEGETABLES AND LEGUMES														
Vegetables														
Raw Vegetables														
Alfalfa Sprouts, fresh	0.5	Cup	16.50	4.79	0.66	0.62	0.41	0.11	0.01	0.01	0.07	0.00	1.32	
Artichokes, Calif, fresh	1	Each	340.00	85.00	6.80	20.40	10.20	0.00	0.00	0.00	0.00	0.00	0.00	
Arugula, chpd, fresh, cup	1	Cup	20.00	5.00	0.52	0.73	0.32	0.13	0.02	0.01	0.06	0.00	23.80	0.00
Asparagus, fresh, cup	0.5	Cup	67.00	13.40	1.47	2.60	1.39	0.08	0.02	0.00	0.05	0.00	25.46	
Asparagus, spears, tips, fresh, 2" long or less	10	Each	35.00	7.00	0.80	1.40	0.70	0.00	0.00	0.00	0.00	0.00	13.30	
Bean Sprouts, navy, mature, fresh	0.5	Cup	52.00	34.84	3.20	6.78	1.99	0.37	0.04	0.02	0.21	0.00	0.10	
Broccoli, bunch, fresh, each	1	Each	608.00	206.72	17.15	40.37	15.81	2.25	0.24	0.07	0.23	0.00	200.64	
Broccoli, florets, fresh	0.5	Cup	35.50	9.94	1.06	1.86	1.03	0.13	0.02	0.01	0.06	0.00	53.25	
Cabbage, fresh harvest, fresh, shredded	0.5	Cup	35.00	8.40	0.42	1.88	0.81	0.06	0.01	0.00	0.03	0.00	2.10	0.00
Cabbage, pickled, Japanese, fresh	0.5	Cup	75.00	22.50	1.20	4.25	2.33	0.08	0.01	0.01	0.04	0.00	6.75	
Cabbage, red, fresh, shredded	0.5	Cup	35.00	10.85	0.50	2.58	0.74	0.06	0.01	0.00	0.04	0.00	19.60	
Cactus, nopales, slices, fresh	0.5	Cup	43.00	6.88	0.57	1.43	0.94	0.04	0.00	0.01	0.02	0.00	9.89	
Carrots, baby, fresh, med	1	Each	10.00	3.50	0.06	0.82	0.18	0.01	0.00	0.00	0.01	0.00	69.00	
Carrots, fresh, chpd	0.5	Cup	64.00	26.24	0.59	6.13	1.79	0.15	0.02	0.01	0.08	0.00	385.28	
Carrots, fresh, med	1	Each	61.00	25.01	0.57	5.84	1.71	0.15	0.02	0.01	0.07	0.00	367.22	
Cauliflower, green, fresh	0.5	Cup	32.00	9.92	0.94	1.95	1.01	0.10	0.02	0.01	0.04	0.00	2.56	
Celery, stalk, sml, 5" long, fresh	1	Each	17.00	2.38	0.12	0.50	0.25	0.03	0.01	0.01	0.01	0.00	3.74	
Chili Peppers, green, hot, fresh, whole	0.5	Cup	75.00	30.00	1.50	7.10	1.12	0.15	0.02	0.00	0.08	0.00	44.25	
Cornsalad, fresh	0.5	Cup	28.00	5.88	0.56	1.01	0.42	0.11				0.00	99.40	
Cucumber, w/skin, fresh, slices	0.5	Cup	52.00	7.80	0.34	1.89	0.26	0.06	0.02	0.00	0.03	0.00	2.60	
Dish, falafel, prep f/recipe, patty, 2 1/4"	1	Each	17.00	56.61	2.26	5.41		3.03	0.41	1.73	0.71	0.00	0.17	
Endive, fresh, chpd	0.5	Cup	25.00	4.25	0.31	0.84	0.78	0.05	0.01	0.00	0.02	0.00	27.00	
Fennel, bulb, fresh, slices	0.5	Cup	43.50	13.48	0.54	3.17	1.35	0.08				0.00	3.04	
Leeks, bulb & lower leaf, fresh, chpd	0.5	Cup	44.50	27.14	0.67	6.30	0.80	0.14	0.02	0.00	0.07	0.00	36.93	
Lemon Grass, fresh	0.5	Cup	33.50	33.17	0.60	8.49		0.16	0.04	0.02	0.07	0.00	0.11	
Lettuce, butterhead, fresh, leaf, med	2	Piece	15.00	1.95	0.20	0.34	0.17	0.03	0.00	0.00	0.02	0.00	24.90	

Vit E (mg)	Vit C	Vit B₁-Thia (mg)	Vit B₂-Ribo (mg)	Vit B₃-Nia (mg)	Fol (mcg)	Vit B₆ (mg)	Vita B₁₂ (mcg)	Sodi (mg)	Pota (mg)	Cal (mg)	Phos (mg)	Magn (mg)	Iron (mg)	Zinc (mg)	Caff (mg)	Alco (g)	Sol Fiber (g)	Insol Fiber (g)
0.02	1.76	0.00	0.02	0.01	2.20	0.00	0.00	6.40	15.40	4.00	3.80	0.80	0.10	0.01	0.00	0.00		
	0.00							0.00		0.00			0.00		0.00	0.00	0.00	0.00
0.03	7.62	0.00	0.02	0.06	1.73	0.03	0.00	4.81	102.33	5.98	8.15	5.00	0.24	0.05	0.00	0.00		
	0.00							0.00		0.00			0.00		0.00	0.00	0.00	0.00
0.01	0.00	0.00	0.00	0.00	1.26	0.00	0.00	0.00	9.66	1.26	1.26	0.70	0.06	0.01	0.00	0.00		
0.00	0.17	0.00	0.00	0.01	0.38	0.00	0.00	5.70	10.26	1.33	1.14	1.14	0.04	0.01	0.00	0.00		
0.00	0.00	0.00	0.00	0.03	0.19	0.01	0.00	0.38	13.49	0.95	1.14	1.14	0.03	0.01	0.00	0.00		
0.01	0.96	0.00	0.01	0.01	1.80	0.00	0.00	11.20	7.40	7.60	0.80	0.40	0.03	0.01	0.00	0.00		
	0.00							0.00		0.00			0.00		0.00	0.00	0.00	0.00
0.00	0.10	0.00	0.06	0.06	2.10	0.00	0.00	0.60	10.50	1.01	1.05	0.42	0.05	0.03	0.00	0.00	0.00	0.00
0.00	0.11	0.00	0.01	0.03	0.42	0.01	0.00	0.85	11.02	1.27	0.85	0.42	0.09	0.05	0.00	0.00		
0.00	0.00	0.01	0.00	0.19	0.00	0.14	0.00	7.58	300.12	42.02	6.35	49.61	0.97	0.06	0.00	0.00	0.00	0.00
0.00	0.00	0.01	0.01	0.22	0.20	0.14	0.00	11.27	510.86	176.30	8.20	44.07	3.59	0.20	0.00	0.00	0.00	0.00
	0.00							0.00		0.00			0.00		0.00	0.00	0.00	0.00
0.00	0.00	0.00	0.00	0.00	0.05	0.00	0.00	1.79	15.92	3.91	1.01	1.33	0.09	0.01	0.00	0.00	0.00	0.00
0.00	0.00	0.00	0.00	0.00	0.00	0.00	0.00	0.02	0.05	0.02	0.00	0.00	0.00	0.00	0.00	0.00	0.00	0.00
0.00	0.00	0.00	0.00	0.00	0.00	0.00	0.00	0.00	0.05	0.03	0.00	0.00	0.00	0.00	0.00	0.00	0.00	0.00
0.00	0.00	0.00	0.00	0.01	0.00	0.00	0.00	63.55	18.04	7.38	4.51	3.28	0.15	0.01	0.00	0.00	0.00	0.00
0.00	0.00	0.00	0.00	0.01	0.00	0.00	0.00	3.60	81.60	26.80	0.80	5.60	0.48	1.67	0.00	0.00	0.00	0.00
0.00	0.00	0.00	0.01	0.00	0.00	0.00	0.00	24.03	2.36	1.97	3.94	0.79	0.03	0.09	0.00	0.00		
0.00	1.35	0.01	0.02	0.08	5.94	0.01	0.00	0.99	13.04	5.28	11.55	4.46	0.16	0.15	0.00	0.00	0.08	0.33
1.36	20.40	0.12	0.12	2.72	136.00	0.12		255.00	578.00	68.00	204.00	136.00	2.44		0.00	0.00		
0.09	3.00	0.01	0.02	0.06	19.40	0.01	0.00	5.40	73.80	32.00	10.40	9.40	0.29	0.09	0.00	0.00		
0.76	3.75	0.09	0.09	0.65	34.84	0.06	0.00	1.34	135.34	16.08	34.84	9.38	1.43	0.36	0.00	0.00		
0.40	2.00	0.10	0.00	0.30	18.20	0.00	0.00	0.70	70.70	8.40	18.20	4.90	0.70	0.20	0.00	0.00		
0.02	9.78	0.20	0.11	0.64	68.64	0.10	0.00	6.76	159.64	7.80	52.00	52.52	1.00	0.46	0.00	0.00		
4.74	542.34	0.43	0.71	3.89	383.04	1.06	0.00	200.64	1921.28	285.76	401.28	127.68	4.44	2.49	0.00	0.00	1.46	14.35
0.16	33.09	0.03	0.04	0.23	25.21	0.06	0.00	9.59	115.38	17.04	23.43	8.88	0.31	0.14	0.00	Alco	0.11	0.91
0.04	17.85	0.02	0.01	0.11	19.95	0.03	0.00	6.30	86.10	16.45	8.05	5.25	0.20	0.06	0.00	Alco	0.27	0.53
0.09	0.53	0.00	0.03	0.13	31.50	0.08	0.00	207.75	639.75	36.00	32.25	9.00	0.37	0.15	0.00	0.00		
0.04	19.95	0.02	0.02	0.15	6.30	0.07	0.00	9.45	85.05	15.75	10.50	5.60	0.28	0.08	0.00	0.00	0.04	0.70
0.00	4.00	0.00	0.02	0.18	1.29	0.03	0.00	9.03	110.51	70.52	6.88	22.36	0.26	0.11	0.00	0.00		
0.04	0.84	0.00	0.00	0.06	3.30	0.01	0.00	7.80	23.70	3.20	2.80	1.00	0.09	0.02	0.00	0.00	0.05	0.13
0.42	3.78	0.05	0.04	0.63	12.16	0.09	0.00	44.16	204.80	21.12	22.40	7.68	0.20	0.15	0.00	0.00	0.75	1.04
0.40	3.60	0.04	0.04	0.60	11.59	0.08	0.00	42.09	195.20	20.13	21.35	7.32	0.18	0.15	0.00	0.00	0.72	0.99
0.01	28.19	0.03	0.03	0.23	18.24	0.07	0.00	7.36	96.00	10.56	19.84	6.40	0.23	0.20	0.00	0.00		
0.05	0.53	0.00	0.01	0.05	6.12	0.01	0.00	13.60	44.20	6.80	4.08	1.87	0.03	0.02	0.00	0.00		
0.52	181.88	0.08	0.08	0.72	17.25	0.20	0.00	5.25	255.00	13.50	34.50	18.75	0.90	0.22	0.00	0.00	0.35	0.80
0.03	10.70	0.02	0.02	0.12	3.92	0.08	0.00	1.12	128.52	10.64	14.84	3.64	0.61	0.17	0.00	0.00		
0.02	1.46	0.01	0.02	0.05	3.64	0.02	0.00	1.04	76.44	8.32	12.48	6.76	0.15	0.10	0.00	0.00	0.03	0.23
0.19	0.27	0.02	0.03	0.18	15.81	0.02	0.00	49.98	99.45	9.18	32.64	13.94	0.58	0.26	0.00	0.00		
0.11	1.62	0.02	0.02	0.10	35.50	0.00	0.00	5.50	78.50	13.00	7.00	3.75	0.21	0.20	0.00	0.00	0.33	0.44
	5.22	0.00	0.02	0.28	11.74	0.02	0.00	22.62	180.09	21.32	21.75	7.40	0.32	0.08	0.00	0.00		
0.41	5.34	0.03	0.02	0.18	28.48	0.10	0.00	8.90	80.10	26.25	15.57	12.46	0.94	0.05	0.00	0.00	0.37	0.43
	0.87	0.02	0.04	0.38	25.13	0.02	0.00	2.01	242.21	21.78	33.84	20.10	2.75	0.74	0.00	0.00		
0.03	0.56	0.01	0.01	0.05	10.95	0.01	0.00	0.75	35.70	5.25	4.95	1.95	0.19	0.03	0.00	0.00		

VEGETABLES AND LEGUMES (continued)

Food Name	Amount	Measure	Weight (g)	Calories	Protein (g)	Total Carb (g)	Dietary Fiber (g)	Total Fat (g)	Sat Fat (g)	Mono Fat (g)	Poly Fat (g)	Chol (mg)	Vit A (mcg RAE)	Vit D (mcg)
Lettuce, iceberg, fresh, leaf, med	2	Piece	16.00	2.24	0.14	0.47	0.19	0.02	0.00	0.00	0.01	0.00	4.00	
Lettuce, looseleaf, fresh, leaf	2	Piece	20.00	3.00	0.27	0.56	0.26	0.03	0.00	0.00	0.02	0.00	74.00	
Lettuce, romaine, fresh, inner leaf	2	Piece	20.00	3.40	0.25	0.66	0.42	0.06	0.01	0.00	0.03	0.00	58.00	
Lettuce, romaine, fresh, leaf Dole Food Company, Inc.	2	Piece	28.33	6.67	0.33	1.00	0.33	0.17	0.00			0.00	16.66	
Mushrooms, crimini, fresh	2	Each	28.00	6.16	0.70	1.15	0.17	0.03	0.00	0.00	0.01	0.00	0.00	
Mushrooms, enoki, lrg, fresh	6	Each	30.00	10.20	0.71	2.11	0.78	0.12	0.01	0.00	0.05	0.00	0.11	0.57
Mushrooms, fresh, pces/slices	0.5	Cup	35.00	7.70	1.09	1.13	0.42	0.12	0.02	0.00	0.05	0.00	0.00	0.67
Mushrooms, oyster, fresh, lrg	1	Each	148.00	54.76	6.13	9.21	3.55	0.75				0.00	2.96	
Mustard Greens, fresh, chpd	1	Cup	56.00	14.56	1.52	2.75	1.85	0.11	0.01	0.05	0.02	0.00	294.00	
Onion, pearl, fresh, chpd	0.5	Cup	80.00	33.60	0.73	8.08	1.12	0.07	0.02	0.01	0.04	0.00	0.08	
Onion, scallions, tops & bulb, fresh, chpd	0.5	Cup	50.00	16.00	0.92	3.67	1.30	0.09	0.02	0.01	0.04	0.00	25.00	
Onion, white, fresh, chpd	0.5	Cup	80.00	33.60	0.73	8.08	1.12	0.07	0.02	0.01	0.04	0.00	0.08	
Onion, yellow, fresh, chpd	0.5	Cup	80.00	33.60	0.73	8.08	1.12	0.07	0.02	0.01	0.04	0.00	0.08	
Parsnips, fresh, slices	0.5	Cup	66.50	49.88	0.80	11.96	3.26	0.20	0.04	0.08	0.03	0.00	0.00	
Peppers, bell, green, sweet, fresh, chpd	0.5	Cup	74.50	14.90	0.64	3.46	1.27	0.13	0.04	0.01	0.05	0.00	13.41	
Peppers, bell, red, sweet, fresh, chpd	0.5	Cup	74.50	19.37	0.74	4.49	1.47	0.22	0.04	0.01	0.12	0.00	116.97	
Peppers, bell, yellow, sweet, fresh, lrg, 3 3/4" long	1	Each	186.00	50.22	1.86	11.76	1.67	0.39	0.06	0.05	0.21	0.00	18.60	0.00
Radicchio, fresh, leaf	2	Each	16.00	3.68	0.23	0.72	0.14	0.04	0.01	0.00	0.02	0.00	0.16	
Radish Sprouts, fresh	0.5	Cup	19.00	8.17	0.72	0.68	0.50	0.48	0.14	0.08	0.22	0.00	3.80	
Radishes, fresh, med, 3/4" to 1"	10	Each	45.00	7.20	0.31	1.53	0.69	0.04	0.01	0.01	0.02	0.00	0.16	
Seaweed, nori, fresh, sheets, Porphyra tenera, for sushi	1	Each	2.60	0.91	0.15	0.13	0.01	0.01	0.00	0.00	0.00	0.00	6.76	
Shallots, chpd, fresh	1	Tablespoon	10.00	7.20	0.25	1.68	0.07	0.01	0.00	0.00	0.00	0.00	6.00	
Soybean Sprouts, mature, fresh	1	Cup	70.00	85.40	9.16	6.70	0.77	4.69	0.65	1.06	2.65	0.00	0.70	
Spinach, fresh, chpd	1	Cup	30.00	6.90	0.86	1.09	0.66	0.12	0.02	0.00	0.05	0.00	140.70	
Squash, summer, all types, fresh, sml	1	Each	118.00	18.88	1.43	3.95	1.30	0.21	0.05	0.02	0.11	0.00	11.80	
Tomatillo, fresh, chpd/diced	0.5	Cup	66.00	21.12	0.63	3.85	1.25	0.67	0.09	0.10	0.28	0.00	3.96	
Tomatoes, red, June-Oct, fresh, chpd	0.5	Cup	90.00	18.90	0.76	4.18	0.99	0.30	0.04	0.04	0.12	0.00	27.90	
Tomatoes, red, stwd f/fresh	0.5	Cup	50.50	39.89	0.99	6.59	0.86	1.35	0.26	0.53	0.44	0.00	16.66	
Tomatoes, roma, fresh, year round avg, fresh	1	Each	62.00	11.16	0.55	2.43	0.74	0.12	0.02	0.03	0.07	0.00	26.04	
Turnips, ckd, drained, cubes	0.5	Cup	78.00	17.16	0.55	3.95	1.56	0.06	0.01	0.00	0.04	0.00	0.00	
Vegetables, stir fry, Oriental, fresh, rtu Frieda's Specialty Produce	3	Ounce-weight	85.05	15.01	1.00	3.00	1.00	0.00	0.00	0.00	0.00	0.00	75.04	

Cooked Vegetables

Food Name	Amount	Measure	Weight (g)	Calories	Protein (g)	Total Carb (g)	Dietary Fiber (g)	Total Fat (g)	Sat Fat (g)	Mono Fat (g)	Poly Fat (g)	Chol (mg)	Vit A (mcg RAE)	Vit D (mcg)
Asparagus, ckd, drained	0.5	Cup	90.00	19.80	2.16	3.70	1.80	0.20	0.06	0.01	0.13	0.00	45.00	
Asparagus, spears, ckd f/fzn, drained	4	Each	60.00	10.80	1.77	1.15	0.96	0.25	0.06	0.01	0.11	0.00	24.00	
Bean Sprouts, mung, mature, stir fried	0.5	Cup	62.00	31.00	2.67	6.56	1.18	0.13	0.02	0.04	0.04	0.00	1.24	
Beets, ckd, drained, sliced	0.5	Cup	85.00	37.40	1.43	8.47	1.70	0.15	0.03	0.03	0.05	0.00	1.70	
Broccoli, chpd, ckd f/fzn w/o salt, drained	0.5	Cup	92.00	25.76	2.86	4.92	2.76	0.11	0.02	0.01	0.05	0.00	51.52	
Broccoli, spears, ckd f/fzn, drained	0.5	Cup	92.00	25.76	2.86	4.92	2.76	0.10	0.02	0.01	0.05	0.00	51.52	
Brussels Sprouts, ckd, drained	0.5	Cup	78.00	28.08	1.99	5.54	2.03	0.39	0.08	0.03	0.20	0.00	30.42	
Cabbage, napa/nappa	0.5	Cup	54.50	6.54	0.60	1.22		0.09				0.00	7.08	
Carrots, ckd f/fzn w/o salt, drained, slices	0.5	Cup	73.00	27.01	0.42	5.64	2.41	0.50	0.09	0.03	0.24	0.00	606.63	
Cauliflower, ckd f/fzn w/o salt, drained, 1" pces	0.5	Cup	90.00	17.10	1.45	3.38	2.44	0.20	0.03	0.01	0.10	0.00	0.46	
Cauliflower, ckd, drained, 1" pces	0.5	Cup	62.00	14.26	1.14	2.55	1.68	0.28	0.04	0.02	0.13	0.00	0.62	
Cauliflower, green, ckd, head	0.2	Each	90.00	28.80	2.73	5.65	2.98	0.28	0.04	0.02	0.13	0.00	6.30	
Celeriac, ckd, drained, pces	0.5	Cup	77.50	20.92	0.75	4.58	0.93	0.15	0.04	0.03	0.08	0.00	0.00	
Collards, chpd, ckd, drained	0.5	Cup	80.00	20.80	1.68	3.92	2.24	0.29	0.04	0.02	0.14	0.00	324.80	
Corn, white, sweet, cob, kernels, ckd f/fzn, drained	0.5	Cup	82.00	77.08	2.55	18.31	1.72	0.61	0.09	0.18	0.29	0.00	0.16	
Corn, yellow sweet kernels ckd f/fzn w/salt drained, pkg	3	Ounce-weight	85.05	68.89	2.17	16.42	2.04	0.57	0.06	0.11	0.17	0.00	8.51	0.00

Vit E (mg)	Vit C	Vit B₁- Thia (mg)	Vit B₂- Ribo (mg)	Vit B₃- Nia (mg)	Fol (mcg)	Vit B₆ (mg)	Vita B₁₂ (mcg)	Sodi (mg)	Pota (mg)	Cal (mg)	Phos (mg)	Magn (mg)	Iron (mg)	Zinc (mg)	Caff (mg)	Alco (g)	Sol Fiber (g)	Insol Fiber (g)
0.03	0.45	0.01	0.00	0.02	4.64	0.01	0.00	1.60	22.56	2.88	3.20	1.12	0.07	0.02	0.00	0.00		
0.06	3.60	0.01	0.02	0.08	7.60	0.02	0.00	5.60	38.80	7.20	5.80	2.60	0.17	0.04	0.00	0.00		
0.03	4.80	0.01	0.01	0.06	27.20	0.01	0.00	1.60	49.40	6.60	6.00	2.80	0.19	0.05	0.00	0.00		
	0.80				13.33			0.00		6.67			0.12		0.00	0.00		
0.03	0.00	0.03	0.14	1.06	3.92	0.03	0.03	1.68	125.44	5.04	33.60	2.52	0.11	0.31	0.00	0.00		
0.02	3.57	0.02	0.03	1.09	9.00	0.01	0.00	0.90	114.30	0.30	33.90	4.80	0.27	0.17	0.00	0.00		
0.00	0.84	0.03	0.14	1.35	5.60	0.04	0.01	1.40	109.90	1.05	29.75	3.15	0.18	0.18	0.00	0.00	0.07	0.35
	0.00	0.08	0.53	5.30	69.56	0.18	0.00	45.88	763.68	8.88	208.68	29.60	2.58	1.15	0.00	0.00		
1.13	39.20	0.05	0.06	0.45	104.72	0.10	0.00	14.00	198.24	57.68	24.08	17.92	0.82	0.11	0.00	0.00	0.88	0.96
0.02	5.12	0.04	0.02	0.07	15.20	0.11	0.00	2.40	115.20	17.60	21.60	8.00	0.15	0.13	0.00	0.00	0.07	1.05
0.28	9.40	0.03	0.04	0.26	32.00	0.03	0.00	8.00	138.00	36.00	18.50	10.00	0.74	0.19	0.00	0.00	0.40	0.90
0.02	5.12	0.04	0.02	0.07	15.20	0.11	0.00	2.40	115.20	17.60	21.60	8.00	0.15	0.13	0.00	0.00	0.07	1.05
0.02	5.12	0.04	0.02	0.07	15.20	0.11	0.00	2.40	115.20	17.60	21.60	8.00	0.15	0.13	0.00	0.00	0.07	1.05
0.99	11.30	0.06	0.04	0.46	44.56	0.06	0.00	6.65	249.38	23.94	47.22	19.28	0.39	0.39	0.00	0.00	1.00	2.26
0.28	59.90	0.04	0.02	0.36	8.20	0.17	0.00	2.24	130.38	7.45	14.90	7.45	0.25	0.10	0.00	0.00	0.15	1.12
1.18	141.55	0.04	0.06	0.73	13.41	0.22	0.00	1.49	157.20	5.22	19.37	8.94	0.32	0.19	0.00	0.00		
1.28	341.31	0.05	0.05	1.66	48.36	0.31	0.00	3.72	394.32	20.46	44.64	22.32	0.86	0.32	0.00	0.00	0.50	1.17
0.36	1.28	0.00	0.00	0.04	9.60	0.01	0.00	3.52	48.32	3.04	6.40	2.08	0.09	0.10	0.00	0.00		
	5.49	0.02	0.02	0.54	18.05	0.06	0.00	1.14	16.34	9.69	21.47	8.36	0.16	0.10	0.00	0.00		
0.00	6.66	0.01	0.02	0.11	11.25	0.03	0.00	17.55	104.85	11.25	9.00	4.50	0.15	0.13	0.00	0.00		
0.03	1.01	0.00	0.01	0.04	3.80	0.00	0.00	1.25	9.26	1.82	1.51	0.05	0.05	0.03	0.00	0.00		
0.01	0.80	0.01	0.00	0.02	3.40	0.03	0.00	1.20	33.40	3.70	6.00	2.10	0.12	0.04	0.00	0.00	0.03	0.04
0.01	10.71	0.24	0.08	0.80	120.40	0.12	0.00	9.80	338.80	46.90	114.80	50.40	1.47	0.82	0.00	0.00		
0.61	8.43	0.02	0.06	0.22	58.20	0.06	0.00	23.70	167.40	29.70	14.70	23.70	0.81	0.16	0.00	0.00		
0.14	20.06	0.06	0.17	0.57	34.22	0.26	0.00	2.36	309.16	17.70	44.84	20.06	0.41	0.34	0.00	0.00		
0.25	7.72	0.03	0.02	1.22	4.62	0.04	0.00	0.66	176.88	4.62	25.74	13.20	0.41	0.15	0.00	0.00		
0.31	23.40	0.05	0.04	0.57	13.50	0.07	0.00	8.10	199.80	4.50	21.60	9.90	0.40	0.08	0.00	0.00	0.23	0.76
0.64	9.19	0.05	0.04	0.56	5.55	0.04	0.00	229.77	124.73	13.13	19.19	7.57	0.54	0.09	0.00	0.00	0.20	0.66
0.33	7.87	0.02	0.01	0.37	9.30	0.05	0.00	3.10	146.94	6.20	14.88	6.82	0.17	0.11	0.00	0.00		
0.02	9.05	0.02	0.02	0.23	7.02	0.06	0.00	12.48	138.06	25.74	20.28	7.02	0.14	0.09	0.00	0.00	0.71	0.85
	21.01							35.02		60.04			0.00		0.00	0.00		
1.36	6.94	0.15	0.13	0.97	134.10	0.07	0.00	12.60	201.60	20.70	48.60	12.60	0.82	0.54	0.00	0.00	0.29	1.51
0.72	14.64	0.04	0.06	0.62	81.00	0.01	0.00	1.80	103.20	10.80	29.40	6.00	0.34	0.25	0.00	Alco	0.16	0.80
0.01	9.92	0.09	0.11	0.74	43.40	0.08	0.00	5.58	135.78	8.06	48.98	20.46	1.18	0.56	0.00	0.00	0.23	0.94
0.03	3.06	0.03	0.03	0.28	68.00	0.06	0.00	65.45	259.25	13.60	32.30	19.55	0.67	0.29	0.00	0.00	0.56	1.14
1.21	36.90	0.05	0.08	0.42	51.52	0.12	0.00	10.12	130.64	30.36	45.08	11.96	0.56	0.26	0.00	0.00	1.46	1.30
1.21	36.90	0.05	0.08	0.42	27.60	0.12	0.00	22.08	165.60	46.92	50.60	18.40	0.56	0.28	0.00	0.00	1.35	1.41
0.34	48.36	0.08	0.06	0.48	46.80	0.14	0.00	16.38	247.26	28.08	43.68	15.60	0.94	0.26	0.00	0.00	0.94	1.09
	1.74	0.00	0.01	0.26	23.43	0.02	0.00	5.99	47.41	15.80	10.35	4.36	0.40	2.05	0.00	0.00		
0.74	1.68	0.03	0.03	0.30	8.03	0.06	0.00	43.07	140.16	25.55	22.63	8.03	0.39	0.26	0.00	0.00		
0.05	28.18	0.03	0.05	0.28	36.90	0.07	0.00	16.20	125.10	15.30	21.60	8.10	0.37	0.12	0.00	0.00	0.94	1.48
0.04	27.47	0.03	0.03	0.26	27.28	0.11	0.00	9.30	88.04	9.92	19.84	5.58	0.20	0.11	0.00	0.00	0.53	1.14
0.03	65.34	0.06	0.10	0.61	36.90	0.19	0.00	20.70	250.20	28.80	51.30	17.10	0.65	0.57	0.00	0.00		
0.15	2.79	0.02	0.03	0.33	2.32	0.08	0.00	47.27	134.07	20.15	51.15	9.30	0.34	0.15	0.00	0.00	0.13	0.80
0.71	14.56	0.03	0.08	0.46	74.40	0.10	0.00	12.80	92.80	112.00	24.00	16.00	0.93	0.19	0.00	0.00	1.01	1.23
0.04	3.94	0.14	0.06	1.24	25.42	0.18	0.00	3.28	205.82	2.46	61.50	23.78	0.50	0.52	0.00	0.00	0.08	1.64
0.06	2.98	0.03	0.05	1.11	29.77	0.08	0.00	208.37	198.17	2.55	67.19	23.81	0.40	0.54	0.00	0.00	0.09	1.96

Food Name	Amount	Measure	Weight (g)	Calories	Protein (g)	Total Carb (g)	Dietary Fiber (g)	Total Fat (g)	Sat Fat (g)	Mono Fat (g)	Poly Fat (g)	Chol (mg)	Vit A (mcg RAE)	Vit D (mcg)
Corn, yellow, sweet, kernels, ckd f/fzn, drained	0.5	Cup	82.00	66.42	2.09	15.83	1.97	0.55	0.08	0.16	0.26	0.00	8.20	
Dasheen, ckd, slices, cup, Tahitian, Colocassia	0.5	Cup	68.50	30.14	2.85	4.69	0.69	0.47	0.10	0.04	0.19	0.00	60.28	
Dish, succotash, ckd f/fzn w/salt, drained	0.5	Cup	85.00	79.05	3.66	16.96	3.48	0.76	0.14	0.14	0.36	0.00	8.50	
Eggplant, ckd, drained, 1" cubes	0.5	Cup	49.50	17.32	0.41	4.32	1.24	0.12	0.02	0.01	0.04	0.00	0.99	
Eggplant, stir fried w/o oil	0.5	Cup	48.00	12.48	0.49	2.92	1.20	0.08	0.02	0.01	0.04	0.00	1.82	0.00
Gobo Root, ckd, drained, 1" pces	0.5	Cup	62.50	55.00	1.31	13.22	1.12	0.09	0.01	0.02	0.04	0.00	0.00	
Gourd, wax, ckd, drained	0.5	Cup	87.50	12.25	0.35	2.66	0.88	0.18	0.01	0.03	0.07	0.00	0.00	
Kale, ckd, drained	0.5	Cup	65.00	18.20	1.24	3.66	1.30	0.26	0.04	0.02	0.12	0.00	442.65	0.00
Kohlrabi, ckd, drained, slices	0.5	Cup	82.50	23.92	1.48	5.52	0.91	0.09	0.01	0.01	0.05	0.00	1.65	
Lambsquarters, ckd, drained	0.5	Cup	90.00	28.80	2.88	4.50	1.90	0.64	0.04	0.12	0.28	0.00	436.50	
Lotus Root, ckd w/salt, drained, slices	0.5	Cup	60.00	39.60	0.95	9.62	1.86	0.04	0.01	0.01	0.01	0.00	0.00	
Mushrooms, batter dipped, fried	5	Each	70.00	155.52	1.91	11.18	0.84	11.80	1.55	3.63	5.99	1.95	5.99	
Mushrooms, shiitake, ckd, pces	0.5	Cup	72.50	39.87	1.13	10.35	1.53	0.16	0.04	0.05	0.03	0.00	0.00	
Mushrooms, stuffed	2	Each	48.00	137.67	5.21	13.08	0.89	7.33	2.18	3.09	1.57	6.11	44.67	0.62
Onion, ckd w/salt, drained	0.5	Cup	105.00	46.20	1.43	10.66	1.47	0.20	0.04	0.02	0.07	0.00	0.11	
Squash, acorn, ckd, mashed	0.5	Cup	122.50	41.65	0.82	10.77	3.18	0.10	0.01	0.01	0.04	0.00	50.22	
Squash, butternut, bkd, cubes	0.5	Cup	102.50	41.00	0.93	10.76	2.87	0.10	0.02	0.01	0.04	0.00	571.95	
Squash, spaghetti, bkd/ckd, drained	0.5	Cup	77.50	20.92	0.51	5.01	1.08	0.20	0.05	0.02	0.10	0.00	4.65	
Squash, summer, all types, ckd, drained, slices	0.5	Cup	90.00	18.00	0.82	3.88	1.26	0.28	0.05	0.02	0.12	0.00	9.90	
Squash, winter, all types, bkd, cubes	0.5	Cup	102.50	37.92	0.92	9.07	2.87	0.36	0.11	0.04	0.22	0.00	267.52	
Swiss Chard, ckd, drained, chpd	0.5	Cup	87.50	17.50	1.64	3.61	1.84	0.07	0.01	0.01	0.02	0.00	267.75	
Vegetables, mixed, broccoli cauliflower carrots, fzn Birds Eye Foods	0.5	Cup	92.00	25.26	1.69	5.37	2.48	0.23	0.05			0.00	250.10	

Frozen, Dehydrated, and Dried Vegetables

Food Name	Amount	Measure	Weight (g)	Calories	Protein (g)	Total Carb (g)	Dietary Fiber (g)	Total Fat (g)	Sat Fat (g)	Mono Fat (g)	Poly Fat (g)	Chol (mg)	Vit A (mcg RAE)	Vit D (mcg)
Artichokes, globe/French, fzn, pkg	3	Ounce-weight	85.05	32.32	2.24	6.60	3.32	0.37	0.08	0.01	0.15	0.00	6.80	
Dish, broccoli, w/cheese flvd sauce, fzn Green Giant	0.5	Cup	84.00	56.28	1.93	7.48		2.10	0.40	0.85	0.22			
Grass, barley, dehyd, pwd	1	Teaspoon	3.50	10.00	0.80	1.30	1.30	0.11					87.50	0.00
Spinach, chpd/leaf, fzn, unprep, pkg	0.5	Cup	78.00	24.18	3.07	3.38	2.42	0.58	0.23	0.00	0.13	0.00	457.08	
Tomatoes, sun dried	0.5	Cup	27.00	69.66	3.81	15.06	3.32	0.80	0.12	0.13	0.30	0.00	11.88	
Tomatoes, sun dried, oil pack, drained	0.5	Cup	55.00	117.15	2.78	12.83	3.19	7.74	1.04	4.76	1.13	0.00	35.20	

Canned Vegetables

Food Name	Amount	Measure	Weight (g)	Calories	Protein (g)	Total Carb (g)	Dietary Fiber (g)	Total Fat (g)	Sat Fat (g)	Mono Fat (g)	Poly Fat (g)	Chol (mg)	Vit A (mcg RAE)	Vit D (mcg)
Artichokes, hearts, marinated, appetizers, cnd Progresso	2	Each	32.00	50.00	0.00	2.00	0.00	5.00	1.00			0.00	0.00	
Asparagus, drained, can	0.5	Cup	121.00	22.99	2.59	2.98	1.82	0.78	0.18	0.03	0.34	0.00	49.61	
Bamboo Shoots, slices, drained, can	0.5	Cup	65.50	12.44	1.12	2.11	0.90	0.26	0.06	0.00	0.12	0.00	0.66	
Beets, julienne, cnd S & W	0.5	Cup	123.00	30.00	1.00	7.00	1.00	0.00	0.00	0.00	0.00	0.00	0.00	
Carrots, cnd, drained, mashed	0.5	Cup	114.00	28.50	0.72	6.32	1.72	0.21	0.04	0.01	0.11	0.00	636.12	
Chili Peppers, green, cnd	0.5	Cup	69.50	14.59	0.51	3.20	1.18	0.19	0.02	0.02	0.12	0.00	4.17	
Chili Peppers, jalapeno, cnd, not drained, chpd	0.5	Cup	68.00	18.36	0.63	3.22	1.77	0.63	0.07	0.05	0.34	0.00	57.80	
Chili Peppers, jalapeno, dices, cnd, drained La Victoria Foods	1	Ounce-weight	28.35	6.75	0.00	1.35	1.35	0.00	0.00	0.00	0.00	0.00	0.00	
Corn, cream style, w/starch, cnd S & W	0.5	Cup	128.00	100.00	2.00	24.00	1.00	1.00	0.00			0.00	0.00	
Corn, yellow, sweet, cream style, can	0.5	Cup	128.00	92.16	2.23	23.21	1.54	0.54	0.08	0.16	0.26	0.00	5.12	
Corn, yellow, sweet, kernels, drained, can	0.5	Cup	82.00	66.42	2.15	15.25	1.64	0.82	0.13	0.24	0.38	0.00	3.28	
Corn, yellow, sweet, kernels, unsalted, cnd, not drained	0.5	Cup	128.00	81.92	2.49	19.72	2.18	0.64	0.10	0.19	0.30	0.00	3.84	
Garlic, crushed, wet McCormick & Co., Inc.	1	Teaspoon	5.00	15.00	0.00	0.00	0.00	0.50				0.00		
Hominy, white, cnd	0.5	Cup	82.50	59.40	1.22	11.77	2.06	0.72	0.10	0.19	0.33	0.00	0.04	
Hominy, yellow, cnd	0.5	Cup	80.00	57.60	1.18	11.41	2.00	0.70	0.10	0.18	0.32	0.00	4.80	

Vit E (mg)	Vit C	Vit B₁-Thia (mg)	Vit B₂-Ribo (mg)	Vit B₃-Nia (mg)	Fol (mcg)	Vit B₆ (mg)	Vita B₁₂ (mcg)	Sodi (mg)	Pota (mg)	Cal (mg)	Phos (mg)	Magn (mg)	Iron (mg)	Zinc (mg)	Caff (mg)	Alco (g)	Sol Fiber (g)	Insol Fiber (g)
0.06	2.87	0.02	0.05	1.08	28.70	0.08	0.00	0.82	191.06	2.46	64.78	22.96	0.39	0.52	0.00	0.00		
1.85	26.03	0.03	0.14	0.33	4.79	0.08	0.00	36.99	426.75	102.06	45.89	34.93	1.07	0.07	0.00	0.00		
0.16	5.01	0.06	0.06	1.11	28.05	0.08	0.00	238.85	225.25	12.75	59.50	19.55	0.76	0.38	0.00	0.00	0.24	3.24
0.20	0.64	0.04	0.01	0.30	6.93	0.04	0.00	0.50	60.88	2.97	7.42	5.44	0.12	0.06	0.00	0.00	0.20	1.04
0.02	0.70	0.02	0.02	0.28	7.30	0.04	0.00	1.44	104.16	3.36	10.56	6.72	0.13	0.06	0.00	0.00	0.48	0.72
0.29	1.62	0.02	0.04	0.20	12.50	0.18	0.00	2.50	225.00	30.62	58.12	24.37	0.48	0.24	0.00	0.00		
0.34	9.19	0.03	0.00	0.34	3.50	0.03	0.00	93.63	4.38	15.75	14.88	8.75	0.33	0.51	0.00	0.00		
0.55	26.65	0.04	0.04	0.32	8.45	0.09	0.00	14.95	148.20	46.80	18.20	11.70	0.58	0.16	0.00	0.00	0.58	0.72
0.43	44.55	0.03	0.02	0.32	9.90	0.13	0.00	17.32	280.50	20.62	37.12	15.67	0.33	0.25	0.00	0.00	0.27	0.63
1.66	33.30	0.10	0.23	0.82	12.60	0.16	0.00	26.10	259.20	232.20	40.50	20.70	0.64	0.28	0.00	0.00		
0.01	16.44	0.08	0.01	0.18	4.80	0.13	0.00	168.60	217.80	15.60	46.80	13.20	0.54	0.20	0.00	0.00	0.72	1.14
2.34	1.20	0.11	0.26	2.25	8.26	0.04	0.03	111.70	154.27	15.30	119.48	6.78	1.22	0.42	0.00	0.00		
0.02	0.22	0.03	0.12	1.09	15.22	0.12	0.00	2.90	84.82	2.17	21.02	10.15	0.32	0.96	0.00	0.00		
0.83	2.81	0.15	0.26	2.64	11.00	0.07	0.10	297.57	208.61	99.82	107.44	14.29	1.49	0.70	0.00	0.08	0.08	0.81
0.02	5.46	0.05	0.02	0.17	15.75	0.14	0.00	250.95	174.30	23.10	36.75	11.55	0.25	0.22	0.00	0.00	0.53	0.95
0.14	7.97	0.13	0.01	0.65	13.47	0.14	0.00	3.67	322.17	31.85	33.07	31.85	0.69	0.13	0.00	0.00	0.32	2.87
1.33	15.48	0.07	0.01	0.99	19.47	0.13	0.00	4.10	291.10	42.02	27.67	29.72	0.61	0.13	0.00	0.00	0.30	2.57
0.09	2.72	0.03	0.02	0.63	6.20	0.07	0.00	13.95	90.67	16.27	10.85	8.52	0.26	0.15	0.00	0.00	0.11	0.98
0.13	4.96	0.04	0.03	0.47	18.00	0.06	0.00	0.90	172.80	24.30	35.10	21.60	0.33	0.35	0.00	0.00	0.48	0.78
0.12	9.84	0.01	0.07	0.51	20.50	0.17	0.00	1.02	447.92	22.55	19.47	13.32	0.45	0.23	0.00	0.00	0.31	2.57
1.65	15.75	0.03	0.08	0.32	7.88	0.07	0.00	156.62	480.38	50.75	28.88	75.25	1.98	0.29	0.00	0.00		
	43.69	0.05	0.07	0.46	49.96	0.15	0.00	27.59	192.28	30.65	38.64	12.88	0.52		0.00	0.00		
0.14	4.51	0.05	0.12	0.73	107.16	0.07	0.00	39.97	210.92	16.16	49.33	22.96	0.43	0.27	0.00	0.00		
	29.74							403.20		45.36			0.54		0.00	0.00		
0.00	11.00	0.01	0.07	0.26	38.00	0.05	1.00	1.00	112.00	18.00	18.00	3.60	2.00	0.02	0.00	0.00		
2.26	18.95	0.08	0.18	0.45	101.40	0.12	0.00	57.72	290.16	120.90	40.56	56.94	1.58	0.35	0.00	0.00		
0.00	10.58	0.14	0.13	2.44	18.36	0.09	0.00	565.65	925.29	29.70	96.12	52.38	2.45	0.54	0.00	0.00	0.84	2.48
0.29	55.99	0.11	0.21	2.00	12.65	0.18	0.00	146.30	860.75	25.85	76.45	44.55	1.47	0.43	0.00	0.00	0.80	2.39
	3.60							110.00		0.00			0.00		0.00	0.00	0.00	0.00
0.37	22.26	0.07	0.12	1.15	116.16	0.13	0.00	347.27	208.12	19.36	52.03	12.10	2.22	0.48	0.00	Alco		
0.42	0.72	0.02	0.02	0.09	1.96	0.09	0.00	4.58	52.40	5.24	16.38	2.62	0.21	0.42	0.00	0.00		
	0.00						0.00	230.00	0.00	0.00			0.72		0.00	0.00		
0.84	3.08	0.03	0.04	0.63	10.26	0.13	0.00	275.88	204.06	28.50	27.36	9.12	0.72	0.30	0.00	0.00	0.87	0.83
	23.77	0.00	0.02	0.44	37.53	0.09	0.00	275.91	78.53	25.02	7.64	2.78	0.93	0.07	0.00	0.00		
0.48	6.80	0.02	0.02	0.27	9.52	0.14	0.00	1136.28	131.24	15.64	12.24	10.20	1.27	0.23	0.00	0.00	0.54	1.22
	1.62							168.75	33.75	0.00			0.00		0.00	0.00		
	1.20						0.00	340.00	0.00	0.00			3.60		0.00	0.00		
0.09	5.89	0.03	0.07	1.23	57.60	0.08	0.00	364.80	171.52	3.84	65.28	21.76	0.48	0.68	0.00	0.00	0.08	1.46
0.03	6.97	0.03	0.06	0.98	40.18	0.04	0.00	175.48	159.90	4.10	53.30	16.40	0.71	0.32	0.00	0.00	0.08	1.56
0.04	7.04	0.03	0.08	1.20	48.64	0.05	0.00	15.36	209.92	5.12	65.28	20.48	0.52	0.46	0.00	0.00	0.10	2.08
								0.00							0.00	0.00	0.00	0.00
0.04	0.00	0.00	0.01	0.03	0.82	0.01	0.00	173.25	7.42	8.25	28.87	13.20	0.51	0.86	0.00	0.00	0.08	1.98
0.08	0.00	0.00	0.01	0.02	0.80	0.01	0.00	168.00	7.20	8.00	28.00	12.80	0.50	0.84	0.00	0.00	0.10	1.90

Food Name	Amount	Measure	Weight (g)	Calories	Protein (g)	Total Carb (g)	Dietary Fiber (g)	Total Fat (g)	Sat Fat (g)	Mono Fat (g)	Poly Fat (g)	Chol (mg)	Vit A (mcg RAE)	Vit D (mcg)
VEGETABLES AND LEGUMES *(continued)*														
Mushrooms, cnd, drained, slices	10	Each	40.00	10.00	0.75	2.04	0.96	0.12	0.02	0.00	0.05	0.00	0.00	
Olives, black, sml, w/o pits, cnd	1	Each	3.20	3.68	0.03	0.20	0.10	0.34	0.05	0.25	0.03	0.00	0.64	
Olives, green, queen, cnd S & W	1	Each	6.50	10.00	0.00	0.50	0.00	1.00	0.00	0.75	0.25	0.00	0.00	
Palm Hearts, cnd	0.5	Cup	73.00	20.44	1.84	3.37	1.75	0.45	0.10	0.07	0.15	0.00	0.00	
Pumpkin, cnd, unsalted	0.5	Cup	122.50	41.65	1.35	9.91	3.55	0.34	0.18	0.05	0.02	0.00	953.05	
Sauerkraut, cnd, drained	0.5	Cup	71.00	13.49	0.65	3.04	1.77	0.10	0.02	0.01	0.04	0.00	0.71	
Spinach, cnd, unsalted, drained	0.5	Cup	107.00	24.61	3.01	3.64	2.57	0.54	0.09	0.01	0.22	0.00	524.30	
Tomatoes, crushed, cnd	0.5	Cup	50.50	16.16	0.83	3.68	0.96	0.14	0.02	0.02	0.06	0.00	17.67	
Tomatoes, puree, cnd	0.5	Cup	125.00	47.50	2.06	11.23	2.37	0.27	0.02	0.02	0.08	0.00	32.50	
Tomatoes, red, cnd, whole, lrg	1	Each	164.00	27.88	1.31	6.41	1.48	0.21	0.03	0.03	0.09	0.00	9.84	
Tomatoes, red, stwd, cnd, not drained	0.5	Cup	127.50	33.15	1.16	7.89	1.27	0.24	0.03	0.04	0.10	0.00	11.47	
Tomatoes, red, w/green chilis, cnd	0.5	Cup	120.50	18.08	0.83	4.36	1.21	0.10	0.01	0.01	0.04	0.00	24.10	
Tomatoes, red, whole, unsalted, can	1	Each	190.00	36.10	1.75	8.30	1.90	0.25	0.04	0.04	0.10	0.00	13.30	
Vegetables, garden medley, cnd Green Giant	0.5	Cup	121.00	40.00	1.00	9.00	2.00	0.00	0.00	0.00	0.00	0.00	100.00	
Vegetables, mixed, cnd, drained	0.5	Cup	81.50	39.94	2.11	7.55	2.45	0.20	0.04	0.01	0.09	0.00	474.33	
Waterchestnuts, Chinese, cnd, not drained, each	4	Each	28.00	14.00	0.25	3.44	0.70	0.02	0.00	0.00	0.01	0.00	0.00	
Legumes														
Bean Cakes, Japanese style	1	Each	32.00	130.46	1.72	15.83	0.91	6.85	1.02	2.90	2.58	0.00	0.00	0.00
Beans, adzuki, mature, ckd w/salt	0.5	Cup	115.00	147.20	8.65	28.48	8.40	0.12	0.04			0.00	0.35	0.00
Beans, black turtle soup, mature, cnd	0.5	Cup	120.00	109.20	7.24	19.87	8.28	0.35	0.09	0.03	0.15	0.00	0.24	
Beans, black, cnd Bush's Best	0.5	Cup	130.00	100.00	7.00	20.00	7.00	0.50	0.00			0.00	0.00	
Beans, black, fermented, Szechuan	0.5	Cup	86.00	164.26	16.60	10.66		6.11						
Beans, blackeyed, immature, ckd, drained	0.5	Cup	82.50	80.03	2.61	16.77	4.13	0.31	0.08	0.03	0.13	0.00	33.00	
Beans, cannellini, cnd Progresso	0.5	Cup	130.00	100.00	5.00	18.00	5.00	0.50	0.00	0.00	0.50	0.00	0.00	
Beans, chickpea, mature, ckd	0.5	Cup	82.00	134.48	7.26	22.49	6.23	2.12	0.22	0.47	0.95	0.00	0.82	
Beans, chickpea/garbanzo, unsalted, cnd	0.5	Cup	130.00	120.00	7.00	19.00	5.00	1.50						
Beans, cowpeas, mature, ckd	0.5	Cup	86.00	99.76	6.65	17.85	5.59	0.46	0.11	0.04	0.19	0.00	0.86	
Beans, fava/broad, cnd Progresso	0.5	Cup	130.00	110.00	6.00	20.00	5.00	0.50	0.00			0.00	0.00	
Beans, fava/broad, mature, cnd, not drained	0.5	Cup	128.00	90.88	7.00	15.89	4.74	0.28	0.04	0.06	0.11	0.00	1.28	
Beans, frijoles, w/cheese, fast food	0.5	Cup	83.50	112.73	5.68	14.36		3.89	2.04	1.31	0.35	18.37	17.54	
Beans, garbanzo, cnd Old El Paso	0.5	Cup	130.00	100.00	6.00	16.00	4.00	1.50	0.00	0.60	0.90	0.00	0.00	
Beans, garbanzo, mature, cnd	0.5	Cup	120.00	142.80	5.94	27.15	5.28	1.37	0.14	0.30	0.61	0.00	1.20	
Beans, great northern, cnd Bush's Best	0.5	Cup	130.00	110.00	7.00	18.00	7.00	0.50	0.00			0.00	0.00	
Beans, great northern, mature, cnd	0.5	Cup	131.00	149.34	9.65	27.55	6.42	0.51	0.16	0.02	0.21	0.00	0.06	
Beans, green, French cut, cnd Green Giant	0.5	Cup	118.00	20.00	1.00	4.00	1.00	0.00	0.00	0.00	0.00	0.00	15.00	
Beans, green, French cut, fzn Birds Eye Foods	0.5	Cup	83.00	25.00	1.33	5.75	1.91	0.15	0.03			0.00	19.04	
Beans, green, snap, fresh	0.5	Cup	55.00	17.05	1.00	3.93	1.87	0.06	0.01	0.00	0.03	0.00	19.25	
Beans, green, whole, deluxe, fzn Birds Eye Foods	10	Each	40.00	10.68	0.60	2.38	0.92	0.09	0.02			0.00	13.73	
Beans, Italian, cut, cnd Del Monte Foods	0.5	Cup	121.00	30.00	1.00	6.00	3.00	0.00	0.00	0.00	0.00	0.00	10.00	
Beans, kidney, dark red, cnd Bush's Best	0.5	Cup	130.00	130.00	8.00	21.00	7.00	1.00	0.00			0.00		
Beans, lentils, ckd f/dry w/o salt	0.5	Cup	99.00	114.84	8.93	19.93	7.82	0.37	0.06	0.07	0.18	0.00	0.40	
Beans, lentils, cnd Westbrae Natural	0.5	Cup	130.00	100.00	8.00	17.00	9.00	0.00	0.00	0.00	0.00	0.00	0.00	
Beans, lima, baby, immature, ckd f/fzn, drained, cup	0.5	Cup	90.00	94.50	5.98	17.50	5.40	0.27	0.06	0.02	0.13	0.00	7.20	
Beans, lima, green, cnd Del Monte Foods	0.5	Cup	126.00	80.00	4.00	15.00	4.00	0.00	0.00	0.00	0.00	0.00	5.00	
Beans, navy, mature, cnd	0.5	Cup	131.00	148.03	9.87	26.78	6.68	0.56	0.15	0.05	0.24	0.00	0.00	
Beans, pinto, cnd Bush's Best	0.5	Cup	130.00	110.00	6.00	19.00	6.00	0.00	0.00	0.00	0.00	0.00		
Beans, refried, fat free, cnd Bush's Best	0.5	Cup	125.00	130.00	9.00	24.00	7.00	0.00	0.00	0.00	0.00	0.00	0.00	
Beans, refried, spicy, cnd Rosarita	0.5	Cup	128.00	100.00	6.00	18.00	6.00	2.00	1.00			0.00	0.00	

Vit E (mg)	Vit C	Vit B$_1$-Thia (mg)	Vit B$_2$-Ribo (mg)	Vit B$_3$-Nia (mg)	Fol (mcg)	Vit B$_6$ (mg)	Vita B$_{12}$ (mcg)	Sodi (mg)	Pota (mg)	Cal (mg)	Phos (mg)	Magn (mg)	Iron (mg)	Zinc (mg)	Caff (mg)	Alco (g)	Sol Fiber (g)	Insol Fiber (g)
0.00	0.00	0.03	0.01	0.64	4.80	0.02	0.00	170.00	51.60	4.40	26.40	6.00	0.32	0.29	0.00	0.00	0.08	0.88
0.05	0.03	0.00	0.00	0.00	0.00	0.00	0.00	27.90	0.26	2.82	0.10	0.13	0.11	0.01	0.00	0.00	0.01	0.10
	0.00						0.00	110.00	0.00	0.00			0.00		0.00	0.00	0.00	0.00
	5.77	0.01	0.04	0.32	28.47	0.02	0.00	310.98	129.21	42.34	47.45	27.74	2.29	0.84	0.00	0.00		
1.30	5.15	0.03	0.07	0.45	14.70	0.07	0.00	6.13	252.35	31.85	42.88	28.18	1.70	0.21	0.00	0.00	0.60	2.95
0.07	10.44	0.01	0.02	0.10	17.04	0.09	0.00	469.31	120.70	21.30	14.20	9.23	1.04	0.13	0.00	0.00	0.80	0.97
2.08	15.30	0.02	0.15	0.42	104.86	0.11	0.00	28.89	370.22	135.89	47.08	81.32	2.46	0.49	0.00	0.00	0.64	1.93
0.27	4.65	0.04	0.03	0.62	6.56	0.08	0.00	66.66	147.96	17.17	16.16	10.10	0.66	0.14	0.00	0.00		
2.46	13.25	0.04	0.10	1.83	13.75	0.17	0.00	498.75	548.75	22.50	50.00	28.75	2.23	0.46	0.00	0.00		
1.16	14.76	0.07	0.08	1.21	13.12	0.15	0.00	209.92	308.32	50.84	31.16	18.04	1.59	0.23	0.00	0.00	0.21	1.26
1.06	10.07	0.06	0.04	0.91	6.37	0.02	0.00	281.77	263.92	43.35	25.50	15.30	1.70	0.22	0.00	0.00	0.32	0.96
0.46	7.47	0.04	0.02	0.77	10.85	0.12	0.00	483.21	128.94	24.10	16.87	13.26	0.31	0.16	0.00	0.00	0.30	0.90
1.52	26.98	0.09	0.06	1.40	15.20	0.17	0.00	19.00	431.30	57.00	36.10	22.80	1.04	0.30	0.00	0.00	0.42	1.48
	0.00							360.00		0.00			0.72		0.00	0.00		
0.28	4.08	0.04	0.04	0.47	19.56	0.06	0.00	121.44	237.17	22.01	34.23	13.04	0.85	0.33	0.00	0.00	0.93	1.52
0.14	0.36	0.00	0.01	0.10	1.68	0.04	0.00	2.24	33.04	1.12	5.32	1.40	0.24	0.11	0.00	0.00		
1.24	0.00	0.08	0.05	0.55	9.10	0.02	0.00	0.53	57.70	3.15	20.86	6.15	0.67	0.16	0.00	0.00		
0.12	0.00	0.13	0.08	0.83	139.15	0.12	0.00	280.60	611.80	32.20	193.20	59.80	2.30	2.03	0.00	0.00		
0.31	3.24	0.17	0.15	0.75	73.20	0.06	0.00	460.80	369.60	42.00	129.60	42.00	2.28	0.65	0.00	0.00	1.16	7.12
	0.00							460.00		40.00			1.80		0.00	0.00		
		0.11	0.21	2.75			0.00			156.52	170.28		4.73		0.00	0.00		
0.18	1.82	0.08	0.12	1.16	104.78	0.06	0.00	3.30	344.85	105.60	42.08	42.90	0.93	0.85	0.00	0.00	0.50	3.63
	0.00							270.00		40.00			1.80		0.00	0.00		
0.28	1.07	0.09	0.05	0.43	141.04	0.12	0.00	5.74	238.62	40.18	137.76	39.36	2.37	1.26	0.00	0.00	1.93	4.30
		0.09	0.07	0.40					250.00	60.00	100.00	60.00	1.44	1.50	0.00	0.00		
0.24	0.34	0.17	0.05	0.43	178.88	0.09	0.00	3.44	239.08	20.64	134.16	45.58	2.16	1.11	0.00	0.00	0.70	4.89
	0.00							250.00		20.00			1.44		0.00	0.00		
0.10	2.30	0.03	0.06	1.22	42.24	0.06	0.00	579.84	309.76	33.28	101.12	40.96	1.28	0.80	0.00	0.00	1.14	3.60
	0.75	0.07	0.17	0.75	55.95	0.10	0.34	440.88	302.27	94.36	87.68	42.59	1.12	0.87	0.00	0.00		
	0.00							340.00		40.00			1.44		0.00	0.00		
0.18	4.56	0.04	0.04	0.17	80.40	0.56	0.00	358.80	206.40	38.40	108.00	34.80	1.62	1.27	0.00	0.00	1.27	4.01
	1.20							400.00		40.00			1.44		0.00	0.00		
0.34	1.70	0.19	0.08	0.60	106.11	0.14	0.00	5.24	459.81	69.43	178.16	66.81	2.06	0.85	0.00	0.00	1.09	5.33
	2.40							390.00		20.00			0.36		0.00	0.00		
	7.59	0.05	0.07	0.25	11.12	0.04	0.00	3.25	141.10	37.61	20.75	18.26	0.79		0.00	0.00		
0.23	8.97	0.05	0.06	0.41	20.35	0.04	0.00	3.30	114.95	20.35	20.90	13.75	0.57	0.13	0.00	0.00	0.77	1.10
	4.34	0.02	0.04	0.12	4.68	0.02	0.00	0.86	70.80	15.43	10.00	8.00	0.31		0.00	0.00		
	2.40							390.00		20.00			0.72		0.00	0.00		
	1.20							260.00		80.00			1.80		0.00	0.00		
0.11	1.49	0.17	0.08	1.05	179.19	0.18	0.00	1.98	365.31	18.81	178.20	35.64	3.30	1.25	0.00	0.00	1.29	6.53
								150.00							0.00	0.00		
0.58	5.22	0.06	0.05	0.69	14.40	0.10	0.00	26.10	369.90	25.20	100.80	50.40	1.76	0.49	0.00	0.00	1.46	3.94
	4.80							390.00		20.00			1.44		0.00	0.00		
1.02	0.92	0.18	0.07	0.63	81.22	0.13	0.00	586.88	377.28	61.57	175.54	61.57	2.42	1.01	0.00	0.00	4.01	2.67
	1.20							390.00		40.00			1.80		0.00	0.00		
	0.00							490.00		60.00			2.70		0.00	0.00		
	0.00							630.00		40.00			1.98		0.00	0.00		

Food Name	Amount	Measure	Weight (g)	Calories	Protein (g)	Total Carb (g)	Dietary Fiber (g)	Total Fat (g)	Sat Fat (g)	Mono Fat (g)	Poly Fat (g)	Chol (mg)	Vit A (mcg RAE)	Vit D (mcg)
VEGETABLES AND LEGUMES *(continued)*														
Beans, refried, vegetarian, cnd Old El Paso	0.5	Cup	118.00	100.00	6.00	17.00	6.00	1.00	0.00	0.00	1.00	0.00	0.00	
Beans, refried/frijoles, cnd	0.5	Cup	126.40	118.82	6.94	19.63	6.70	1.59	0.60	0.70	0.20	10.11	0.00	
Beans, white, sml, cnd S & W	0.5	Cup	122.00	80.00	7.00	19.00	6.00	0.50	0.00			0.00	0.00	
Beans, yardlong, ckd, drained	0.5	Cup	52.00	24.44	1.32	4.77	2.60	0.05	0.01	0.01	0.02	0.00	11.96	
Beans, yellow, snap, fresh	0.5	Cup	55.00	17.05	1.00	3.93	1.87	0.07	0.01	0.00	0.03	0.00	2.75	
Jicama, fresh, chpd	0.5	Cup	65.00	24.70	0.47	5.74	3.19	0.06	0.02	0.00	0.03	0.00	0.65	
Peas, edible pod, ckd, drained	0.5	Cup	80.00	33.60	2.62	5.64	2.24	0.19	0.04	0.02	0.08	0.00	41.60	
Peas, green, ckd, drained	0.5	Cup	80.00	67.20	4.29	12.51	4.40	0.18	0.03	0.02	0.08	0.00	32.00	
Peas, green, drained, can	0.5	Cup	85.00	58.65	3.76	10.69	3.48	0.29	0.05	0.03	0.14	0.00	22.95	
Peas, pigeon, mature, ckd w/salt	0.5	Cup	84.00	101.64	5.68	19.53	5.63	0.32	0.07	0.00	0.17	0.00	0.13	0.00
Peas, split, mature, ckd w/salt	0.5	Cup	98.00	115.64	8.17	20.68	8.14	0.38	0.06	0.08	0.16	0.00	0.35	
Soybeans, edamame, in pods, edible parts only Seapoint Farms	0.5	Cup	75.00	100.00	8.00	9.00	4.00	3.00	0.00			0.00	22.50	
Soybeans, edamame, shelled Seapoint Farms	0.5	Cup	75.00	100.00	8.00	9.00	4.00	3.00	0.00			0.00	22.50	
Soybeans, green, ckd w/salt, drained	0.5	Cup	90.00	126.90	11.11	9.94	3.78	5.76	0.67	1.09	2.71	0.00	7.20	
Soybeans, mature, dry rstd	0.5	Cup	86.00	387.86	34.04	28.14	6.97	18.60	2.69	4.11	10.50	0.00	0.00	
Vegetables, peas & carrots, ckd f/fzn, drnd, pkg	3	Ounce-weight	85.05	40.82	2.63	8.61	2.64	0.36	0.07	0.03	0.17	0.00	398.03	
Vegetables, peas & carrots, cnd, not drained	0.5	Cup	127.50	48.45	2.77	10.81	2.55	0.34	0.06	0.03	0.17	0.00	368.47	
Potatoes														
Dish, baked potato & bacon, w/cheese sauce	1	Each	299.00	451.49	18.42	44.43		25.89	10.13	9.71	4.75	29.90	188.37	
Dish, baked potato & broccoli, w/cheese sauce	1	Each	339.00	403.41	13.66	46.58		21.42	8.51	7.68	4.18	20.34	267.81	
Dish, baked potato, w/cheese sauce	1	Each	296.00	473.60	14.62	46.50		28.74	10.56	10.70	6.04	17.76	251.60	
Dish, baked potato, w/cheese sauce & chili	1	Each	395.00	481.90	23.23	55.85		21.84	13.04	6.84	0.90	31.60	185.65	
Dish, baked potato, w/sour cream & chives	1	Each	302.00	392.60	6.67	50.01		22.32	10.01	7.87	3.32	24.16	265.76	
Dish, mashed potatoes, granules prep w/milk water margarine	0.5	Cup	105.00	121.80	2.30	16.88	1.36	5.03	1.27	2.05	1.41	2.10	49.35	0.23
Dish, mashed potatoes, w/whole milk & margarine	0.5	Cup	105.00	118.65	2.10	17.76	1.57	4.40	1.05	1.83	1.27	1.05	43.05	0.15
Dish, potatoes au gratin, prep f/dry w/water milk&butter svg	1	Each	137.00	127.41	3.15	17.59	1.23	5.64	3.54	1.61	0.18	20.55	71.24	
Dish, potatoes o'brien, fzn	0.5	Cup	97.09	73.79	1.78	16.96	1.84	0.14	0.03	0.01	0.06		6.80	
Dish, scalloped potatoes, prep f/dry w/whl milk & butter svg	1	Each	137.00	127.41	2.90	17.49	1.51	5.89	3.61	1.66	0.27	15.07	47.95	
Potatoes, baked, peeled, unsalted, 2 1/3" × 4 3/4"	1	Each	156.00	145.08	3.06	33.62	2.34	0.16	0.04	0.00	0.07	0.00	0.00	
Potatoes, baked, unsalted, lrg, 3" to 4 1/4"	1	Each	298.90	277.98	7.47	63.22	6.58	0.39	0.10	0.01	0.17	0.00	2.99	
Potatoes, ckd in skin, peeled, unsalted, 2 1/2", each	1	Each	136.00	118.32	2.54	27.38	2.45	0.14	0.04	0.00	0.06	0.00	0.20	
Potatoes, french fries, heated f/fzn w/o salt	10	Each	50.00	100.00	1.58	15.60	1.60	3.78	0.63	2.38	0.39	0.00	0.12	0.00
Potatoes, hash browns, plain, fzn, pkg	0.5	Cup	105.00	86.10	2.16	18.61	1.47	0.65	0.17	0.01	0.28	0.00	0.00	
Potatoes, peeled, ckd, lrg, 3" to 4 1/4"	1	Each	299.60	257.66	5.12	59.95	5.39	0.30	0.08	0.01	0.13	0.00	0.45	
Potatoes, red, w/skin, baked, med, 2 1/4" to 3 1/4"	1	Each	173.00	153.97	3.98	33.89	3.11	0.26	0.04	0.00	0.07	0.00	1.73	
Potatoes, skin, bkd	1	Each	58.00	114.84	2.49	26.71	4.58	0.06	0.02	0.00	0.02	0.00	0.58	
Potatoes, w/skin, baked, lrg, 3" to 4 1/4"	1	Each	299.00	281.06	6.28	63.03	6.28	0.45	0.07	0.01	0.11	0.00	2.99	
Potatoes, wedges, USDA, fzn	3	Ounce-weight	85.05	104.61	2.30	21.69	1.70	1.87	0.47	1.23	0.09	0.00	0.00	

Vit E (mg)	Vit C	Vit B₁-Thia (mg)	Vit B₂-Ribo (mg)	Vit B₃-Nia (mg)	Fol (mcg)	Vit B₆ (mg)	Vita B₁₂ (mcg)	Sodi (mg)	Pota (mg)	Cal (mg)	Phos (mg)	Magn (mg)	Iron (mg)	Zinc (mg)	Caff (mg)	Alco (g)	Sol Fiber (g)	Insol Fiber (g)
	0.00							490.00		40.00			1.80		0.00	0.00		
0.00	7.58	0.03	0.01	0.39	13.90	0.18	0.00	377.94	337.49	44.24	108.70	41.71	2.09	1.47	0.00	0.00	2.54	4.16
	0.00							440.00	350.00	60.00			1.44		0.00	0.00		
0.12	8.42	0.05	0.05	0.33	23.40	0.01	0.00	2.08	150.80	22.88	29.64	21.84	0.51	0.18	0.00	0.00		
0.05	8.96	0.05	0.05	0.42	20.35	0.04	0.00	3.30	114.95	20.35	20.90	13.75	0.57	0.13	0.00	0.00	0.41	1.45
0.30	13.13	0.02	0.02	0.13	7.80	0.03	0.00	2.60	97.50	7.80	11.70	7.80	0.39	0.11	0.00	0.00		
0.31	38.32	0.10	0.06	0.43	23.20	0.11	0.00	3.20	192.00	33.60	44.00	20.80	1.57	0.29	0.00	0.00	0.96	1.28
0.11	11.36	0.21	0.12	1.62	50.40	0.17	0.00	2.40	216.80	21.60	93.60	31.20	1.23	0.95	0.00	0.00	1.20	3.20
0.03	8.16	0.10	0.07	0.62	37.40	0.05	0.00	214.20	147.05	17.00	56.95	14.45	0.80	0.60	0.00	0.00	0.34	3.14
0.09	0.00	0.12	0.05	0.65	93.24	0.04	0.00	202.44	322.56	36.12	99.96	38.64	0.93	0.76	0.00	0.00	2.53	3.10
0.03	0.39	0.18	0.06	0.88	63.70	0.05	0.00	233.24	354.76	13.72	97.02	35.28	1.27	0.98	0.00	0.00	2.77	5.37
	5.40							30.00		50.00			1.62		0.00	0.00		
	5.40							30.00		50.00			1.62		0.00	0.00		
0.01	15.30	0.23	0.14	1.12	99.90	0.05	0.00	225.00	485.10	130.50	142.20	54.00	2.25	0.82	0.00	0.00		
3.96	3.96	0.37	0.65	0.91	176.30	0.19	0.00	1.72	1173.04	120.40	558.14	196.08	3.39	4.10	0.00	0.00	2.99	3.98
0.44	6.89	0.19	0.05	0.98	22.11	0.07	0.00	57.83	134.38	19.56	41.67	13.61	0.80	0.38	0.00	0.00	0.21	2.42
0.24	8.41	0.10	0.07	0.75	22.95	0.11	0.00	331.50	127.50	29.32	58.65	17.85	0.95	0.74	0.00	0.00	0.23	2.32
	28.70	0.27	0.24	3.98	29.90	0.75	0.33	971.75	1178.06	307.97	346.84	68.77	3.14	2.15	0.00	0.00		
	48.48	0.27	0.27	3.59	61.02	0.78	0.34	484.77	1440.75	335.61	345.78	77.97	3.32	2.03	0.00	0.00		
	26.05	0.24	0.21	3.34	26.64	0.71	0.18	381.84	1166.24	310.80	319.68	65.12	3.02	1.89	0.00	0.00		
	31.60	0.28	0.36	4.19	47.40	0.95	0.24	699.15	1572.10	410.80	497.70	110.60	6.12	3.79	0.00	0.00		
	33.82	0.27	0.18	3.71	33.22	0.79	0.21	181.20	1383.16	105.70	184.22	69.46	3.11	0.91	0.00	0.00		
0.54	6.82	0.09	0.09	0.91	8.40	0.17	0.10	180.60	162.75	33.60	65.10	21.00	0.22	0.25	0.00	0.00		
0.44	11.02	0.10	0.05	1.23	9.45	0.26	0.07	349.65	342.30	21.00	50.40	19.95	0.27	0.31	0.00	0.00		
1.64	4.25	0.03	0.11	1.29	9.59	0.05	0.00	601.43	300.03	113.71	130.15	20.55	0.44	0.33	0.00	0.00	0.25	0.99
0.17	10.97	0.05	0.04	1.10	7.77	0.20	0.00	32.04	241.75	12.62	47.57	17.48	1.00	0.28	0.00	0.00		
0.21	4.52	0.03	0.08	1.41	13.70	0.06	0.00	467.17	278.11	49.32	76.72	19.18	0.52	0.34	0.00	0.00	0.30	1.21
0.06	19.97	0.16	0.03	2.18	14.04	0.47	0.00	7.80	609.96	7.80	78.00	39.00	0.55	0.45	0.00	0.00	0.56	1.78
0.12	28.69	0.19	0.14	4.21	83.69	0.93	0.00	29.89	1599.11	44.83	209.23	83.69	3.23	1.08	0.00	0.00	1.64	4.93
0.01	17.68	0.14	0.03	1.96	13.60	0.41	0.00	5.44	515.44	6.80	59.84	29.92	0.42	0.41	0.00	0.00	0.54	1.90
0.10	5.05	0.06	0.01	1.04	6.00	0.15	0.00	15.00	209.00	4.00	41.00	11.00	0.62	0.20	0.00	0.00	0.27	1.33
0.18	8.61	0.10	0.01	1.75	4.20	0.09	0.00	23.10	299.25	10.50	49.35	11.55	1.03	0.22	0.00	0.00		
0.03	22.17	0.29	0.06	3.93	26.96	0.81	0.00	14.98	982.69	23.97	119.84	59.92	0.93	0.81	0.00	0.00	2.04	3.36
0.07	21.80	0.12	0.09	2.76	46.71	0.37	0.00	13.84	942.85	15.57	124.56	48.44	1.21	0.69	0.00	0.00		
0.02	7.83	0.07	0.06	1.78	12.76	0.36	0.00	12.18	332.34	19.72	58.58	24.94	4.08	0.28	0.00	0.00		
0.12	37.67	0.14	0.13	4.57	113.62	0.63	0.00	20.93	1626.56	29.90	224.25	80.73	1.91	1.05	0.00	0.00		
	9.53	0.09	0.03	1.31		0.30	0.00	41.67	335.10	12.76	73.99	16.16	0.60	0.31	0.00	0.00		

Food Name	Amount	Measure	Weight (g)	Calories	Protein (g)	Total Carb (g)	Dietary Fiber (g)	Total Fat (g)	Sat Fat (g)	Mono Fat (g)	Poly Fat (g)	Chol (mg)	Vit A (mcg RAE)	Vit D (mcg)
VEGETABLES AND LEGUMES *(continued)*														
Sweetpotatoes, bkd in skin, unsalted, peeled	0.5	Cup	100.00	90.00	2.01	20.71	3.31	0.15	0.05	0.00	0.09	0.00	961.00	
Sweetpotatoes, candied, prep f/recipe, 2 1/2" × 2" pce	1	Piece	105.00	151.20	0.92	29.25	2.52	3.41	1.42	0.66	0.16	8.40	0.00	
Yams, orange, bkd in skin, unsalted, peeled	0.5	Cup	100.00	90.00	2.01	20.71	3.31	0.15	0.05	0.00	0.09	0.00	961.00	
WEIGHT LOSS BARS & DRINKS														
Weight Loss Bars														
Bar, diet, banana nut, low carb, snack Slim Fast Low Carb	1	Each	32.00	120.00	6.00	18.00	1.00	3.00	2.00			5.00		1.50
Bar, diet, chewy trail mix, granola Slim Fast	1	Each	56.00	220.00	8.00	33.00	2.00	5.00	1.00			5.00		3.50
Bar, diet, chocolate chip Carb Options	1	Each	50.00	200.00	16.00	17.00	0.50	8.00	4.00			3.00		3.50
Bar, diet, chocolate chip, granola Slim Fast	1	Each	56.00	220.00	8.00	35.00	1.00	6.00	3.50			5.00		3.50
Bar, diet, hi prot & low carbohydrate, chocolate banana Optimum Nutrition Complete Protein Diet	1	Each	50.00	180.00	21.00	3.00	0.50	4.50	3.00			0.00		
Bar, diet, hi prot, chocolate raspberry Optimum Nutrition Pro-Complex	1	Each	70.00	260.00	31.00	11.00	1.00	5.00	3.50			0.00		
Bar, diet, honey peanut	1	Each	56.00	220.00	8.00	34.00	2.00	5.00	3.50			3.00		3.50
Bar, diet, Metabolift, chocolate coconut Twin Laboratories	1	Each	35.00	120.00	12.00	7.00	5.00	4.00	2.00					
Bar, diet, milk chocolate peanut Slim Fast Meal on the Go	1	Each	56.00	220.00	8.00	36.00	2.00	5.00	3.00			3.00		3.50
Bar, diet, toasted oats & spice Slim Fast Meal on the Go	1	Each	56.00	220.00	8.00	37.00	2.00	5.00	3.50			3.00		3.50
Weight Loss Drinks														
Drink, diet, café mocha, soy prot, pwd scp Slim Fast Ultra	2	Each	48.00	170.00	15.00	26.00	5.00	1.50	0.50	0.50	0.50	0.00		3.50
Drink, diet, choc fudge, milk base, rtd can Slim Fast	1	Each	345.00	220.00	10.00	42.00	5.00	3.00	1.00	1.50	0.50	5.00		3.50
Drink, diet, hi prot & low carbohydrate, choc, dry pkt Optimum Nutrition Complete Protein Diet	1	Each	49.00	200.00	35.00	3.00	0.00	5.00	1.00			20.00		4.00
Drink, diet, straw cream, milk base, rtd can Slim Fast	1	Each	345.00	220.00	10.00	40.00	5.00	2.50	0.50	1.50	0.50	5.00		3.50
Drink, diet, vanilla cream, low carb, rtd can Slim Fast Low Carb	1	Each	350.00	190.00	20.00	7.00	5.00	9.00	1.50	6.00	1.50	15.00		3.50
MISCELLANEOUS														
Baking Chips, Chocolates, Coatings, and Cocoas														
Baking Bar, chocolate, semi sweet Hershey Foods	0.5	Ounce-weight	14.18	70.88	1.01	9.11		4.05	2.53				0.00	
Baking Chips, chocolate morsels, semi sweet Toll House	1	Tablespoon	14.18	70.00	1.00	9.00	1.00	4.00	2.50			0.00	0.00	
Baking Chips, M & M's, milk chocolate, mini bits	1	Tablespoon	14.20	70.72	0.68	9.56	0.38	3.31	2.05	1.08	0.10	2.13		
Baking Chips, M & M's, semi sweet chocolate, mini bits	1	Tablespoon	14.00	72.52	0.62	9.23	0.94	3.68	2.19	1.23	0.12	0.42	0.56	
Baking Chips, Reese's peanut butter Hershey Foods	1	Tablespoon	15.00	80.00	3.00	7.00		4.00	4.00			0.00	0.00	
Baking Chips, white morsels, premier Toll House	1	Tablespoon	14.18	80.00	1.00	9.00	0.00	4.00	3.50			0.00	0.00	

Vit E (mg)	Vit C	Vit B₁-Thia (mg)	Vit B₂-Ribo (mg)	Vit B₃-Nia (mg)	Fol (mcg)	Vit B₆ (mg)	Vita B₁₂ (mcg)	Sodi (mg)	Pota (mg)	Cal (mg)	Phos (mg)	Magn (mg)	Iron (mg)	Zinc (mg)	Caff (mg)	Alco (g)	Sol Fiber (g)	Insol Fiber (g)
0.71	19.60	0.11	0.11	1.48	6.00	0.28	0.00	36.00	475.00	38.00	54.00	27.00	0.69	0.32	0.00	0.00		
3.99	7.04	0.02	0.04	0.41	11.55	0.04	0.00	73.50	198.45	27.30	27.30	11.55	1.18	0.16	0.00	0.00	1.03	1.49
0.71	19.60	0.11	0.11	1.48	6.00	0.28	0.00	36.00	475.00	38.00	54.00	27.00	0.69	0.32	0.00	0.00		
2.05	9.00	0.23	0.26	3.00	60.00	0.30	0.90	80.00	20.00	250.00	100.00		2.70			0.00		
4.77	21.00	0.23	0.60	7.00	60.00	0.70	2.10	150.00	400.00	300.00		140.00	2.70	2.25	0.00	0.00		
4.77	21.00	0.23	0.60	7.00	60.00	0.70	2.10	200.00	400.00	300.00	400.00	140.00	2.70	2.25		0.00		
4.77	21.00	0.23	0.60	7.00	60.00	0.70	2.10	270.00	400.00	300.00	400.00	140.00	2.70	2.25		0.00		
								95.00		60.00	100.00		0.72			0.00		
							0.60	130.00		200.00	200.00		1.08			0.00		
4.77	21.00	0.53	0.60	7.00	120.00	0.70	2.10	160.00	170.00	300.00	250.00	140.00	2.70	2.25	0.00	0.00		
								80.00		256.00			0.50		5.00	0.00		
4.77	21.00	0.53	0.60	7.00	120.00	0.70	2.10	125.00	160.00	300.00	250.00	140.00	2.70	2.25		0.00		
4.77	21.00	0.53	0.60	7.00	60.00	0.70	2.10	160.00	65.00	300.00	250.00	140.00	2.70	2.25	0.00	0.00		
13.64	60.00	0.53	0.60	7.00	200.00	2.00	6.00	270.00	400.00	600.00	400.00	120.00	6.30	5.25		0.00		
13.64	60.00	0.53	0.60	7.00	120.00	0.70	2.10	220.00	600.00	400.00	400.00	140.00	2.70	2.25		0.00		
8.18	60.00	0.90	0.85	20.00	200.00	1.20	3.00	70.00	380.00	490.00	290.00	148.00	0.20	6.00		0.00	0.00	0.00
13.64	60.00	0.53	0.60	7.00	120.00	0.70	2.10	220.00	600.00	400.00	400.00	140.00	2.70	2.25	0.00	0.00		
13.64	60.00	0.53	0.60	2.00	120.00	0.20	0.60	200.00	400.00	400.00	400.00	140.00	2.70	2.25	0.00	0.00		
	0.00							0.00		0.00			0.36			0.00		
	0.00	0.01		0.06				0.00	45.23	0.00	22.40		0.00		7.66	0.00		
0.13	0.09	0.01	0.03	0.03	0.71	0.00	0.04	9.66	41.61	16.47	23.57	6.53	0.17	0.15	2.51	0.00		
0.15	0.00	0.01	0.01	0.06	3.92	0.01	0.00	0.42	47.04	4.76	17.08	14.84	0.41	0.21	9.10	0.00		
	0.00							35.00		0.00			0.00			0.00	0.00	
	0.00							20.00		20.00			0.00			0.00	0.00	0.00

Food Name	Amount	Measure	Weight (g)	Calories	Protein (g)	Total Carb (g)	Dietary Fiber (g)	Total Fat (g)	Sat Fat (g)	Mono Fat (g)	Poly Fat (g)	Chol (mg)	Vit A (mcg RAE)	Vit D (mcg)
Baking Chocolate, Mexican, square	1	Each	20.00	85.20	0.73	15.48	0.80	3.12	1.72	1.01	0.23	0.00	0.00	
Baking Chocolate, unswntd, liquid	1	Tablespoon	15.00	70.80	1.82	5.09	2.72	7.16	3.79	1.38	1.61	0.00	0.15	
Cocoa Powder, unswtnd, w/alkali, dry	0.25	Cup	21.50	47.73	3.89	11.78	6.41	2.82	1.67	0.95	0.09	0.00	0.00	
Baking Ingredients														
Baking Powder, double acting, sodium aluminum sulfate	1	Teaspoon	4.60	2.44	0.00	1.27	0.01	0.00	0.00	0.00	0.00	0.00	0.00	
Baking Soda	1	Teaspoon	4.60	0.00	0.00	0.00	0.00	0.00	0.00	0.00	0.00	0.00	0.00	
Yeast, baker's, dry active, pkg	1	Each	7.00	20.65	2.66	2.66	1.47	0.35	0.07	0.21	0.00	0.00	0.00	
Condiments														
Bacon Bits, Bac O Bits General Mills, Inc.	1	Tablespoon	6.00	24.96	2.46	1.62		0.96				0.00		
Catsup	1	Tablespoon	15.00	15.00	0.26	3.87	0.14	0.07	0.01	0.01	0.03	0.00	7.05	
Catsup, low sod	1	Tablespoon	15.00	15.60	0.23	4.09	0.20	0.05	0.01	0.01	0.02	0.00	7.80	
Horseradish, prep, tsp	1	Teaspoon	5.00	2.40	0.06	0.56	0.17	0.03	0.00	0.01	0.02	0.00	0.01	
Ketchup, pkt	1	Each	6.00	6.00	0.10	1.55	0.05	0.03	0.00	0.00	0.01	0.00	2.82	
Mustard, deli Hebrew National	1	Teaspoon	5.00	4.00	0.00	0.00	0.00	0.00	0.00	0.00	0.00	0.00		
Mustard, yellow Westbrae Natural	1	Teaspoon	5.00	0.00	0.00	0.00	0.00	0.00	0.00	0.00	0.00			
Pepperoncini, Greek GL Mezzetta	1	Ounce-weight	28.35	7.65	0.21	1.42	0.38	0.13	0.04	0.02	0.08	0.00		
Pickles, bread & butter	1	Each	8.00	6.16	0.07	1.43	0.12	0.02	0.00	0.00	0.01	0.00	0.56	
Pickles, dill, slices	5	Piece	35.00	6.30	0.22	1.45	0.40	0.07	0.01	0.00	0.02	0.00	3.15	
Pickles, sour, slices	5	Piece	35.00	3.85	0.12	0.79	0.42	0.07	0.02	0.00	0.02	0.00	2.45	
Pickles, sour, spears	1	Piece	30.00	3.30	0.10	0.68	0.36	0.06	0.02	0.00	0.02	0.00	2.10	
Pickles, sweet, lrg, 3" long	1	Each	35.00	40.95	0.13	11.13	0.38	0.09	0.02	0.00	0.03	0.00	3.15	
Relish, cranberry orange, cnd, cup	0.25	Cup	68.75	122.38	0.21	31.76	0.00	0.07	0.01	0.01	0.04	0.00	2.75	
Sauce, hot dog chili, rts, pkg Chef-Mate	0.25	Cup	63.00	69.30	2.69	9.23	1.70	2.38	0.97	0.97	0.22	4.41		
Sauce, hot, jalapeno, svg	1	Each	14.00	4.94	0.00	0.99	0.00	0.00	0.00	0.00	0.00	0.00	0.00	
Sauce, soy, f/soy & wheat	2	Tablespoon	32.00	16.96	2.01	2.44	0.26	0.01	0.00	0.00	0.01	0.00	0.00	
Sauce, steak Carb Options	1	Tablespoon	16.00	5.00	0.00	1.00	0.00	0.00	0.00	0.00	0.00	0.00	0.00	
Sauce, tabasco, rts	1	Teaspoon	4.70	0.56	0.06	0.04	0.03	0.04	0.00	0.00	0.02	0.00	3.85	
Sauce, taco, green, mild La Victoria Foods	2	Tablespoon	30.18	9.05	0.24	1.76	0.18	0.11				0.00	1.21	
Sauce, taco, hot Old El Paso	2	Tablespoon	30.00	10.00	0.00	2.00	0.00	0.00	0.00	0.00	0.00	0.00	0.00	
Sauce, worcestershire	1	Tablespoon	17.00	11.39	0.00	3.31	0.00	0.00	0.00	0.00	0.00	0.00	0.85	
Vinegar, balsamic, 60 grain Fleischmann's Vinegars&Wines	1	Tablespoon	15.00	21.00	0.00	5.33	0.00	0.00	0.00	0.00	0.00	0.00		
Salsas														
Salsa La Victoria Foods	2	Tablespoon	30.00	10.00	0.00	2.00	0.00	0.00	0.00	0.00	0.00	0.00	0.00	
Salsa, chili, chunky, cnd La Victoria Foods	2	Tablespoon	30.00	9.30	0.24	1.96	0.15	0.05					3.30	
Salsa, green, Jalapena La Victoria Foods	2	Tablespoon	30.16	9.65	0.28	1.42	0.27	0.33				0.00	4.22	
Sauce, picante Pace	2	Tablespoon	32.40	10.00	0.00	2.00	0.83	0.00	0.00	0.00	0.00	0.00		
Sauce, picante, rts, pkg Ortega	2	Tablespoon	30.00	10.20	0.37	2.00	0.00	0.07	0.01	0.01	0.03	0.00		

Vit E (mg)	Vit C	Vit B$_1$-Thia (mg)	Vit B$_2$-Ribo (mg)	Vit B$_3$-Nia (mg)	Fol (mcg)	Vit B$_6$ (mg)	Vita B$_{12}$ (mcg)	Sodi (mg)	Pota (mg)	Cal (mg)	Phos (mg)	Magn (mg)	Iron (mg)	Zinc (mg)	Caff (mg)	Alco (g)	Sol Fiber (g)	Insol Fiber (g)
0.07	0.02	0.01	0.02	0.37	1.00	0.01	0.00	0.60	79.40	6.80	28.40	19.00	0.44	0.25	2.80	0.00		
0.91	0.00	0.01	0.04	0.32	2.85	0.01	0.00	1.80	174.90	8.10	51.00	39.75	0.62	0.55	7.05	0.00		
0.02	0.00	0.02	0.10	0.52	6.88	0.03	0.00	4.08	539.43	23.86	156.52	102.34	3.34	1.37	16.77	0.00		
0.00	0.00	0.00	0.00	0.00	0.00	0.00	0.00	487.60	0.92	270.30	100.79	1.24	0.51	0.00	0.00	0.00		
0.00	0.00	0.00	0.00	0.00	0.00	0.00	0.00	1258.56	0.00	0.00	0.00	0.00	0.00	0.00	0.00	0.00	0.00	0.00
0.00	0.00	0.14	0.35	2.80	163.80	0.14	0.00	3.50	140.00	4.48	90.30	6.86	1.19	0.42	0.00	0.00		
		0.52	0.02	0.11				102.60	163.80	13.20			0.40		0.00	0.00		
0.22	2.27	0.00	0.07	0.23	1.50	0.02	0.00	166.50	56.55	2.70	4.80	2.85	0.08	0.04	0.00	0.00	0.03	0.10
0.24	2.27	0.01	0.01	0.21	2.25	0.03	0.00	3.00	72.15	2.85	5.85	3.30	0.11	0.03	0.00	0.00	0.05	0.15
0.00	1.25	0.00	0.00	0.02	2.85	0.00	0.00	15.70	12.30	2.80	1.55	1.35	0.02	0.04	0.00	0.00		
0.09	0.91	0.00	0.03	0.09	0.60	0.01	0.00	66.60	22.62	1.08	1.92	1.14	0.03	0.01	0.00	0.00	0.01	0.04
								65.00							0.00	0.00	0.00	0.00
								75.00							0.00	0.00	0.00	0.00
	1.83							368.55		10.75			0.17		0.00	0.00		
0.01	0.72	0.00	0.00	0.00	0.32	0.00	0.00	53.84	16.00	2.56	2.16	0.16	0.03	0.00	0.00	0.00		
0.03	0.66	0.00	0.01	0.02	0.35	0.00	0.00	448.70	40.60	3.15	7.35	3.85	0.19	0.05	0.00	0.00		
0.02	0.35	0.00	0.00	0.00	0.35	0.00	0.00	422.80	8.05	0.00	4.90	1.40	0.14	0.01	0.00	0.00	0.00	0.42
0.02	0.30	0.00	0.00	0.00	0.30	0.00	0.00	362.40	6.90	0.00	4.20	1.20	0.12	0.01	0.00	0.00	0.00	0.36
0.03	0.42	0.00	0.01	0.06	0.35	0.00	0.00	328.65	11.20	1.40	4.20	1.40	0.21	0.02	0.00	0.00	0.00	0.38
0.03	12.38	0.02	0.01	0.07	2.06	0.02	0.00	22.00	26.13	7.56	5.50	2.75	0.14	0.06	0.00	0.00	0.00	0.00
0.29	0.06	0.05	0.05	0.66	22.05	0.07	0.13	398.79	149.31	19.53	39.69	12.60	0.98	0.55	0.00	0.00		
	0.00							108.64						0.00	0.00	0.00	0.00	0.00
0.00	0.00	0.01	0.05	0.70	4.48	0.05	0.00	1803.84	69.44	6.08	40.00	13.76	0.62	0.17	0.00	0.00		
	0.00							200.00		0.00			0.00		0.00	0.00	0.00	0.00
	0.21	0.00	0.00	0.01	0.05	0.01	0.00	29.75	6.02	0.56	1.08	0.56	0.05	0.01	0.00	0.00		
	1.45							191.34		2.41			0.02		0.00	0.00		
	0.00							180.00		0.00			0.00		0.00	0.00	0.00	0.00
0.01	2.21	0.01	0.02	0.12	1.36	0.00	0.00	166.60	136.00	18.19	10.20	2.21	0.90	0.03	0.00	0.00	0.00	0.00
	0.15	0.15	0.15	0.15				3.00	10.50	1.80	3.00		0.15		0.00	0.00	0.00	0.00
	2.40							115.00	55.00	0.00			0.00		0.00	0.00	0.00	0.00
	3.15							147.90		4.20			0.01		0.00	Alco		
	3.62							180.96		4.83			0.12		0.00	0.00		
	0.00							230.00		0.00			0.00		0.00	0.00		
0.37	0.57	0.02	0.01	0.29	3.00	0.04	0.00	252.00	80.40	12.60	8.40	4.50	0.15	0.05	0.00	0.00	0.00	0.00

Total Carb = Total Carbohydrates	**Sodi** = Sodium
Sat Fat = Saturated Fat	**Pota** = Potassium
Mono Fat = Monosaturated Fat	**Cal** = Calcium
Poly fat = Polyunsaturated Fat	**Phos** = Phosphorus
Chol = Cholesterol	**Magn** = Magnesium
RAE = Retinol Activity Equivalents	**Caff** = Caffeine
Thia = Thiamin	**Alco** = Alcohol
Ribo = Riboflavin	**Sol Fiber** = Water Soluble Fiber
Nia = Niacin	**Insol Fiber** = Water Insoluble Fiber
Fol = Folate	

Are You Properly Insured?

The right supplements—along with a healthy diet—will ensure that you live well and run strong

◆ BY LIZ APPLEGATE, PH.D.

Sure, healthy eating would be a lot easier if we could skip food altogether and pop a few well-formulated pills. (Remember the Jetsons?) But relying on vitamin and mineral pills to stay healthy and run well is just not an option. That's why they're called supplements. They should *supplement* an already healthy diet of whole foods.

So which supplements should you consider? Check out the nine I outline, and, while you're at it, think about your diet as well. If it's lacking in any of these areas, it might be time to improve some of your eating habits *and* invest in some supplemental insurance.

LUTEIN SAVES EYESIGHT

Lutein, a pigment found in green leafy vegetables, has been shown to protect eyes from macular degeneration, the leading cause of blindness in people over 65. Luckily, many multivitamins now come with added lutein (and its cousin, zeaxanthin). Check the label on your multi and aim for 6 to 10 milligrams every day.

CALCIUM BOOSTS BONE HEALTH

It should come as no surprise that calcium is the star bone-building supplement. Aim for 1,000 milligrams every day (1,500 milligrams for the over-50 crowd). You already know that the best food sources are dairy products, calcium-fortified beverages and foods, and green leafy vegetables. But taking a calcium supplement can help you reach your daily goal. For maximum absorption, don't take more than 500 milligrams

at a time, and look for easily absorbed supplemental forms of calcium such as calcium carbonate or calcium citrate.

ZINC BOLSTERS IMMUNITY

Zinc sits at the top of the list of nutrients that strengthen the immune system. Research shows that even a mild zinc deficiency weakens immunity, which can make you more susceptible to invading bacteria, viruses, and other organisms. But too much zinc can hamper copper absorption, another mineral needed for a healthy immune system. So aim for 15 to 20 milligrams of zinc a day. Good food sources include seafood, meats, and beans. Or a multivitamin with added minerals should do the trick. Just check the label for the desired amount of zinc.

VITAMINS C AND E PROTECT AGAINST CANCER

A number of nutrients have been shown to offer protection from this age-related disease. Antioxidants such as vitamins C and E

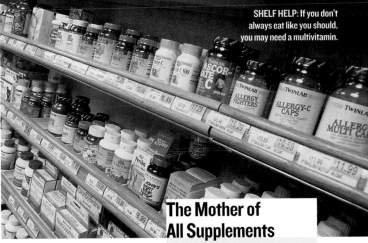

SHELF HELP: If you don't always eat like you should, you may need a multivitamin.

The Mother of All Supplements

If you pick the right multivitamin, you may not need to take any other supplements. So look for a multi that provides:

■ 100 to 200 percent of the Daily Value for water-soluble vitamins such as the eight B vitamins (B_1, B_2, niacin, B_6, folic acid, B_{12}, biotin, and pantothenic acid), and vitamin C.

■ No more than 100 percent of the Daily Value for the fat-soluble vitamins A, D, and K, because these vitamins can be toxic in high doses.

■ 100 percent of the Daily Value for the trace minerals iron, zinc, copper, selenium, and manganese.

■ 20 to 45 percent of the Daily Value for calcium, 20 to 50 percent for magnesium, and 35 percent for phosphorus. Multis can't contain 100 percent of the Daily Value for these minerals because they are too bulky to fit into one tablet.

■ If you're over 50, your multi can provide up to 200 percent of the Daily Value for vitamin D, since your need for this vitamin increases with age. And because you don't need as much iron after 50, choose a low-iron formula.

MITCH MANDEL

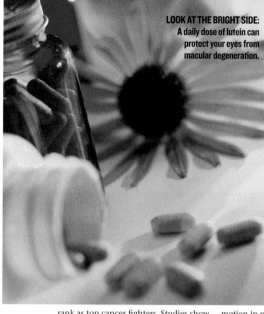

LOOK AT THE BRIGHT SIDE:
A daily dose of lutein can protect your eyes from macular degeneration.

rank as top cancer fighters. Studies show that eating an antioxidant-rich diet (you know, lots of fruits and vegetables) helps ward off all kinds of cancers. Supplement studies show less convincing results, but for those times when you skimp on fruits and vegetables, taking an antioxidant supplement is a good idea. Aim for 200 I.U.s of vitamin E and 250 to 500 milligrams of vitamin C every day.

GINGKO BILOBA ENHANCES SEXUAL PERFORMANCE

Poor circulation causes impotence in many men over 50. For women, circulation problems can cause a lack of sexual desire and satisfaction. Some research has shown that the herb ginkgo biloba can enhance circulation and improve sexual performance in both men and women. (This herb also shows promise in slowing age-related memory loss.) Keep your daily dose below 120 milligrams. And because ginkgo biloba can thin the blood, talk to your doctor before taking it.

GLUCOSAMINE STRENGTHENS JOINTS

To help protect the cartilage that keeps your joints strong, look to glucosamine. This supplement has been shown to ease joint pain and stiffness, and improve range of motion in people with osteoarthritis. And while glucosamine won't prevent joint injuries, it may speed recovery. Take 1,500 milligrams divided into three 500-milligram doses over the course of the day.

FIBER ACCELERATES WEIGHT LOSS

Because exercise—the best way to lose excess weight and keep it off—doesn't come in a pill, what's the next best aid? Forget dangerous metabolic stimulants such as ephedrine. Rather, simple fiber is the answer. Yes, the roughage in whole grains, vegetables, and fruits fills you up and helps squelch your appetite. Studies show that people who eat 25 grams of fiber or more a day weigh significantly less than those who eat a low-fiber diet. Fiber is easy to get from foods, but when you need some help reaching the recommended 25-gram minimum, a fiber supplement made with vegetable or grain fiber can help fill out your total.

OMEGA-3 FATS KEEP HEARTS HEALTHY

There are many nutrients that can boost your heart health, and omega-3 fats are some of the most potent. These essential fats, found primarily in seafood, but also in flaxseed oil, not only lower your risk of heart disease, but may also stave off a number of age-related diseases, including Alzheimer's. If you don't eat seafood or omega-3-rich seeds regularly, consider an omega-3 supplement of 1,000 to 3,000 milligrams a day.

CAFFEINE INCREASES ENERGY LEVELS

For the best stimulant around, look no further than your morning cup of coffee. That's right. Caffeine works. Countless studies have shown that 200 to 300 milligrams of caffeine (the equivalent in 2 to 3 cups of coffee) will improve alertness, reaction time, and even make an exercise session feel easier. And if you keep your intake under 300 milligrams a day, there are no side effects or long-term health implications associated with caffeine also.

Added bonus: Caffeine may help protect against Parkinson's disease. You can find caffeine in teas, coffee, colas, and energy drinks, such as Red Bull. (Although sodas and energy drinks also contain a lot of extra calories.) If you want to take caffeine in pill form, check the label amounts, because some doses may exceed the 300-milligram limit. ℞

Supplement Savvy

Dietary supplements include vitamins, minerals, amino acids, herbs, and more. And they can come in many forms—pills, capsules, powders, and even foods and beverages (think energy drinks). But dietary supplements are not considered foods, so they're not regulated by the Food and Drug Administration. Bottom line: Be careful. Here's what to watch out for:

1. Don't believe everything you read. Supplement manufacturers can make big claims on their labels, such as "boosts energy levels" or "promotes healthy blood cholesterol," without providing any proof to support them. So take supplements based on your own knowledge and research, not because of the promises on the label.

2. Look closely. Most supplements contain a number of ingredients, so be sure to read the label carefully. And be aware that while supplement labels must list major ingredients and their amounts, some manufacturers don't list contaminants such as lead and steroids that may also be present. So stick with major, reputable brands when choosing a supplement.

3. Talk to a professional. Many dietary supplements, particularly herbal products, can interact with medications. And taking excessive amounts of supplements can be risky, especially for people with certain medical conditions. So be sure to talk to your doctor about any supplements you take. Your local pharmacist can also advise you about potentially risky supplement and medication combinations.

4. Reach for food first. Research shows that the nutrients you get from foods can provide a host of health benefits. But the evidence from supplement studies is less conclusive. Why is this? Many experts believe that it's not just the nutrient alone that promotes good health but the interaction of the nutrient with other substances found in food. The deal is this: A good diet is the best way to stay healthy and strong. Only use supplements to fill in the gaps.

KURT WILSON

NUTRITION

BY LIZ APPLEGATE, PH.D.

Raising the Bar

With so many energy bars around, it's tough to know which are best. Till now

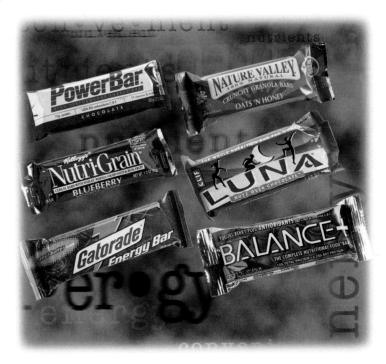

Fewer choices make for easier decisions, I always say. If you believe this too, then we're both out of luck when it comes to choosing the right energy bar.

Talk about choices! The energy/snack bar market now totals $1.5 billion a year, with options ranging from basic workout snacks to meal replacements, weight-loss aids to muscle builders, even bars designed specifically for women. And while energy bars were once relegated to the dark corners of running shops and health-food stores, you can now find them in just about any grocery store, often right next to the candy bars.

But which bar is right for you? That depends on your needs. So to prep you for your very own bar exam, here's a rundown of the major energy bar categories, plus my recommendations on the best bar for you.

High-Carbohydrate Bars

In the mid-1980s, PowerBar made a big splash in the energy-bar market, as it was specifically designed with runners' high-carbohydrate needs in mind. Since then, many other bars have followed suit.

High-carbohydrate bars generally supply about 200 to 260 calories, with over 70 percent of those calories coming from carbohydrates. They are also moderate in protein (usually 10 grams or less) and low in fat (check the label to make sure), because both can slow digestion during exercise. Main ingredients include sugars, such as corn syrup and brown rice syrup, and grains such as oats and rice. Some bars also contain dried fruit, which is another source of easily digestible carbohydrates for your working muscles.

MITCH MANDEL

Most bars in this category come fortified with an array of vitamins and minerals as well. This extra boost of nutrients may be important if you tend to skip meals or avoid nutritious fruits, vegetables, and whole grains. But if you eat fortified breakfast cereals and other fortified foods, or take a daily multivitamin, these extra vitamins and minerals are not essential.

So how do these high-carbohydrate energy bars stack up against other high-carbohydrate foods such as Fig Newtons, bananas, or bagels when eaten before or during exercise? Only a few studies have been done, but so far the science suggests that energy bars work as well as whole foods in fueling endurance workouts.

USES: Most high-carbohydrate bars work fine before, during, or after workouts. For a great preworkout snack, eat a bar about 1 to 2 hours before exercise, and make sure you drink 16 ounces of water with it. For fueling during a long workout or race, eat about one energy bar per hour—aiming for 30 to 60 grams of carbohydrate for every hour of exercise—and make sure you also take in between 5 and 12 ounces of water every 15 to 20 minutes. Following a workout, these high-carbohydrate bars make a convenient choice along with some fresh fruit and a cup of milk, soymilk, or yogurt for added carbohydrates and protein.

High-Protein Bars

First developed for bodybuilders in search of easy-to-eat gym food, high-protein bars have recently surged in popularity as many dieters take to high-protein/low-carbohydrate fare in an effort to lose weight. These bars have also become the bars of choice for vegetarians and other athletes trying to boost protein intake.

Most high-protein bars supply anywhere from 15 to more than 35 grams

continued on page 79

BAR*	Calories	Protein (g)	Carbs (g)	Fat (g)
High-Carbohydrate				
Clif Bar	240	10	41	4
Gatorade Energy Bar	260	8	46	5
Odwalla Bar!	250	7	38	7
PowerBar Performance	230	10	45	3
Tiger's Milk	140	7	18	5
High-Protein				
Atkins Advantage	220	18	2.5**	11
EAS Myoplex HP	240	20	29	5
PowerBar ProteinPlus	290	24	38	5
Promax Bar	270	20	39	5
40-30-30				
Balance	200	14	22	6
Ironman Hi Energy Bar	230	16	26	8
PR Bar	200	13	22	6
ZonePerfect	210	14	24	7
Women Only				
EAS Results	200	11	28	6
Luna	180	10	24	4.5
PowerBar Pria	110	5	16	3
Balance Oasis	180	8	28	3
Meal Replacement				
Opti-Pro Meal	290	20	40	5
Slim-Fast Meal On-The-Go	220	8	34	5
Others:				
Nature Valley Granola Bar (2)	180	4	29	6
Nutri-Grain Cereal Bar	140	2	27	3
Fig Newtons (4)	220	2	44	5

*Bar sizes vary—see label.

**Does not include glycerine and other sugar alcohols that count as carbohydrates.

Values listed for each bar may vary slightly for different flavors.

of protein. Keep in mind that the Daily Value for protein is 50 grams, yet runners require about 60 to 100 grams daily, depending on their individual body size and mileage.

It's important to check the source of protein on the ingredient label. Look for high-quality protein sources such as soy, whey, casein, and egg. These proteins supply your body with crucial amino acids for muscle repair. Steer clear of bars containing hydrolyzed proteins (you'll see this word on the label), as these are poor-quality proteins made from animal hooves and connective tissue.

Also, be wary of protein bars labeled "low-carbohydrate." They often contain sugar alcohols such as manitol, and fillers including glycerine, which sweeten the bars and bulk up their size. Some manufacturers don't include these ingredients in the carbohydrate count, but they should, because these sugars are processed much like regular carbohydrates. The FDA has recently warned some bar makers to revamp their labels and include these ingredients for a more honest carbohydrate count.

Like many other bars, high-protein versions are often vitamin- and mineral-fortified, and some contain amino acids and creatine. All fine, but not necessarily essential. Take note of the fat content as well, since several high-protein bars enhance their flavor with extra, artery-clogging saturated fat.

USES: High-protein bars can be helpful for folks who don't take in enough protein, such as some vegetarian athletes as well as high-mileage runners who find it difficult to keep their weight up. Most people can easily meet their protein needs by eating fish, soy, lean meats, beans, and eggs, but an occasional high-protein bar may help on those days when you don't get enough from your usual diet.

40-30-30 Bars

These bars are derived from the popular 1995 book *Enter the Zone* by Barry Sears, Ph.D., which touts a 40-30-30 ratio of carbohydrates, protein, and fat for weight loss and optimal athletic performance. The bars are typically higher in fat and protein, and lower in fiber than their high-carbohydrate counterparts. The higher fat content makes many of these bars taste just like candy bars. Most come fortified with an array of vitamins and minerals, with some bars containing well over 100 percent of the Daily Value for certain nutrients. If you already take supplements or eat fortified foods, you won't need all this extra fortification.

Some 40/30/30 bar manufacturers claim their products help burn body fat, yet the few research studies performed with these bars fail to support such statements. That said, the extra fat in these bars may help stave off hunger.

USES: The higher-fat and lower-carbohydrate content of these bars makes them less desirable for use during exercise. But when combined with high-carbohydrate foods such as fresh fruit or whole-grain bread, these bars can become a tasty and effective recovery meal.

Women-Only Bars

Women had long clamored for energy bars that suited their nutritional needs without all the calories. Bar makers have responded with lots of "petite" versions of earlier bars (usually under 200 calories) that are packed with the nutrients women typically lack. Many, such as Luna bars, use heart-healthy soy protein, and come fortified with calcium, folic acid, and iron. They also contain the same amount of protein as a glass of milk.

USES: These bars make a tasty snack when there's no fresh fruit or other foods around. If you eat them in place of a meal (as some women tell me they do), try to include other foods such as a cup of yogurt and fruit, or bowl of bean soup. Men can also enjoy these less-filling, smaller bars.

Meal-Replacement Bars

This is a growing category, as many people enjoy the convenience of a prepackaged bar rather than preparing a complete meal. And in an effort to trim waistlines, many people turn to bars to help them control calories and portion sizes.

Slim-Fast Meal On-The-Go bars may, in fact, assist in weight loss when used in place of a meal. A recent study showed that overweight women who replaced two of their three daily meals with a Slim-Fast bar (or drink) experienced greater success with weight loss and maintenance than women who didn't incorporate meal replacements. Not that there's anything magical in these bars. It's simply that some people are able to control their portion sizes better (and, consequently, eat fewer calories) when opting for a bar than when eating regular food.

USES: Many bars, especially high-protein types, can substitute for a meal on occasion. But keep in mind that no single bar supplies the wealth of nutrients and health-boosting substances found in whole foods. So don't belly up to a bar for a meal on a regular basis. *R*

NUTRITION

BY LIZ APPLEGATE, PH.D.

Race Ready

Different race distances call for different eating plans. Here's the rundown

A meal for every distance: Be sure to tailor your prerace meal to the distance you'll be racing.

When people ask me for the best eating plan for runners, I always respond with the question: "What type of runner are you—a 5- or 10-K'er, half-marathoner, or marathoner?" You see, sports nutrition doesn't offer a one-size-fits-all plan. Your caloric and nutritional needs change according to your body size, gender, and especially your training program.

Your eating plan should closely relate to your weekly mileage, which you typically adjust based on your racing aspirations for the season. Based on what I've designed for myself and my runner-clients, here are three individual plans—one for 5- or 10-K runners, half-marathoners, and marathoners.

I based the number of calories and food quantities on a 150- to 160-pound runner. Calorie and meal amounts may vary based on your weight. If you weigh less, you should eat the smaller quantities suggested. If you weigh more, you should eat the larger ones. If

you're not planning a season of races but simply want to know what to eat for your regular, recreational runs, pick the plan that most closely matches your weekly mileage.

5- and 10-K

As a 5- or 10-K runner, you need more calories, carbohydrate, and protein than your average Joe. A training run of 2 to 5 miles burns an extra 200 to 500 calories. On top of that, running bumps up your protein needs by an additional 15 to 25 grams. You need the extra protein to rebuild muscle and produce new blood cells. If longer runs are part of your training program, you should include more carbohydrate on your long-run day for a faster recovery.

Sample Meal Plan

Breakfast: 1 cup oatmeal with ¾ cup 1-percent milk or fortified soy milk; one whole-grain English muffin spread with 2

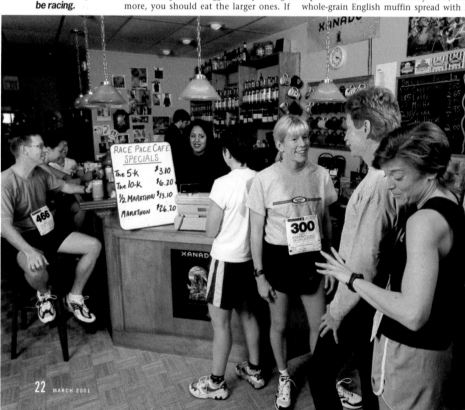

22 MARCH 2001

ERIK RUSSO

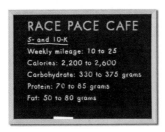

RACE PACE CAFE

5- and 10-K

Weekly mileage: 10 to 25
Calories: 2,200 to 2,600
Carbohydrate: 330 to 375 grams
Protein: 70 to 85 grams
Fat: 50 to 80 grams

tablespoons jam and 2 teaspoons soft margarine; one banana

Morning snack: ¼ cup trail mix (made with soy nuts, nuts, and raisins); 1 cup green tea flavored with 2 teaspoons honey

Lunch: One bean burrito (made with one tortilla, 1 cup black beans, ½ cup rice, 1 ounce cheese, salsa); one sliced tomato; 1 cup fresh fruit salad; two oatmeal cookies

Snack: One energy bar with water

Dinner: 1 cup pasta topped with ¾ cup red sauce (made with 3 ounces ground turkey or soy substitute); 2 cups green salad with 2 tablespoons reduced-fat dressing; two 1-ounce pieces of chocolate

Prerace meal: Eat a small meal before your race to top off your fuel tank and help you stay alert (especially if the start is early in the morning). Aim for 300 to 500 calories, 2 to 4 hours before the start. Your meal should be high in carbohydrate, modest in protein, and low in fat. For example, try one energy bar and 1 cup of sports drink or one whole-wheat bagel spread with jam, half a banana, and water.

During the race: Because you're finishing your race within an hour, plain water is your best bet. Cruise into at least one water station during your 10-K to down ½ cup of fluid. (Drink more if it's hot or humid.)

Half-Marathon

As a half-marathoner, you'll need more calories, carbohydrate, protein, and a host of other nutrients than people who run only 5- and 10-Ks. The extra carbohydrate will fuel your training, and the extra protein will help repair small muscle-fiber tears. Also, as you bump up your mileage, you'll need more healthful fats—especially omega-3 fats—to help boost your immunity.

Sample Meal Plan

Breakfast: Egg pita (two scrambled eggs and 2 tablespoons salsa inside a whole-wheat pita); 1 cup fresh fruit salad; 1 cup cranberry juice

Morning Snack: One carton of low-fat yogurt with 1 tablespoon honey and 2 tablespoons chopped almonds

Lunch: One salmon-salad sandwich (two slices whole-oat bread, 2 ounces canned salmon with 2 teaspoons reduced fat mayo, ½ cup chopped celery, one chopped dill pickle, and ¼ cup chopped cilantro); one apple sliced and spread with 1 tablespoon chunky peanut butter; two fig bars

Snack: Four dried pear halves; 2 cups sports drink

Dinner: 3 ounces grilled chicken served over 1 cup brown rice; 1 cup steamed cauliflower and broccoli with 1 tablespoon grated Parmesan cheese; ½ cup boiled red potatoes tossed with ¼ cup chopped parsley and 1 teaspoon olive oil; ½ cup low-fat frozen yogurt topped with 1 cup fresh strawberries and 2 tablespoons chocolate sauce

Prerace meal: Your 13.1-mile effort will probably take anywhere from 75

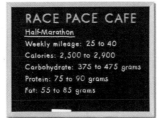

RACE PACE CAFE

Half-Marathon

Weekly mileage: 25 to 40
Calories: 2,500 to 2,900
Carbohydrate: 375 to 475 grams
Protein: 75 to 90 grams
Fat: 55 to 85 grams

minutes to more than 2 hours, which is enough to tax your glycogen stores. Therefore, you'll need to beef up your prerace eating as well as fuel up with carbohydrates during your run. Aim for 400 to 800 high-carbohydrate calories about 3 hours before the race. For example, try two 6-inch pancakes spread with 3 teaspoons jam, 1 cup sports drink, and half an energy bar.

During the race: You need to replenish fluids and calories. Aim for ½ to ¾ cup of water or sports drink every 15 to 20 minutes and about 100 calories every half-hour. Don't forget to count the calories in your sports drink as part of your carbohydrate intake (about 50 to 70 calories per cup). Other good high-carbohydrate choices include gels, energy bars, and fruit.

The Marathon

Training for a marathon seriously increases your nutritional needs. Not only does the extra mileage boost your calorie needs, but you'll need to eat even more carbohydrate to recover from training runs, especially those exceeding 90 minutes. Studies show that you need to eat at least 3 to 5 grams of carbohydrate per pound of body weight to fully restock your glycogen stores within 24 hours, making running the day after a long run more comfortable.

You must also pay special attention to eating wholesome foods that are rich in vitamins and minerals such as iron, zinc, and B vitamins. Taking a daily multi-vitamin/mineral supplement or eating fortified foods, such as breakfast cereal, is good nutritional insurance.

Sample Meal Plan

Breakfast: 2 cups fortified cereal with 1 cup 1-percent milk or fortified soy milk; one whole-grain bagel spread with 1 tablespoon almond butter; 12 ounces orange juice

Morning snack: Four fig bars; 12 ounces tomato juice

Lunch: One roasted turkey sandwich (3 ounces roasted turkey meat, two hearty slices whole-grain bread, ⅙ of an avocado sliced, 2 teaspoons reduced-fat mayo, four tomato slices, 2 teaspoons mustard, 1 ounce provolone cheese); 1 cup vegetable soup; 1 cup red grapes; four ginger snap cookies

Snack: 1 cup cold rice mixed with ¼ cup vanilla-flavored soy milk, a dash of cinnamon, 3 tablespoons raisins, and 2 tablespoons chopped pecans

Dinner: 3 ounces lean beef stir-fried with 1½ cups of mixed baby spinach, corn, snow peas, and broccoli and served over 1½ cups whole-wheat soban noodles; three potstickers; three fortune cookies

Evening snack: 3 cups air-popped popcorn; 12 ounces cranberry-grapefruit juice

Prerace meal: Since you'll be pounding the pavement for 3 or more hours, your muscles need a hefty prerace meal. Aim for 500 to 1,000 high-carbohydrate calories about 3 to 4 hours before the start. If your race starts late (at noon, for example) try eating two meals to keep

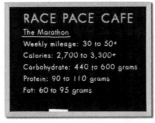

RACE PACE CAFE

The Marathon

Weekly mileage: 30 to 50+
Calories: 2,700 to 3,300+
Carbohydrate: 440 to 600 grams
Protein: 90 to 110 grams
Fat: 60 to 95 grams

your body and brain fueled (important for a positive attitude). Try 1 cup cream of wheat topped with 2 tablespoons honey and one sliced banana, one plain toasted bagel spread with 2 tablespoons jam, and a before-race snack of one can of a meal replacement (such as Boost, Ensure, or GatorPro).

During the race: Start replacing fluids and carbohydrate by mile 5 or 6. Drink ½ to ¾ cups of fluid every 15 to 20 minutes and consume 100 calories per half hour in the form of sports drink, energy gel, energy bar, or dried or fresh fruit. **R**

Reach for a Cold One

With a tidal wave of new sports beverages available, we'll tell you which are right for you

◆ BY LIZ APPLEGATE, PH.D.

Thirsty? No problem. Take a stroll down any beverage aisle, and you'll soon be drowning in choices. ◆ But all those choices aren't equal. To help you figure out which drink best suits your hydration needs during the day or during a marathon, I've outlined the five major sports beverage categories below. So grab a cup and some ice, and let's get started.

WATER, PLAIN OR FANCY

Whether bottled or straight from the tap, water is great for meeting your hydration needs. Sure, bottled waters are advertised as tasting better than what flows from the kitchen sink, but research doesn't show any difference between the two when it comes to hydration. Both work fine. And while some bottled water is purified, there are strict government safety regulations on tap water. So rest assured that your local water supply is safe.

Depending on the source of the water, it likely contains small amounts of calcium, magnesium, and other beneficial minerals that can add to your daily nutrient total.

Best uses: Throughout the day, drink 8 to 10 cups of water to meet your basic hydration needs. (And even though caffeinated beverages such as some sodas, coffees, and teas contain water, they should not be counted toward this water total.) During runs lasting less than an hour, drink 5 to 12 ounces of water every 15 to 20 minutes.

FITNESS WATERS

If you're looking for a great-tasting beverage with next-to-no calories, you're in luck. Fitness waters have arrived. Despite the newness of this category, there are already a number of products from which to choose.

Gatorade's Propel and Reebok's Fitness Water offer a mere handful of calories with a dash of vitamins and minerals in several tasty flavors. There's also ChampionLyte, which is sweetened with sucralose and contains a splash of electrolytes (important minerals that we lose through our sweat when we run).

Then there's the newest thing in fitness water—super-oxygenated water. Manufacturers of super-O_2 waters claim the extra oxygen added to the water gets into the body and boosts both performance and recovery. However, research from the University of Wisconsin has shown that athletes performed equally well on a treadmill test while drinking either plain water or the oxygen-juiced variety.

Best uses: If you're bored with plain water, fitness waters are an excellent choice during workouts lasting less than an hour. Just keep in mind that the small amount of carbohydrate in these drinks won't help refuel your muscles. So during longer workouts, be sure to include solid carbohydrate sources such as fruit or energy bars and gels. Or switch to a sports drink. Aim for 5 to 12 ounces every 15 to 20 minutes of exercise.

SPORTS DRINKS

Designed with both hydration and proper fueling in mind, sports drinks are perfect for workouts or races where both fluids and carbohydrates are crucial. Most sports drinks are a blend of water and carbohydrates—usually sucrose, glucose, fructose, or maltodextrins—along with a smattering of electrolytes such as sodium and potassium. And they usually contain between 13 and 21 grams of carbohydrate per cup of fluid, which is ideal for replenishing spent carbohydrates as well as supplying ample water to cover sweat loss. Drinks with higher concentrations of carbohydrate per cup of fluid, such as energy drinks and sodas, hamper fluid absorption, giving you that sloshing feeling in your stomach.

A new sports drink called G-Push contains a different carbohydrate source—galactose, a sugar derived from milk and other foods. The manufacturers of galactose claim it offers an advantage over other sugars because insulin isn't required to process

STAY LIQUID: To keep yourself well-hydrated, try this simple plan: About 2 hours before you run, drink 16 ounces of fluid. Then drink 5 to 12 ounces every 15 to 20 minutes during the run. Afterward, drink 16 to 24 ounces for every pound lost as sweat.

MITCH MANDEL

Drink Up

To help you stay hydrated this summer, here are a few examples of each of the five major sports-beverage categories, along with their calorie and carbohydrate counts based on an 8-ounce serving.

	Calories	Carbohydrate (g)	Extras
Waters			
Tap water	0	0	Minerals—vary by source
Dasani	0	0	Spring source
Fiji	0	0	Artesian source
Penta	0	0	Purified
Fitness Waters			
ChampionLyte	0	0	Electrolytes
Life O_2	0	0	10 times O_2 as tap water
Propel	10	3	Electrolytes, vitamins
Reebok	12	3	Electrolytes, vitamins, trace minerals
Sports Drinks			
All Sport	70	20	No longer carbonated, vitamins B and C
G-Push (G²)	70	18	Electrolytes, vitamins
Gatorade	50	14	Electrolytes
GU₂O	50	14	Electrolytes
Powerade	72	19	Electrolytes, vitamins
Simple Sports Drink	80	21	Electrolytes, vitamin C
Recovery Drinks			
Endurox R⁴	180	35	Electrolytes, vitamins
G-Push (G⁴)	110	27	Electrolytes, vitamins, trace minerals
Gatorade Energy Drink	207	41	Vitamins
Energy Drinks			
Red Bull	109	27	Taurine, caffeine, vitamins
SoBe Adrenaline Rush	135	35	Taurine, ribose, caffeine

galactose in the body. Sounds great, but more research is needed to support these claims. G-Push is also offered in different carbohydrate concentrations depending on the intensity or duration of your workout.

Other hot trends in the sports-drink arena: colorless flavors such as Gatorade Ice in strawberry, lime, and orange. Also, Odwalla, which makes fresh-squeezed juice products, has just released a drink called Simple Sports Drink. It's a refreshing sports drink made from pure fruit juice and honey, spiked with vitamin C and electrolytes. And All Sport has changed its formula by taking out the carbonation and adding vitamins B and C. Finally, the makers of GU, an energy gel, now offer GU₂O, a low-acid sports drink that's light tasting and said to be easy on the stomach during exercise.

Best uses: Drink sports drinks before a workout for an extra carbohydrate kick, or during your longer runs. Aim for 5 to 12 ounces every 15 to 20 minutes during workouts lasting more than 60 minutes.

RECOVERY DRINKS

Eating and drinking after a workout is key for a quick recovery. But sometimes after a hot, long run, solid food is the last thing you want. During that crucial 30- to 60-minute window when you need to refuel, try a high-carbohydrate recovery drink. These drinks contain more carbohydrate than sports drinks. Some also come with added protein, which may help rebuild your muscle glycogen (carbohydrate) stores faster.

Best uses: Recovery drinks can be used in place of food immediately following a workout. Aim for 40 to 60 grams of carbohydrate during the first 30 to 60 minutes after a run. Along with your recovery drink, take in additional fluids. Aim for 16 to 24 ounces for every pound lost due to sweating.

ENERGY DRINKS

New age energy drinks (the ones in those funky-looking cans) are loaded with carbohydrates. Too loaded, in fact, for use before or during exercise. Many of these drinks also come laced with stimulants such as caffeine, which may leave you feeling jittery, and can also increase urination.

Best uses: With all the other fluid options available, you'll do best to drink these beverages only on occasion, and never before or during a run. ℞

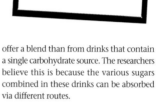

Get Your Carbs Here

There are more ways than ever to fuel up on the run. Time for a user's guide to drinks, gels, bars, and nature's own sports food

◆ BY LIZ APPLEGATE, PH.D.

On a recent flight to New York City, I met an impressive athlete. Nope, it wasn't a New York Yankee. It was the head flight attendant, Cindy. Despite her international travel schedule, Cindy is an ultrarunner who logs more than 70 miles per week. To stay properly fueled for her taxing job and grueling running schedule, Cindy downs sports drinks, carbohydrate gels, and energy bars as part of her daily fare. And they help. That's because they've been specially formulated by some very smart, sports-minded people to meet the nutritional (and convenience) needs of people on the go.

Whether you run 70 miles per week like Cindy does, or closer to 10, sports-nutrition products, when used wisely, fuel your body for optimal performance. Here's what you need to know.

RUNNING ON "E"

Just like a car, the human body can't run on empty. Running performance is limited by four fueling factors:

1. Loss of body fluids. Losing more than 2 percent of your weight as sweat during a run can hamper your performance. In a nutshell, dehydration hurts your running, because it thickens the blood, decreases the heart's efficiency, increases heart rate, and raises body temperature.

2. Drop in blood sugar levels. Your brain relies heavily on a steady supply of sugar (glucose) for fuel. Running drains your blood glucose stores, which eventually gives you that lightheaded, woozy feeling.

3. Depletion of muscle carbohydrate stores. Your muscles also suck up stored glucose (glycogen) as fuel. Depending on the intensity and distance of your run, you'll deplete your glycogen stores in as little as 60 minutes. Once this happens, you get that lead-like feeling in your legs.

4. Altered amino acid levels. Researchers also believe there is a chemical component to fatigue. For example, levels of circulating amino acids have been shown to change during endurance exercise. And research shows that endurance may be improved with specially formulated foods or beverages that modify amino acid levels and, in a sense, keep your brain thinking you're not tired.

FILL 'ER UP

Fortunately, it's never been easier to fuel up properly before and during a run thanks to all the sports foods and drinks available today. Just keep in mind that you need to take in 20 to 60 grams of carbohydrate per hour of exercise (the longer and harder you exercise, the more you need). Here's a rundown of the different fueling options and how to use each for the best results.

SPORTS DRINKS: With their mix of water and carbohydrates, sports drinks are an excellent on-the-run source of fuel. For exercise lasting anywhere from 60 minutes to several hours, they significantly boost your endurance compared with quaffing plain water.

Most sports drinks offer a blend of carbohydrates such as the sugars sucrose, glucose, fructose, and galactose. A few beverages also add maltodextrin, a complex carbohydrate made of several different glucose units. New research suggests that the body can absorb more carbohydrates from sports drinks that offer a blend than from drinks that contain a single carbohydrate source. The researchers believe this is because the various sugars combined in these drinks can be absorbed via different routes.

Sports drinks also come with added electrolytes (the vital minerals we lose when we sweat). Sodium is the most important of these, as studies show that drinks with added sodium help maintain fluid balance in the body and also promote the uptake of fluid in your intestines. In plain English: You stay better hydrated when you drink beverages that contain sodium.

For optimum fueling: Stick with sports drinks that contain 13 to 19 grams of carbohydrate per 8 ounces. Drinks with higher carb concentrations hamper fluid absorption, and will give you that sloshing feeling in your stomach. Drinks with lower carb concentrations won't refuel your muscles fast enough.

Aim to drink 1½ to 4 cups of sports drink per hour of exercise (the bigger you are and the faster you run, the more you need) to get both the fluid and carbohydrates required for endurance.

ENERGY GELS: Carbohydrates don't get any more convenient than this. Gels come in small, single-serve plastic packets that can fit in that tiny key pocket in most running shorts. (Go ahead and try that with a sports drink. Actually, you better not.)

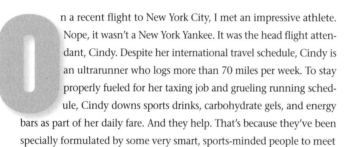

Gels contain mainly sugars and maltodextrins, which make them similar to sports drinks without the water. Some newer gels, such as e-Gel, also come with added electrolytes. There are also gels with extras such as ginseng and other herbs, amino acids, vitamins, and Coenzyme

KURT WILSON

NUTRITION

Q10 (a non-essential substance found in the body).

Caffeine is also in some gels. Check the label or consult the manufacturer's Web site for specific amounts as some gels contain as much caffeine as a half-cup of coffee. This won't be a problem if you normally use products with caffeine, but it can cause nervousness in folks not accustomed to it.

If you're a fan of honey—nature's original carbohydrate gel—but not into fitting that little plastic bear in your running shorts, check out Honey Stinger gel packs. Research by Richard Kreider, Ph.D., of Baylor University in Texas, suggests that honey boosts endurance just as well as the high-tech carb gels.

For optimum fueling: Most carbohydrate gels contain about 100 calories and 25 grams of carbohydrate. Depending on the intensity and duration of your run, you take in one to three gels for every hour you're out there. Remember to wash each down with ample water.

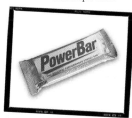

ENERGY BARS: With all the new bars on the market, you might need to eat one for some quick energy before you try to figure out which is best for you. Given all the

versions, including women-only, high-protein, and meal-replacement bars, try to read labels carefully if you want to fuel up properly.

The standard high-carbohydrate bars, such as PowerBar and Clif Bar, are great for fueling both before and during a run because, as with sports drinks and gels, they facilitate a rapid release of carbohydrate into the bloodstream. About 70 percent of their carbohydrate calories come from sugars (brown-rice syrup and sucrose) and grains (oats and rice crisps). Some bars also contain fruit, which is another source of easily digestible carbohydrates for your working muscles.

For optimum fueling: The best bars for before and during a run contain about 25 grams of carbohydrate and less than 15 grams of protein, which is not a crucial fuel source during exercise. Also, check the label for fat content. Some bars can pack a hefty fat dose, which will slow your digestion. Eat one bar about an hour before a run. If you're running for more than an hour, eat one high-carb bar per hour of running, along with ample water.

FRUIT: While prepackaged, specially-formulated sports foods and drinks are a great way to stay properly fueled for your runs, you can go *au naturel* if you prefer. Fruit, whether dried or fresh, is easily digestible and supplies a good shot of carbohydrate. And dried fruit is simple to transport (dried banana chips are indestructible compared with the real thing).

Many runners avoid eating fruit before or

during a run because they fear it will cause gastrointestinal upset thanks to its fiber content. Recent research should put those fears to rest.

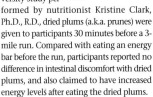

As part of a Penn State University study performed by nutritionist Kristine Clark, Ph.D., R.D., dried plums (a.k.a. prunes) were given to participants 30 minutes before a 3-mile run. Compared with eating an energy bar before the run, participants reported no difference in intestinal discomfort with dried plums, and also claimed to have increased energy levels after eating the dried plums.

For optimum fueling: Most fruit provides about 15 grams of carbohydrate per serving, which for fresh fruit is about the size of a tennis ball. For dried fruit, a serving is equal to about ¼ cup. Aim for one to two servings of fruit before a workout and one to two servings during every hour of running. Drink plenty of water to wash it all down. **R**

Visit lizapplegate.com for more nutrition and fitness tips from Liz, and for information on her new book, *Bounce Your Body Beautiful*.

KURT WILSON

The Choice is Yours

As long as you take in 20 to 60 grams of carbohydrate per hour of exercise, you'll be properly fueled for optimal performance. But should you get those carbs from sports drinks, gels, bars, or old-fashioned food? That's a tough question, since what works best for one runner doesn't always work for another. Below are the pros and cons of each for the different categories of sports foods. Experiment as needed.

	PROS:	CONS:
SPORTS DRINKS	• They hydrate in addition to providing carbs. • Liquids are easy to digest and well-tolerated on a run.	• Bottles can be bulky to carry when running. • Some runners dislike the salty taste of certain drinks.
GELS	• They fit in any pocket or can be pinned to the waistband of your shorts. • They come in a concentrated form, so you get a lot of carbs in one or two swallows.	• Some runners can't tolerate the consistency. • You need to take them with water.
ENERGY BARS	• They're more substantial than a drink or gel, so they give you a feeling of sustenance. • They can serve as a meal-replacement when you're pressed for time before or after a workout.	• They can be bulky to carry on a run. • They need to be washed down with water.
FRUIT	• Fresh fruit supplies you with water as well as carbs. • It's a less expensive, natural alternative to prepackaged sports foods.	• Can be messy or bulky to carry on a run. • Dried fruit must be washed down with water.

Effective Nutritional Ergogenic Aids

Elizabeth Applegate

Athletes use a variety of nutritional ergogenic aids to enhance performance. Most nutritional aids can be categorized as a potential energy source, an anabolic enhancer, a cellular component, or a recovery aid. Studies have consistently shown that carbohydrates consumed immediately before or after exercise enhance performance by increasing glycogen stores and delaying fatigue. Protein and amino acid supplementation may serve an anabolic role by optimizing body composition crucial in strength-related sports. Dietary antioxidants, such as vitamins C and E and carotenes, may prevent oxidative stress that occurs with intense exercise. Performance during high-intensity exercise, such as sprinting, may be improved with short-term creatine loading, and high-effort exercise lasting 1–7 min may be improved through bicarbonate loading immediately prior to activity. Caffeine dosing before exercise delays fatigue and may enhance performance of high-intensity exercise.

Key Words: dietary supplements, carbohydrate, protein, amino acids, antioxidants, creatine

Athletes of all competitive levels speak about embracing the ideal of sport: the quest for success through hard work and unaided effort, or simply doing the best with what you have. This ideal, however, does not match reality in competitive sports. Beyond genetic endowment and training, many athletes turn to extrinsic methods, such as the use of ergogenic aids, to enhance performance.

The use of performance-enhancing aids has been documented since ancient times (2, 19), and such practices are not reserved for elite or Olympic-level athletes. Back-of-the-pack runners and "weekend warriors" also quest for success at their own levels and look for means of achieving success beyond their own abilities and efforts. Since many athletes are looking for ergogenic aids that do not have side effects and cannot be detected during drug testing, nutritional ergogenic aids, including carbohydrate, creatine, and dietary antioxidants, are promising alternatives.

Nutritional ergogenic aids encompass a broad range of substances that include standard dietary constituents such as carbohydrate and protein as well as atypical dietary constituents such as sodium bicarbonate and creatine. Often, nutritional ergogenic aids must be consumed in amounts that would be unachievable through food consumption alone and thus require users to take supplemental quantities for the purported benefits. For example, creatine, a popular nutritional ergogenic aid among strength athletes, is consumed in powder or pill form. Amounts of

Elizabeth Applegate is with the Nutrition Department, University of California, Davis, 1 Shields Ave., Davis, CA 95616.

229

Reprinted by permission from Applegate, 1999, "Effective Nutritional Ergogenic Aids," *International Journal of Sport Nutrition,* Vol. 9 (No. 2): 229–239.

creatine shown to be ergogenic would require astronomical daily consumption of raw meat, a source of creatine (49). A brief listing of nutritional ergogenic aids follows:

Acetyl choline	Inosine
Amino acids	MCT oils
(individual/combinations)	Octacosanol
Bee pollen	Omega-3 fatty acids
Caffeine	Royal jelly
Carnitine	Spirulina
Chromium picolinate	Sodium bicarbonate
CoQ_{10}	Sodium phosphate
Creatine	Vitamins (individual/
Eicosanoids	combinations)
Ginseng	Wheat germ oil
Hydroxy methylbutryrate (HMB)	

As described by Butterfield (8) and Williams (55), nutritional aids can be divided into four categories: (a) products representing an energy source (e.g., carbohydrate); (b) substances that may enhance anabolism, thereby favorably altering body composition (e.g., amino acids); (c) products that act as cellular components, playing a role in exercise metabolism (e.g., sodium bicarbonate); and (d) products that may enhance recovery or an aspect of recovery from physical exertion (e.g., dietary antioxidants). This discussion focuses on the documented ergogenic potential of several nutritional performance aids: carbohydrate, protein and amino acids, dietary antioxidants, creatine, sodium bicarbonate, and caffeine.

Evaluation of Ergogenic Aids

Health food/supplement retail outlets carry numerous nutritional aids purported to enhance performance, and most fitness-related consumer magazines are full of advertisements for such products. Athletes often request fitness professionals to evaluate claims made about ergogenic aids. Several challenges arise when evaluating nutritional ergogenic aids, including the lack of regulation regarding health and performance claims about products. Many athletes fall prey to the colorful advertisements and the testimonials made by successful athletes who "owe" their victories to a particular product. Fitness professionals and others who advise athletes must probe beyond the advertisements and product literature provided by manufacturers.

In a recent article, Butterfield (8) described problems and solutions in evaluating performance-enhancing claims made about nutritional ergogenic aids. Three steps can be taken to evaluate claims. The first is to investigate the performance claim based upon a physiological and biochemical understanding of exercise. In essence, does the performance claim make sense? This requires knowledge in a variety of applicable fields such as nutrition, exercise physiology, and biochemistry. The second step is to investigate supportive evidence and use care when the evidence is not published research from peer-reviewed journals. For further reading on this subject, refer to a review by Sherman and Lamb (46). The third step is to determine the safety, ethical, and legal consequences of taking the ergogenic aid.

For example, excessive intake of a nutrient may impair the absorption or action of another nutrient. It is also crucial to examine ethical and legal issues particularly as they relate to the International Olympic Committee (IOC) doping rule, which states that "the use of a physiological substance taken in abnormal quantity . . . with the intention of increasing [performance] in an artificial and unfair manner. . . is to be regarded as doping" (57, p. 122). However, difficulty lies in establishing what constitutes "abnormal quantities" of specific cellular components or energy substrates.

Nutritional Performance Aids

Carbohydrate

For several decades, carbohydrate has been viewed as an effective ergogenic aid. Scandinavian researchers in the 1930s and 1960s demonstrated that high-carbohydrate diets improved endurance performance (4, 10). Their work became the foundation for the dietary regimen that many athletes use today to modify carbohydrate intake prior to, during, and following prolonged endurance exercise. This dietary regimen boosts muscle glycogen stores, delays fatigue, and enhances recovery. This brief discussion is limited to carbohydrate intake prior to and following exercise as an ergogenic aid.

Because fatigue during prolonged exercise is associated with muscle glycogen depletion, athletes are recommended to consume diets that provide 9–10 g carbohydrate/kg body weight (15). Carbohydrate consumption as a percentage of total caloric intake for an endurance athlete should be at least 60% (52). For the several days prior to competition, the literature suggests increasing carbohydrate intake to approximately 70% of total energy intake. Supercompensating muscle glycogen stores by increasing carbohydrate intake and tapering training enhances performance when practiced several days prior to competition or prolonged exercise (31, 45).

Although glycogen loading regimens are considered effective for endurance athletes participating in events longer than 90 min, some research suggests that a similar loading regimen may improve performance in high-intensity, short-duration exercise. In a random crossover design, Pizza et al. (42) compared runners on a mixed diet (4.0 g/kg body weight) to those on a high-carbohydrate diet (8.2 g/kg body weight) consumed for several days prior to an exhaustive run at VO_2max. Subjects completed a 15-min submaximal treadmill run at 75% of VO_2max. Following a 5-min rest, the subjects ran a performance run to exhaustion at their VO_2max workload. Time to exhaustion on the performance run was longer (approximately 23 s) and carbohydrate oxidation greater following the high-carbohydrate diet.

Preexercise feedings of carbohydrate have also been suggested to affect performance, with the timing of intake and possibly the form of carbohydrate (e.g., glycemic index) as determining factors. Carbohydrate ingested 3–6 hr before exercise enhances performance (14, 27, 44) most likely by "topping off" liver and muscle glycogen stores and increasing glucose availability via the circulation. The literature contains mixed findings regarding carbohydrate ingested 30–60 min prior to exercise; it has been shown to improve performance (47), impair performance (22), and have no impact (23).

The glycemic index (GI) of carbohydrate-containing foods consumed prior to exercise has been suggested to affect performance by maintaining blood glucose levels (51). The GI of a food reflects the magnitude of the blood glucose rise following the ingestion of that food. Low-GI foods (e.g., lentils, milk, apples) may have potential benefits over high-GI foods (e.g., raisins, bagel, or banana) consumed 30–60 min prior to endurance exercise. The literature suggests that low-GI foods may increase fat oxidation and potentially spare glycogen by minimizing hypoglycemia that occurs at the start of exercise following consumption of high-GI carbohydrate (53).

An adequate carbohydrate intake is essential in repleting glycogen stores following prolonged exercise (4, 16). The literature suggests that a carbohydrate intake of 7–10 g/kg body weight within 24 hr after prolonged exercise normalizes muscle glycogen levels. Limited research has been performed that links this rapid normalization of glycogen stores following exercise to improved endurance capacity or exercise time to exhaustion. Fallowfield and Williams (21) reported improved endurance capacity 22.5 hr after a bout of prolonged exercise in runners consuming a high-carbohydrate diet (8.8 g/kg body weight) versus a mixed diet (5.8 g/kg body weight). Burke et al. (7) and others (53) have suggested that high-GI foods are more beneficial than low-GI foods following prolonged exercise, because high-GI foods enhance glycogen resynthesis. To date, however, research does not support the idea that consumption of high-GI foods following exercise provides a performance benefit over low-GI foods in subsequent endurance events.

Protein and Amino Acids

The lure of protein as a potential ergogenic aid has been documented for several decades. Initially, athletes turned to supplemental dietary protein to enhance muscle mass (33), and in the last 20 years they have focused on protein powders, isolates, and individual amino acid supplements (48). Many athletes look to protein to optimize body composition. For strength athletes such as football players, increased muscle mass may enhance strength and power. Runners and other endurance athletes, on the other hand, want to reduce body fat levels while maintaining lean body mass. Optimizing body composition, or lean body mass, requires sufficient energy and protein intake (36).

The literature suggests that both strength and endurance athletes' protein needs are greater than the Recommended Dietary Allowance (RDA), which is 0.8 g/kg body weight daily. Lemon (35, 36) and others (56) recommend an intake of 1.5–2.0 g/kg body weight daily for strength athletes. Since protein catabolism may account for 5 to 10% or more of the energy requirements during prolonged exercise, particularly if glycogen stores are low (37), endurance athletes are recommended to consume about 1.2–1.4 g/kg body weight daily provided energy intake is adequate (36).

These protein recommendations for both strength and endurance athletes are easily achieved through dietary intake of typical foods. Athletes are recommended to consume 12–15% of their total energy intake as protein. For a 70-kg runner consuming 14.7 MJ (3,500 kcal) daily, a protein intake of 105–131 g represents 12–15% of the total energy intake and translates to 1.5–1.9 g/kg body weight daily, well within the recommended range.

The ergogenic potential of individual amino acids to stimulate muscle growth, enhance strength, and perhaps delay fatigue is less clear and requires further exploration with well-controlled research studies. While several studies suggest that individual amino acid supplementation may stimulate protein synthesis and in turn enhance lean body mass gains and muscle strength by elevating human growth hormone and insulin secretion (6, 20), others do not support this effect (for review, see 34 and 36).

Supplementation of branched-chain amino acids (BCAA) during prolonged exercise has been hypothesized to delay fatigue (17). The theory is that an increased serum ratio of free tryptophan to BCAA may cause fatigue through increased production of the brain neurotransmitter serotonin. To date, several studies have shown that BCAA supplementation during exercise may delay fatigue (17), but further research is needed for a conclusive recommendation.

Dietary Antioxidants

Antioxidant nutrients including carotenes and vitamins C and E do not appear to directly affect exercise performance. Instead, these and other antioxidants may enhance performance indirectly by enhancing recovery from exercise; enhanced recovery comes from their ability to detoxify free radicals that are produced during strenuous exercise such as intense aerobic exercise or resistance training. There is growing evidence that free radicals mediate skeletal muscle damage, soreness, and/ or inflammation following strenuous exercise. As a result of increased oxygen use by mitochondria during exercise, lipid peroxidation increases. These peroxides, according to the literature, are then detoxified by dietary antioxidants, along with antioxidant enzymes (for review, see 13, 18, and 30). In theory, supplemental dietary antioxidants may reduce oxidative stress and skeletal muscle damage associated with strenuous exercise.

Several research studies suggest that supplemental dietary antioxidants, singularly and in combination, reduce indices of oxidative stress, such as lipid and protein peroxidation (18). One group of researchers who employed 5 months of vitamin E supplementation in competitive cyclists found reduced indices of oxidative stress compared to controls following a performance cycling test (43). In a recent study, runners who consumed an antioxidant-fortified (commercially available) food bar for several weeks experienced less oxidative stress following an exhaustive treadmill run compared to the control condition of an unfortified bar (9). In addition to elevated levels of circulating antioxidants, runners also experienced less lipid and protein oxidation. Also, low-density lipoprotein oxidation was reduced following fortified bar consumption. Such protection from oxidative damage may have implications for preventing or reducing the risk of chronic diseases such as vascular disease and cancer.

Several researchers and health professionals have recommended that athletes and active individuals would benefit from supplemental intake of dietary antioxidants (5). Some have made specific recommendations ranging from 600 to 3,000% RDA for vitamins C and E and beta carotene. While further studies are needed for specific recommendations for levels of dietary antioxidant intake, evidence thus far supports that supplemental intake protects against oxidative stress due to exercise and perhaps enhances recovery and minimizes muscle soreness.

Creatine

Currently one of the most popular ergogenic aids used by a wide variety of athletes, creatine has been reported to improve performance in certain exercise protocols (25, 50). In the muscle, creatine phosphate (CP) is necessary to maintain adenosine triphosphate (ATP) levels and thus support muscle contractions during high-intensity exercise. CP depletion has been implicated as a primary factor in fatigue during high-intensity exercise (11). In theory, then, increasing muscle levels of CP via supplementation may delay fatigue and enhance performance in exercise requiring force maintenance, but not during prolonged submaximal exercise.

Studies show that creatine supplementation of approximately 20–25 g/day for several days increases creatine levels in the skeletal muscle by 20% (28). Several studies show that following this brief period of supplementation, work output is increased in exercise protocols involving repeated bouts of short-duration activity such as maximal knee extensions, cycling ergometry, and repeated short treadmill runs (26, 40, 49). However, when protocols involve a single session of maximal-effort exercise, such as a swim or run sprint, creatine supplementation is not beneficial.

To date, few studies have focused on the impact of creatine supplementation on submaximal exercise lasting more than 5 min. In one study, performance time on a 6-km terrain run was impaired following creatine supplementation (3). As suggested by these authors, the longer running time may be a consequence of weight gain experienced by the runners while on creatine supplements. Several other researchers have reported increased body weight following several days of creatine supplementation (26, 50). Most speculate that the increase in body weight is due to greater water content of the muscles following creatine loading. More research is needed that involves longer periods of creatine supplementation to determine if creatine increases protein synthesis and lean body mass.

While anecdotal evidence suggests that muscle cramping and intestinal discomfort are possible side effects of creatine supplementation, published research does not support these effects. Additionally, "field" use of creatine supplementation is often in a cyclic pattern of loading—several days of creatine loading followed by several days of no supplementation. Research is needed to determine if this type of supplementation regimen enhances performance particularly during the periods without supplemental creatine. With the popularity of this ergogenic aid and the broad use of creatine, much more research is needed to determine effective doses, maintenance doses, and possible detrimental side effects. Athletes should also consider that creatine supplementation may be considered a violation of the IOC doping rule.

Sodium Bicarbonate

Athletes who engage in high-intensity exercise such as sprint cycling and swimming along with track events in the 400 to 800 m range are interested in ergogenic aids that buffer against lactic acid. Sodium bicarbonate, or baking soda, is a popular buffering agent. During near-maximal exercise efforts lasting more than approximately 60 s, muscles rely on the anaerobic breakdown of glucose to lactic acid. This metabolic by-product, however, increases muscular [H+]. One of the body's natural buffering agents is bicarbonate, which helps offset this drop in pH that contributes significantly to muscular fatigue. The drop in pH as a result of lactic acid accumulation is thought to inhibit the resynthesis of ATP as well as inhibit muscle contraction (29,30).

Bicarbonate loading (ingestion of sodium bicarbonate), in theory, would increase the body's capacity to buffer lactic acid, thereby delaying fatigue during high-intensity exercise. According to the literature, including a meta-analytical review (39), sodium bicarbonate is an effective ergogenic aid during exercise lasting approximately 1 to 7 min, particularly when repeated sprints or an interval-style exercise protocol is used. In those studies that measured time to exhaustion, performance was enhanced approximately 30% (39). Most studies indicate an effective dose of 300 mg/kg body weight taken 1 to 2 hr prior to high-intensity exercise (29, 38, 39). However, it is not clear whether the ergogenic benefit of sodium bicarbonate is a result of buffering or perhaps the sodium ion itself, which some suggest may be an ergogenic aid (32).

Athletes consume sodium bicarbonate as baking soda mixed with water or take gelatinlike capsules marketed as buffering agents. These sometimes contain other buffering agents such as sodium citrate and sodium phosphate. Athletes are encouraged not to exceed recommended dosages, because severe alkalosis may result. Additionally, side effects may occur such as gastrointestinal discomfort, bloating, and diarrhea, particularly if sufficient water (at least a liter) is not taken with the sodium bicarbonate. While sodium bicarbonate is not currently banned by the IOC, athletes should consider that bicarbonate loading may violate the IOC doping rule.

Caffeine

Perhaps because of caffeine's availability and social acceptance, it has become the most casually and widely used ergogenic aid by a wide variety of athletes ranging from elite competitors to weekend warriors. Caffeine occurs naturally in several foods, such as chocolate, coffee, and tea, and is added to others, such as soft drinks and medications. The ergogenic potential of caffeine has been noted for some time, and currently caffeine is on the IOC's list of restricted substances. Yet the legal limit of 12 μg/ml of urine allows athletes to consume caffeine without fear of disqualification. In fact, doses of caffeine of 3–9 mg/kg body weight enhance athletic performance without exceeding the "legal" limit (12, 24). Although generally thought to be of value in endurance events, caffeine has recently been suggested to improve anaerobic, high-intensity efforts.

Caffeine is theorized to improve performance in two ways. As a central nervous system stimulant, caffeine affects perception of effort, wards off drowsiness, and increases alertness. Most likely these effects involve stimulation of the sympathetic nervous system (41). Caffeine is also thought to improve performance through altering fuel utilization, specifically, increasing fat oxidation and reducing carbohydrate use. This effectively spares glycogen and helps delay fatigue during prolonged exercise sessions (24).

Well-controlled studies have demonstrated that 3–13 mg caffeine/kg body weight taken 1 hr prior to exercise improves endurance performance (12, 24) by prolonging time to exhaustion. Exercise protocols typically involve cycling or running at approximately 80% VO$_2$max. Although the ergogenic potential of caffeine has been demonstrated in laboratory settings, few well-controlled studies have assessed the effectiveness of caffeine in the field. Anecdotally, countless runners and other athletes, elite and recreational, ritualistically drink coffee or other caffeinated beverages prior to exercise.

Recently, caffeine has been touted as an ergogenic aid during high-intensity exercise. One study investigated the effect of a moderate caffeine dose on run time for a 1,500-m simulated race. Ingestion of caffeine improved run time and the speed of the "finishing burst" (54). The ability of caffeine to enhance short-term exercise performance does not appear to be related to glycogen sparing but perhaps is due to direct action on the muscle or the central nervous system (1).

More research is needed to establish if the ergogenic effect of caffeine is gender specific, because most studies have included only male subjects. Additionally, since caffeine also acts as a diuretic, hydration status following caffeine use should be explored more fully, particularly in older recreational athletes, on whom very few studies have been performed.

Summary

Athletes use several effective nutritional ergogenic aids to enhance performance. Included in this discussion are standard dietary constituents, such as carbohydrate and protein along with atypical dietary aids such as bicarbonate and creatine. Use of these nutritional ergogenic aids has proven effective under certain conditions. In the search for a competitive edge, however, athletes and coaches must consider both ethical and legal issues when using a substance in abnormal quantities with the expressed intent to improve performance. Additionally, one must consider safety issues surrounding use of dietary ergogenic aids. Insufficient research exists on the safety of many of theses dietary aids.

References

1. Anselme, F., K. Collomp, B. Mercier, S. Ahmaidi, and C. Prefaut. Caffeine increases maximal anaerobic power and blood lactate concentration. *Eur. J. Appl. Physiol.* 65:188-191, 1992.
2. Applegate, E.A., and L.E. Grivetti. Search for the competitive edge: A history of dietary fads and supplements. *J. Nutr.* 127:869S-873S, 1997.
3. Balsom, P.D., S.D.R. Harridge, K. Soderlund, B. Sjodin, and B. Ekblom. Creatine supplementation per se does not enhance endurance exercise performance. *Acta Physiol. Scand.* 149:521-523, 1993.
4. Bergstrom, J., L. Hermansen, E. Hultman, and B. Saltin. Diet, muscle glycogen and physical performance. *Acta Physiol. Scand.* 71:140-150, 1967.
5. Brainin-Rodriquez, L. Antioxidants and exercise: Do they affect recovery and performance? *SCAN Pulse Newsletter* 13:3-5, 1994.
6. Bucci, L., J.F. Hickson, J.M. Pivarnik, I. Wolinsky, and J.C. McMahon. Ornithine ingestion and growth hormone release in body builders. *Nutr. Res.* 10:239-245, 1990.
7. Burke, L.M., M. Hargreaves, and G.R. Collier. Muscle glycogen storage after prolonged exercise: Effect of the glycemic index of carbohydrate feedings. *J. Appl. Physiol.* 74:1019-1023, 1993.
8. Butterfield, G. Ergogenic aids: Evaluating sport nutrition products. *Int. J. Sport Nutr.* 6:191-197, 1996.
9. Camplen, L.M., K.L. Olin, H.H. Schmitz, E.A. Applegate, J.B. German, D. Pearson, J.D. Shaffrath, C. Emenhiser, S.J. Schwartz, M.E. Gershwin, and C.L. Keen. Nutritional status during strenuous exercise and training: Changes in plasma micronutrient concentrations and indices of oxidative stress after chronic supplementation with a fortified energy bar in healthy males. *J. Am. Diet. Assoc.* In press.
10. Christensen, E.H., and O. Hansen. Respiratorischen quitient und O2-aufnahme. *Skandinavisches Archiv. Fur Physiolgie* 81:180-189, 1939.
11. Clark, J.F. Creatine and phosphocreatine: A review of their use in exercise and sport. *J. Athl. Train.* 32:45-50, 1997.

12. Clarkson, P.M. Nutritional ergogenic aids: Caffeine. *Int. J. Sport Nutr.* 3:103-111, 1993.
13. Clarkson, P.M. Antioxidants and physical performance. *Critical Rev. Food Sci. Nutr.* 35:131-141, 1995.
14. Coggan, A.R., and S.C. Swanson. Nutritional manipulations before and during endurance exercise: Effects on performance. *Med. Sci. Sports Exerc.* 24:S331-S335, 1992.
15. Costill, D.L. Carbohydrates for exercise: Dietary demands for optimal performance. *Int. J. Sports Med.* 9:1-18, 1988.
16. Costill, D.L., W.M. Sherman, W.J. Fink, C. Maresh, M. Witten, and J.M. Miller. The role of dietary carbohydrates in muscle glycogen resynthesis after strenuous running. *Am. J. Clin. Nutr.* 35:1831-1836, 1981.
17. Davis, J.M., and S.P. Bailey. Possible mechanisms of central nervous system fatigue during exercise. *Med. Sci. Sports Exerc.* 29:45-57, 1997.
18. Dekkers, J.C., L.J.P. vanDooren, and H.C.G. Kemper. The role of antioxidant vitamins and enzymes in the prevention of exercise-induced muscle damage. *Sports Med.* 21:213-238, 1996.
19. Eichner, E.R. Ergogenic aids: What athletes are using—and why. *Physician Sportsmed.* 25:70-83, 1997.
20. Elam, R.P., D.H. Hardin, R.A.L. Sutton, and L. Hagen. Effects of arginine and ornithine on strength, lean body mass and urinary hydroxyproline in adult males. *J. Sports Med. Phys. Fit.* 28:35-39, 1988.
21. Fallowfield, J.L., and C. Williams. Carbohydrate intake and recovery from prolonged exercise. *Int. J. Sports Nutr.* 3:150-164, 1993.
22. Foster, C., D.L. Costill, and W.J. Fink. Effects of preexercise feedings on endurance performance. *Med. Sci. Sports* 11:1-5, 1979.
23. Glesson, M., R.J. Maughan, and P.L. Greenhaff. Comparison of the effects of pre-exercise feeding of glucose, glycerol, and placebo on endurance and fuel homeostasis in man. *Eur. J. Appl. Physiol.* 55:6645-6653, 1986.
24. Graham, T.E., and L.L. Spriet. Caffeine and exercise performance. *Gatorade Sports Science Exchange* 9(1), 1996.
25. Greenhaff, P.L. Creatine and its application as an ergogenic aid. *Int. J. Sport Nutr.* 5:S100-S110, 1995.
26. Greenhaff, P.L., K. Bodin, K. Soderlund, and E. Hultman. Effect of oral creatine supplementation on skeletal muscle phosphocreatine resynthesis. *Am. J. Physiol.* 266:E725-E730, 1994.
27. Hargreaves, M., D.L. Costill, W.J. Fink, D.S. King, and R.A. Fielding. Effect of pre-exercise carbohydrate feedings on endurance cycling performance. *Med. Sci Sports Exerc.* 19:33-36, 1987.
28. Harris, R., K. Soderlund, and E. Hultman. Elevation of creatine in resting and exercised muscle of normal subjects by creatine supplementation. *Clin. Sci.* 83:367-374, 1992.
29. Horswill, C.A. Effects of bicarbonate, citrate, and phosphate loading on performance. *Int. J. Sport Nutr.* 5:S111-S119, 1995.
30. Kanter, M.M., and M.H. Williams. Antioxidants, carnitine, and choline as putative ergogenic aids. *Int. J. Sport Nutr.* 5:S120-S131, 1995.
31. Karlsson, J., and B. Saltin. Diet, muscle glycogen and endurance performance. *J. Appl. Physiol.* 31:203-206, 1971.
32. Kozak-Collins, K., E.R. Burke, and R.B. Schoene. Sodium bicarbonate ingestion does not improve performance in women cyclists. *Med. Sci. Sports Exerc.* 26:1510-1515, 1994.

33. Kraut, H., E.A. Müller, and H. Müller-Wecker. Die abhangigkeit des muskeitrainings und eiweissbestand des korpers. *Biochem. Z.* 324:280-294, 1953.
34. Kreider, R.B., V. Miriel, and E. Bertun. Amino acid supplementation and exercise performance. *Sports Med.* 16:190-209, 1993.
35. Lemon, P.W.R. Effect of exercise on protein requirements. *J. Sports Sci.* 9:53-70, 1991.
36. Lemon, P.W.R. Protein and amino acid needs of the strength athlete. *Int. J. Sport Nutr.* 1:127-145, 1991.
37. Lemon, P.W.R. and J. Mullin. Effect of initial muscle glycogen levels on protein catabolism during exercise. *J. Appl. Physiol.* 48:624-629, 1980.
38. Linderman, J.K., and K.L. Gosselink. The effects of sodium bicarbonate ingestion on exercise performance. *Sports Med.* 18:75-80, 1994.
39. Matson, L.G., and Z.V. Tran. Effects of sodium bicarbonate ingestion on anaerobic performance: A meta-analytic review. *Int. J. Sport Nutr.* 3:2-28, 1993.
40. Maughan, R.J. Creatine supplementation and exercise performance. *Int. J. Sport Nutr.* 5:94-101, 1995.
41. Nehlig, A., and G. Debry. Caffeine and sports activity: A review. *Int. J. Sports Med.* 15:215-223, 1994.
42. Pizza, F.X., M.G. Flynn, B.D. Duscha, J. Holden, and E.R. Kubitz. A carbohydrate loading regimen improves high intensity, short duration exercise performance. *Int. J. Sport Nutr.* 5:110-116, 1995.
43. Rokitzki, L., E. Logemann, G. Huber, E. Keck, and J. Kuel. Alpha-tocopherol supplementation in racing cyclists during extreme endurance training. *Int. J. Sport Nutr.* 4:253-264, 1994.
44. Sherman, W.M., G. Brodowicz, D.A. Wright, W.K. Allen, J. Simonsen, and A. Dernbach. Effects of 4 h pre-exercise carbohydrate feedings on cycling performance. *Med. Sci. Sports Exerc.* 21:598-604, 1989.
45. Sherman, W.M., D.L. Costill, W.J. Fink, and J.M. Miller. The effect of exercise and diet manipulation on muscle glycogen and its subsequent use during performance. *Int. J. Sports Med.* 2:114-118, 1981.
46. Sherman, W.M., and D.R. Lamb. Introduction to ergogenic aids supplement. *Int. J. Sport Nutr.* 5:Siii-Siv, 1995.
47. Sherman, W.M., M.C. Peden, and D.A. Wright. Carbohydrate feedings 1 h before exercise improve cycling performance. *Am. J. Clin. Nutr.* 54:866-870, 1991.
48. Short, S.H., and L.F. Marquart. Sports nutrition fraud. *N.Y. State J. Med.* 93:112-116, 1993.
49. Volek, J.S. Creatine supplementation and its possible role in improving physical performance. *ACSM's Health Fit. J.* 1(4):23-29, 1997.
50. Volek, J.S., W.J. Kraemer, J.A. Bush, M. Boetes, T. Incledon, K.L. Clark, and J.M. Lynch. Creatine supplementation enhances muscular performance during high-intensity resistance exercise. *J. Am. Diet. Assoc.* 97:765-770, 1997.
51. Walberg-Rankin, J. Glycemic index and exercise metabolism. *Gatorade Sports Science Exchange* 10(1), 1997.
52. Walberg-Rankin, J. Dietary carbohydrate as an ergogenic aid for prolonged and brief competitions in sport. *Int. J. Sport Nutr.* 5:S13-S28, 1995.
53. Walton, P., and E.C. Rhodes. Glycemic index and optimal performance. *Sports Med.* 23:164-172, 1997.
54. Wiles, J.D., S.R. Bird, J. Hopkins, and M. Riley. Effect of caffeinated coffee on running speed, respiratory factors, blood lactate and perceived exertion during 1500-m treadmill running. *Br. J. Sport Med.* 26:116-120, 1992.

55. Williams, M.H. Nutritional ergogenics in athletics. *J. Sports Med.* 13:S63-S74, 1995.
56. Williams, M.H. Nutritional supplements for strength trained athletes. *Gatorade Sports Science Exchange* 6(6), 1993.
57. Williams, M.H. The use of nutritional ergogenic aids in sports: Is it an ethical issue? *Int. J. Sport Nutr.* 4:120-131, 1994.

Manuscript received: November 17, 1997
Accepted for publication: March 24, 1998

Wander Award on Biochemistry of Exercise

Honour Award on Biochemistry of Exercise

The Wander Award, presented every 3 years by Isostar Sport Nutrition Foundation and the Research Group on Biochemistry of Exercise (ICSSPE-UNESCO), is given in recognition of the best study (in English) on (a) muscle energy metabolism and exercise or (b) sports and nutrition. Potential participants are currently invited to submit unpublished papers or those published between January 1, 1997 and June 30, 1999. For a subscription form, contact the Isostar Sport Nutrition Foundation, Attention: Rien Peeters, P.O. Box 1350, NL-6201 BJ Maastricht, The Netherlands (Fax: +31 43 367 06 76; E-mail: ISNF@novartis.unimass.nl).

The Honour Award, also presented every 3 years by ICSSPE-UNESCO, is designed to honor a scientist who had made substantial contributions to the development of research on the biochemistry and nutrition of exercise. Nominations must be submitted by December 31, 1999. Candidates can be nominated by writing to Martina Brouns, P.O. Box 1350, NL-6201 BJ Maastricht, The Netherlands (Fax: +31 43 367 06 76; E-mail: M.Brouns@novartis.unimass.nl).

The 2000 Awards will be presented during the 11th International Biochemistry of Exercise Conference in Little Rock, AK, June 3-7, 2000.

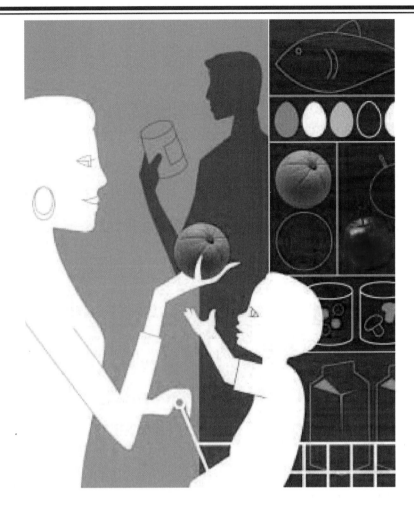

Finding Your Way to a Healthier You:

Based on the
*Dietary Guidelines
for Americans*

U.S. Department of Health and Human Services
U.S. Department of Agriculture
www.healthierus.gov/dietaryguidelines

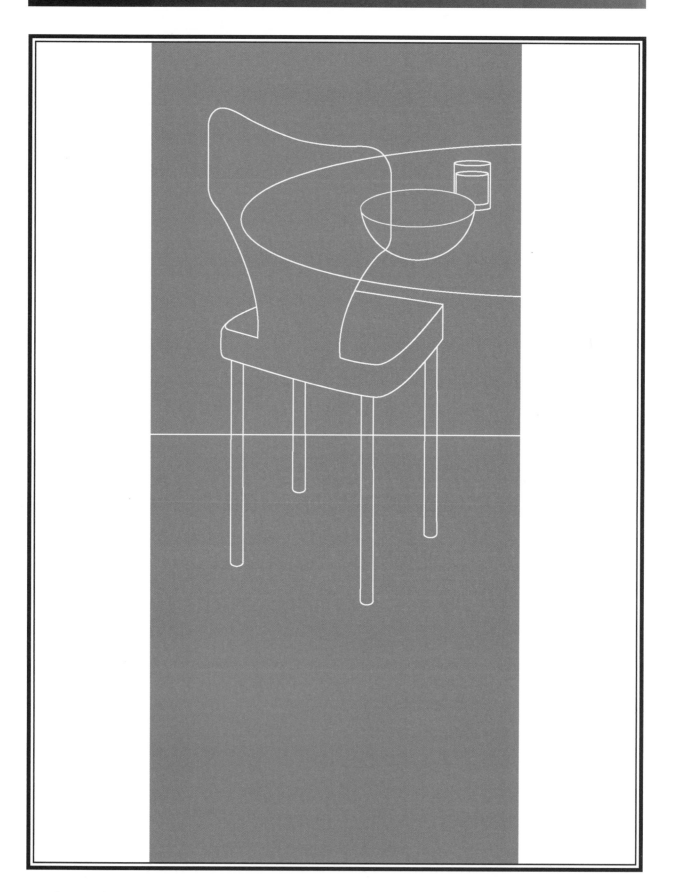

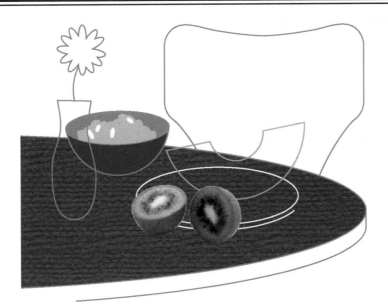

Feel better today.
Stay healthy for tomorrow.

Here's how: The food and physical activity choices you make every day affect your health—how you feel today, tomorrow, and in the future. The science-based advice of the *Dietary Guidelines for Americans,* 2005 in this booklet highlights how to:

- Make smart choices from every food group.
- Find your balance between food and physical activity.
- Get the most nutrition out of your calories.

You may be eating plenty of food, but not eating the right foods that give your body the nutrients you need to be healthy. You may not be getting enough physical activity to stay fit and burn those extra calories. This booklet is a starting point for finding your way to a healthier you.

Eating right and being physically active aren't just a "diet" or a "program"—they are keys to a healthy lifestyle. With healthful habits, you may reduce your risk of many chronic diseases such as heart disease, diabetes, osteoporosis, and certain cancers, and increase your chances for a longer life.

The sooner you start, the better for you, your family, and your future. Find more specific information at www.healthierus.gov/dietaryguidelines.

Make smart choices from every food group.

The best way to give your body the balanced nutrition it needs is by eating a variety of nutrient-packed foods every day. Just be sure to stay within your daily calorie needs.

A healthy eating plan is one that:
- Emphasizes fruits, vegetables, whole grains, and fat-free or low-fat milk and milk products.
- Includes lean meats, poultry, fish, beans, eggs, and nuts.
- Is low in saturated fats, *trans* fats, cholesterol, salt (sodium), and added sugars.

DON'T GIVE IN WHEN YOU EAT OUT AND ARE ON THE GO

It's important to make smart food choices and watch portion sizes wherever you are—at the grocery store, at work, in your favorite restaurant, or running errands. Try these tips:

- At the store, plan ahead by buying a variety of nutrient-rich foods for meals and snacks throughout the week.
- When grabbing lunch, have a sandwich on whole-grain bread and choose low-fat/fat-free milk, water, or other drinks without added sugars.
- In a restaurant, opt for steamed, grilled, or broiled dishes instead of those that are fried or sautéed.
- On a long commute or shopping trip, pack some fresh fruit, cut-up vegetables, string cheese sticks, or a handful of unsalted nuts—to help you avoid impulsive, less healthful snack choices.

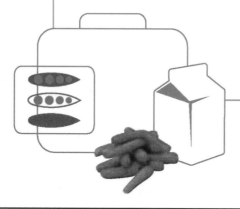

Mix up your choices within each food group.

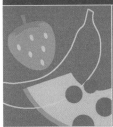

Focus on fruits. Eat a variety of fruits—whether fresh, frozen, canned, or dried—rather than fruit juice for most of your fruit choices. For a 2,000-calorie diet, you will need 2 cups of fruit each day (for example, 1 small banana, 1 large orange, and ¼ cup of dried apricots or peaches).

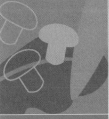

Vary your veggies. Eat more dark green veggies, such as broccoli, kale, and other dark leafy greens; orange veggies, such as carrots, sweetpotatoes, pumpkin, and winter squash; and beans and peas, such as pinto beans, kidney beans, black beans, garbanzo beans, split peas, and lentils.

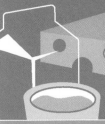

Get your calcium-rich foods. Get 3 cups of low-fat or fat-free milk—or an equivalent amount of low-fat yogurt and/or low-fat cheese (1½ ounces of cheese equals 1 cup of milk)—every day. For kids aged 2 to 8, it's 2 cups of milk. If you don't or can't consume milk, choose lactose-free milk products and/or calcium-fortified foods and beverages.

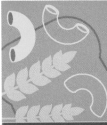

Make half your grains whole. Eat at least 3 ounces of whole-grain cereals, breads, crackers, rice, or pasta every day. One ounce is about 1 slice of bread, 1 cup of breakfast cereal, or ½ cup of cooked rice or pasta. Look to see that grains such as wheat, rice, oats, or corn are referred to as "whole" in the list of ingredients.

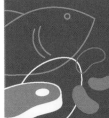

Go lean with protein. Choose lean meats and poultry. Bake it, broil it, or grill it. And vary your protein choices—with more fish, beans, peas, nuts, and seeds.

Know the limits on fats, salt, and sugars. Read the Nutrition Facts label on foods. Look for foods low in saturated fats and *trans* fats. Choose and prepare foods and beverages with little salt (sodium) and/or added sugars (caloric sweeteners).

Find your balance between food and physical activity.

Becoming a healthier you isn't just about eating healthy—it's also about physical activity. Regular physical activity is important for your overall health and fitness. It also helps you control body weight by balancing the calories you take in as food with the calories you expend each day.

- Be physically active for at least 30 minutes most days of the week.
- Increasing the intensity or the amount of time that you are physically active can have even greater health benefits and may be needed to control body weight. About 60 minutes a day may be needed to prevent weight gain.
- Children and teenagers should be physically active for 60 minutes every day, or most every day.

CONSIDER THIS:

If you eat 100 more food calories a day than you burn, you'll gain about 1 pound in a month. That's about 10 pounds in a year. The bottom line is that to lose weight, it's important to reduce calories and increase physical activity.

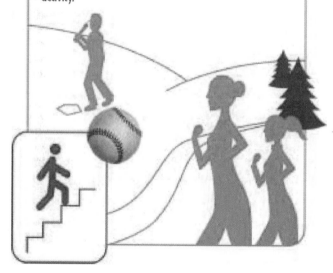

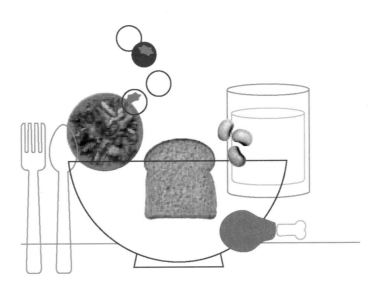

Get the most nutrition out of your calories.

There is a right number of calories for you to eat each day. This number depends on your age, activity level, and whether you're trying to gain, maintain, or lose weight.* You could use up the entire amount on a few high-calorie items, but chances are you won't get the full range of vitamins and nutrients your body needs to be healthy.

Choose the most nutritionally rich foods you can from each food group each day—those packed with vitamins, minerals, fiber, and other nutrients but lower in calories. Pick foods like fruits, vegetables, whole grains, and fat-free or low-fat milk and milk products more often.

* 2,000 calories is the value used as a general reference on the food label. But you can calculate your number at www.healthierus.gov/dietaryguidelines.

NUTRITION:
To know the facts...

Most packaged foods have a Nutrition Facts label. For a healthier you, use this tool to make smart food choices quickly and easily. Try these tips:

- Keep these low: saturated fats, *trans* fats, cholesterol, and sodium.
- Get enough of these: potassium, fiber, vitamins A and C, calcium, and iron.
- Use the % Daily Value (DV) column when possible: 5% DV or less is low, 20% DV or more is high.

Check servings and calories. Look at the serving size and how many servings you are actually consuming. If you double the servings you eat, you double the calories and nutrients, including the % DVs.

Make your calories count. Look at the calories on the label and compare them with what nutrients you are also getting to decide whether the food is worth eating. When one serving of a single food item has over 400 calories per serving, it is high in calories.

Don't sugarcoat it. Since sugars contribute calories with few, if any, nutrients, look for foods and beverages low in added sugars. Read the ingredient list and make sure that added sugars are not one of the first few ingredients. Some names for added sugars (caloric sweeteners) include sucrose, glucose, high fructose corn syrup, corn syrup, maple syrup, and fructose.

Know your fats. Look for foods low in saturated fats, *trans* fats, and cholesterol to help reduce the risk of heart disease (5% DV or less is low, 20% DV or more is high). Most of the fats you eat should be polyunsaturated and monounsaturated fats. Keep total fat intake between 20% to 35% of calories.

Reduce sodium (salt), increase potassium. Research shows that eating less than 2,300 milligrams of sodium (about 1 tsp of salt) per day may reduce the risk of high blood pressure. Most of the sodium people eat comes from processed foods, not from the saltshaker. Also look for foods high in potassium, which counteracts some of sodium's effects on blood pressure.

...use the label.

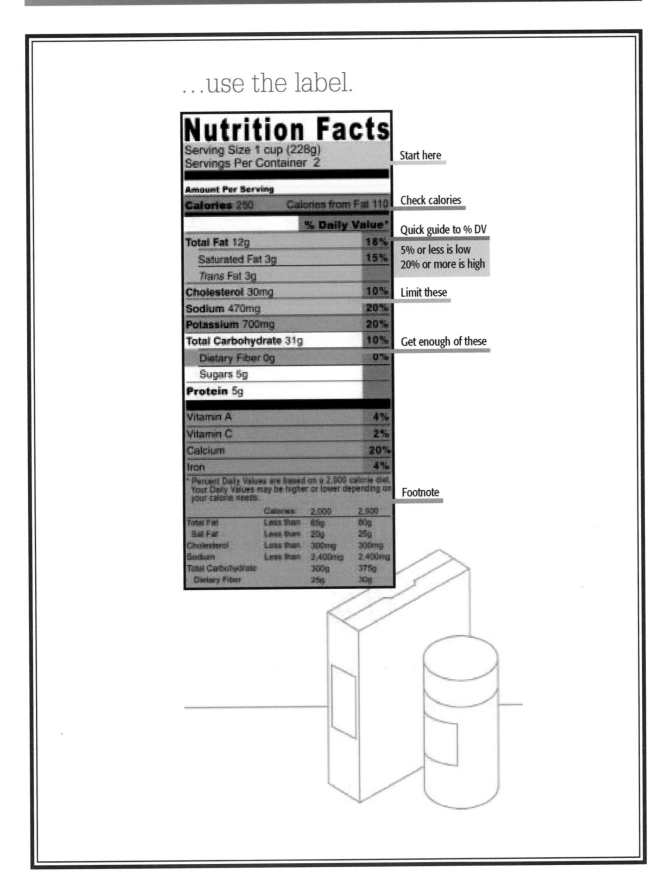

Nutrition Facts

Serving Size 1 cup (228g)
Servings Per Container 2

Start here

Amount Per Serving

Calories 250   Calories from Fat 110

Check calories

	% Daily Value*
Total Fat 12g	**18%**
Saturated Fat 3g	**15%**
Trans Fat 3g	
Cholesterol 30mg	**10%**
Sodium 470mg	**20%**
Potassium 700mg	**20%**
Total Carbohydrate 31g	**10%**
Dietary Fiber 0g	**0%**
Sugars 5g	
Protein 5g	
Vitamin A	**4%**
Vitamin C	**2%**
Calcium	**20%**
Iron	**4%**

Quick guide to % DV

5% or less is low
20% or more is high

Limit these

Get enough of these

* Percent Daily Values are based on a 2,000 calorie diet. Your Daily Values may be higher or lower depending on your calorie needs.

Footnote

	Calories:	2,000	2,500
Total Fat	Less than	65g	80g
Sat Fat	Less than	20g	25g
Cholesterol	Less than	300mg	300mg
Sodium	Less than	2,400mg	2,400mg
Total Carbohydrate		300g	375g
Dietary Fiber		25g	30g

Play it safe with food.

Know how to prepare, handle, and store food safely to keep you and your family safe:

- Clean hands, food-contact surfaces, fruits, and vegetables. To avoid spreading bacteria to other foods, meat and poultry should *not* be washed or rinsed.
- Separate raw, cooked, and ready-to-eat foods while shopping, preparing, or storing.
- Cook meat, poultry, and fish to safe internal temperatures to kill microorganisms.
- Chill perishable foods promptly and thaw foods properly.

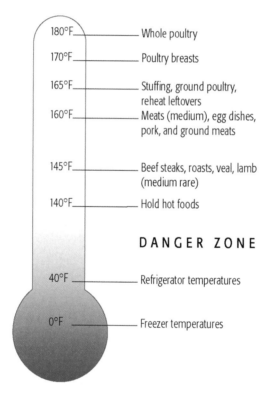

180°F	Whole poultry
170°F	Poultry breasts
165°F	Stuffing, ground poultry, reheat leftovers
160°F	Meats (medium), egg dishes, pork, and ground meats
145°F	Beef steaks, roasts, veal, lamb (medium rare)
140°F	Hold hot foods
	DANGER ZONE
40°F	Refrigerator temperatures
0°F	Freezer temperatures

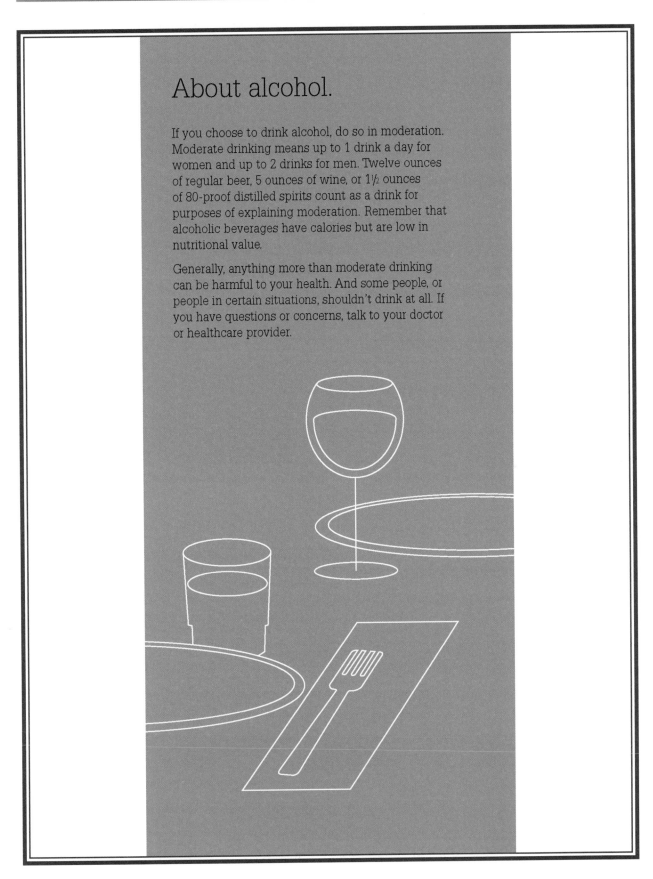

About alcohol.

If you choose to drink alcohol, do so in moderation. Moderate drinking means up to 1 drink a day for women and up to 2 drinks for men. Twelve ounces of regular beer, 5 ounces of wine, or 1½ ounces of 80-proof distilled spirits count as a drink for purposes of explaining moderation. Remember that alcoholic beverages have calories but are low in nutritional value.

Generally, anything more than moderate drinking can be harmful to your health. And some people, or people in certain situations, shouldn't drink at all. If you have questions or concerns, talk to your doctor or healthcare provider.

These are the basic guidelines for eating a healthy diet and being physically active. For more information about the food groups and nutrition values, or to pick up some new ideas on physical activity, go to www.healthierus.gov/dietaryguidelines.

This booklet, as well as *Dietary Guidelines for Americans, 2005,* 6th Edition, may be viewed and downloaded from the Internet at www.healthierus.gov/dietaryguidelines.

To purchase single printed copies of this booklet, call the Federal Citizen Information Center toll-free at (888) 878-3256. To purchase bulk copies, 100 copies per pack (Stock Number 001-000-04718-3), call the U.S. Government Printing Office toll-free at (866) 512-1800, or access the GPO Online Bookstore at http://bookstore.gpo.gov.

To purchase printed copies of the complete 80-page *Dietary Guidelines for Americans,* 2005 (Stock Number 001-000-04719-1), call the U.S. Government Printing Office at (866) 512-1800, or access the GPO Online Bookstore at http://bookstore.gpo.gov.

  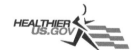

HHS Publication number: HHS-ODPHP-2005-01-DGA-B

USDA Publication number: Home and Garden Bulletin No. 232-CP

MyPyramid Worksheet

Check how you did today and set a goal to aim for tomorrow

MyPyramid.gov
STEPS TO A HEALTHIER YOU

Food Group	Tip	Goal Based on a 1400 calorie pattern.	List each food choice in its food group*	Estimate Your Total
GRAINS	Make at least half your grains whole grains	**5 ounce equivalents** (1 ounce equivalent is about 1 slice bread, 1 cup dry cereal, or ½ cup cooked rice, pasta, or cereal)		ounce equivalents
VEGETABLES	Try to have vegetables from several subgroups each day	**1 ½ cups** Subgroups: Dark Green, Orange, Starchy, Dry Beans and Peas, Other Veggies		cups
FRUITS	Make most choices fruit, not juice	**1 ½ cups**		cups
MILK	Choose fat-free or low fat most often	**2 cups** (1 ½ ounces cheese = 1 cup milk)		cups
MEAT & BEANS	Choose lean meat and poultry. Vary your choices—more fish, beans, peas, nuts, and seeds	**4 ounce equivalents** (1 ounce equivalent is 1 ounce meat, poultry, or fish, 1 egg, 1 T. peanut butter, ½ ounce nuts, or ¼ cup dry beans)		ounce equivalents
PHYSICAL ACTIVITY	Build more physical activity into your daily routine at home and work.	At least **30 minutes** of moderate to vigorous activity a day, 10 minutes or more at a time.	*Some foods don't fit into any group. These "extras" may be mainly fat or sugar—limit your intake of these.	minutes

Write in Your Choices for Today

How did you do today? ☐ Great ☐ So-So ☐ Not so Great

My food goal for tomorrow is:

My activity goal for tomorrow is:

MyPyramid Worksheet

Check how you did today and set a goal to aim for tomorrow

Food Group	Tip	Goal Based on a 1800 calorie pattern.	List each food choice in its food group*	Estimate Your Total
GRAINS	Make at least half your grains whole grains	**6 ounce equivalents** (1 ounce equivalent is about 1 slice bread, 1 cup dry cereal, or ½ cup cooked rice, pasta, or cereal)		_____ ounce equivalents
VEGETABLES	Try to have vegetables from several subgroups each day	**2 ½ cups** Subgroups: Dark Green, Orange, Starchy, Dry Beans and Peas, Other Veggies		_____ cups
FRUITS	Make most choices fruit, not juice	**1 ½ cups**		_____ cups
MILK	Choose fat-free or low fat most often	**3 cups** (1 ½ ounces cheese = 1 cup milk)		_____ cups
MEAT & BEANS	Choose lean meat and poultry. Vary your choices—more fish, beans, peas, nuts, and seeds	**5 ounce equivalents** (1 ounce equivalent is 1 ounce meat, poultry, or fish, 1 egg, 1 T. peanut butter, ½ ounce nuts, or ¼ cup dry beans)		_____ ounce equivalents
PHYSICAL ACTIVITY	Build more physical activity into your daily routine at home and work.	At least **30 minutes** of moderate to vigorous activity a day. 10 minutes or more at a time.		_____ minutes

*Some foods don't fit into any group. These "extras" may be mainly fat or sugar—limit your intake of these.

Write in Your Choices for Today

How did you do today? ☐ Great ☐ So-So ☐ Not so Great

My food goal for tomorrow is: _____

My activity goal for tomorrow is: _____

MyPyramid.gov
STEPS TO A HEALTHIER YOU

MyPyramid Worksheet

Check how you did today and set a goal to aim for tomorrow

MyPyramid.gov
STEPS TO A HEALTHIER YOU

Write in Your Choices for Today	Food Group	Tip	Goal Based on a 2000 calorie pattern.	List each food choice in its food group*	Estimate Your Total
	GRAINS	Make at least half your grains whole grains	**6 ounce equivalents** (1 ounce equivalent is about 1 slice bread, 1 cup dry cereal, or ½ cup cooked rice, pasta, or cereal)		ounce equivalents
	VEGETABLES	Try to have vegetables from several subgroups each day	**2 ½ cups** Subgroups: Dark Green, Orange, Starchy, Dry Beans and Peas, Other Veggies		cups
	FRUITS	Make most choices fruit, not juice	**2 cups**		cups
	MILK	Choose fat-free or low fat most often	**3 cups** (1 ½ ounces cheese = 1 cup milk)		cups
	MEAT & BEANS	Choose lean meat and poultry. Vary your choices—more fish, beans, peas, nuts, and seeds	**5 ½ ounce equivalents** (1 ounce equivalent is 1 ounce meat, poultry, or fish, 1 egg, 1 T. peanut butter, ½ ounce nuts, or ¼ cup dry beans)		ounce equivalents
	PHYSICAL ACTIVITY	Build more physical activity into your daily routine at home and work.	At least **30 minutes** of moderate to vigorous activity a day, 10 minutes or more at a time.	*Some foods don't fit into any group. These "extras" may be mainly fat or sugar—limit your intake of these.	minutes

How did you do today? ☐ Great   ☐ So-So   ☐ Not so Great

My food goal for tomorrow is: _____

My activity goal for tomorrow is: _____

MyPyramid Worksheet

Check how you did today and set a goal to aim for tomorrow

Food Group	Tip	Goal Based on a 2400 calorie pattern.	List each food choice in its food group*	Estimate Your Total
GRAINS	Make at least half your grains whole grains	**8 ounce equivalents** (1 ounce equivalent is about 1 slice bread, 1 cup dry cereal, or ½ cup cooked rice, pasta, or cereal)	_____ _____ _____ _____	_____ ounce equivalents
VEGETABLES	Try to have vegetables from several subgroups each day	**3 cups** Subgroups: Dark Green, Orange, Starchy, Dry Beans and Peas, Other Veggies	_____ _____ _____	_____ cups
FRUITS	Make most choices fruit, not juice	**2 cups**	_____ _____	_____ cups
MILK	Choose fat-free or low fat most often	**3 cups** (1 ½ ounces cheese = 1 cup milk)	_____ _____	_____ cups
MEAT & BEANS	Choose lean meat and poultry. Vary your choices—more fish, beans, peas, nuts, and seeds	**6 ½ ounce equivalents** (1 ounce equivalent is 1 ounce meat, poultry, or fish, 1 egg, 1 T. peanut butter, ½ ounce nuts, or ¼ cup dry beans)	_____ _____ _____	_____ ounce equivalents
PHYSICAL ACTIVITY	Build more physical activity into your daily routine at home and work.	At least **30 minutes** of moderate to vigorous activity a day, 10 minutes or more at a time.	*Some foods don't fit into any group. These "extras" may be mainly fat or sugar—limit your intake of these.	_____ minutes

Write in Your Choices for Today

How did you do today? ☐ Great ☐ So-So ☐ Not so Great

My food goal for tomorrow is: _____

My activity goal for tomorrow is: _____

MyPyramid.gov
STEPS TO A HEALTHIER YOU

Web Site References

Center for Nutrition Policy and Promotion, USDA
www.usda.gov/cnpp

Food and Nutrition Information Center
www.fns.usda.gov/fns

Healthfinder®—Gateway to Reliable Consumer Health Information
www.healthfinder.gov

American Institute for Cancer Research
www.aicr.gov

National Heart, Lung, and Blood Institute Information Center
www.nhlbi.nih.gov

National Institute of Diabetes and Digestive and Kidney Diseases
www.niddk.nih.gov

National Institute on Alcohol Abuse and Alcoholism
www.niaaa.nih.gov

Berkeley Wellness Letter
www.berkeleywellness.com

Food and Drug Administration
www.fda.gov

Centers for Disease Control and Prevention
www.cdc.gov

Anorexia Nervosa and Related Eating Disorders, Inc.
www.anred.com

American Council on Exercise (ACE)
www.acefitness.org

American College of Sports Medicine (ACSM)
www.acsm.org

Coalition for a Healthy and Active America
www.chaausa.org

WebMD
www.webmd.com

CNN Health
www.cnn.com/HEALTH/

Index

amylase, 77f
android obesity, 168
anemia, 206, 210, 233, 234
  hemolytic, 248
anorexia nervosa
  malnutrition and, 187
  nutritional problems with, 187–188
  symptoms of, 186
antioxidants, 238–239, 265
  beta-carotene, 243f, 244, 265
  cancer risk and, 265
  honey, 72
  vitamin C, 238–241
  vitamin E, 247–249
arcuate nucleus (ARC), 175
arteries, normal, 142f
artery walls, 142
  lipoproteins and, 149
ascorbic acid, 238–241
Asians
  alcohol and, 260
  mineral content in, 192
  aspirin, 110
atherosclerosis, 143f
athletes, body fat in, 3–4, 4f

B

bacteria, 242
  vitamin K produced by, 250
barley, 236, 257
Basal Metabolic Rate (BMR), 56, 182
  activity profile as percentage of, 59–60
  age and, 58
  calculating, 60–61
  computing calorie costs of, 57–58
  exercise and, 58
  fasting and, 58
  in females, 57–58
  in males, 57–58
  supplements and, 59
beef protein, 17–18, 17f, 18
beer, 257, 301f

behavior modification, 180
  cognitive restructuring, 182
  of eating patterns, 181–182
  environmental cues and, 182
beriberi, 227–228
beta-carotene, 243f, 244, 265
bile, 121, 121f
  cholesterol as precursor to, 132
binge eating, 187
bioavailability, 193–194, 194f
  calcium, 199
  iron, 207–209
  nutrient requirements and, 194
  potassium, 203
  sodium, 203
  zinc, 212
bioelectrical impedance fat measurement, 164
birth defects, vitamin A and, 244–245
blindness, 215, 242
bloating, 79
  olestra and, 119
blood, 10
  alcohol levels, 259
  cells, 2, 94
  high cholesterol in, 148–149, 169
  protein, 14
  sugar levels in, 6
  vessels, 19, 24, 81
body
  cholesterol sources in, 134
  composition, 258
  fluids, 6
  hair, 2
  how it copes, 6–7
  mass index, 164–166, 165f, 166f, 167f, 292f
  protein content of, 19
  temperature, 6
body fat, 3, 164, 166–169
  alcohol and, 258
  athletes and, 3–4, 4f
  distribution, 166–169
  visceral, 168, 169f

Body Mass Index (BMI), 164–166, 165f, 166f, 167f, 292f
body proteins, turnover rate of, 26f
body water, 3, 6, 6f, 202f
  alcohol and, 258
  content, 6
body weight, 6
  desirable, 163–164
  healthy, 162–163
bolus, 7
bomb calorimeter, 51–52, 51f
bone(s), 2, 3, 4, 294
  calcium in, 19
  growth, 241–242
bowel movement, 80, 81
brain, 91, 97, 99, 175f
  centers, 175
  tissue, 3
breast-feeding, 171, 176
breath vapor, 7f
bulimia, 186
  nutritional problems associated with, 187–188
  symptoms of, 187

C

calcium, 4, 193, 289, 294
Adequate Intake and, 199
  bioavailability, 199
  in bones, 19
  deficiency, 195–199
  excess, 200, 201f
  food sources of, 199–200, 200f
  function of, 195
  homeostasis of, 195–196, 196f
  requirements, 199, 199f
  supplementation, 200
calorie(s), 4, 19, 27
  balance, 162f, 291
  carbohydrates and, 51
  college student's annual intake of, 1
  definition of, 50–51
  empty, 261–262